V. Schumpelick · A.N. Kingsnorth (Eds.)

Incisional Hernia

Springer

Berlin
Heidelberg
New York
Barcelona
Hong Kong
London
Milan
Paris
Singapore
Tokyo

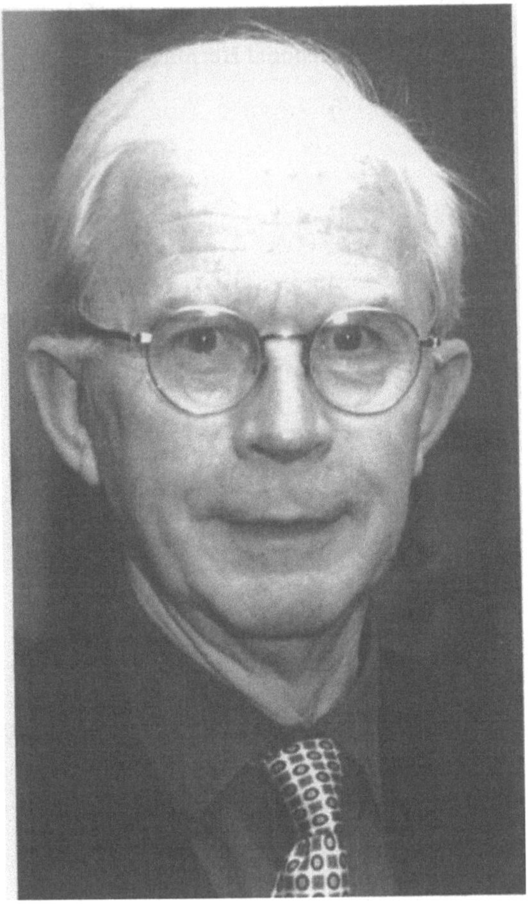

H Brendan Devlin 1932–1998

This book is dedicated to the memory of our friend H Brendan Devlin. Born in Lancashire, England, into a medical family Brendan was educated in Waterford, Ireland and qualified from Trinity College, Dublin in 1957. He received his surgical training in Ireland and later London (St. Thomas' Hospital) England and moved to practice in Stockton, England in 1970. He achieved international recognition in Day Case surgery, Audit (he also had a BA in Public Administration and Political Science) and Hernia Surgery and had delivered prestigious lectures worldwide. His influence on the surgical fraternity, particularly in the field of hernia was profound. His courtesy and keen intelligence were his hallmark and our inspiration. The surgical society has lost a great surgeon and scientist. we will miss our friend and mentor, whose extraordinary personality was of uncomparable formative influence on the Suvretta II meeting, March 98, our last common congress.

V. Schumpelick A. N. Kingsnorth

V. Schumpelick · A.N. Kingsnorth (Eds.)

Incisional Hernia

With 167 Figures, 19 in colour and 80 Tables

Springer

Volker Schumpelick
Prof. Dr. med. Dr. h.c.
Chirurgische Universitätsklinik und Poliklinik
der RWTH Aachen
Pauwelsstr. 30
52074 Aachen, Germany

Andrew N. Kingsnorth
Prof. M. D.
Plymouth Postgraduate Medical School,
Surgical University Clinic
Level 07, Derriford Hospital, Plymouth,
Devon PL6 SDH, U.K.

ISBN-13:978-3-642-64267-8

Die Deutsche Bibliothek - CIP-Einheitsaufnahme
Incisional hernia : with 80 tables / V. Schumpelick ; A. N. Kingsnorth (ed.). - Berlin ; Heidelberg ; New York ; Barcelona ; Hong Kong ; London ; Milan ; Paris ; Singapore ; Tokyo : Springer, 1999
ISBN-13:978-3-642-64267-8 e-ISBN-13:978-3-642-60123-1
DOI: 10.1007/978-3-642-60123-1

Softcover reprint of the hardcover 1st edition 1999

Cover design: E. Kirchner, Heidelberg

Typesetting: cicero Lasersatz, Dinkelscherben

SPIN: 10714897 24/3135 - 5 4 3 2 1 0 – Printed on acid-free paper

Contents

Part II Wound Healing

Part III Abdominal Wall Defects

Part IV Principles of Repair

Part VII Repair of Incisional Hernia

Part X Conclusion

Contributors

Amid, Parviz K., M.D., FACS
Lichtenstein Hernia Institute, Inc., 9201 Sunset Boulevard, Suite 505, Los Angeles, California 90069, USA

Arlt, Georg, Priv.-Doz. Dr. med.
Surgical Department, Park-Klinik Weißensee, Schönstraße 80, D-13086 Berlin

Bendavid, R., M.D., FACS
Shouldice Hospital and Department of Surgery, University of Toronto, Toronto, Ontario, Canada

Bennet, Dr.
Surgical University Clinic, Plymouth Postgraduate Medical School, Plymouth Devon Pl6 8DH, GB

Berger, A., Prof. Dr. med.
Clinic for Plastic, Hand- and Reconstructive Surgery, Hannover Medical School, Podbielskistr. 380, 30659 Hannover, Germany

Bruch, H.-P., Prof. Dr. med.
Dept. of Surgery, University of Luebeck, Medical School, Ratzeburger Allee 160, D-23538 Lübeck, Germany

Carlson, Mark A., M.D.
Department of Surgery, University of Texas Southwestern, 5323 Harry Hines Boulevard, Dallas, TX 75235-9160

Chevrel, J. P., Prof. Dr. med.
Department of General and Gastrointstinal Surgery, Hopital Avicenne, F-93009 Bobigny Cedex, France

Conze, J., Dr. med.
Surgical University Clinic of RWTH Aachen, Pauwelsstraße 30, D-52074 Aachen, Germany

Decurtins, M., P. D.
Chir. Klinik, Kantonsspital, CH-8401 Winterthur

Devlin, H. Brendan, M.D. FRCS
North Tees General Hospital, Hardwick, Stockton-on-Tees TS19 8PE, UK

Filipi, Ch. J., M.D., FACS
Department of Surgery, Suite 3740, Creighton University,
St. Joseph Hospital 601 N. 30th Street, Omaha Ne 68131-2197/USA

Fischer, Eva, M.D.
Assistant Professor of Surgery, Cornell University Medical College

Flament, J. B., Prof. Dr. med.
Hopital Robert-Debre Avenue du Général Koenig, F-51092 Reims Cedex

Gislason, Hjörtur, M.D.
Department of Surgery, Haukeland Hospital, N-5021 Bergen, Norway

Hartel, Wilhelm, Prof. Dr. med.
Generalsekretär der Deutschen Gesellschaft für Chirurgie,
Steinhölzle 16, D-89190 Westerstetten, Germany

Herszage, L., Dr. med.
Viamonte 1620 2°C, 1055 Buenos Aires, Argentinien

Israelsson, Leif, M.D. PhD
Kirurgkliniken, Sundsvalls Sjukhus, S-85186 Sundsvall, Sweden

Kingsnorth, A. N., Prof. of Surgery
Postgraduate Medical School, Derriford Hospital, Level 7, Plymouth PL6 8 DH, UK

Klaiber, Ch., Dr. med.
Spital Aarberg, Department of Surgery, Ch-3270 Aarberg

Klinge, U., Dr. med.
Surgical University Clinic of RWTH Aachen,
Pauwelsstraße 30, D-52074 Aachen, Germany

Klosterhalfen, B., Priv.-Doz. Dr. med.
Surgical University Clinic of RWTH Aachen, Institute for Pathology,
Pauwelsstraße 30, D-52074 Aachen, Germany

Muschaweck, Ulrike, Dr. med.
Arabella-Klinik, Arabellastraße 5, D-81925 München, Germany

Nilsson, Erik, Prof. Dr. med.
Department of Surgery, Motala Hospital, 59185 Motala, Sweden

Osther, P. J., M.D. PhD
Department of Urologic Surgery, Skejby Hospital, University of Aarhus,
DK-8200 Aarhus N, Denmark

Peiper, Christian, Dr. med.
Surgical University Clinic of RWTH Aachen,
Pauwelsstraße 30, D-52074 Aachen, Germany

Prescher, A., Priv.-Doz. Dr. med.
Institute of Anatomy I der RWTH-Aachen, Universitätsklinikum,
Pauwelsstraße 30, D-52057 Aachen, Germany

Read, Raymond C., M.D.
Surgical Service (II2LR), John L. McClellan Memorial Veterans' Hospital,
General Thoracic Surgery,
4300 West Seventh, Room 2C100, Little Rock, Arkansas 72205

Roblick, U. J., Dr. med.
Dept. of Surgery, University of Luebeck, Medical School,
Ratzeburger Allee 160, D-23538 Lübeck, Germany

Schimmelpennig, H., Dr. med. Dr. S. C. I.
Dept. of Surgery, University of Luebeck, Medical School,
Ratzeburger Allee 160, D-23538 Lübeck, Germany

Schippers, Ekkehard, Prof. Dr. med.
Julius-Spital, Dept. of Surgery, Juliuspromenade 19, D-97070 Würzburg, Germany

Schumpelick, Volker, Prof. Dr. med. Dr. h.c.
Surgical University Clinic of RWTH Aachen,
Pauwelsstraße 30, D-52074 Aachen, Germany

Simmermacher, R. K. J., M. D., Ph. D.
Dept. of Surgery, University Hospital Utrecht, 3508 GA Utrecht, The Netherlands

Skandalakis, John E., M. R., Ph. D., FACS
Emory University School of Medicine, The Robert W. Woodruff Health Sciences Center,
1462 Clifton Road, N.E., Suite 303, Atlanta, Georgia 30322

Stoppa, R., Prof. Dr.
Clinique Chirurgical de l'Université, Centre Hospitalier Universitaire d'Amiens,
Hospital Nord, place Victor-Pauchet, F-80054 Amiens Cedex 1, France

Töns, Christian, Priv.-Doz. Dr. med.
Surgical University Clinic of RWTH Aachen,
Pauwelsstraße 30, D-52074 Aachen, Germany

Treutner, Karl-Heinz, Priv.-Doz. Dr. med.
Surgical University Clinic of RWTH Aachen,
Pauwelsstraße 30, D-52074 Aachen, Germany

Truong, S. N., Prof. Dr. med.
Surgical University Clinic of RWTH Aachen,
Pauwelsstraße 30, D-52074 Aachen, Germany

Wantz, George E., M.D., FACS
Clinical Professor of Surgery, Cornell University Medical College

Willis, S., Dr. med.
Surgical University Clinic of RWTH Aachen,
Pauwelsstraße 30, D-52074 Aachen, Germany

Preface

The worldwide debate on inguinal hernias seems to have overshadowed the substantial surgical problem of incisional hernia using both the conventional and the laparoscopic approach. Whereas the difference in outcome obtained by various techniques of inguinal hernia repair, as reflected by the 5-year recurrence rate, ranges from 1% to 4%, the results in incisional hernia are at least ten times worse, with worldwide recurrence rates of 40%–50%. In half of all incisional hernia repairs, a repeat operation has to be performed because the technique has failed, and the majority of these reoperations are not successful. No other benign disease has such bad surgical results.

Incisional hernia is defined as an abdominal wall defect at the site of abdominal wall closure, and repairing such defects requires many problems to be overcome: a multilayered wall structure of different tissue properties in constant motion has to be sutured, positive abdominal pressure has to be dealt with, and tissues with impaired healing properties, reduced perfusion, and connective tissue deficiencies have to be joined.

In abdominal wall repair in particular, the use of synthetic material has a long tradition. However, the results obtained are not always acceptable, because meshes can lead to abdominal stiffness, loss of elasticity and mobility, and sometimes pronounced foreign body reactions and infections. Many years ago, the French surgical school was the first to demonstrate that it is only by using synthetic meshes that good results can be obtained in incisional hernia repair. However, these techniques are not generally known among surgeons or their use is controversial.

With these facts in mind, most of the world's leading herniologists took part in a seminar designed to reach a state-of-the-art consensus on the management of incisional hernia. Four years after the first Suvretta meeting on inguinal hernia, this second meeting focused on incisional hernia as the most demanding problem in herniology today. We defined incisional hernia as a hernia in any incision of the abdominal wall including the groin, and the term therefore includes recurrent inguinal hernia. Interactive sessions included topics on anatomy, physiology, function, pathogenesis, wound healing, and methods of repair. In the course of a week spent in the seclusion of this remote hotel in the Swiss Alps, a combination of presentations, discussions, videos, and other demonstrations resulted in a number of definitive and accepted conclusions. We hope that the written proceedings of this Suvretta II-meeting will allow surgeons a better understanding of why, when, and how to prevent or treat incisional hernias successfully.

V. Schumpelick
A. N. Kingsnorth

March 1999

Part I Anatomy of the Abdominal Wall

CHAPTER 1

Descriptive Anatomy

J.E. Skandalakis, G.L. Colborn, P.N. Skandalakis, L.J. Skandalakis

The bare accounts, for example, of the regions concerned in Hernia I have left to the systematic treatises, and have dealt only with the bearings of the anatomy of the parts upon the circumstances of practice. (Frederick Treves 1883)

The abdominal wall from superficial to deep is formed by several layers (Fig. 1):
- Skin
- Subcutaneous tissue
- Innominate fascia of the external oblique muscle
- External oblique aponeurosis and muscle
- Internal oblique aponeurosis and muscle
- Transversus abdominis aponeurosis and muscle
- Anterior lamina of the fascia transversalis
- Posterior lamina of the fascia transversalis
- Preperitoneal fat
- Peritoneum

Some of these layers form spaces, such as the vascular space and the space of Bogros.

1.1 Skin

The skin is more mobile in older individuals. It has a rich blood supply, very good but peculiar lymphatic drainage, and very good innervation. All these blood vessels, lymphatics, and nerves are related to similar structures of the subcutaneous fat. For all practical purposes, these entities cannot be described without describing the same entities of the subcutaneous fat. The only difference between the skin of males and females is at the lower abdominal wall, where the skin of the scrotum and the skin of the labia majora differ considerably.

1.1.1 Surgical Applications

The following points should be noted:
- Parallel incisions, angles between vertical and transverse or subcostal incisions, and incisions in irradiated tissues should be avoided.
- If possible, a preexisting incision should be extended or reused.
- Avoid undermining skin flaps.

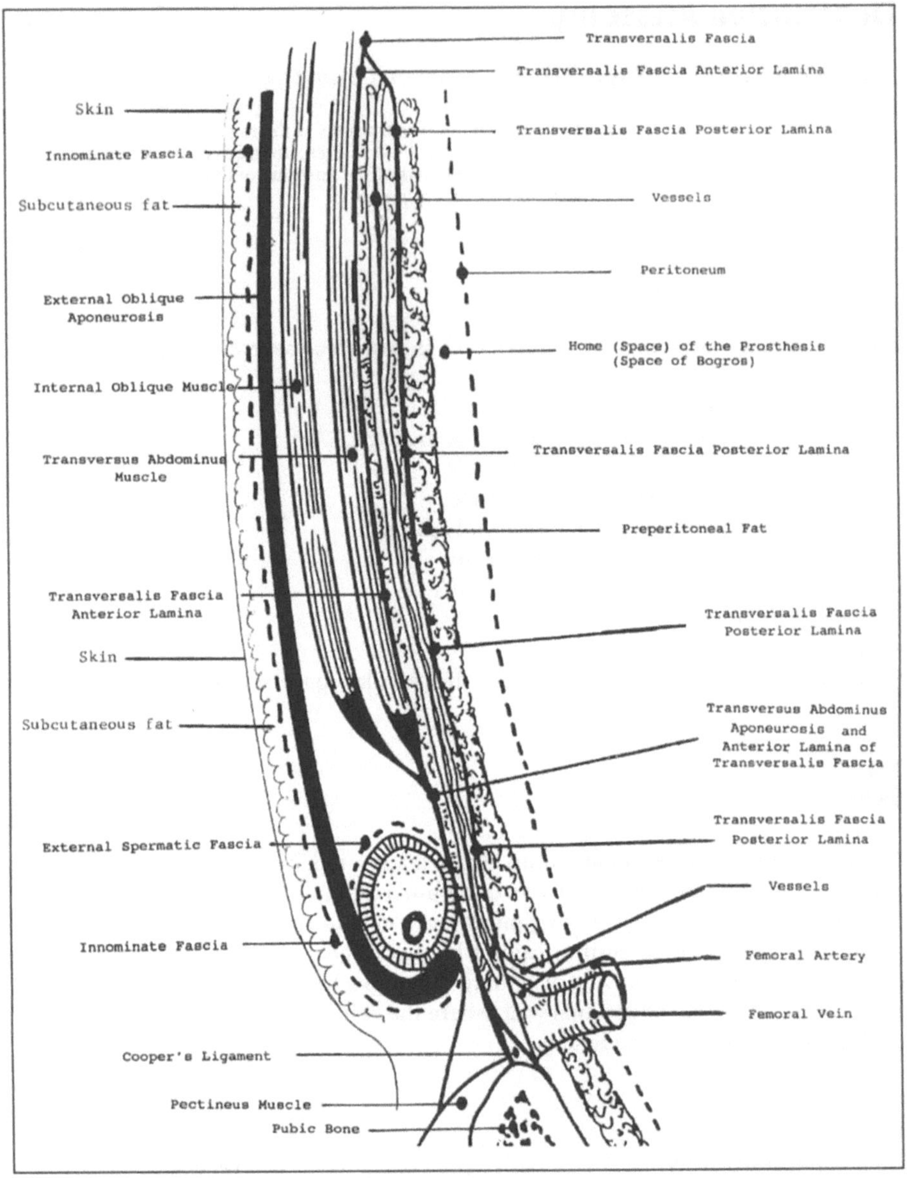

Fig. 1. Layers and spaces of the anterior abdominal wall. (Modified from [32], with permission)

1.2 Subcutaneous Tissue

The subcutaneous tissue consists of two portions: a superficial layer (Camper's fascia) and a deep layer (Scarpa's fascia). The superficial fascia consists of subcutaneous fat, and the deep layer is thin and membranous (Fig. 2). These two layers are well developed in the inguinal area and are clearly defined in most cases. Scarpa's fascia is so well developed in the inguinal area that the surgeon may mistake it for the aponeurosis of the external oblique muscle. This may lead to treating a superficial ectopic testicle as an inguinal cryptorchidism. There may be a layer of fat between the fascia and the aponeurosis. White states that as long as fat is encountered, the external oblique fascia has not been reached [1].

However, the downward continuation of Camper's and Scarpa's fasciae, especially in the scrotum, raises some questions. Experts agree to disagree regarding the penile fascia. Scarpa's and Camper's fasciae essentially merge and intermingle on the penis as its superficial fascia. Buck's fascia, the deep fascia of the penis, is separate from the superficial fascia in structure and appearance.

We agree, however, with Wendell-Smith (personal communication, 1997) that the term "superficial fascia" should be replaced by the term "subcutaneous tissue."

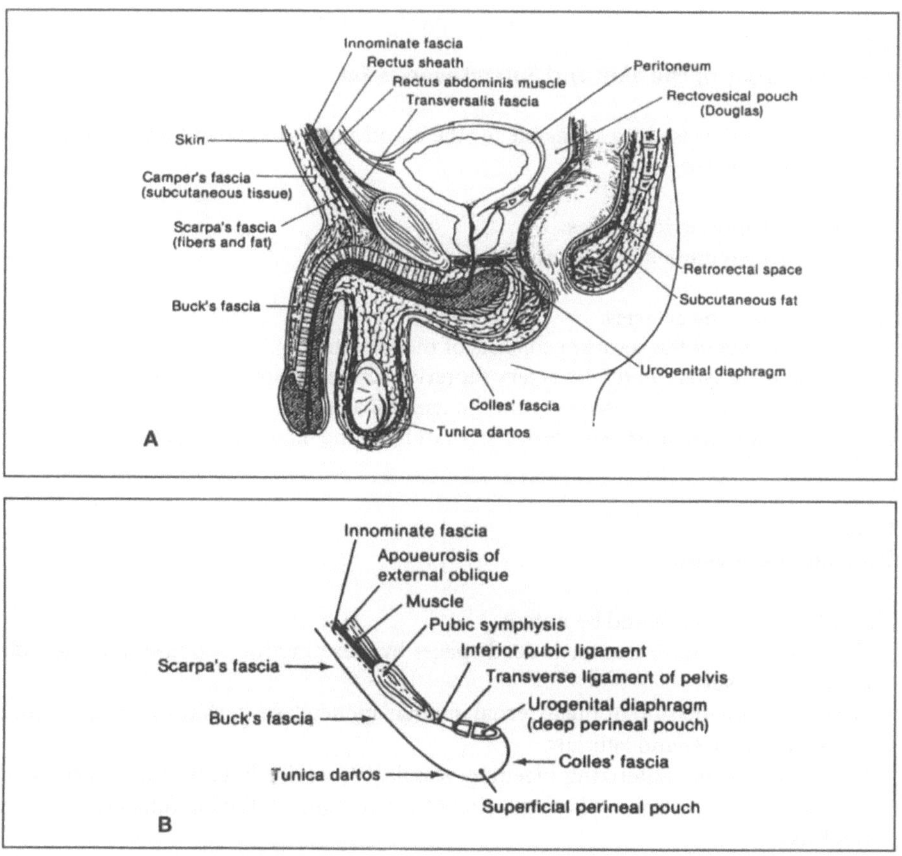

Fig. 2A, B. *A* Note the downward continuation of Scarpa's fascia, Buck's fascia, tunica dartos, and Colles' fascia. Also note the formation of the superficial and deep perineal pouch. *B* Formation of the superficial and deep perineal pouch. (From [33], with permission)

Interesting anatomic features of the perineum include those of the superficial perineal cleft and the superficial perineal pouch. The cleft is continuous with the potential space deep to Scarpa's fascia on the abdominal wall, and it is situated between Colles' fascia and the fascia that covers the muscles of the superficial perineal pouch. The pouch is bounded superiorly by the perineal membrane, inferiorly by the external perineal fascia, and laterally by the ischiopubic rami. This area may be the site of urine or blood extravasation from urethral injury, which will then pass from the superficial pouch into the cleft and may continue downward in the scrotum or anterior abdominal wall.

From the surgical viewpoint in the male, both the superficial and deep (Buck's) fascial layers, as well as the scrotum (dartos) and perineal fascia (Colles'), extend from the abdominal wall downward, with Colles' fascia ending at the urogenital diaphragm. In the female, a similar situation exists.

The superficial perineal pouch is closed posteriorly and open anteriorly because of the union of Colles' fascia and the perineal membrane. Urine can reach both axillae after rupture of the urethra, especially when the bladder is full.

1.2.1 Vascular Supply of the Skin and Subcutaneous Fat

The following arteries are responsible for the blood supply of the abdominal wall:
- Lower intercostals
- Lumbar arteries
- Superficial epigastric arteries
- Superficial circumflex iliac arteries

The veins follow the arteries.
The blood supply of the scrotum consists of the following:
- Superficial external pudendal artery (anterior scrotal) from the femoral artery
- Deep external pudendal artery from the femoral artery
- Internal pudendal artery (posterior scrotal) from the internal iliac artery

1.2.2 Surgical Applications

The following points should be noted:
- To avoid seromas, do not form dead spaces by elevating the two layers of the subcutaneous tissue.
- Clean only the incision of the external oblique aponeurosis perhaps 1 cm above and below, or medially and laterally.
- If possible, avoid cauterizing bleeding vessels. We advise ligating the vessels with the suture of your choice. The formation of a hematoma in the inguinal area is quite unpleasant.
- Urine can reach both axillae after rupture of the urethra, especially when the bladder is full, because the superficial perineal pouch or cleft is closed posteriorly by the union of Colles' fascia and the perineal membrane.

- It is important for any incision in the inguinal area to be located parallel to and at least one or two fingers above the inguinal ligament.

1.3 Surgical Anatomy of the Umbilical Region

The three anatomic entities of the umbilicus are the following:
- Umbilical ring
- Round ligament
- Umbilical fascia

In a study of the umbilical region, Orda and Nathan [2] found that, in most individuals (74%), the round ligament of the liver passed over the superior margin of the umbilical ring and crossed the ring to attach to the inferior margin (Fig. 3A). In about one fourth of subjects, the round ligament bifurcated and attached to the superior margin of the ring (Fig. 3B). In such cases, the floor of the ring was formed by fascia transversalis and peritoneum only. In fewer than 1% of subjects, the round ligament branches before reaching the umbilical ring (Fig. 3C). Each branch continues with the medial umbilical ligament without attaching to the umbilical ring.

The floor of the umbilical ring may be further strengthened by a thickening of the fascia transversalis in this area, the fascia umbilicalis. This thickened fascia may cover the umbilical ring entirely (Fig. 3D) or partially (Fig. 3E, F). It may fail to cover the ring (Fig. 3G), and it was completely absent in 15% of specimens.

There are thus two structures, the round ligament and the fascia umbilicalis, that protect the umbilical area. If both are absent (Fig. 3B, F), the floor of the umbilical ring is relatively unsupported. Herniation through such a ring has been referred to as direct umbilical hernia by Orda and Nathan [2].

Where the umbilical fascia partly covers the ring (Fig. 3E, F), the superior or inferior edge may form a fold or recess through which a hernia may occur. Such an "indirect" umbilical hernia descends into the umbilical ring from a superior fascial fold or ascends into the ring from an inferior fold. A combination of the variations shown in Fig. 3B and Fig. 3E or Fig. 3F would appear to predispose to herniation through the umbilical ring. Far from supporting the ring in such cases, the umbilical fascia may predispose to hernia.

1.4 Flat Muscles of the Anterior Abdominal Wall and the Rectus Abdominis and Pyramidalis Muscles

It is not within the scope of this paper to present well-known descriptions of the flat muscles or the rectus abdominis and pyramidalis muscles. We will emphasize only a few points from a surgical standpoint; the pyramidalis muscle is of no surgical importance.

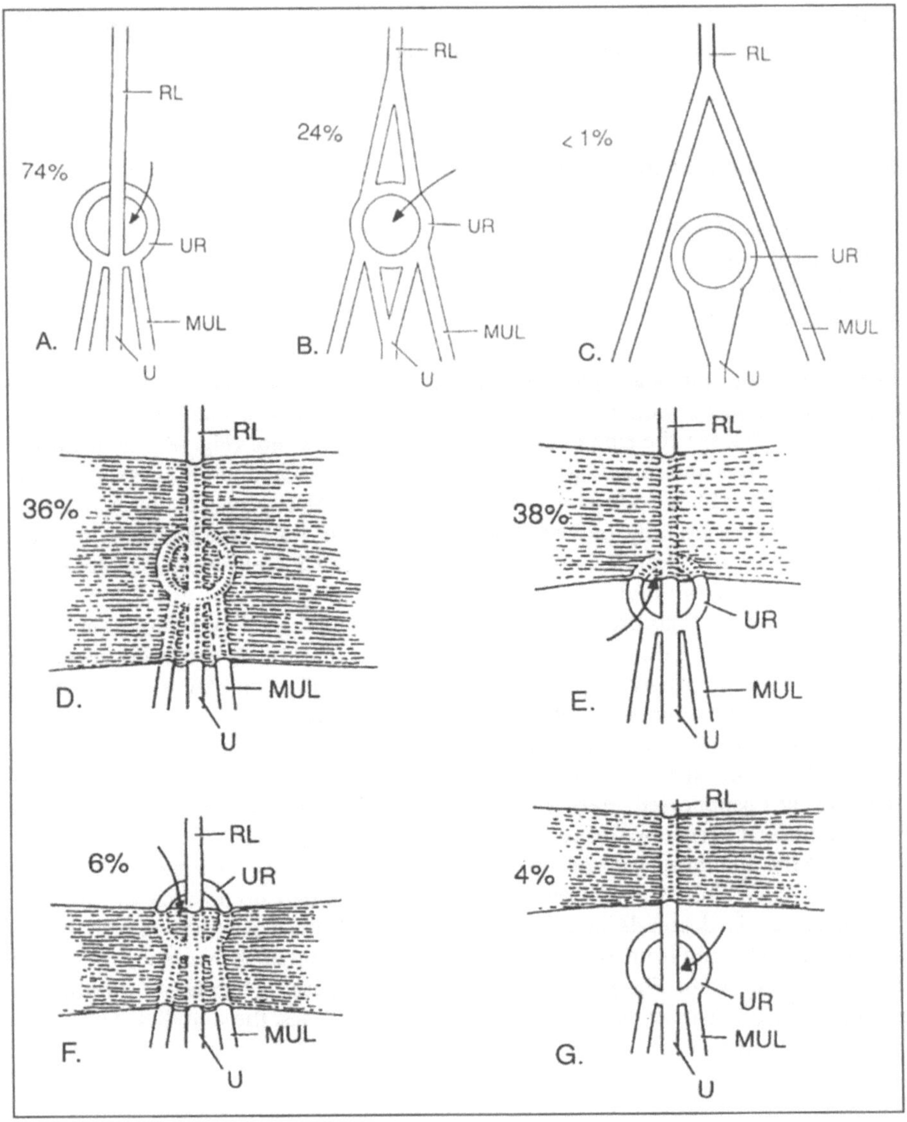

Fig. 3A–G. Variations in the disposition of the umbilical ligaments as seen from the posterior (peritoneal) surface of the body wall. Arrows indicate: *A* Usual relations (74%) of the umbilical ring (UR), the round ligament (RL), the urachus (U), and the medial umbilical ligaments (MUL). The round ligament crosses the umbilical ring to insert on its inferior margin. *B* Less common configuration (24%). The round ligament splits and is attached to the superior margin of the umbilical ring. *C* Rare configuration (less than 1%). The round ligament branches before reaching the umbilical ring. Each branch continues with the medial umbilical ligament without attaching to the umbilical ring. *D–G* Variations in the presence and form of the insertions of the umbilical fascia as seen from the posterior (peritoneal) surface of the body wall. *D* The thickened fascia transversalis forms the umbilical fascia covering the umbilical ring (36%). Arrows indicate: *E* The umbilical fascia covering only the superior portion of the umbilical ring (38%). *F* The umbilical fascia covering only the inferior portion of the umbilical ring (6%). *G* Though present, the umbilical fascia does not underlie the umbilical ring (4%). In another variant (not shown), the fascia is entirely absent (16%). (From [34], with permission)

1.4.1
External Oblique Fascia (Innominate Fascia of Gallaudet)

The innominate fascia is a thin, tissue-like membrane that covers the external oblique muscle and aponeurosis. In the superficial ring, it forms the intercrural fibers between the crura on its way down to the scrotum, following the spermatic cord, and forms the external spermatic fascia.

It should be remembered that the external oblique aponeurosis does not extend down to the scrotum and is not a covering of the spermatic cord.

1.4.2
External Oblique Aponeurosis

According to Rizk [3] and Askar [4], the external oblique aponeurosis is formed by two layers, superficial and deep, which, together with the bilaminar internal oblique and transversus abdominis aponeuroses, form the rectus sheath and, finally, the linea alba by linear decussation. If one acknowledges these results, then at the lower abdominal wall, the anterior rectus sheath (since there is no posterior one) is formed by six aponeurotic layers, two from each flat muscle all fused together.

The "touchdown" point where the bilaminar external oblique aponeurosis enters ("touches down" on) the anterior rectus sheath is never at the linea alba or at the lateral border of the rectus sheath; it is always between the two (Fig. 4). This should be remembered, when a relaxing incision is necessary.

The external oblique aponeurosis ends with the formation of the inguinal ligament. This extends from the anterior superior iliac spine to the pubic tubercle, where the lacunar ligament and the reflected inguinal ligament also are formed.

The superficial inguinal "ring" is a triangular opening of the external oblique aponeurosis 1–1.5 cm above and lateral to the pubic tubercle. The opening is formed by a splitting of the external oblique aponeurosis, creating the crura of the subcutaneous ring. The inferior crus (lateral crus) inserts into the tubercle and pecten; the superior crus (medial crus) inserts anterior to the pubic bone and symphysis. The insertion of the inferior crus is, in part, by way of the lacunar ligament. Fibers from the superior crus cross the midline to insert on the opposite tubercle.

It should be remembered that, in the inguinal area, there are three regional modifications of the external oblique aponeurosis: the inguinal ligament, the lacunar ligament, and the reflected inguinal ligament.

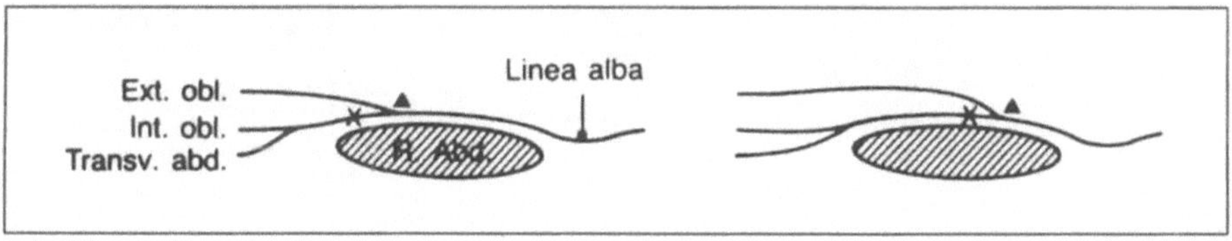

Fig. 4. Relaxing incision. The X point of the relaxing incision is at the anterior lamina of the rectus sheath. Triangles mark the "touchdown" of the external oblique aponeurosis, always between the linea alba and semilunar line. (From [33], with permission)

1.4.3 Inguinal (Poupart's) Ligament

The inguinal ligament (Fig. 5) is the lower edge of the external oblique aponeurosis extending from the anterior superior iliac spine to the pubic tubercle. The inguinal ligament (or ligament of Poupart) is related to the following: iliopsoas muscle and its fascia, femoral vessels (indirectly), femoral ring, iliopubic tract, and other thickenings of the fascia transversalis. On the way to the pubic tubercle and prior to its insertion, Gimbernat's ligament and the reflected inguinal ligament are formed.

1.4.4 Ligament of Gimbernat (Lacunar Ligament)

The lacunar ligament (Fig. 5) can, according to Madden [5], be demonstrated only when "the pyriform fossa is completely exposed," because the ligament practically forms the floor of the fossa.

The ligament of Gimbernat is a triangular extension of the inguinal ligament before its insertion to the pubic tubercle. It is inserted at the pecten pubis, and its lateral end meets the proximal end of the ligament of Cooper (Fig. 5). Condon [6] states that "it (the ligament of Gimbernat) never forms the medial border of the normal femoral canal." Other investigators, however, hold the opposite view.

The reflected inguinal ligament originates from the inferior crus of the superficial inguinal ring and travels up to the linea alba.

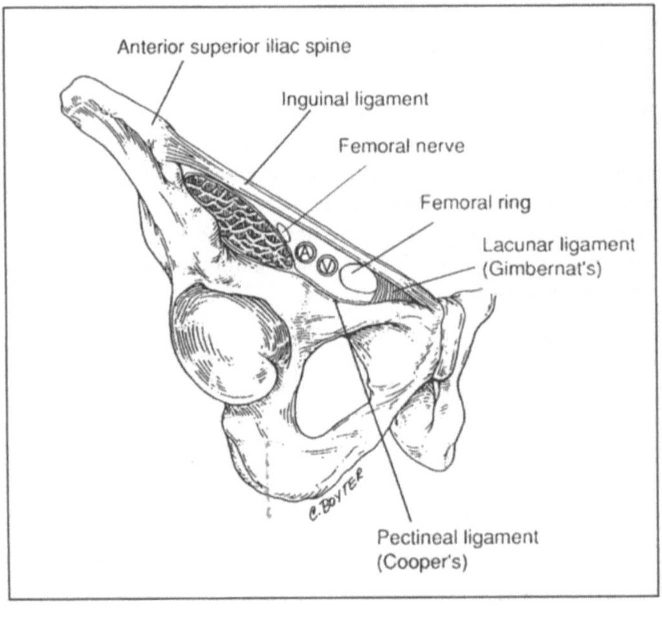

Fig. 5. The inguinal ligament, lacunar ligament (Gimbernat's), and pectineal ligament (Cooper's). (Modified from [35], with permission)

1.4.5
Internal Oblique Muscle and Aponeurosis

The relationship of the internal oblique muscle to other entities in the inguinal region is a subject of disagreement. McVay [7] regarded the iliopsoas muscle fascia as the actual origin of the muscle. We observed this arrangement in fresh, slender cadavers. The origin of the internal oblique muscle from the iliopsoas fascia could be seen when the fascial attachments of the internal oblique muscle were easily separated from the inguinal ligament with the knife handle.

The medial termination of the internal oblique muscle is also a subject of debate. Anatomists are in accord regarding its participation in the anterior rectus lamina, yet they disagree on the formation of the conjoined tendon, a topic to be covered later.

The fibers of the internal oblique muscle do not add to the lower portion of the posterior inguinal wall, because they do not have an insertion into Cooper's ligament [7]. The internal oblique aponeurosis is formed by two layers, anterior and posterior, which are fused and, together with the two other bilaminar aponeuroses (external oblique and transversus abdominis), help form the anterior rectus sheath and linea alba.

1.4.6
Transversus Abdominis Muscle and Aponeurosis

There is debate also about the origin of the transversus abdominis muscle. Instead of quoting several authors, we again voice our agreement with McVay [7] that this muscle in the inguinal area arises from the iliopsoas fascia and not from the inguinal ligament.

In the environment of the internal ring, the internal oblique is muscular and the transversus abdominis is aponeurotic. The transversus abdominis muscle inserts on Cooper's ligament. Moreover, medially in the inguinal area, all the aponeurotic layers of the three flat muscles pass anterior to the rectus muscle to form the anterior lamina of the sheath.

It is the integrity of the transversus abdominis muscle that prevents the formation of hernia. Thus we agree again with McVay [7] that, in this sense, it is the most important layer of the abdominal wall. Accepting Rizk's [7] and Askar's [4] findings that the aponeurosis of this muscle is bilaminar, then both laminae (anterior and posterior) fuse together or there is some attenuation of the posterior layer, as Rizk reported. To summarize, Rizk described each abdominal aponeurosis as bilaminar and each wall of the rectus sheath as trilaminar (like plywood) [3].

1.4.7
Arch of the Internal Oblique and Transversus Abdominis Muscles

The transversus abdominis arch is the lower part of the transversus abdominis muscle. In most, if not all, cases, it is quite aponeurotic. It is formed by the free aponeurotic and muscular lower margin of the muscle. Medially, the arch is aponeurotic; however, toward the internal ring, it is both muscular and aponeurotic.

The internal oblique muscle practically covers the arch and occasionally is fixed with the arch in such a way that elevation of the internal oblique muscle will also produce elevation of the arch.

1.4.8
Conjoined Area

By definition, the conjoined tendon is the fusion of lower fibers of the internal oblique aponeurosis with similar fibers from the aponeurosis of the transversus abdominis just as they insert on the pubic tubercle and superior ramus of the pubis.

The anatomic configuration thus described is rare. Hollinshead [8] found it to exist in only 5% of bodies; Condon [9] determined 3%; McVay [7] believed it to be only an artifact of dissection.

It is because of the number of structures juxtaposed in this area and because the term "conjoined tendon" is extensively used that we propose that the concept of the area of the conjoined tendon be replaced by that of "conjoined area" (Fig. 6). The area can be easily identified by the inexperienced surgeon who understands that it is occasionally tendinous. In other words, this is the area in which there would be a conjoined tendon if there were a conjoined tendon. We trust this will accommodate both the myth and the facts.

The following are a few other definitions to clarify the local anatomy:

- The ligament of Henle was originally termed "falx inguinalis." This term is preferred since the falx has become confused with the conjoined tendon. The ligament of

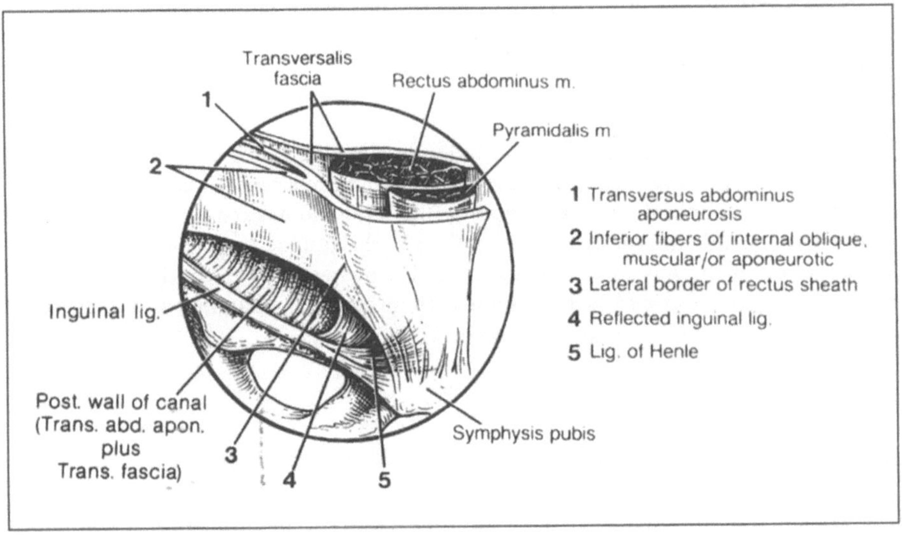

Fig. 6. The "conjoined area." (Modified from [36], with permission)

Henle is the lateral expansion of the tendon of the rectus abdominis or an expansion of the rectus sheath that inserts on the pecten of the pubis. This ligament is present in 30%–50% of patients and is fused with the fascia transversalis. Because of this, it may be seen occasionally in the surgical field and the surgeon's needle may penetrate it once or twice in the course of hernia repair.
- The interfoveolar ligament (of Hesselbach) is an apparent thickening of the fascia transversalis at the medial side of the internal inguinal ring. It lies in front of the inferior epigastric vessels like a spiderweb. When well developed, it gives the impression that it is only a lateral condensation of the ligament of Henle, but it is not a true ligament.
- The reflected inguinal ligament is composed of aponeurotic fibers from the inferior crus of the external inguinal ring reaching medially upward toward the linea alba. This is the "posterior crus" of the French anatomists.

The following points should be noted:
- The transversus abdominis layer is the most important of the three flat muscles. The integrity of this layer prevents herniation.
- If the transversus abdominis layer and transverse fascia are intact, neither inguinal nor femoral herniation can develop.
- External and internal obliques are of only secondary importance.
- Only fascial attachments – no muscles – originate from or insert into the inguinal ligament [10]. The internal oblique and transversus abdominis are related approximately to the lateral half of inguinal ligament.

1.4.9 Rectus Abdominis Muscle and its Sheath

The rectus muscle is enclosed in a stout sheath. This sheath is formed by the bilaminar aponeurosis of the three flat muscles that split and pass anteriorly and posteriorly around the muscle. They start at the lateral border of the rectus abdominis, form the linea alba, and continue in a complicated way to pass to the opposite side [3, 4]. In several publications, both Risk [3] and Askar [4] independently reported findings that radically changed the traditional view of the formation of the anterior and posterior rectus sheath and that of the linea alba [3, 4, 11–13].

It is in the lower fourth of the abdominal wall that the aponeuroses pass anteriorly to the rectus muscle, which is bounded posteriorly by the fascia transversalis. The dividing line is the linea semicircularis of Douglas, which marks the lower level where the rectus sheath loses its posterior wall. If the change is gradual, it is poorly defined; if the change is abrupt, the line is well marked.

A comparison of the structures of the upper three fourths to the lower fourth of the abdominal wall, which is closely related to the inguinal area, is illustrated in Table 1. It was Rizk's [3] belief that the linea alba might be considered less the insertion of the abdominal muscles than the common area of decussation of their intermediate aponeuroses.

Medial retraction of the rectus muscle should be avoided [14].

Table 1. Structures of the abdominal wall as related to the inguinal area. Reprinted with permission from [31]

Upper midline	Lower midline
Linea alba well developed	Linea alba poorly developed
Right and left recti well separated	Right and left recti close together
Anterior and posterior layers of sheath present	Only anterior layer of sheath present
Aponeurosis of external oblique weak or absent	Aponeurosis of external oblique strong and well developed

1.4.10 Linea Alba

In Askar's [4] understanding of the linea alba formed by decussating aponeurotic fibers of the rectus sheath, he found the following: in 30% of cases, there was a single decussation of fibers of the anterior and posterior rectus sheath; in 10% of cases, there was a single decussation of anterior and triple decussation of posterior rectus sheath; in 60% of cases, there was a triple decussation of aponeurotic fibers of both anterior and posterior rectus sheaths. Subjects in the 30% group with single fibrous crossings may be more susceptible to linea alba herniation.

Rizk [3] believed that the most destructive incision is the vertical midline, and the least destructive, the subcostal.

1.5 Fascia Transversalis

Sir Astley Cooper [15] reported the fascia transversalis as follows:

When the lower portions of the internal oblique and transversalis muscles are raised from their subjacent attachments, a layer of fascia is found to be interposed between them and the peritoneum, through which the spermatic vessels emerge from the abdomen. This fascia, which I have ventured to name "fascia transversalis" varies in density, being strong and unyielding towards the ilium, but weak and more cellular towards the pubes.

The term "fascia transversalis" formerly was applied to the deep fascia covering the internal surface of the transversus abdominis muscle and is now applied to the entire connective tissue sheet lining the musculature of the abdominal cavity. In some areas, this fascial layer is given a specific name such as "iliacus" or "psoas" fascia where it covers those specific muscles.

The old concept of fascia transversalis is illustrated in Fig. 7A, and the new concept in Fig. 7B.

The fascia transversalis varies in nature. It is thin and closely adherent in the portion covering the transversus abdominis aponeurosis; however, in other areas, it is thick and discrete [15].

By itself, the fascia transversalis is a weak layer that is useless for hernia repair. Yet when it is fused with the transversus abdominis aponeurosis, "good stuff" for repair is formed.

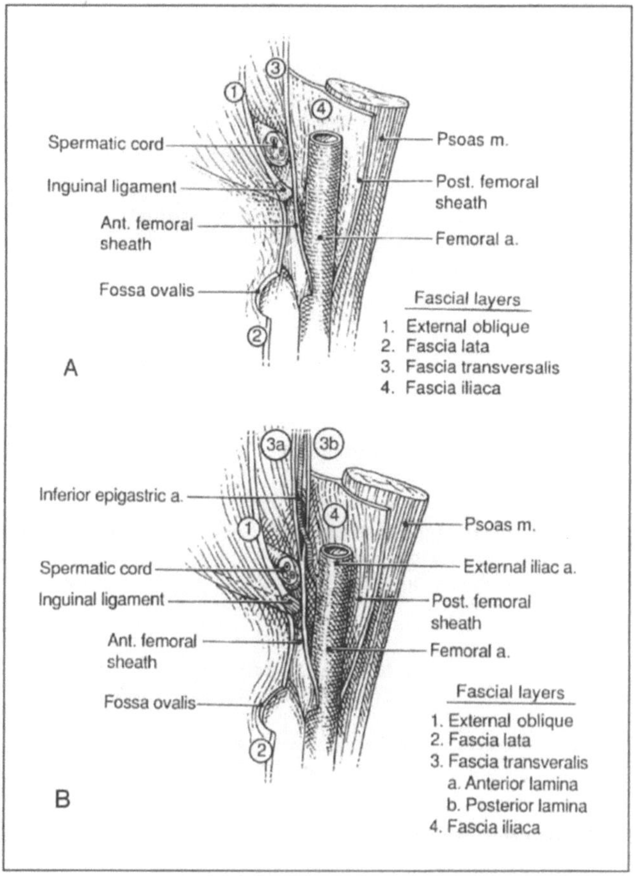

Fig. 7A, B. *A* Fascia transversalis and femoral sheath (old concept). *B* Fascia transversalis and femoral sheath (new concept), emphasizing the bilaminar nature of the fascia transversalis in the inguinal area. (From [32], with permission)

1.5.1 Thickenings of the Fascia Transversalis

1.5.1.1 Fascia Transversalis Crura

The fascia transversalis forms a sling around the internal ring, an incomplete ring that consists of a thickening forming two crura: a long anterior crus and a short posterior crus (Fig. 8). Characteristically, the anterior crus is fixed to the transversus abdominis muscle or aponeurosis above and to the internal ring medially. The posterior crus is fixed to, or inserts on, the iliopubic tract. This arrangement forms an inverted U-shaped sling. By contraction of the transversus abdominis muscle, the sling closes the internal ring under the muscular edge of the internal oblique muscle.

The fascia transversalis should not be sutured to the shelving edge of the inguinal ligament, as such a suture might not permit sphincteric action of the transversus abdominis muscle.

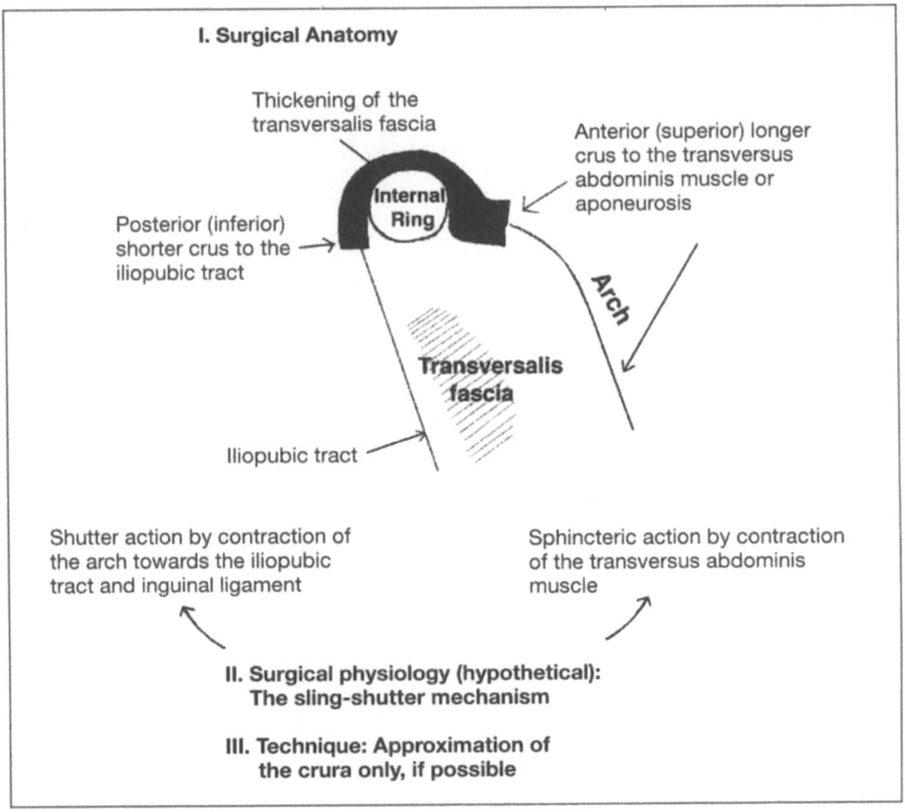

Fig. 8. Fascia transversalis crura

1.5.1.2
Iliopubic Tract

Described by Alexander Thomson in 1836, the iliopubic tract is an aponeurotic band that extends from the iliopectineal arch to the superior ramus of the pubis. It creates the inferior margin of the deep musculoaponeurotic layer made up of the transversus abdominis muscle and aponeurosis and the fascia transversalis (Fig. 9).

Medical students and students of anatomy are confused by the many names used to refer to the iliopubic tract, such as the following:
- Ligament of Thomson
- Deep crural arch
- Deep femoral arch
- Anterior femoral sheath
- Bandelette iliopubienne

(If Hesselbach was the first to report this ligament in 1814, then perhaps it should be named the ligament of Hesselbach).

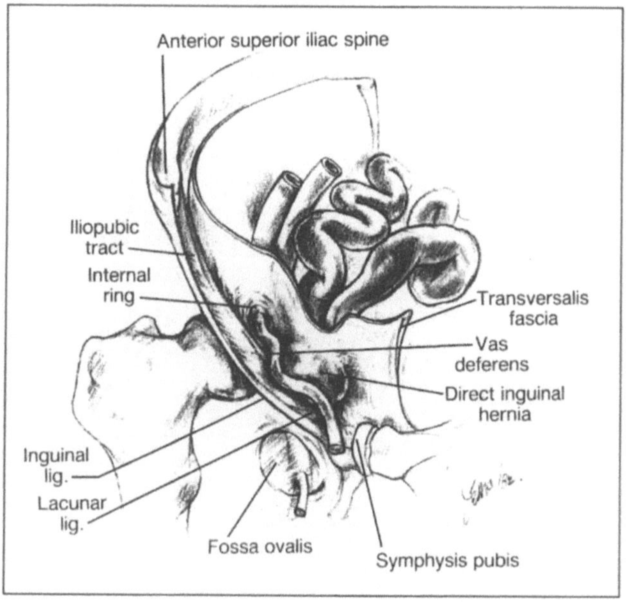

Fig. 9. The iliopubic tract. Note the direct inguinal hernia. (From [36], with permission)

The tract is attached laterally to the iliacus and psoas fascia and continues more laterally to the anterior superior spine of the ilium. Medially, it forms the lower border of the internal inguinal ring, crossing the femoral vessels to form the anterior margin of the femoral sheath and composing part of the fascia transversalis. In reality, perhaps, all these anatomic entities originate from the fascia transversalis. The tract curves around the medial surface of the femoral sheath to attach to the pectineal ligament.

Condon [9] found the iliopubic tract present in 98% of dissections. He points out that it has frequently been confused with the inguinal ligament, which, although nearby, belongs to the anterior lamina (superficial musculoaponeurotic layer), and the iliopubic tract is part of the deep layer (postlaminar structures). According to Madden [5], the iliopubic tract is the inferior segment of the posterior wall of the inguinal; we agree.

We disagree, however, with Gray's Anatomy [16], in which the iliopubic tract is called the "deep crural arch." As there is no "superficial crural arch," we see no reason to call it that. Wendell-Smith agrees with us (personal communication, 1997).

The shelving edge of the inguinal ligament is located anterior to the iliopubic arch, so the iliopubic arch can be seen by a special anterior dissection. The iliopubic tract is therefore related to the direct inguinal hernia inferiorly, but it is not related to the classic external supravesical hernia.

The following points should be remembered:

- The cremaster vessels and the genital branch of the genitofemoral nerve are located very close to the iliopubic tract at the posterior wall of the inguinal canal (Figs. 10, 11)
- According to Condon [17], the iliopubic tract is visible along the inferior margin of the deep inguinal ring, but is covered partially by the inguinal ligament.
- The fascia transversalis crura may be approximated with care.

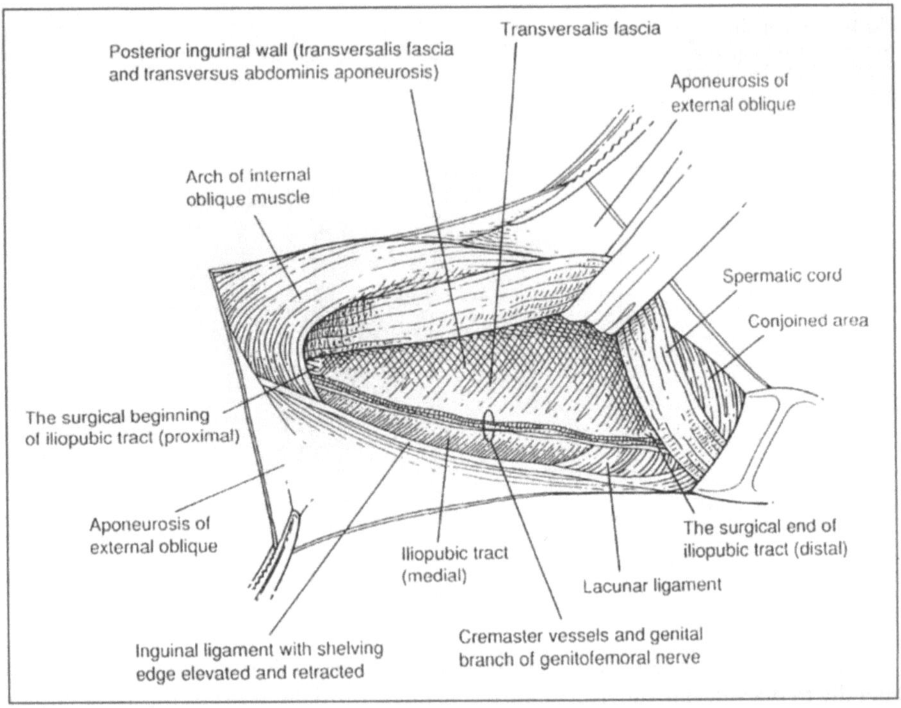

Fig. 10. The iliopubic tract and its relation to the genital branch of the genitofemoral nerve. (From [37], with permission)

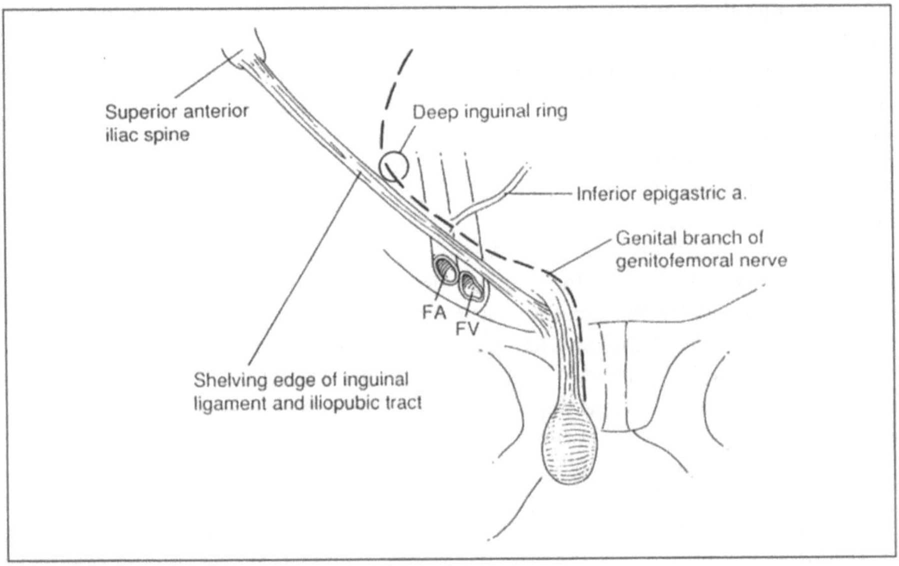

Fig. 11. Pathway of the genital branch of the genitofemoral nerve from the deep inguinal ring to the medial side of the spermatic cord. FA, femoral artery; FV, femoral vein. (From [37], with permission)

1.6 Spaces

1.6.1 Vascular Space (Fig. 1)

The vascular space is situated between the two laminae of the fascia transversalis and contains the inferior epigastric vessels.

1.6.2 Space of Bogros (Fig. 1)

Fat and other connective tissue, either thick or thin, lie within a space between the peritoneum and the fascia transversalis. Fibrous bands are present, and lipomata similar to those in the spermatic cord are occasionally found. The preperitoneal space is exposed by the reflection of parietal peritoneum toward the iliac fossa before it reaches the pubic bone [7].

According to Stoppa (personal communication, 1992), Bogros was a French anatomist and surgeon who wrote a thesis in 1823 about the surgical anatomy of the iliac region. He described a triangular space with the following boundaries: laterally, iliac fascia; anteriorly, fascia transversalis; and medially, parietal peritoneum.

Stoppa wisely stated that this cleavable interparietoperitoneal space is considered to be the lower prolongation of the great posterior paraurinary space. Hureau et al. [18, 19], after radiologic and anatomic studies of this area, considered the posterior paraurinary area as follows: (a) Gerota's fat anteriorly and (b) a cellular space posteriorly that most likely incorporates the space of Bogros in the internal iliac fossa.

According to Bendavid [20], the space of Bogros is a lateral extension of the retropubic space of Retzius and may be explored by incising the fascia transversalis from the internal ring to the pubic crest. He also reported that a venous network is probably located at the lower anterior part of the space of Bogros with fixation of the network to the anterior wall. The Bendavid "venous circle," located at the subinguinal space of Bogros, is a network composed of the following veins: deep inferior epigastric, iliopubic, rectusial, retropubic, and communicating rectusioepigastric. This circular network, again according to Bendavid, is variable (Figs. 12, 13). He advised familiarity with this venous circle, particularly by those surgeons using prosthetic material.

1.7 Vascularization of the Muscles

The following arteries vascularize the muscles:
- Superior epigastric
- Inferior epigastric
- Several other branches from the blood supply of the fat

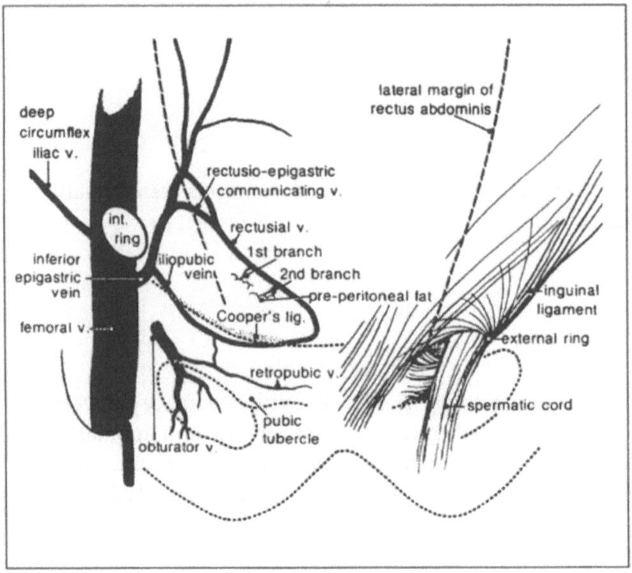

Fig. 12. The deep inguinal vasculature within the space of Bogros. (From [38], with permission)

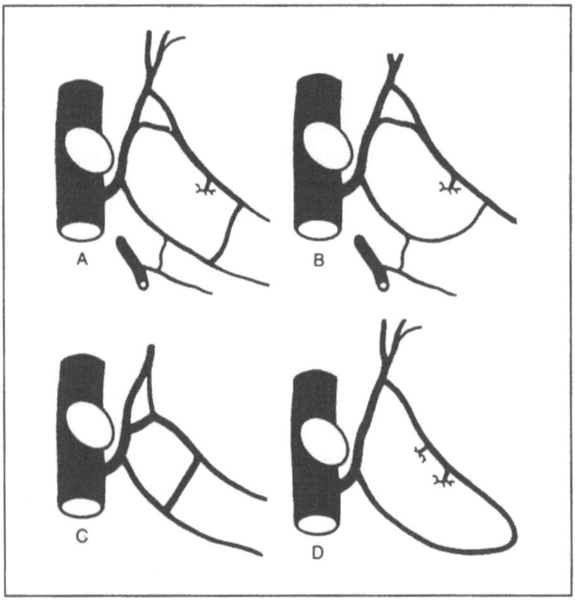

Fig. 13A–D. Variations in the vasculature of the deep inguinal venous system. (From [38], with permission)

- Superficial circumflex
- Deep circumflex.

The veins follow the arteries (characteristically each artery has two veins).

1.8 Innervation of the Abdominal Wall

1.8.1 Thoracoabdominal Nerves

Thoracoabdominal nerves (7–12) supply the upper abdominal wall. The lower wall is supplied by the ilioinguinal and iliohypogastric nerves. It should be remembered that the thoracoabdominal nerves traveling between the internal oblique and transversus abdominis muscles are responsible for the three flat muscles, rectus abdominis muscle, and pyramidalis muscle.

The 12th nerve is the subcostal. It supplies partially the internal oblique, transversus abdominis pyramidalis, and rectus muscle.

The observations of the nerves most commonly encountered and their relations are summarized below, based on 99 cadaveric dissections by Skandalakis et al. [21].

1.8.2 Ilioinguinal Nerve (Fig. 14)

The results were as follows: typical (ilioinguinal nerve resting on the spermatic cord), 72%; nerve within the spermatic cord, 26%; and nerve absent or not found, 2%.

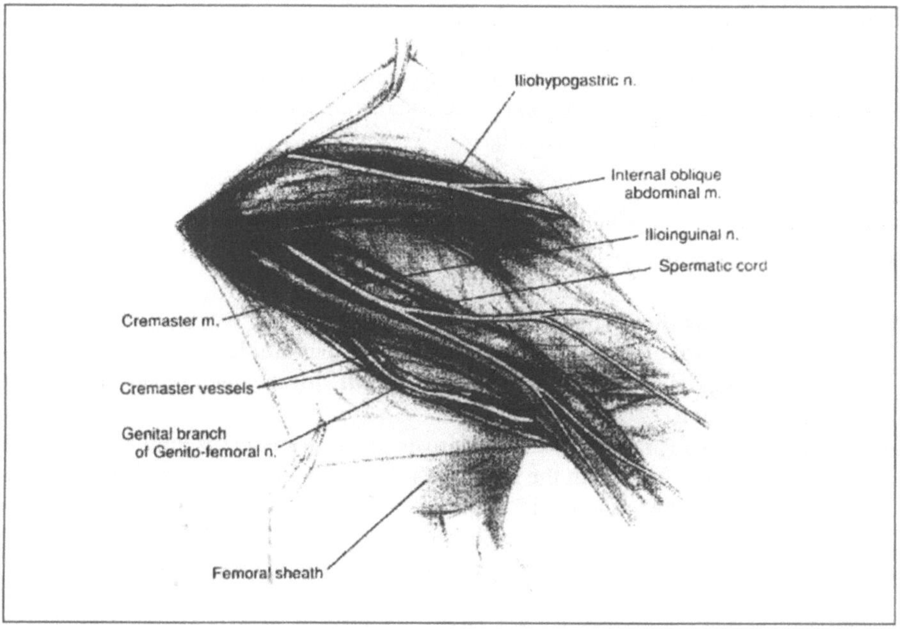

Fig. 14. Sensory nerves of the groin. (Modified from [23], with permission)

1.8.3
Iliohypogastric Nerve (Fig. 14)

The iliohypogastric nerve was always present, although in many cases the ilioinguinal nerve was (for all practical purposes) combined with it. In such instances, the ventral primary ramus of L1 (primarily) courses between the transversus abdominis and the internal oblique muscle just above the iliac crest, piercing the internal oblique just medial to the anterior superior iliac spine. At a variable distance from the anterior spine, this nerve divides into iliohypogastric and ilioinguinal nerves. It is typical that, when such a combined nerve divides, it does so just superior to the external inguinal ring, and the ilioinguinal nerve then descends across the spermatic cord before reaching its typical exit position from the inferolateral margin of the external ring. Needless to say, incisions of the external inguinal ring must allow for the possibility of this variation to avoid unnecessary injury.

1.8.4
Genitofemoral Nerve (Figs. 10, 11, 14)

The femoral branch of the genitofemoral nerve, which is usually distributed to the skin of the femoral (Scarpa's) triangle of the proximal thigh, in some cases communicated with, or was replaced by, an intermediate femoral cutaneous nerve arising in the iliac fossa. The genital branch in most cases exited the abdomen in the inferomedial angle of the deep ring, in company with the cremasteric branches of the inferior epigastric vessels. Lying deep to the cremaster, it was distributed to that muscle by three or more branches and also supplied twigs to the skin of the scrotum. The genital branch was rather often combined with the ilioinguinal nerve (7.7%) in the present study.

An anterior femoral cutaneous or accessory femoral nerve was present and visible in some cases. When it is present, this nerve usually passes through the iliopubic tract 2–4 cm lateral to the deep inguinal ring.

1.8.5
Surgical Applications

The following points should be noted:

- Despite the fact that the inguinal ligament is considered of less than prime importance, it is categorized by the authors as "good stuff" for the open repair of inguinofemoral herniation.
- The arch that is formed by the aponeurosis of the transversus abdominis and is sometimes heavily fixed with the muscular part of the internal oblique also belongs to the category of the "good stuff."
- The conjoined area should be remembered.
- The lacunar ligament occasionally may be used for hernia repair in the open method.
- The relaxing incision must be done at the anterior lamina of the rectus sheath medial to the conjoined tendon after elevation of the external oblique muscle.

- The relaxing incision or prosthesis is recommended if the posterior wall is defective or the arch is displayed medially.

1.9 Peritoneum

The peritoneum is the innermost layer of the abdominal wall and, consequently, of the inguinal area. It is connected loosely with the posterior lamina of the fascia transversalis in most areas except at the internal ring, where the connection is stronger. The processus vaginalis, a peritoneal diverticulum, is related embryologically to the deep inguinal ring.

1.10 Fossae of the Anterior Abdominal Wall

The posterior surface of the anterior abdominal wall above the inguinal ligament is divided into three shallow fossae (from lateral to medial): lateral, medial, and supravesical. These are located on either side of the midline and are marked by the obliterated embryonic urachus that extends from the dome of the bladder to the umbilicus (median umbilical ligament). Laterally, the fossae are separated by the medial umbilical ligaments (obliterated umbilical arteries) and the lateral umbilical ligaments (inferior or deep epigastric arteries), as shown in Fig. 15. From lateral to medial, the fossae are as follows: The lateral fossa, lateral to the inferior epigastric arteries, contains the

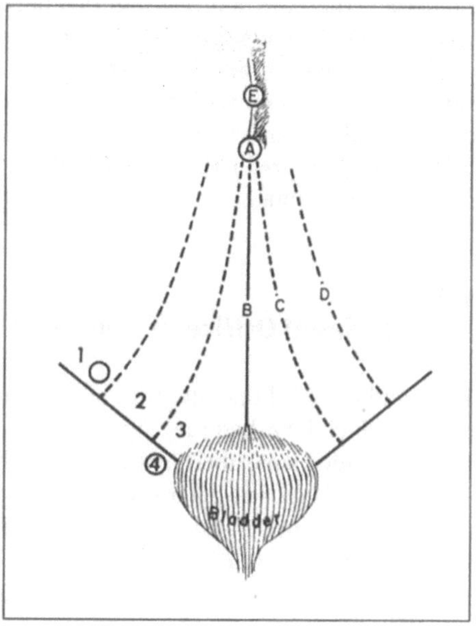

Fig. 15. Fossae of the anterior abdominal wall and their relation to the sites of groin hernias. A, umbilicus; B, median umbilical ligament (obliterated urachus); C, medial umbilical ligament (obliterated umbilical arteries); D, lateral umbilical ligament containing inferior (deep) epigastric arteries; E, falciform ligament. Sites of possible hernias: 1, lateral fossa (indirect inguinal hernia); 2, medial fossa (direct inguinal hernia); 3, supravesical fossa (supravesical hernia); 4, femoral ring (femoral hernia). (From [39], with permission)

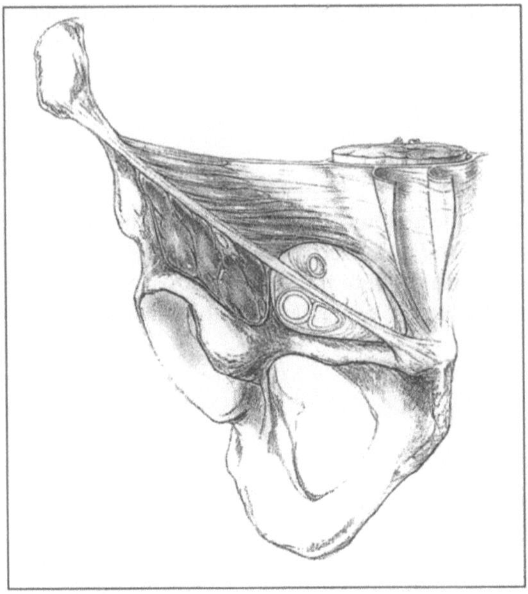

Fig. 16. Anterior view of Fruchaud's myopectineal orifice. (From [23], with permission)

internal inguinal ring, the site of indirect inguinal hernias. The medial fossa, between the inferior epigastric artery and the medial umbilical ligament, is the site of direct inguinal hernia. The supravesical fossa, between the medial and median umbilical ligaments, is the site of external supravesical hernia.

The supravesical fossa partially overlies Hesselbach's triangle so that the medial umbilical ligament lies within it. A hernia through either the medial or the supravesical fossa is therefore a direct inguinal hernia. A direct hernia may also be inguinal (in the medial fossa) or supravesical (in the supravesical fossa).

The termination of the aponeurosis of the internal oblique muscle and the transversus abdominis muscle meet to form the "conjoined tendon" (see Sect. 4.8 above) in only a small percentage of patients. In most individuals, this tendon is absent. Skandalakis et al. [22] prefer the lateral border of the rectus sheath as the landmark for a supravesical hernia.

1.11 Myopectineal Orifice of Fruchaud

Fruchaud believed that all groin hernias began in a single weak area within the groin, an area which he called the "myopectineal orifice" (Fig. 16) [23]. The myopectineal orifice is bounded superiorly by the arch of the internal oblique muscle and the transversus abdominis muscle, laterally by the iliopsoas muscle, medially by the lateral border of the rectus muscle and its anterior lamina, and inferiorly by the pubic pecten. The inguinal ligament spans and divides this framework. The area is transversed by the spermatic cord and femoral vessels and is bridged on its inner surface by the fascia transversalis only.

According to Madden [5], the "pyriform fossa" of Fruchaud forms part of the posterior wall ("floor") of the inguinal canal. This potential structure is a semiovoid space filled with fibrofatty tissue located at the medial part of the floor. It is defined as follows: The iliopubic tract, which inserts into Cooper's ligament, is its superior border; the shelving edge of the inguinal ligament is its inferior border; the ligament of Gimbernat is its medial border and "floor"; and the medial wall of the femoral sheath is its lateral border.

1.12 Cooper's Ligament

Cooper [15] described this "ligament" almost 200 years ago (in 1804). What is the ligament of Cooper (Fig. 17)? The following few notes may help the reader understand it.

According to Nyhus and Bombeck [24], "periosteum of the pelvis ... is intimately fused with another condensation of the transversalis fascia and iliopubic tract to form Cooper's ligament."

An excellent description by Neidhardt [25] states that the pectineal ligament is formed by three layers: (1) the deep layer is in continuity with the periosteum of the superior pubic ramus, (2) the middle, muscular layer is formed by the pectineus muscle, and (3) the superficial aponeurotic layer is formed by the pectineal aponeurosis.

Hollinshead [26] wrote that the ligament of Cooper is the lateral continuation of the ligament of Gimbernat. However, if this statement is correct, the ligament of Cooper belongs to the anterior lamina of the abdominal wall and, more specifically, is the product – together with the ligament of Gimbernat – of the aponeurosis of the external oblique muscle. This assumption, however, is dangerous, because it will destroy the well-accepted philosophy of the anterior and posterior lamina.

What, then, is the ligament of Cooper? In all honesty, we do not know, but we feel that both the ligament of Cooper and the ligament of Gimbernat are good neighbors and perhaps the point of their union is the meeting point of the anterior and posterior lamina.

The ligament of Cooper may include elements of the following anatomic entities:

- Periosteum
- Lateral continuation of the lacunar ligament (which is fused to the periosteum)
- Fibers originating from the upper part of the pectineal fascia in such a way that the fascia is located under the periosteum and the lacunar ligament (this might be said to be the origin and not the insertion)
- Aponeurotic fibers from the insertion of the transversus abdominis
- Insertion of the fascia transversalis and its iliopubic tract
- Occasionally, fibers from the insertion of the rectus tendon or the internal oblique.

However, for all practical purposes, Cooper's ligament consists of the following: (a) the periosteum of the pectineal line, (b) the insertion of the iliopubic tract from above to the periosteum, (c) the insertion of the lacunar ligament from below to the periosteum, and (d) the insertion or origin of the pectineal fascia from below (Fig. 17).

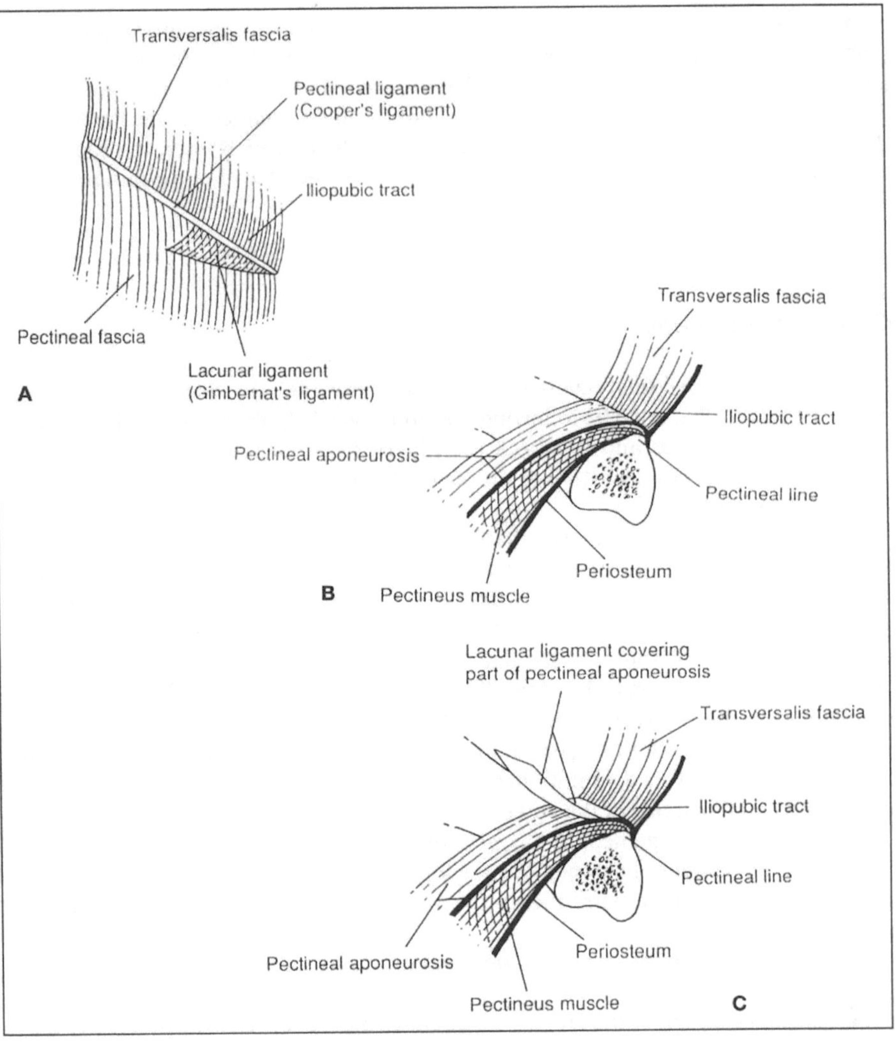

Fig. 17A–C. *A* Anatomic entities participating in the formation of the pectineal ligament (Cooper's). *B* Insertion of the iliopubic tract into the ligament of Cooper and perhaps the origin of the pectineal aponeurosis. *C* The lacunar ligament (Gimbernat's) partially covers the pectineal aponeurosis. (From [37], with permission)

The following points should be remembered:
- The iliopubic tract is inserted into the ligament of Cooper from above (superiorly).
- The ligament of Gimbernat is inserted partially into the ligament of Cooper from below (inferiorly).
- The pectineus tendon originates from the ligament of Cooper from below (inferiorly), and its medial part is covered by the ligament of Gimbernat.

However, each time I (J.E.S.) dissect the ligament of Cooper, I change my mind about its real formation.

1.13 Femoral Canal and Femoral Sheath

Between the inguinal ligament and the linea terminalis (iliopectineal line), which is that part of the pelvic brim extending from the ala of the sacrum to the pubic tubercle, is a space organized into three compartments (Fig. 18). The most lateral of these is the neuromuscular compartment, which contains the iliopsoas muscle, the femoral nerve, and the lateral femoral cutaneous nerve. Medial to this, the vascular compartment contains the femoral artery and vein. Still more medial is the compartment of the femoral canal. The femoral sheath, an extension of the fascia transversalis of the abdomen, envelops the femoral artery, vein, and femoral canal.

As previously described, the femoral sheath is formed anteriorly and medially by the fascia transversalis, posteriorly by the pectineus and psoas fasciae, and laterally by the iliacus fascia. The most medial of the three compartments of the sheath is the femoral canal, through which a femoral hernia may pass.

The femoral canal is conical, approximately 1.25–2 cm in length. At its apex is the fossa ovalis, the opening for the great saphenous vein. Thus a femoral hernia may present as a bulge of the skin over the fossa ovalis.

The femoral ring is inflexible. McVay [27] states that the transverse diameter ranges from 8 to 27 mm, with 70% lying between 10 and 14 mm. The anteroposterior diameter ranges from 9 to 19 mm, with 70% lying between 12 and 16 mm. The lateral boundary is the femoral vein and connective tissue. The posterior boundary is the pectineal ligament (Cooper's). The iliopubic tract or inguinal ligament, or both, form the anterior boundary. The fascia transversalis, the aponeurotic insertion of the transversus abdominis muscle, and, more medially, the lacunar ligament form the medial boundary.

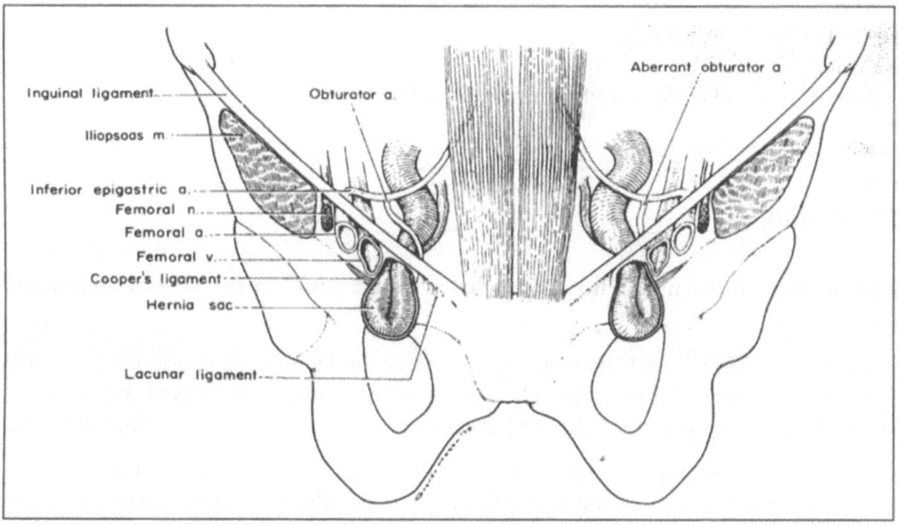

Fig. 18. Cooper's ligament and the ligament of Gimbernat *(left)* in a patient with an incarcerated femoral hernia with the presence of an aberrant obturator artery *(right)*. (From [30], with permission)

McVay [7] located the lacunar ligament at the medial margin of the femoral ring in only eight of 362 subjects. He believed the transversus abdominis aponeurosis to be the usual boundary. Condon [28] believes that either the aponeurosis or the recurved iliopubic tract may form the medial boundary.

The exit of the femoral canal is as follows: anteriorly, the fascia lata; posteriorly, the pectineal fascia; laterally, the femoral sheath; and medially, the iliopubic tract and occasionally the lacunar ligament.

The formation of a femoral hernia is an enigma to us.

Where is the site of obstruction in an incarcerated or strangulated femoral hernia? The femoral ring or a point 1.5 cm below the ring? Lytel [29] believes the latter and advises partial transection of the ligament of Gimbernat. We prefer partial transection of the inguinal ligament for two reasons:

1. To avoid injury to an aberrant obturator artery passing medial to the hernial sac
2. It is the easy way to transect partially the inguinal ligament [30].

1.14 "Good Stuff"

The previous pages have described anatomic entities which, when used for anchoring sutures, are useful for the repair of inguinofemoral herniation; we call these entities the "good stuff." To summarize, the following entities are "good stuff":

- Inguinal ligament
- Lacunar ligament (Gimbernat's)
- Pectineal ligament (Cooper's)
- Fascia transversalis and transversus abdominis aponeurosis
- Iliopubic tract
- Anterior femoral sheath
- Fascia transversalis crura
- Conjoined area
- Arch of internal oblique and transversus abdominis muscle.

1.15 Discussion

Schumpelick: In the inguinal region, what is "good stuff" in the ventral abdominal wall?

Skandalakis: The inguinal ligament, occasionally the lacunar ligament, the pectineal ligament of Cooper of course, the fascia transversalis, the aponeurosis of the transverse muscle, the ileopubic tract, the conjoined area, and the oblique abdominal muscles.

Kingsnorth: On the topic of the linea alba, Professor Chevrel, I know that you have made very good studies of the strength of the linea alba with tensiometers and you have looked in detail at the laminae of the linea alba. Can you tell us more about these studies and the differential strength of the upper region, the mid region, and the lower region of the linea alba?

Chevrel: In the upper part of the linea alba, the anterior sheath is made with the external oblique tendon and part of the internal tendon and in the inferior part all the tendons of flat muscles before the rectus muscles. I think the most important point is that the linea alba must be considered as an actual tendon of flat muscles. That is how Professor John Rives and my friend Flament regard it.

Schumpelick: Dr. Skandalakis, please could you explain to us again the construction of the linea alba as shown in the figure.

Skandalakis: With regard to the studies by Askar, in 70% there are three cross-sections, and only in 30% are there less.

Hartel: The metabolism and blood supply of fascia is very low, and during an operation this is maybe transected. Are there any special points that should be preserved during an operation?

Skandalakis: I don't know.

Simmermacher: I have a question about Ramirez' component separation technique. We are told to divide the lateral sides of the external abdominal from the internal, and this is supposed to be a bloodless area. In an article in Hernia, Meyer from Strasbourg tells us to divide the transversus from the internal; is there a bloodless area as well?

Skandalakis: I don't know.

Bendavid: In Miami, I said that the fascia transversalis is a trilaminar structure under the microscope and is not in fact a condensation of the so-called endopelvic fascia. This thin fascia suddenly became thick in the inguinal region. Cooper himself spoke about two layers. In fact, three layers can be seen: fascia of internal oblique, fascia of the transversus, and the endopelvic fascia. The continuation becomes the ileopubic tract, and the normal external oblique aponeurosis then joins it; then you have the so-called Gimbernat's ligament, which inserts again into the ligament of Cooper. I think we should perhaps start thinking of the fascia transversalis as a three-layered structure.

Skandalakis: I don't know.

Filipi: I very much appreciate the amount of work you have done and your dedication to the topic; I think it is outstanding. I hope that you will present this material again, especially at laparoscopic meetings. We have dissected a few cadavers, but not anywhere close to the number that you have. One question is, where are these lateral nerves located in relation to the iliopubic tract, and how often are the lateral and anterior femorocutaneous nerves anterior to the iliopubic tract?

Skandalakis: I have not seen that. They are always posterior between the cremasteric vessels, between the inguinal ligament and the iliopubic tract. They are just a small distance apart. My advice to the laparoscopist is therefore not to make deep incisions between the iliopubic tract below and the arch above.

Filipi: Another entity that I am not aware of is the vesical umbilical fascia you mentioned in one of your slides. I wonder what significance it might have for laparoscopic surgeons.

Skandalakis: I don't think honestly that it has anything to do with laparoscopic surgery. You can open and sacrifice and do anything you want with this fascia, because it is covered with peritoneum above, so somehow we are protected in this area.

Filipi: One final question. Did you have any cadavers with indirect hernias? I am interested in the anatomical relationships of the vas and the spermatic vessels to indirect hernia sacs at the internal ring level.

Skandalakis: We created some in our cadavers. The hernia sac is practically just above the spermatic cord; sometimes it is fixed and sometimes not. We practically saw the same thing that we saw with the typical orthodox procedure from above. Our philosophy is to present the real anatomy and not the anecdotal anatomy that was presented in the past.

Schumpelick: I am interested in the genital branch of the genitofemoral nerve. How often is it located in the ring?

Skandalakis: It is always there. In most cases, it is fixed with the spermatic vessels and is below the iliopubic tract. I call this "the enemy below," because sometimes you can take this with your sutures and you get a post-traumatic neuralgia.

Schumpelick: And within the channel, now coming from the other side in the inguinal canal, where is it located?

Skandalakis: It is located in the inferior and medial part close to the lateral crest, which is fixed to the iliopubic tract. Fortunately, it is very deep, and when we take sutures there, we do not injure the nerve. However, it is sometimes superficial. We always have to elevate the lateral crest with mosquitoes and see what goes up there. If we prepare this area very well, we can see a silver-like cord formation, which is nothing else but the nerve.

References

1. White RR: Atlas of Pediatiric Surgery, 2nd edition, New York, McGraw-Hill, 1978
2. Orda R, Nathan H: Surgical anatomy of the umbilical structures. Int Surg 58(7):454–64, 1973
3. Rizk NN. A new description of the anterior abdominal wall in man and mammals. J Anat 131(3):373–385, 1990
4. Askar OM. Aponeurosis hernias: recent observations upon paraumbilical and epigastric hernias. Surg Clin North Am 64:315–333, 1984
5. Madden JL. Abdominal Wall Hernias . Philadelphia: Saunders, 1989
6. Condon RE. Surgical anatomy of the transversus abdominis and transversalis fascia. Ann Surg 173:1, 1971
7. McVay CB. Surgical Anatomy, 6th Ed. Philadelphia: WB Saunders, 1984, pp. 484–584
8. Hollinshead WH. The abdominal wall and inguinal region. In: Anatomy for Surgeons: The Thorax, Abdomen and Pelvis, Vol 2. New York: Paul B. Hoeber, 1956, pp.216–268
9. Condon RE. The anatomy of the inguinal region and it's relationship to groin hernia, 2nd Ed. Philadelphia: Lippincott, 1978, pp. 14–78
10. McVay CB. The anatomic basis for inguinal and femoral hernioplasty. Surg Gynecol Obstet 139:931, 1974
11. Askar OM. Surgical anatomy of the aponeurotic expansions of the anterior abdominal wall. Ann R Coll Surg Engl 59:313–321, 1977
12. Askar OM: A new concept of the aetiology and surgical repair of paraumbilical and epigastric hernias. Ann R Coll Surg Engl 60:42–48, 1978
13. Rizk NN. A new description of the anterior abdominal wall. Anat Rec 184:515, 1976

14. Nahai F, Brown RG, Vasconez LO. Blood supply to the abdominal wall as related to planning abdominal incisions. Am Surg 42:691–695, 1976
15. Cooper A. The Anatomy and Surgical Treatment of Abdominal Hernia. Philadelphia: Lea & Blachard, 1804, pp. 26–27
16. Williams PL. Gray's Anatomy, 38th Ed. New York: Churchill Livingstone, 1995, p. 829
17. Condon RE. The anterior iliopubic tract repair. In Nyhus LM, Condon RE (eds). Hernia, 4th Ed. Philadelphia: Lippincott, 1995, pp. 136–152
18. Hureau J. Agossou-Voyeme AK, Germain M, Pradel J. Les espaces interparieto-peritoneaux posterieurs ou espaces retroperitoneaux: Anatomie topographique normale. J Radiol 72:101–116, 1991
19. Hureau J, Pradel J, Agossou-Voyeme AK, Germain M. Les espaces interparieto-peritoneaux posterieurs ou espaces retroperitoneaux: Anatomie tomodensitometrique pathologique. J Radiol 72:205–227, 1991
20. Bendavid R. The Space of Bogros and the deep inguinal venous circulation. Surg Gynecol Obstet 174:355, 1992
21. Skandalakis JE, Skandalakis LJ, Colborn GL: Testicular atrophy and neuropathy in herniorrhaphy. Am Surg 9:775–782, 1996
22. Skandalakis JE, Gray SW, Rowe JS Jr. Hernias. In: Anatomical Complications in General Surgery. New York: McGraw-Hill, 1983, pp. 252–268
23. Wantz GE. Atlas of Hernia Surgery. New York: Raven Press, 1991, pp. 4–5
24. Nyhus LM, Bombeck CT. Hernias. In: Sabiston DC (ed). Textbook of Surgery, 13th Ed. Philadelphia: WB Saunders, 1986, pp. 1231–1252
25. Neidhardt JPH. Surgical anatomy of the anterolateral and posterior abdominal walls and points of weakness. In: Chevrl JP (ed). Surgery of the Abdominal Wall. Berlin: Springer-Verlag, 1987, pp. 3–26
26. Hollinshead WH. Anatomy for Surgeons, Vol 2. New York: Hoeber-Harper, 1961, p. 243
27. McVay CB. The anatomic basis for inguinal and femoral hernioplasty. Surg Gynecol Obstet 139:931, 1974
28. Condon RE. Surgical anatomy of the transversus abdominis and transversalis fascia. Ann Surg 173:1, 1971
29. Lytle WJ. Special comment: The low operation for femoral hernia. In: Nyhus LM, Harkins HN (eds). Hernia. Philadelphia: JB Lippincott, 1964, pp. 208–211
30. Skandalakis JE, Gray SW, Akin JT Jr. The surgical anatomy of hernial rings. Surg Clin North Am 54(6), 1974, p. 1230
31. Skandalakis JE, Colborn G, Gray S, Skandalakis L, Pemberton LB. The surgical anatomy of the inguinal area. Contemp Surg 1991;38(1,2):20–34
32. Skandalakis JE, Colborn GL, Androulakis JA, LJ Skandalakis, Pemberton LB. Embryologic and anatomic basis of inguinal herniorrhaphy. Surg Clin North Am 73(4), 1993
33. Skandalakis JE, Colborn GL, Gray SW, Skandalakis LJ, Pemberton LB. The surgical anatomy of the inguinal area – Part I. Contemp Surg 38:20–34, 1991
34. Skandalakis LJ, Gadacz TR, Mansberger AR Jr, Mitchell WE Jr, Colborn GL, Skandalakis JE. Modern hernia repair: the embryological and anatomical basis of surgery. New York: Parthenon, 1996
35. Skandalakis JE, Gray SW, Mansberger AR, Colborn GL, Skandalakis LJ. Hernia: Surgical anatomy and technique. New York: McGraw-Hill, 1989
36. Gray SW, Skandalakis JE, McClusky DA. Atlas of surgical anatomy for general surgeons. Baltimore: Williams & Wilkins, 1985
37. Colborn GL, Skandalakis JE. Importance of the iliopubic, Cooper's and Gimbernat's ligaments. Problems in General Surgery 12(1):35–40, 1995
38. Bendavid R. The space of Bogros and the deep inguinal venous circulation. Surg Gynecol Obstet 174:356–357, 1992
39. Rowe JS Jr, Skandalakis JE, Gray SW. Multiple bilateral inguinal hernias. Am Surg 39:269, 1973

CHAPTER 2

Functional Anatomy

B. Devlin†

The anterior abdominal wall can be divided into two structural/functional zones, the upper "parachute area" aiding respiratory movement and a lower "belly support" area. These two functional layers are reflected in anatomical structure. Functional failure in the abdomen may lead to epigastric and umbilical hernia in the upper zone and to indirect inguinal hernia in the lower abdomen.

2.1 Upper Abdominal Zone Herniation

The anatomy of the midline aponeurosis is related to epigastric and umbilical (para-umbilical) hernia formation. Epigastric herniation is found exclusively in patients having a single anterior and single posterior line of decussation; this was found in only 30% of cadaver specimens examined by Askar in 1984 [1]. Uncoordinated tearing strains on the aponeurotic fibres of the linea alba, e.g. in vigorous sports, coughing or vomiting, will stretch the decussations and allow the development of fatty protrusions between their bundles (Fig. 1). Obesity and multiparity contribute to the development

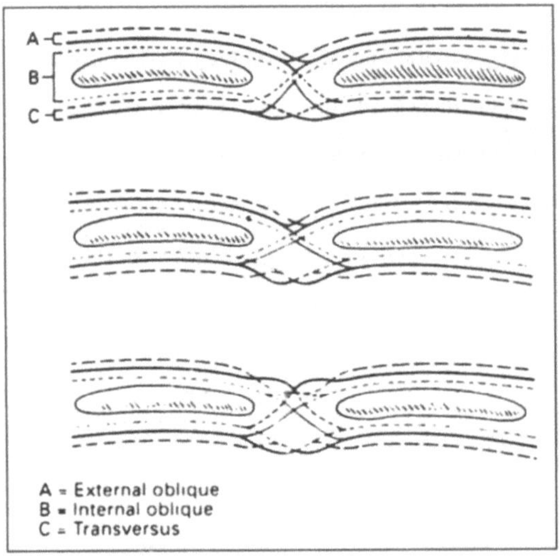

Fig. 1. Decussation of antero-lateral fibres of the aponeurotic layers at the linea alba. (From [6])

of umbilical hernias. Stretching of the umbilicus in laparoscopic procedures is a new iatrogenic cause of umbilical herniation [2].

2.2 Incidence

The population incidence of epigastric hernia has not been determined. These hernias are infrequent in infants and young children. They occur in children in their teens or in young adults. They are more frequent in males than females in a ratio of 3:13. They account for 3.4% of external hernias in a series from Nigeria [4]; in the U.S. Armed Forces they account for 5.0% of external abdominal hernias, but this figure may be an underestimate, because these small, fatty hernias are often not classified separately in official data [5]. Other authors record a similarly low incidence. They are frequently found in young men taking up physical exercise, such as athletes or those doing military service.

Umbilical hernias in adults account for 0.03% of hernias operated on in the United Kingdom. They have no racial characteristics, unlike umbilical hernias in childhood. In the United Kingdom, umbilical hernias most frequently occur in females who are overweight and usually multiparous [6].

2.3 Pathological Anatomy

The linea alba is an area of decussation of the three tendinous aponeurotic muscle strata of the anterior abdominal wall. At the midline, these three aponeuroses, the external oblique, the internal oblique and the transverse abdominis, are formed of fine tendinous fibres invested in loose areolar tissue.

The fibres of the external oblique aponeurosis have a downward, forward and medial inclination and additionally – especially around the umbilicus – describe a gentle upward curve. Above the umbilicus, most aponeurotic fibres cross the midline and appear as the superficial fibres of the opposite side; they thus form the superficial layer of a double-strata external oblique aponeurosis. When they make the crossover from one side to the other, they decussate with the fibres of the opposite side; in 40%, the fibres decussate only once at the midline ("single decussation"), whereas in 60% of abdominal walls they decussate another twice to give three decussations ("triple decussation"). This triple decussation is seen only above the umbilicus and never below. In single decussation, the fibres of the deep strata of one side appear superficial at the midline and then deep again after crossing the midline and decussating again. Below the umbilicus, except for a small area immediately adjacent to the umbilicus, this pattern of triple decussation is not seen; all the fibres of the external oblique aponeurosis invariably passed downwards and medially in a single stratum, and all the fibres then cross the midline in a single decussation to give the external oblique aponeurosis a clearly defined pattern [1].This pattern of single or triple decussation with interlocking fibres gives the external oblique aponeurosis a very fine reinforced mesh structure around and above the umbilicus (Fig. 1).

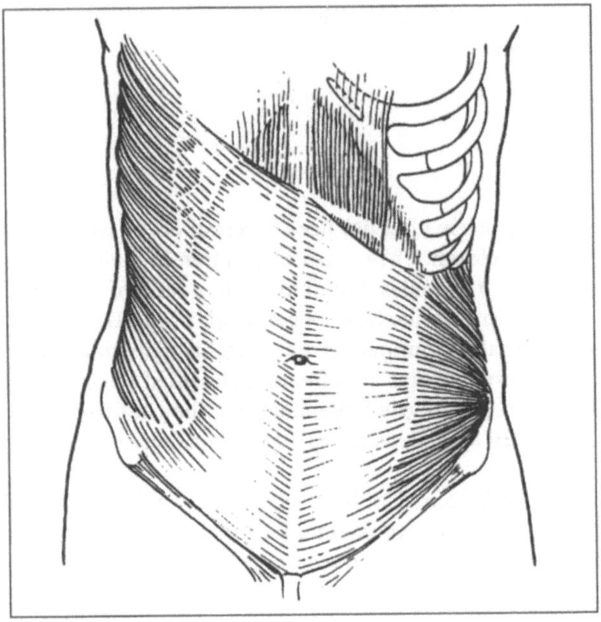

Fig. 2. The fibres of the external oblique muscle. (From [6])

The internal oblique muscle consists of fan-shaped muscle bundles laterally; the upper fibres are directed upwards and medially, the middle horizontally and the lower arch downwards and medially. The aponeurotic bundles in both the superficial and deep strata follow the same direction. At the midline, the linea alba, the anterior lamina fibres fuse with and are continuous with the fibres of the contra-lateral external oblique aponeurosis (Fig. 2).

The deepest layer of abdominal musculature, the transverse abdominal muscle, consists of fleshy bundles which are not strictly transverse; the upper bundles run horizontally and upwards, and the lowermost ones are horizontal. In 5% of specimens, all the fibres run medially towards each other. The lowermost fibres of the transverse muscle are directed downwards and medially and are often parallel to the inguinal ligament (Fig. 3).

These various muscle bundle and aponeurotic fibre directions give the anterior abdominal wall a reinforced criss-cross "plywood" structure, particularly in the upper abdomen [1] (Fig. 4).

2.4 Repair Techniques

All epigastric hernias should be repaired surgically. The only cure for the sometimes disabling and troublesome symptoms is surgery, and exploration is always advisable. In 1936, Pemberton and Curry reviewed the patients from the Mayo Clinic and noted the pleomorphic symptoms caused by umbilical and epigastric hernias [7].The sym-

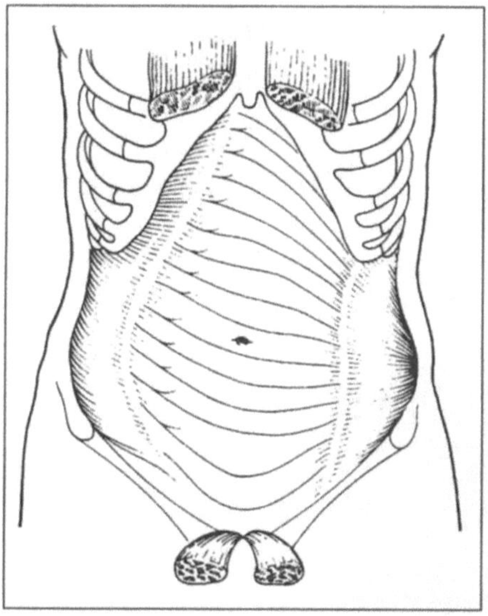

Fig. 3. The fibres of the internal oblique muscle. (From [6])

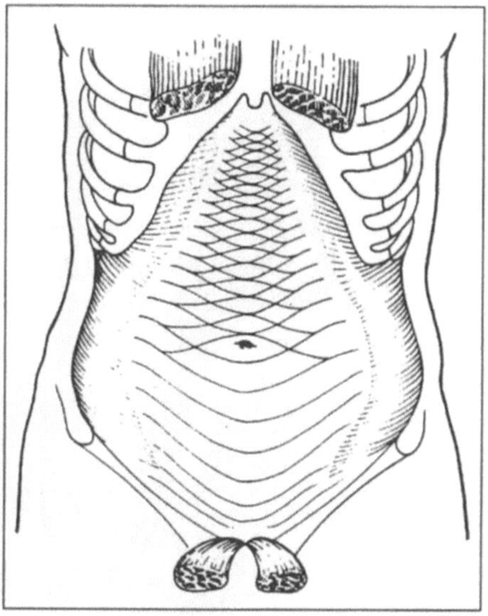

Fig. 4. The fibres of the transversus abdominis muscle. (From [6])

ptoms of an epigastric hernia can mimic almost any intraperitoneal pathology. Simple excision of small, partly strangulated, fatty hernias suffices, and only when there is a demonstrable aponeurotic deficit is suturing or mesh repair required [6].

2.5 Condensation and Sling of the Fascia Transversalis

The other aspect of functional anatomy we should dwell on is the function of the sling of the deep ring of the fascia transversalis. This was described by Astley Cooper in 1812, but more particularly by Lytle in 1970 [8, 9] and by Fruchaud in 1956 [10].

Lytle was principally concerned with the anatomy and shutter mechanism of the deep inguinal ring. He dissected the deep ring and made a remarkable film to demonstrate its protective mechanism in indirect herniation. He was concerned to preserve the mechanism of the ring and at the same time to reinforce its patulous medical margin in indirect herniation. He emphasised that manoeuvres which damaged the lateral "pillars of the ring" inevitably compromised the physiological shutter mechanism [8] (Fig. 5). In a subsequent study, he clearly described the embryological anatomy of the ring and how it could be repaired, in the fascia transversalis layer, without losing its function [9] (Fig. 6).

Fruchaud published two books in Paris in 1956, *L'Anatomie Chirurgicale de la Region de l'Aine* ("Surgical anatomy of the groin region") [10] and *Le Traitement Chirurgical des Hernies de l'Aine* ("Surgical treatment of groin hernias") [11]. He combined traditional anatomical studies of the groin, the work of Cooper, Bogros and Madden, with his own extensive anatomical and surgical experience (Fig. 7). He invented an

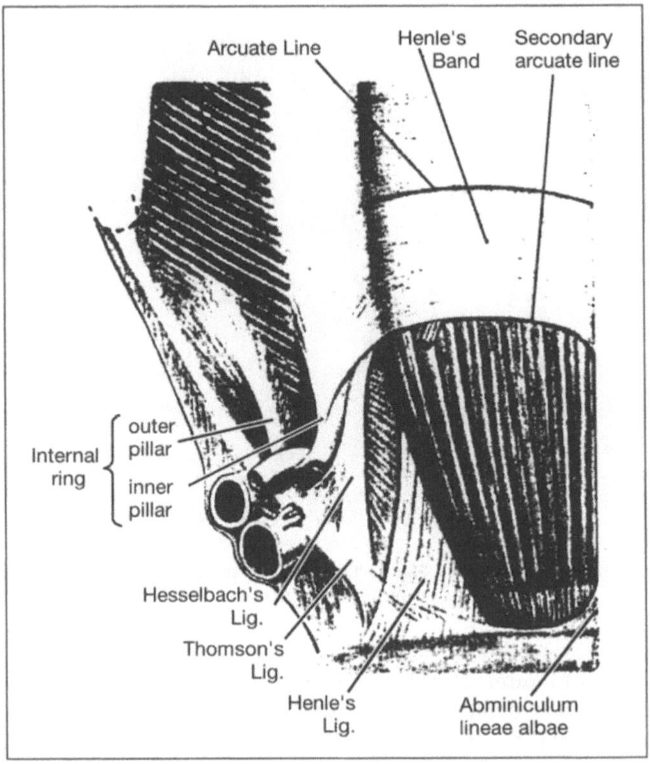

Fig. 5. "Physiological shutter" of the deep ring. (From [8])

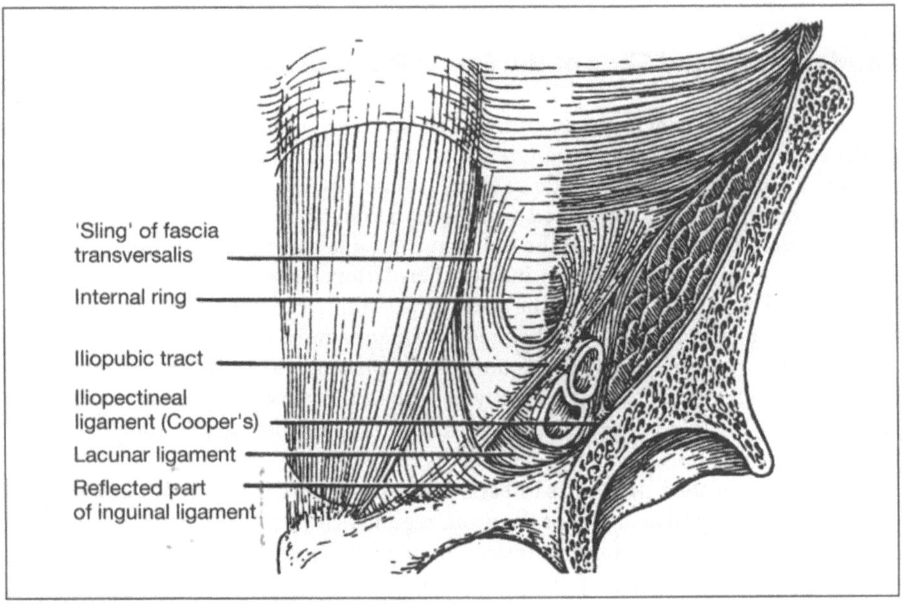

Fig. 6. The fascia transversalis at the deep ring, the shutter mechanism and sling. (From [6])

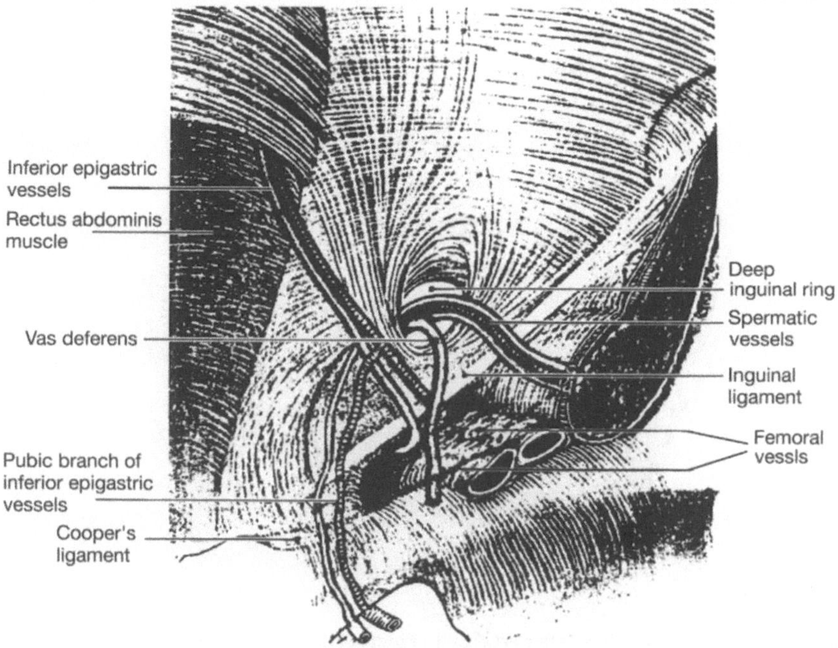

Fig. 7. The deep ring described by Fruchaud. (From [10])

entirely new concept, "the myopectineal orifice", which combined the traditionally separate inguinal and femoral canals together to form a unified highway from the abdomen to the thigh. The abdomino-crural tunnel of fascia transversalis extended through this myopectineal orifice, through which all inguinal and femoral hernias pass, as do the iliofemoral vessels. Based on this anatomical concept, Fruchaud recommended complete reconstruction of the endofascial wall (fascia transversalis) of the myopectineal orifice. This concept forms the basis for all extra-peritoneal mesh repairs, open or laparoscopic, of groin hernias [12] (Fig. 8).

The dissection of both the layers of fascia transversalis from the cord structures at the deep inguinal ring is an important component of hernioplasty, allowing the dissection of an indirect peritoneal sac and the divided peritoneal stump to retract at the deep ring in a classical Bassini and Shouldice operation for indirect hernias.

This U-shaped fold, the fascia transversalis sling, is the functional basis of the inguinal shutter mechanism; as the transverse muscle contracts during coughing or straining, the column/pillars of the ring are pulled together and the entire sling is drawn upwards and laterally. This motion increases the obliquity of exit of the spermatic cord structures through the ring and provides protection from forces tending to cause an indirect hernia. The reconstruction of this sling medially with preservation of the function of the ring laterally is the rationale of anterior inguinal hernioplasty. In front of the ring lies the lower border of the transverse muscle and the internal oblique muscle. Each of these structures supports the internal ring, and together they provide

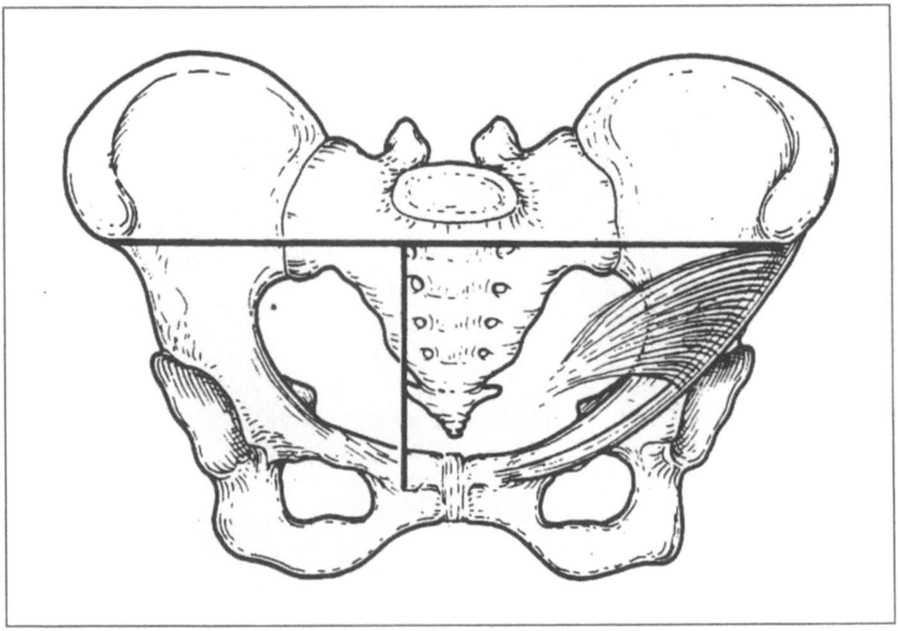

Fig. 8. The "myopectineal orifice" after Fruchaud. (From [10])

a very effective valve when the intra-abdominal pressure rises [8]. The origin of the internal oblique muscle from the inguinal ligament varies and may be deficient in some African subjects, leading to the increased frequency of indirect herniation observed in Negroes [6] (Fig. 9).

The shutter action of the internal ring, the fascia transversalis sling, can be demonstrated readily at operation under local anaesthetic. If the patient is asked to cough, the ring is suddenly pulled upwards and laterally behind the lower margin of the transverse muscle. In an adult with an obliterated processus vaginalis, a flat lid of peritoneum covers the ring internally for the spermatic vessels and the vas deferens lies extraperitoneally. The spermatic vessels pass down almost vertically retroperitoneally on the psoas muscle. As they enter the narrow gutter of the groin, they are joined by the vas deferens: the spermatic cord thus formed turns obligingly upwards and then hooks around the fascia transversalis sling to enter the deep ring, acquiring an investment of internal spermatic fascia as it traverses the ring.

The inferior border of the internal ring abuts a condensation of the fascia transversalis, the iliopubic tract or bandelette iliopubienne of Thomson. This small fascial band extends from the anterior superior iliac spine laterally to the pubis medially.

The band is a condensation of and integral part of the fascia transversalis; it lies on a plane somewhat deeper than the inguinal ligament and can be readily demonstrated as distinct from it at operation. The iliopubic tract bridges the femoral canal medially and then curves inferiorly and posteriorly to spread out like a fan to its attachment to a broad area of the superior ramus of the pubis along the iliopectineal line (Cooper's ligament). The iliopubic tract thus forms the inferior margin of the defect in the fascia

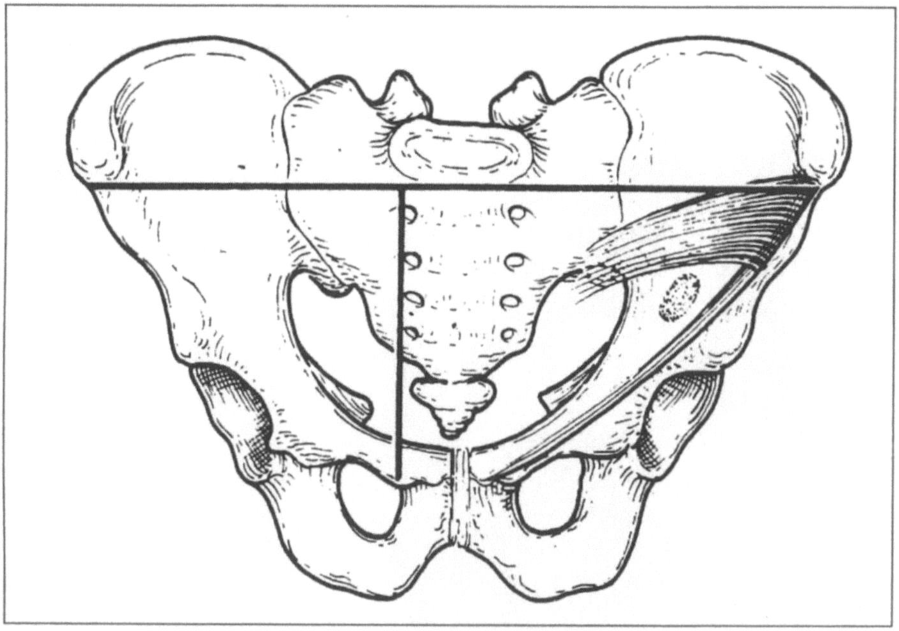

Fig. 9. The origin of the internal oblique muscle from the lateral inguinal ligament in European people. (From [6])

transversalis in an indirect inguinal hernia and in a direct hernia; it is anterior to the peritoneal sac of a femoral hernia (Fig. 10).

The fascia transversalis superior to the iliopubic tract extends over the posterior wall of the inguinal canal up to and posterior to the arch of the transverse muscle. Medially, the fascia transversalis merges into the rectus sheath and aponeurosis of the transverse muscle or conjoint tendon. The fascia transversalis in the posterior wall of the inguinal canal is supported to a variable extent by the aponeurosis of the transverse muscle as it arches down to its attachment to the pubis and iliopectineal line. Medial to the deep inguinal ring and deep to the fascia transversalis, lying in the extra-peritoneal fat between the peritoneum and the fascia, the deep epigastric vessels follow an oblique course upward and medially to the deep aspect of the rectus muscle. This triangular area, bounded by the deep epigastric vessels laterally, the lateral margin of the rectus muscle medially and the inguinal ligament below, is known to surgeons as Hesselbach's triangle; this is the area through which a direct inguinal hernia protrudes.

More exactly, a direct hernia explodes through the fascia transversalis in the area bounded by the iliopubic tract inferiorly, the medial limb of the fascia transversalis sling laterally and the lower margin of the arch of the transversus aponeurosis superiorly.

Condon (1971) investigated the anatomy of the fascia transversalis using a technique of transillumination of fresh tissue. He clearly showed these anatomic details and defined the margins of the aponeurotic deficiency in the posterior inguinal canal wall

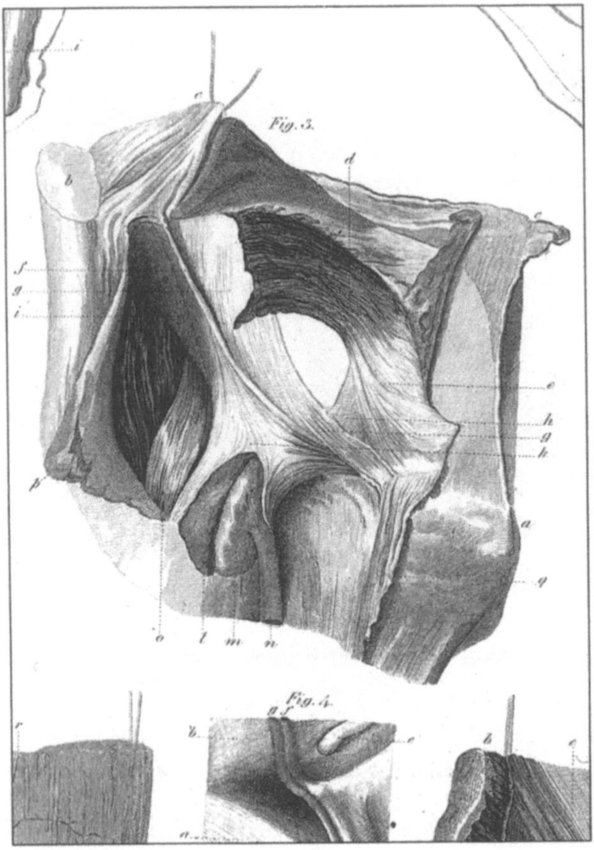

Fig. 10. The fascia transversalis envelopes the femoral vessels. From [6])

through which direct hernia protrude. This area of fascia transversalis is buttressed anteriorly to a greater or lesser degree by the aponeurosis of the transverse muscle as it inserts into the iliopectineal line. At operation, these features – the iliopubic tract, the deep ring and the "line" of the arch of the transverse aponeurosis – are easily identifiable if the fascia transversalis is adequately dissected. Indeed, the identification of all these features is an essential prerequisite for adequate anterior inguinal hernioplasty [13].

The fascia transversalis in the groin is but a segment of the endo-abdominal fascia. This fascia is distinct in the lower abdomen, the functional "belly support" zone of anterior abdominal wall, but is fused into the fascia on the deep surface of the transverse abdominal muscle superiorly. This composite layer, the transverse muscle and its fascia (the fascia transversalis), is the most important of the abdominal wall strata in solving the problem of inguinofemoral hernia, as the integrity of this layer prevents herniation. Defects in it, congenital or acquired, are the aetiology of all groin hernias [14].

Inferior to the inguinal ligament, the fascia transversalis attaches to the iliopectineal line medially and posteriorly to the femoral vessels.

This funnel of fascia transversalis extends into the thigh as the sheath surrounding the femoral vessels, as far as the fossa ovalis in the deep fascia. This anatomic arrangement allows for a small "space" medial to the femoral vein through which some lymphatics pass. When a femoral hernia develops, this space is expanded.

The anatomy and surgery of these hernias is extensively reviewed elsewhere [6].

2.6 Discussion

Schumpelick: What happens to the abdominal wall in pregnancy? Is it a flexible system or is it a relaxative system?

Devlin: The upper part of the abdominal wall at least is elastic.

Kingsnorth: Some extra information on that was provided by the American Hernia Association and by Rutkow. He told us that there are 700,000 inguinal hernias per year in the United States – only 25,000 femoral hernias, but 110,000 are umbilical hernias. So it is actually a very important entity. I think we really need to discuss the anatomy around the umbilical area. Our two French anatomists have done some very important work on the linea alba, particularly around the umbilicus, on its width and tensile strength. At the umbilicus, the linea alba is 1.5 cm wide, and it is therefore very susceptible to any herniation. Its tensile strength is also weakest around the umbilicus compared to its supra- and infraumbilical tensile strength.

Chevrel: It is important, when we repair incisional hernias, to reconstruct the linea alba, but if mesh is used, the function of the transverse muscle is not good and there will be respiratory disturbance.

Schumpelick: To what extent do we need the abdomen for respiration? Are there any percentages available on the extent to which people ventilate using the abdomen?

Devlin: I do not know, but if you put your hand on the epigastric region, the abdominal wall does not move.

Schumpelick: And what happens if you create an artificial pneumoperitoneum such as the Moreno type? Does it flatten the wall or is it relaxation? What is it? It works, and after a few weeks, the abdomen has a different size. What happens to the abdominal wall in functional terms?

Devlin: It works, but I doubt whether anybody knows the exact mechanism.

Kingsnorth: You said that susceptibility to hernia in the midline is connected with to the way the lamina are formed. We know that there is probably a large problem of ineffective technical repairs of the epigastric and umbilical hernias. Should we be abandoning sutured repairs of these midline hernias? Again, I know that some good work has been done by our French anatomists suggesting that sutured repairs at the midline, such as the Mayo repair of umbilical hernia, have a very high failure rate; perhaps for the reasons you have mentioned, we should be rethinking the way we go about doing these operations.

Bendavid: We perform a lot of hernias – 7500 a year – and about 300 of them are umbilical. I do not see the failure rates that have been suggested, but certainly wherever there is what looks much like a punched-up area we would use prosthetic measures for repair. I have rarely seen the failure of a primary umbilical repair using the Mayo method.

Wantz: We do not carry out repair using the Mayo method any more; we just put one layer of sutures to close the umbilicus and have no recurrences at all. If they are big enough, we use a prosthesis. In the vast majority of cases, we can use a small, simple polypropylene suture.

Simmermacher: A paper was presented years ago about the Mayo repair method suggesting that it should not be carried out vertically but horizontally, because otherwise you would use sutures which cut through the transversally oriented collections, and this would give bad results.

Another question I had, follows on from your question. What should we do with a woman who is 8 months pregnant and has a groin hernia? Should we repair it? And if so, how? Or should we leave it, hoping it will resolve itself after delivery?

Devlin: It is a rare problem, but I would wait.

Schumpelick: Can you tell us something about the innervation of the abdominal wall? Is there any relaxation or paralysis of the abdominal wall? What do we know about the function of the abdominal wall? Does a destruction of nerves take place? Is relaxation as in the diaphragm possible here, for example?

Devlin: Not during pregnancy, I don't think.

Schumpelick: What about innervation and the direction of our incisions? Some say that it is better to make them transversal and others say we should make them vertical because of the innervation ? Does it make sense?

Skandalakis: Even if you only just destroy two nerves, there will be some muscular deficit. If the 11th and tenth nerves are destroyed, for example.

Klaiber: Is rectal diastasis a defect or is it genetically preconditioned? Do you see differences in your diagrams concerning diathesis?

Berger: We try to leave the posterior wall and the innervation intact. This is all being discussed in plastic surgery. Should you protect the nerve and leave it untouched on the lateral side? In the lower part it is not so problematic as in the upper part, because of the close innervation, but there is the problem of the rectus muscle in the lower part. Our advise is to protect the nerve.

Schumpelick: I think the important point is that of innervation. What would you suggest to us as abdominal surgeons? What type of incision would be better – a transverse vertical one?

Berger: In terms of the nerve, a vertical incision would be advisable. In my experience, if you use a transverse incision between both areas, the lower part of the innervation and the mixed innervation in the upper part of the abdomen, no problems are encountered. However, if it goes into the umbilicus area, some parts of the innervation are destroyed, and I have seen it repaired. There were three cases which we repaired, because one side of the rectus muscle was completely denervated and there was no chance of repairing this abdominal wall using classical methods. We just had to use a reinnervated muscle.

Hartel: On the subject of rectal diastasis, suturing it under tension is a risk factor. Experimental work has been done on that. Hudstrom found that, in sutures under tension, there is a great accumulation of neutrophils, which probably lowers the breaking strength. So there should be no suture under tension.

Amid: Since we are talking about abdominal plasty, we see quite a number of patients after TRAM – reconstruction of breasts after mastectomy, where the rectus muscle is transferred for a breast construction. If the rectus muscle is missed, patients obviously develop a bulge in that area. Some people would consider this a hernia and would attempt to repair it. I reviewed a case in which a plastic surgeon decided to carry out abdominal plastic surgery with mesh after a TRAM operation. During the operation, he injured the femoral artery. The patient now has a major problem. It is really a reason to consider these bulges as a true hernia and do something about it.

Osther: You showed us the three ways that the linea alba may appear and told us about the significance of these structures and the development of linea alba hernias. Could you comment on the significance of any of these layers in the development of postoperative incisional hernias?

Devlin: No, I do not know.

Bendavid: I am surprised that no one has mentioned the area where the commonest problem occurs. It is really a flank incision, and in such cases you would often see a bulge and not necessarily a hernia in a couple of cases, because you have to anchor the mesh and make use of the muscles that are not affected by the previous incision. This sometimes means anchoring sutures right up to the psoas, and interiorly you have to pass the midline in order to anchor your mesh to a structure that is still innervated.

Wantz: About 5% of the TRAM procedures in the United States result in hernias big enough for us to fix. It is an easy thing to fix. Our plastic surgeons are now almost routinely carrying out a prosthetic procedure such as this for all TRAM procedures. They expose the wound to infection and other possible problems, it is being discussed whether or not they should do that. However, we have taught them how to fix them. They are easy defects, just like the flank hernias are.

References

1. Askar Om. Aponeurotic hernias. Recent observations upon para-umbilical and epigastric hernias. Surgical Clinics of North America 1984; 64: 315–354
2. De Giuli M, Festa V, Denoye GC, Morino M. Large post-operative umbilical hernia following laparoscopic cholecystectomy: a case report. Surgical Endoscopy 1998; 8: 904–905
3. Robin AP. Epigastric Hernia. Hernia, 4th ed. Eds LM Nyhus, RE Condon. Philadelphia: Lippincott, 1995.
4. Elechi EN. External abdominal wall hernias: experiences with elective and emergency repairs in Nigeria. British Journal of Surgery 1987; 74: 834–835
5. Heydorn WH, Velanovich V. A five year U.S. Army experience with 36,250 abdominal hernia repairs. American Surgeon 1990; 56: 596–600

6. Devlin HB and Kingsnorth AN. Management of Abdominal Hernias. 2nd Edition, 1998. London Chapman and Hall
7. Pemberton J, De J, Curry FS. The symptomatology of epigastric hernia: analysis of 196 cases. Minnesota Medicine 1936; 19: 109–112
8. Lytle WJ Internal inguinal ring. British Journal of Surgery, 1945; 32: 441–446
9. Lytle WJ. The deep inguinal ring, development, function and repair. British Journal of Surgery, 1970; 57: 531–536
10. Fruchaud H. Le traitement chirurgicale des hernies de l'Aine chez l'adulte. Paris: G Doin, 1956
11. Fruchaud H. L'Anatomie Chirurgicale de l'Aine. Paris: C Doin & Co, 1956
12. Stoppa RF, Warlaumont Cr. The preperitoneal approach and prosthetic repair of groin hernia. Hernia, 3rd ed. Eds LM Nyhus, RE Condon. New York: Lippincott, 1989
13. Condon RE. Surgical anatomy of the transversus abdominis and transversalis fascia. Annals of Surgery, 1971; 173: 1–5
14. Cannon DJ, Read RC. Metastatic emphysema. A mechanism for acquiring inguinal herniation. Annals of Surgery, 1981; 194: 270–276

CHAPTER 3

Surgical Anatomy

A. Prescher

3.1 Introduction

A large gap in the structure of the skeleton exists between the lower edge of the thorax and the upper edge of the pelvis. According to August Rauber, this gap is referred to as the lacuna sceleti sterno-pubica. This considerable gap is closed by the soft abdominal wall, which is exclusively composed of broad muscles and aponeuroses. The soft abdominal wall allows not only the motility of the chest, but also of the entire trunk. The simultaneously reduced protective function for the abdominal viscera is compensated for by an elevated and pronounced excitability of the muscles of the abdominal wall by means of reflexes.

The muscular base of the abdominal wall is formed by autochthonous muscles only, which are subdivided into the lateral (m. obliquus externus abdominis, m. obliquus internus abdominis and m. transversus abdominis), the anterior (m. rectus abdominis and m. pyramidalis) and the deep abdominal muscles (m. quadratus lumborum and m. psoas major).

These muscles extend across a bony frame formed by the thorax, the pelvis and the processus costarii of the lumbar vertebrae and are complemented by characteristic fascias, systems of connective tissues and intercalated segmental nerves and vessels.

Functionally, the abdominal wall not only retains the weight of the intra-abdominal organs, but experiences additional loads by bending or stretching of the body. In this respect, surgical incisions should always be considered as resulting in local damage and disturbances and in a defective healing of this complex system. Finally, in approximately 10% of cases, hernias develop at the scars of the abdominal wall (Klinge et al. 1997).

3.2 Skin and Subcutis

Comparison of the courses of the cleavage lines, also called Langer's lines after Karl von Langer, with the location and the direction of surgical incisions shows a lack of congruence in many places. The surgical incisions can therefore be considered as the cause of major traumatizations of the skin.

After careful removal of the cutis, the differences between the distribution of the cutaneous ligaments in the upper abdominal area and in the lower abdominal area become immediately evident. In the upper abdominal area, a closely packed distribution of the cutaneous ligaments can be seen on the back of the dermal flap (Fig. 1a), whereas in the region below the umbilicus, a coarse distribution can be observed (Fig. 1b). This difference in the distribution of the cutaneous ligaments is closely related to the lobulation of the subcutaneous fatty tissue and its connective tissue architecture. In the upper abdominal region, the deposits of fat are subdivided into much smaller fatty lobules than in the lower abdominal region.

Upon removal of the subcutaneous fatty tissues, the superficial fascia of Scarpa appears directly in the upper abdominal range, while below the umbilicus the yellowish fascia subcutanea superficialis of Camper (Fig. 2) becomes visible. From this fascia with its honeycomb-like architecture, the lig. suspensorium penis in men and the lig. suspensorium clitoridis in women arises.

Some authors (e.g. Forster 1937) deny this concept of two different fasciae, and indeed it is often difficult to demonstrate the two fascial layers by gross preparation. Furthermore, it must be said that the innominate fascia of Gallaudet (Gallaudet 1931) does not meet the criteria for a fascia. It is only a layer of somewhat condensed connective tissue of no importance for surgery.

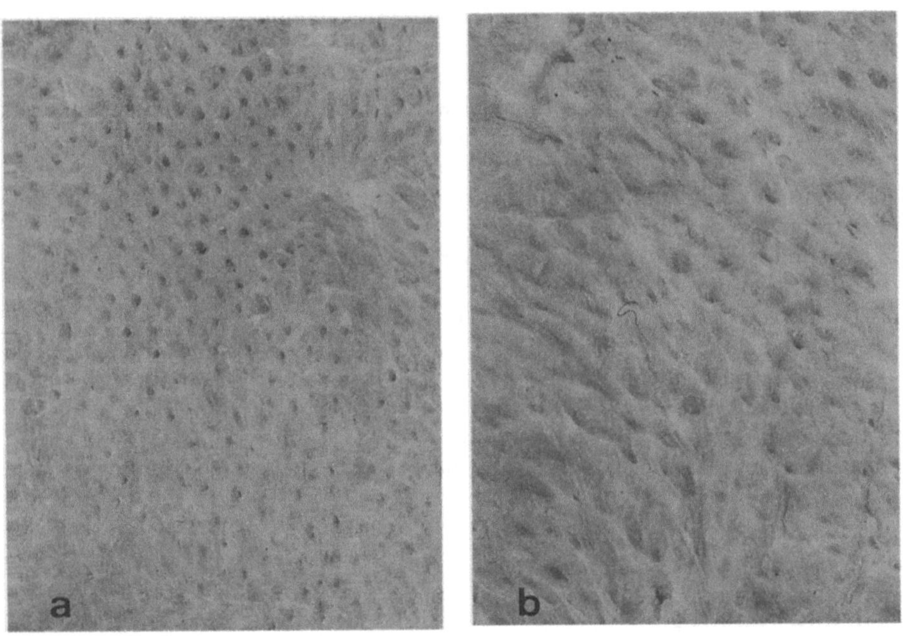

Fig. 1a, b. *a* Dorsal aspect of a dermal flap from the upper abdominal wall. The closely packed distribution of the cutaneous ligaments can be seen. *b* Dorsal aspect of a dermal flap from the lower abdominal wall. The coarse distribution of the cutaneous ligaments can be observed

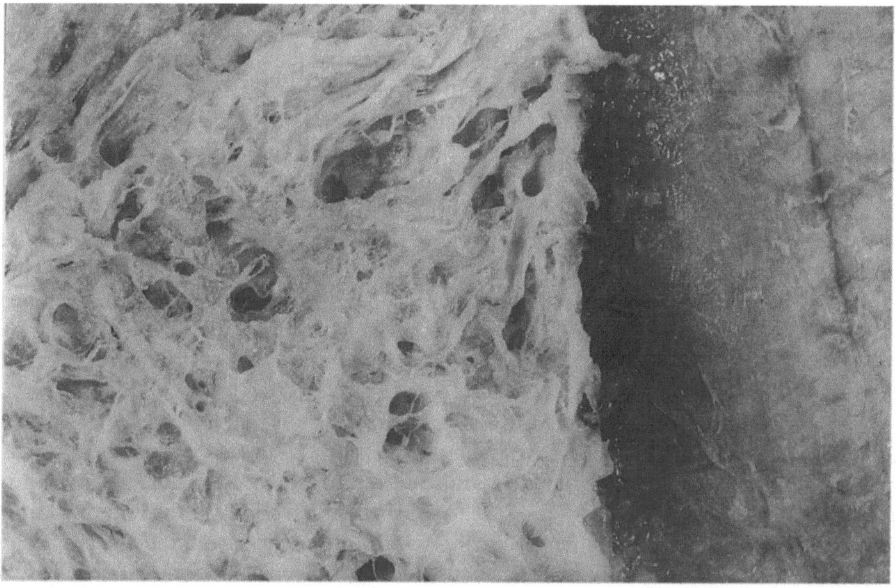

Fig. 2. The honeycomb-like architecture of the fascia subcutanea superficialis (fascia of Camper) can be recognised (*left*). A step deeper (*right*), the superficial fascia of Scarpa can be seen

3.3 Muscles of the Abdominal Wall

3.3.1 Rectus Abdominis Muscle (Fig. 3)

The wide, paired m. rectus abdominis originates at three points (Fig. 3) from the anterior surface of the costal cartilages of the fifth to seventh rib and can therefore be considered as a thoraco-abdominal muscle. The lateral point is the widest and originates at the anterior surface of the costal cartilage of the fifth rib up to the transition from the cartilaginous to the bony part of that rib. The fibres at this point have an inclined caudal direction in many places. The intermediate point originates at the anterior surface of the costal cartilage of the sixth rib, and the medial point from the anterior surface of the costal cartilage of the seventh rib and the anterior surface of the xiphoid process. The medial point extends around the rising edge of the costal cartilage of the seventh rib and even attaches itself to the dorsal area, a noteworthy detail. Up to the first tendinous intersection, the direction of the fibres in the intermediate and the medial point is exclusively longitudinal.

The insertion of the rectus abdominis muscle is achieved by means of a strong, flat tendon at the upper edge of the pubic symphysis and the adjacent parts of the superior ramus of the pubic bone. The detailed structures of the lateral and the medial part of the tendon are quite different: laterally, the tendon has an average length of 4–5 cm, medially a length of only 2–3 cm (Fig. 3). The transition does not take place along a continuous line extending from the lateral to the medial part, but occurs abruptly at a single point (Fig. 3). This point also marks the otherwise hardly noticeable subdivision into a lateral and a medial part of the muscle. The lateral part of the tendon inserts at the anterior edge of the superior ramus of the pubic bone, the medial part at the pubic tubercle. A certain contingent of fibres extends across the midline to the contralateral pubic tubercle (Fig. 3). There, mixing and crossing of the fibres takes place. Some fibres stray into the suspensory ligament of the penis. In addition, an insertion of the medial margin of the rectus abdominis muscle takes places at the linea alba. This "medial insertion" is particularly pronounced below the umbilicus and becomes stronger caudally. The strong attachment of the rectus abdominis muscle at the linea alba protects the two rectal muscles from giving way laterally, the so-called diastasis of the rectus.

The overall structure of the rectus abdominis muscle is subdivided by tendinous intersections, resulting in a four-sectioned muscle (Fig. 3). The tendinous intersections are true tendons with longitudinally arranged fibres, firmly fused to the anterior lamina of the rectus sheath. The fusion of the tendinous intersections to the anterior lamina prevents the entire muscle from shifting within the rectus sheath and permits the isolated function of the individual parts of the rectus muscle. The cranialmost one is located at the level of the tip of the eighth rib, the next at the level of the lower edge of the tenth rib, and the third at the level of the umbilicus. The facultatively caudalmost one (the fourth) is found at the level of the arcuate line of Douglas (Fig. 3). These tendinous intersections are up to 1 cm wide, show a serrated or inclined course and are medially firmly fused to the linea alba.

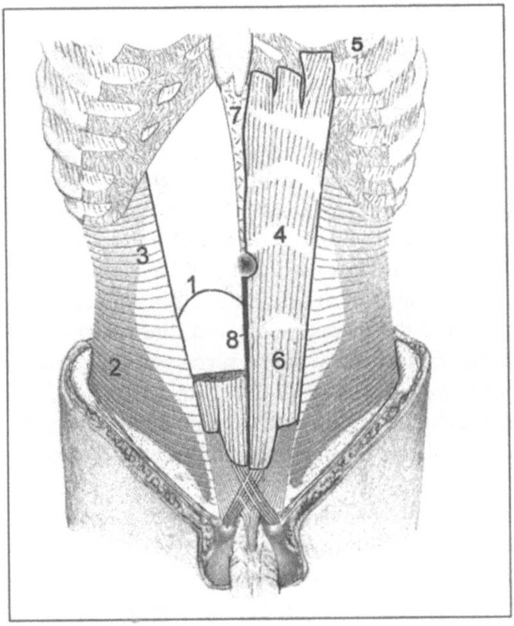

Fig. 3. Rectus abdominis muscle, the transversus abdominis muscle and the rectus sheath. 1, arcuate line of Douglas; 2, transversus abdominis muscle; 3, semilunar line of Spieghel; 4, tendinous intersection of the rectus abdominis muscle; 5, fifth rib; 6, rectus abdominis muscle; 7, linea alba, seen as a broad tendinous strip in the cranial part; 8, linea alba, seen as a condensed tendinous strip in the caudal part

The arterial supply to the m. rectus abdominis is provided by the superior and inferior epigastric artery. The blood vessels are located in a distinct groove at the dorsal side of the muscle.

The nerve supply is provided by the ventral rami of T7 to T12, frequently supplemented by accessory branches from T6 and L1 (Eisler 1912). The individual muscular rami enter the muscle at the dorsal area. Due to this topography, a lateral incision (pararectal incision) will destroy the innervation (Braus and Elze 1954; Hollinshead 1971). Furthermore, the motoric branches of the segmental nerves interweave and exchange fibres before entering the muscle, something which should be borne in mind.

3.3.2 Oblique External Muscle of the Abdomen (Fig. 4)

Of the lateroventral abdominal muscles, the external oblique muscle of the abdomen merits particular attention. It originates from the fifth to the 12th rib, exhibiting a characteristic line of origin. This line extends from the cartilaginous-bony junction of the fifth rib to the rudimentary cartilaginous part of the 12th rib. There, the muscle develops dentations, which interdentate with the serratus anterior and the latissimus dorsi muscle (Fig. 4). The resulting line, which is also distinctly visible in living subjects, is called Gerdy's line. From the cranial area to the eighth rib, the dentations of the external oblique muscle of the abdomen increase in size, subsequently becoming smaller again, but thicker. The ventral delimiting line (the transition to the aponeuro-

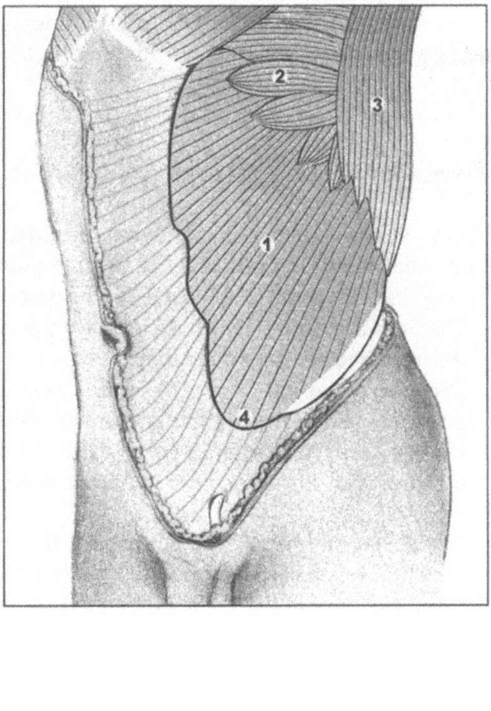

Fig. 4. External oblique muscle of the abdomen. 1, external oblique muscle of the abdomen; 2, serratus anterior muscle; 3, Latissimus dorsi muscle; 4, Gaupp's corner

sis) is smooth in the cranial section, but wavy in the lower section (Fig. 4). At approximately the level of the anterior superior iliac spine, it deflects at a right angle into the caudal margin of the muscle and forms Gaupp's corner (Fig. 4). The external oblique muscle is inserted at the external lip of the iliac crest and at the pubic tubercle as well as at the linea alba. In the area of the iliac crest, the insertion is made by means of a short but strong tendon.

The direction of the fibres of the external oblique muscle is particularly important in the field of surgery. Within the muscular part, fibres diverging in the mediocaudal direction predominate, with the upper fibres still extending almost horizontally and the inclination of the fibres increasing in the caudal direction. The collagenous fibres of the aponeurosis run in the same direction. The fibres of the external oblique aponeurosis transgress the midline and interweave with fibres of the contralateral internal oblique muscle of the abdomen.

Furthermore, the aponeurotic fibres originating from the caudal margin of the muscle from the anterior superior iliac spine up to Gaupp's corner require particular attention. These fibres form a tight train of fibres, laterally attached to the anterior superior iliac spine and medially at the pubic tubercle. Above the iliopsoas muscle, this strip is inseparably fused to the iliac fascia. This typical, strong strip of aponeurotic tissue is called the inguinal ligament of Poupart.

At the external surface of the external oblique muscle, a well-developed muscular fascia can be found. This layer is strongly developed above the muscle, but clearly thins above the aponeurosis. Inspection of the texture of this fascia shows that the direction of the fibres corresponds to that of the muscle fibres. Following transition across the costal arch, this texture changes in the subcostal region, with the direction of the fibres becoming more horizontal, i.e. almost perpendicular to their previous direction. After removal of the external oblique muscle, the lack of direct attachment to the costal arch becomes evident. The muscle here is fixed solely by means of tender fibres of connective tissue. A thin dorsal muscular fascia, which can easily be prepared, shows the same direction of the fibres as the muscle itself.

3.3.3 **Oblique Internal Muscle of the Abdomen** (Fig. 5)

The m. obliquus internus abdominis originates at the intermediate line of the iliac crest, from the superficial sheet of the lumbodorsal fascia and from the lateral part of the inguinal ligament. The muscle can be described as a five-sided plate (Fig. 5):

- The *lateral* margin (Fig. 5, *A*) includes the origin of the internal oblique muscle at the intermediate line of the iliac crest.
- The *caudal margin (Fig. 5,* B) of the muscle, extending mostly in the mediocaudal direction, is the shortest margin and exhibits numerous varieties. Fibres frequently emerge from this often poorly definable margin and join the spermatic cord together with fibres of the transversus abdominis muscle, forming the cremasteric muscle.
- The *dorsal margin (Fig. 5,* C) extends from the iliac crest vertically in the cranial direction to enter the cranial margin of insertion, which ranges from the tip of the costal cartilage of the tenth rib to the tip of the costal cartilage of the 12th rib.

- The *cranial* margin (Fig. 5, *D*) of insertion is not straight, but shows a variable stepwise course, depending on the configuration of the ribs.
- The *anterior* margin (Fig. 5, *E*) of the internal oblique muscle is the longest one and also serves for insertion, describing a line ranging from the pubic tubercle to the tip of the tenth rib. The formation of small dentations at the caudal part of the anterior margin is typical of this region.

The direction of the fibres has to be mentioned separately for the individual muscular parts: the fibres originating from the range between the anterior superior iliac spine and the glutaeal tubercle show great divergence. The fibres of this part of the muscle following caudally run in a parallel direction, whereas in the dorsal part fibres running cranially and parallel occur.

The above-mentioned cranial margin of the muscle with a course containing steps (Fig. 5) serves for insertion of the muscle at the ribs. The ventral margin simultaneously forms the transition into the wide aponeurosis of the internal oblique muscle. The direction of the collagenous fibres of the aponeurosis corresponds to the direction of the muscle fibres, and there are thus three parts with different directions.

The internal oblique muscle is enclosed in a thin, superficial (ventral) fascia and a thick deep (dorsal) fascia. The deep, thick layer of connective tissue contains the segmental nerves (T8 to L1) and blood vessels and is inseparably fused with the anterior fascia of the transversus abdominis muscle. According to Eisler (1912), the internal oblique muscle is supplied by T10 to L2.

The aponeurosis of the internal oblique muscle is also enclosed in a tender fascia. This fascia is extremely thin and therefore cannot be prepared. It serves as a connective tissue layer facilitating sliding motion.

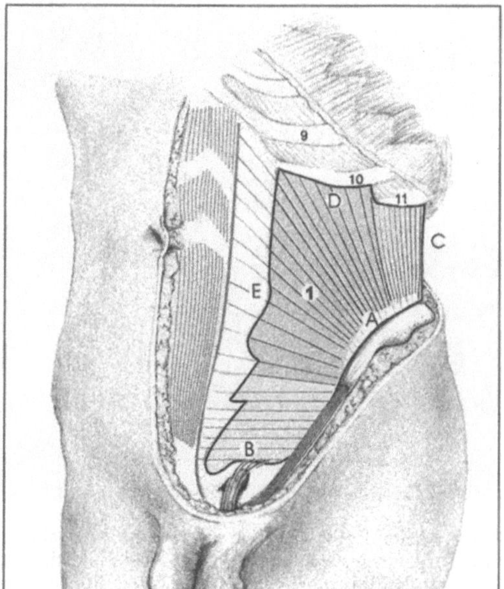

Fig. 5. Internal oblique muscle of the abdomen. 1, internal oblique muscle of the abdomen; A, lateral border; B, caudal border; C, dorsal border; D, cranial border; E, anterior border; 9–11, ninth to 11th rib

3.3.4
Transverse Muscle of the Abdomen (Fig. 3)

Of the three lateroventral abdominal muscles, the transversus abdominis muscle is the deepest. It originates from the six lower ribs, from the deep sheet of the lumbodorsal fascia and from the internal lip of the iliac crest. It usually also reaches the lateral section of the inguinal ligament (Fig. 3). The transversus abdominis muscle inserts at the linea alba, at the xiphoid process, at the cranial edge of the pubic symphysis and at the neighbouring medial parts of the pubic bone.

The fibres of the transversus abdominis muscle run parallel and have a horizontal direction (Fig. 3). In the caudal region, the course of the fibres bends to take a caudal direction. At this ventral margin, there is a transition of the transversus abdominis muscle into its aponeurosis. The line of transition is referred to as the semilunar line of Spieghel (Fig. 3). The horizontal direction of the muscular fibres continues in the horizontal direction of the aponeurotic fibres.

On the outside, the muscle is enclosed by its external muscular fascia, which is inseparably fused with the dorsal fascia of the internal oblique muscle. The fibres of this fascia run horizontally. This fascia can easily be prepared and extends above the costal arch into the region of the chest (Fig. 6). The external fascia of the transverse muscle

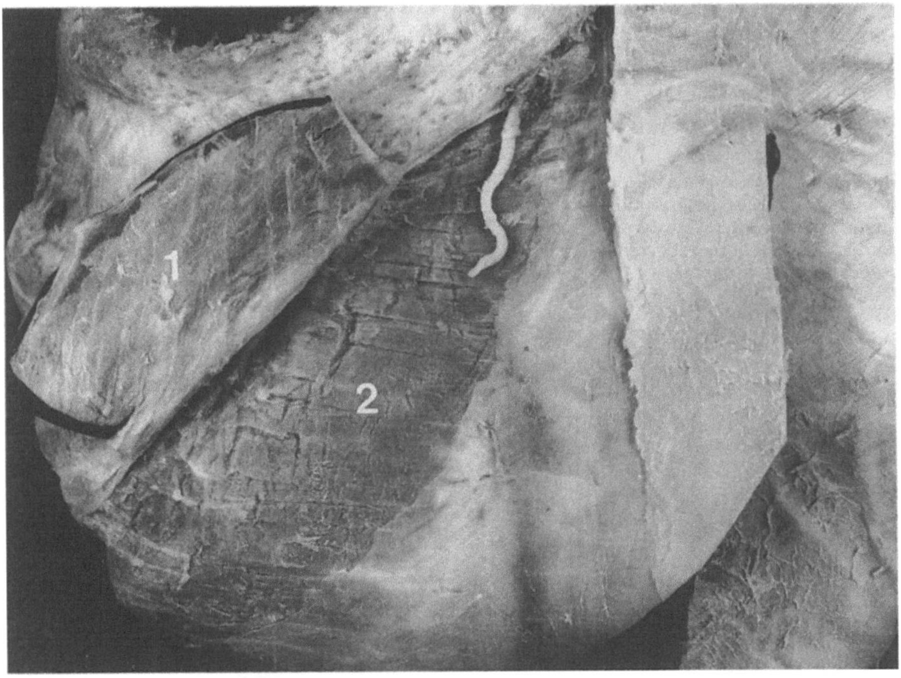

Fig. 6. Anatomical preparation of the transversus abdominis muscle in the subcostal region. 1, ventral fascia of the transverse muscle, extending above the costal arch into the region of the chest; 2, transversus abdominis muscle, extending below the costal arch into the region of the origin of the diaphragm

adheres to the costal arch, but is easily detachable. The transverse muscle itself extends below the costal arch (Fig. 6) and interdentates with the diaphragm in the area of its costal origin. The dorsal aspect of the transverse muscle is covered by the transverse fascia and the peritoneum. In the region of the costal arch, these two layers are inseparable. It is also easy to separate the transverse muscle from the ribs. As the external fascia of the transverse muscle is the only structure which is more sturdily attached to the costal arch, it is understandable that incisions located close to the costal arch create unstable conditions and increase the risk of an incisional hernia at this point.

The innervation of the transversus abdominis muscle is provided by T5(6), and the iliohypogastric and the ilioinguinal nerves are also involved.

3.4 Fascial Structures

3.4.1 Sheath of Rectus Abdominis Muscle (Fig. 3)

The paired sheath of the rectus abdominis muscles forms a flat tube of connective tissue for the rectus abdominis muscle. This tube is formed by the anterior and the posterior lamina, which are fused both medially and laterally. There is no posterior lamina in the cranial range, where the rectus abdominis muscle rests on the thorax. As far as the level of the costal cartilage of the ninth rib, the posterior lamina consists almost exclusively of the aponeurosis of the transversus abdominis muscle, since the dorsal sheet of the aponeurosis of the internal oblique muscle is quite thin. The typical structure of the posterior lamina does not develop until below the level of the costal cartilage of the ninth rib. The posterior lamina is then composed of the transverse fascia, the transversus abdominis muscle and the dorsal sheet of the aponeurosis of the internal oblique muscle. The posterior lamina thus formed then takes on the upper two thirds of the rectus sheath and undergoes a substantial transformation caudally. Approximately 4–6 cm below the umbilicus, the dorsal sheet of the aponeurosis of the internal oblique muscle and the aponeurosis of the transversus abdominis muscle are also positioned anterior to the rectus muscle and are therefore components of the anterior lamina. In the zone of transition (area arcuata), a concave line becomes visible and is referred to as the semicircular line of Douglas (Fig. 3). Numerous varieties are possible (Monkhouse and Khalique 1986; Rizk 1991). Below the semicircular line, the posterior lamella consists solely of the transverse fascia and is consequently very thin and delicate. This caudal part is fused to the linea alba and finally inserts at the pubic bone.

The anterior lamina of the rectus sheath also consists of two parts with different structures. Up to the level of the line of Douglas, the anterior lamina is composed of the aponeurosis of the external oblique muscle of the abdomen and the ventral sheet of the aponeurosis of the internal oblique muscle. Below the arcuate line, it is composed of the aponeurosis of the external oblique muscle, both sheets of the aponeurosis of the internal oblique muscle and the aponeurosis of the transversus abdominis muscle.

The space within the rectus sheath is divided into a frontal and a dorsal part. The frontal part is located in front of the rectus abdominis muscle and is further subdivided by the fusion of the tendinous intersections with the anterior lamina. At the lateral margin of the rectus abdominis muscle, the anterior space does not communicate with the space behind the rectus abdominis muscle, since fibres of connective tissue originating from the lateral margin of the muscle are firmly attached to the lateral zone of the rectus sheath. This division of the internal space of the rectus sheath is important for the spread of pathological processes.

3.4.2 Linea Alba

The linea alba is a strip of connective tissue resulting from the medial union of the bilateral aponeuroses of the abdominal muscles. With a length of approximately 35–40 cm, the linea alba starts at the ventral aspect of the xiphoid process. Caudally, the linea alba inserts at the pubic tubercles and radiates with numerous fibres into the fascia of the adductor muscles. At the linea alba, two large sections exhibiting different textures can be identified (Eisler 1912):

- The cranial section, extending up to 4–5 cm caudal to the umbilicus, can be seen as a tendinous tract 1–2.5 cm wide, in which both a sagittal and a frontal transitional crossing of the fibres of the aponeuroses takes place. This criss-cross architecture of the linea alba is a complex system and was carefully investigated by Askar (1977).
- The caudal section, extending to the pubic symphysis, is characterized by the absence of the sagittal component of the crossing fibres (Eisler 1912) and is therefore seen only as a small, condensed, tendinous tract.

The adminiculum lineae albae is a special structure of the linea alba in the caudal region. This structure starts at the level of the semicircular line of Douglas and then become increasingly wider in the caudal direction, resulting in a triangular plate of fibres (triangular ligament of the linea alba). Two important details of this ligament located dorsal to the rectus abdominis muscles must be mentioned: Firstly, the ligament is attached dorsal to the tendons of the rectus muscle to the superior ramus of the pubic bone. Furthermore, the ventromedial crest of the triangular ligament enters between the two rectus muscles and becomes firmly attached to the linea alba.

The cranial, wide part of the linea alba forms the umbilical ring. Accessory openings above the umbilicus may also occur. The resulting rectangular openings are then rounded by arched fibres extending in a circular direction. A plug of fat, related to the subperitoneal fatty tissue, can be found in the accessory openings only located cranial to the umbilicus. These accessory gaps are gaps through which linea alba hernias or umbilical hernias may occur.

Surgical incisions should never touch the xiphoid process, as heterotopic ossifications might develop on that part (Chevrel 1998). Figure 7 shows such a case, which was observed in a 78-year-old woman.

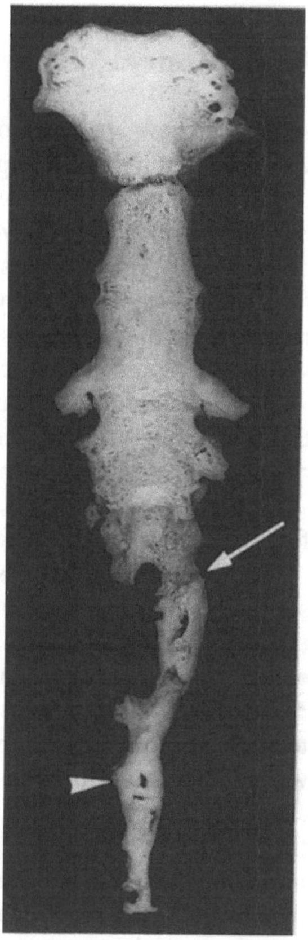

Fig. 7. Macerated sternum (78-year-old female) showing an exhaustive heterotopic ossification (*arrowhead*) in a scar resulting from a midline incision. The *arrow* points to the former lower edge of the xiphoid process

3.4.3 Fascia Transversalis

The transverse fascia is a layer of connective tissue varying considerably in thickness. According to Lierse (1996), this fascia can be interpreted in different ways: it can be interpreted as an aponeurosis, as a membrane, as a layer of adipose tissue or as a border lamella of the peritoneum. The transverse fascia is firmly fused to the subserous connective tissue of the peritoneum and is located on the inner surface of the transversus abdominis muscle and its aponeurosis. Slightly above the umbilicus, the transverse fascia turns into the firmer and more tightly woven umbilical fascia. This structure is therefore a particularly conspicuous part of the transverse fascia, and its fibres run in a horizontal direction. The umbilical fascia tapers off in the cranial direction, while its caudal edge frequently forms a sharp concave arch. Special conditions exist for the transverse fascia in the caudal region. In this region, it is fused to the total length of the inguinal ligament and constitutes the iliopubic tract. Furthermore, it participates in the formation of the dorsal wall of the inguinal canal and the deep inguinal ring. At the entry of the spermatic cord into the inguinal canal, the transverse fascia continues as a tender layer of connective tissue in the spermatic cord and is referred to as the internal spermatic fascia.

3.5 Preperitoneal Space

A short review of the topographical conditions at the inner aspect of the abdominal wall would appear to be appropriate here, as these features are particularly important in the genesis and interpretation of direct hernias. In the midline, the median umbilical fold extends from the vertex of the bladder to the umbilicus. This fold contains the obliterated urachus. At a short distance laterally, a second fold, the medial umbilical fold, can be seen bilaterally. These folds contain the obliterated former umbilical arteries. At a further short distance laterally, the inferior epigastric vessels can be observed, seen as lateral umbilical or epigastric folds.

Finally, according to Hammond et al. (1941), there are four different possibilities for the morphology of the embryological relicts just mentioned. The variety most frequently observed is twisting of the structures towards the plexus of Luschka.

The supravesical fossa, the medial inguinal fossae and, lateral to the epigastric folds, the lateral inguinal fossae are located between the string-like structures.

The lateral inguinal fossa is located laterally to the epigastric umbilical fold and should be mentioned as the location of the deep inguinal ring. As indirect hernias enter the inguinal canal at this point, the location of these hernias lateral to the inferior epigastric vessels is evident.

The medial inguinal fossa, the weakest point of the anterior abdominal wall, is located between the medial umbilical and the epigastric umbilical fold. This considerable weakness results from the absence of muscles at that point. In addition, the aponeurosis of the external oblique muscle of the abdomen located on the outside divides into the medial and lateral crus of the superficial inguinal ring. Reinforcement of this important locus minoris resistentiae may be made using the conjoined tendon, the interfoveolar ligament or the variable interfoveolar muscle, which is formed by aberrant fibres of the transversus abdominis muscle. The medial inguinal fossa is the inner area of entry of direct hernias, which become manifest on the outside at the superficial inguinal ring and are located medial to the inferior epigastric vessels. Likewise, the important inguinal triangle of Hesselbach with its borders (arcade of the transversus muscle, inguinal ligament of Poupart and the lateral edge of the rectus muscle) can be easily identified (Fig. 8).

After the peritoneum and the transverse fascia (Eisler 1912) have been removed from the anterior abdominal wall, two structures are exposed, which are described in the literature in different ways and often only superficially: the conjoined tendon (falx inguinalis) and the interfoveolar ligament of Hesselbach.

3.6 Falx Inguinalis (or Conjoined Tendon or Henle's Ligament)

The conjoined tendon is part of the aponeurosis of the transversus abdominis muscle and rests on the dorsal area of the aponeurosis, reinforcing that structure. It is a triangular sheet of connective tissue with a sickle-shaped lateral border, is fused medially to the lateral margin of the rectus muscle and inserts caudally with its base at the inguinal ligament. It should be mentioned that many different opinions exist concer-

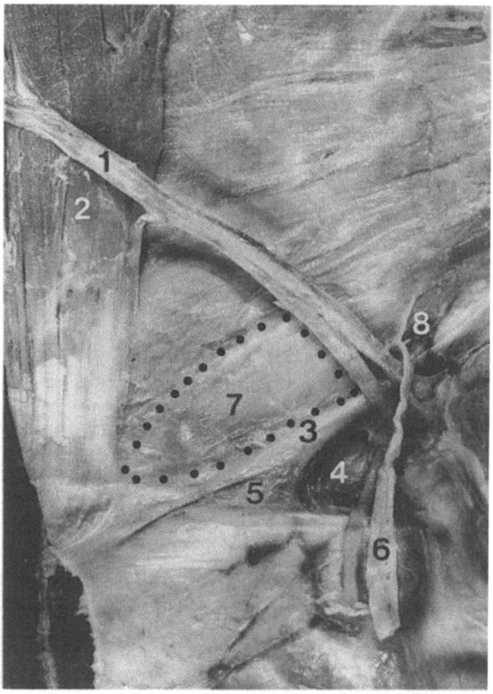

Fig. 8. Dorsal aspect of the lower part of the abdominal wall. 1, inferior epigastric vessels; 2, rectus abdominis muscle; 3, tractus iliopubicus and, behind this structure, the inguinal ligament of Poupart; 4, femoral septum of Cloquet; 5, lacunar ligament of Gimbernat; 6, round ligament of uterus; 7, Hesselbach's triangle (the borders are *dotted*); 8, deep inguinal ring

ning the definition of the conjoined tendon (e.g. Douglas 1890; Eisler 1912; Cherner 1939; Chandler and Schadewald 1944; Clark and Hashimoto 1946; Anson et al. 1960), and this is not the place to enumerate, discuss and evaluate all the different opinions.

3.7 Interfoveolar (Hesselbach's) Ligament

The interfoveolar ligament of Hesselbach constitutes a tendinous fibrous tract that branches out into the arcuate region from the posterior area of the aponeurosis of the transversus abdominis muscle, extending in the caudal direction and inserting at the inguinal ligament, at the pecten of the pubic bone and at the lacunar ligament of Gimbernat.

The interfoveolar ligament separates the deep inguinal ring located laterally from the medial inguinal fossa. The inferior epigastric vessels rest dorsally on the train of the ligament. If well developed, the fibres of the interfoveolar ligament may continue up to the dorsal part of the rectus sheath. The appearance of the interfoveolar ligament is linked to the appearance of the conjoined tendon and the iliopubic tract. If the latter two structures are well developed, they substitute for the interfoveolar ligament, and vice versa (Braus and Elze 1954). Both the conjoined tendon and the interfoveolar ligament can be considered as additional and rudimentary insertions of the transversus abdominis muscle to the pelvis.

The space anatomically defined as the preperitoneal Retzius space is only a small space delimited by the medial umbilical folds. The surgical definition of the preperitoneal space should include all the preperitoneally located structures of the dorsal aspect of the abdominal wall discussed, since important interventions for the repair of hernias, e.g. the placement of meshes (Schumpelick 1996; Chevrel 1998), are performed in this region.

3.8 Discussion

Simmermacher: First, I would like to congratulate you on this superb anatomical work, which I do not think I have ever seen or heard before.

Skandalakis: Do you believe in the innominate fascia of Gallaudet?

Prescher: I think it is a layer of connective tissue that is not strictly defined and which does not fit the definition of a fascia. It is only a layer of connective tissue. Similar fasciae are found in other places.

Skandalakis: The reasons for this question is that many anatomical books state that the aponeurosis of the external oblique muscle continues down to the inguinal area as an external spermatic fascia surrounding the chord. Perhaps you agree with them.

Prescher: I do.

Skandalakis: And the external spermatic fascia is nothing but the downward continuation of the fascia of Gallaudet.

Prescher: Yes, you could say that.

Read: You mentioned that the inferior epigastric vessels run in the preperitoneal space. The evidence now available shows that, soon after their origin, the inferior epigastric vessels enter the abdominal wall by passing through the fascia transversalis and run in the abdominal wall all the way. Although all the textbooks say that inferior epigastric vessels run in the preperitoneal space, I think that is wrong. I think there is evidence in the old anatomical textbooks that the inferior epigastric vessels enter the abdominal wall long before they enter the rectus sheath.

Prescher: I suppose they do not enter the abdominal wall at the beginning.

Klaiber: In laparoscopic surgery, we have found a new kind of fascia. There is always a difference between anatomy in cadavers and in live subjects, and when we use the microscope to look into the peritoneal space, after the linea alba, we find a special kind of fascia that has no name; it makes it difficult to divide the anterior wall (the muscle) from the peritoneum. It is below the arcuate line, and it varies greatly. Sometimes it is very tough tissue, like a fascia, and sometimes it is a kind of a layer that you have to cut through before you reach the real peritoneum. I wonder whether anyone knows about this fascia. Did you recognise this fascia? It is very common in endoscopic preperitoneal preparations. Laparoscopic surgeons seem to report this very frequently.

Bendavid: Laparoscopic surgeons often talk about this. Regi talks about this layer actually being completely separate from the transverse fascia. Perhaps Filipi could comment on this.

Filipi: I had not appreciated the fact that anatomical structures seem very easy to dissect the preperitoneal space without any need to divide a tissue. It is a blunt dissection. There is a fine fibrillous tissue. The dissection can be performed with a balloon, but there does not seem to be a need for any dissection using scissors at all.

Schumpelick: Dr. Prescher, I was very impressed by the heterotopic ossification. We only find that in the midline. Perhaps you could explain why that is so. And my second question is: Are there other animals with a spine that goes down to the pubic bone? Do all mammals have a free-floating belly, or do they have bones in there?

Prescher: I remember, that Manis species present a very long xiphoid process, because this sceletal element is the origin of the long sternoglossal muscles. Furthermore, Ungulates have a large xiphoid process which supports the ventral abdominal wall.

Schumpelick: The second thing is that the different layers of the muscles and fasciae are not so firmly connected. They can slide over each other. Is that true?

Prescher: Yes, it is. There is no direct attachment for these muscle layers.

Schumpelick: And is the same true of the attachment to the ribs?

Prescher: Yes, the attachment to the ribs is very loose. The only structure that is more firmly attached is the fascia of the transverse muscle.

Simmermacher: Continuing on from the question by Dr. Schumpelick, I would like to ask, when you say that all these lateral muscles can move freely over each other, does that mean that there are no crossing fasciae from one transverse muscle to the other? Does it mean that all these muscles are vascularized individually?

Prescher: Yes, we have seen it. Only very few vessels enter the muscle layers.

Simmermacher: So they do not go through different layers.

Schumpelick: Would it make any difference in anatomy if we had a bone in the middle of the abdomen? Because you say all are fixed at this point and there is no crossing of the linea alba at the point of fixation.

Prescher: There is crossing at the linea alba, but not very much.

Hartel: I have a question about the substernal bone. Is it not possible that they might be calcified haematomas because they always occur after operations? And what happens when we remove them? I think we all remove them, but I do not know what the outcome is.

Prescher: These bones cannot come from haematomas. Ossified haematomas have a different architecture and structure. I think it is heterotopic ossification.

Schumpelick: Why are so few anatomists interested in this field? Is it not fashionable to be interested in macroscopic anatomy? They are all in molecular biology and only a few are working in this field. I think there are a lot of unsolved questions.

Kingsnorth: That is very true. I think we have to read this in anatomy at least once in a generation, because we have abandoned things such as paramedian incisions in favour of midline incisions, but now that people like you have contributed more to our anatomical understanding, perhaps we need to revise that, particularly now that new materials are available. I think it is important to read this on a regular basis.

Skandalakis: I feel very sad every time I speak about anatomy, because we human anatomists are the most educated bastards in the United States. We do not know anything about medicine and surgery. If you are not a cell biologist in the United States, you are good for nothing. So I beg you all, we have to talk about anatomy in every session. We are scientists and not technicians who are only doing something without knowing what they are doing.

References

Anson, B. J., Morgan, E. H., McVay, C. B.: Surgical anatomy of the inguinal region based upon a study of 500 body halves. Surg. Gynec. Obstet. 111, 707–725 (1960)
Askar, O.M.: Surgical anatomy of the aponeurotic expansions of the anterior abdominal wall. Ann. R. Coll. Surg. Engl. 59, 313–321 (1977)
Braus, H., Elze, C.: Anatomie des Menschen. 3. Aufl. Bd 1. 1954
Chandler, S. B., Schadewald, M.: Studies on the inguinal region. 1: The conjoined aponeurosis versus the conjoined tendon. Anat. Rec. 89: 339–343 (1944)
Chevrel, J. P. (ed.): Hernias and surgery of the abdominal wall. Paris [etc.]: Springer 1998
Cherner, M.: Direct and indirect hernia in the light of the newer interpretation of the anatomy of the anterior abdominal wall. Am. J. Surg. 44, 593–599 (1939)
Clark, J. H., Hashimoto, E. I.: Utilization of Henle's ligament, iliopubic tract, aponeurosis transversus abdominis and Cooper's ligament in inguinal herniorrhaphy: A report of 162 consecutive cases. Surg. Gynec. Obstet. 82, 480–484 (1946)
Douglas, K. M.: The anatomy of the transversalis muscle and its relation to inguinal hernia. J. Anat. Physiol. 24, 220–226 (1890)
Eisler, P.: Die Muskeln des Stammes. In: Handbuch der Anatomie des Menschen. Hrsg. von K. von Bardeleben. Bd 2, Abt. 2, T. 1.1. Jena: G. Fischer 1912
Forster, D. S.: A note on Scarpa's fascia. J. Anat. 72, 130–131 (1937)
Gallaudet, B. B.: A description of the planes of fascia of the human body with special reference of the fascia of the abdomen, pelvis and perineum. New York: Columbia Univ. 1931
Hammond, G., Yglesias, L., Davis, J.E.: The urachus, its anatomy and associated fasciae. Anat. Rec. 80, 271–287 (1941)
Hollinshead, W. H.: The thorax, abdomen and pelvis. In: Hollinshead: Anatomy for Surgeons. Vol. 2. 2. ed. New York [etc.]: Harper & Row 1971
Klinge, U., Prescher, A., Klosterhalfen, B., Schumpelick, V.: Entstehung und Pathophysiologie der Bauchwanddefekte. Chirurg 68, 293–303 (1997)
Lierse, W.: Anatomie. In: Schumpelick, V.: Hernien. 3. ed. Stuttgart: Enke 1996
Monkhouse, W. S., Khalique, A.: Variations in the composition of the human rectus sheath: a study of the anterior abdominal wall. J. Anat. 145, 61–66 (1986)
Rizk, N. N.: The arcuate line of the rectus sheath – does it exist? J. Anat. 175, 1–6 (1991)
Schumpelick, V.: Hernien. 3. ed. Stuttgart: Enke 1996

Part II Wound Healing

CHAPTER 4

Fascial Metabolic Defects

R.C. Read

4.1 Introduction

Modern herniology began during the golden age of anatomy (1750–1850), the underlying assumption being that the tissues lining the various abdominal defects were normal and would stay so. Causation was attributed to a mechanical disparity between visceral pressure and the resistance of the musculature. Cooper [1] not only described the fascia transversalis and its role in preventing groin herniation, but listed factors which increase intra-abdominal pressure – cough, obesity, constipation, pregnancy, ascites, and unusual exertion, i.e., heavy lifting. The strength of the abdominal wall was considered to be diminished by congenital deficiency, debility, or ageing. Rupture of the peritoneum or abdominal musculature (Galen) was disproved as a significant factor by dissection and the fact that trauma, unless massive, did not result in herniation.

Even though it was well known [2] that, at autopsy, persistence of a patent processus vaginalis did not equate with herniation, surgical thought regarding etiology became dominated by Russel's saccular theory [3] which rejects the view that hernia can ever be 'acquired' in the pathological sense ... the presence of a developmental diverticulum is a necessary antecedent in every case and we may have an open funicular peritoneum with perfectly formed muscles: We may have congenitally weak muscles with a perfectly closed funicular peritoneum and we may have them separately or together in infinitely variable gradations.

In 1922, Harrison [4] was the first to question this dictum:

When we consider the dozens and hundreds of men who first show a hernia at 50 or 60, after their active life is over, the (saccular) hypothesis becomes improbable to say the least. However, the main objection to the theory is that even if true, it gives us no useful guidance. In and of itself, the persistence of a more or less elongated narrow processus vaginalis should not predispose to a future hernia if all elements of strength present in the wall of the abdomen were also present in the wall of the processus ... the muscles, however, appeared to be normal ... The natural conclusion is that the cause of an indirect hernia as of a direct hernia is the failure of the transversalis fascia to withstand the intra-abdominal pressure to which it is subjected.

The following year, Sir Arthur Keith [5] dealt another blow to the saccular concept, stating that

We are so apt to look on tendons, fascial structures and connective tissues as dead passive structures. They are certainly alive, and the fact that hernias are so often multiple in middle-aged and old people leads me to suspect that a pathological change in the connective tissues of the belly wall may render certain individuals particularly liable to hernia.

It is most important that surgeons should form a just and true opinion concerning the manner in which hernias arise. If they occur only in those who have hernial sacs already formed during fetal life, then we must either excise the sacs at birth or stand by and do nothing but trust to luck. But if ... the occurrence of hernia is due to circumstances over which we have control, then the prevention of hernia is a matter worthy of our serious study.

Andrews [6] followed in 1924, suggesting that atrophy of the conjoined tendon played a role. In 1964, Wirtschafter and Bentley [7] pointed to connective tissue abnormalities as a possible cause of herniation in humans. They cited an increased incidence of hernia in patients with lathyrism coupled with its experimental induction in animals using lathyrogens.

Nevertheless, little attention was paid to these pioneers. Zimmermann and Anson, in their 1967 textbook [8], continued to state that inguinal herniation developed as a result of a congenital anatomical predisposition. Indirect hernias were ascribed to the presence of a performed sac; direct herniation was explained by the absence of the lowermost fibers of the internal oblique muscle, leaving the transversalis fascia floor of the inguinal floor unsupported.

4.2 Personal Observations

My interest in the role of metabolic factors in the causation of hernia was stimulated by a finding made in the late 1960s [9] during the development of a modified McEvedy posterior preperitoneal approach to the repair of groin hernias. The rectus sheath some centimeters above the defects appeared thinner than normal [10] and felt greasy. Samples of constant size weighed significantly less than those taken from matched controls operated upon for other conditions. Patients with direct or bilateral hernias showed more attenuation than those with indirect defects [11]. Atrophy was unrelated to age or muscle mass [12]. Hydroxyproline content and therefore collagen, which comprises 80% of the rectus sheath, was strikingly decreased. Collagen showed altered salt precipitability and impaired hydroxylation, with decreased amounts of mature insoluble (polymeric) collagen [13]. Cultured fibroblasts proliferated less and had reduced uptake of radioactive proline. Collagen fibrils on electron microscopy showed irregular periodicity, variable diameters, and some intracellular positioning. Similar findings were obtained in pericardial and skin biopsies [14]. Since, as McVay [15] emphasized, the anterior rectus sheath is continuous with the fascia transversalis (as demonstrated historically by the success of relaxing incisions in the former to reduce suture tension after herniorrhaphy), the data reflect changes in the floor of the inguinal canal unaffected by scarring, secondary to the protrusion itself.

4.3 Hypothesis

Thus veterans were presenting in late middle age with a surprisingly high incidence of primary inguinal herniation, almost half having direct or bilateral defects. They showed evidence of widespread damage to connective tissue, different to that seen in lathyrism, because cross-linking of collagen was unaffected. Almost all smoked heavily, having become addicted to nicotine when, during World War II, cigarettes were sent up with the rations. Many had already suffered the consequences, e.g., emphysema, lung cancer, accelerated atheroscelerosis. Since the collagen changes in their skin biopsies (similar to those in the groin) resembled those seen in the skin and lungs of patients with pulmonary emphysema, with or without deficiency of α_1-antitrypsin [16], it seemed likely that smoke was not only damaging their lungs, but also, by a systemic effect, the abdominal wall. This thereby allowed herniation through a locus minoris resistentiae, the inguinal canal. The conclusion was that excessive long-term exposure to tobacco smoke was a risk factor for groin herniation. To ascertain the mechanism involved, we first considered what was known about how smoking damages the lung.

4.4 Pulmonary Emphysema

Prior to 1962, clinicians speculated that destruction of alveoli in pulmonary emphysema resulted from mechanical factors (cough and forced expiration against resistance) similar to those once ascribed for hernia. However, the report by Laurell and Eriksson [17] of predisposition to this disease secondary to an inherited deficiency of α_1-antitrypsin, coupled with its experimental production by Gross using tracheal installation of proteolytic enzymes [18], led to the now accepted protease–antiprotease imbalance theory. Smoking stimulates a neutrophil–macrophage response. Their five- to tenfold concentration in the lungs, with activation and release of zymogen elastase, is the prime mover. Further, oxidant combustion products of tobacco damage antiprotease defenses [19].

4.5 Metastatic Emphysema

To explain the systemic effects of smoking and, in particular, the effect on connective tissue, we envisaged that the chronic inflammatory response in the lungs was spilling over into the systemic circulation. Uninhibited proteolytic activity and large numbers of activated neutrophils and macrophages, along with products of tobacco combustion, were causing collagenolysis and inhibiting repair [20]. The process would be analogous to metastatic damage to the lung and skin seen in acute pancreatitis or the secondary pulmonary effects of visceral or extremity ischemia [21].

4.6 Supporting Data

Our patients with inguinal herniation, 18% of whom had associated pulmonary emphysema, had leukocytosis with elevated circulating elastolytic activity and a reduced antiproteolytic inhibitory capacity. Neutrophils showed enlarged zymogen granules and were primed for proteolysis. The changes were more marked in direct herniation and in those with bilateral defects [22]. Thus the data suggested that the presence of a preformed indirect sac allowed indirect herniation with less attenuation of the fascia transversalis than seen with direct protrusions. The age distribution of 2500 hernia patients admitted to our surgical service resembled that of 500 patients treated for lung cancer and another 3000 patients with cardiovascular diseases related to chronic smoking. The changes in collagen that we observed in our patients resemble those previously described in the skin of smokers (wrinkles) [23]. Peacock, while maintaining that the connective tissue changes in adults with groin herniation are restricted to the groin, did allow that the pathology was also present on the clinically normal side [24]. In 1988, the use of tobacco was reported to be significantly more common in patients presenting with hernia, especially women [25]. The year before, Weitz and his colleagues [26] had provided independent support for the metastatic emphysema hypothesis when they unequivocably recovered the "fingerprints" of free active neutrophil elastase (increased fivefold) from the plasma of cigarette smokers by measuring a specific fibrinopeptide cleavage product of fibrinogen identified by radioimmunoassay. They concluded that "our findings raise the possibility that other systemic complications of cigarette smoking (for example, atherosclerotic disease) may be the result of uncontrolled neutrophil elastase activity."

4.7 Proteolysis in Patients with Aneurysm

Yet another abdominal protrusion, aortic aneurysm, was once blamed on mechanical factors, turbulence, hypertension, and ageing, abetted by atherosclerosis. Nevertheless, smoking was shown to be a risk factor in 1968 [27]. Auerbach [28] later found nonsmokers to be outnumbered eight to one, while Cronenwett [29] determined that the presence of obstructive pulmonary disease was the best predictor of rupture. In 1980, Swanson et al. [30] invoked for the first time a metabolic factor, endogenous collagenase, in the pathogenesis of ruptured aneurysm. In the same year, Busuttil et al. [31] reported that elastase caused aneurysm with a 70%–80% loss of elastin, but prevented occlusive disease. They suggested that the enzyme originated in neutrophils or monocytes. Two years later, we [32] reported that smokers with aortic aneurysm, but not Leriche syndrome, demonstrated leukocytosis with elevated serum and leukocyte elastase activity (later to be confirmed, even after excision of the aneurysm) [33] and reduced antiproteolytic capacity. Smoking was then shown to increase aortic elastase content experimentally [34].

Since these findings were similar to those previously described by us in patients with hernia, we investigated the possibility of an association between the two conditions. We found inguinal herniation to be twice as common in patients with aneurysm compared to those with Leriche syndrome. In addition, the former had more severe fascial attenuation with earlier and larger, mainly direct, recurrent or bilateral hernial defects [21]. A similar relationship was later shown [35] and repeatedly confirmed [36, 37] to hold with incisional herniation after resection of an aneurysm, but not for occlusion with aortofemoral prosthetic interposition. In 1984, Brown et al. [38] reported increased serum monocyte circulating elastase activity persisting long after the aneurysm had been excised, proving again that these proteases do not originate in the aortic wall. In 1988, Rizzo et al. [39] described inflammatory cell infiltrates permeating the wall of aneurysms.

Cigarette smoking has also been correlated with the formation, expansion, and rupture of saccular aneurysms arising in the intracerebral arteries, previously thought to be congenital [40]. The fact that pancreatic trypsins and elastase have also been identified in the blood of smokers and may contribute to the development of abdominal aortic aneurysm emphasizes the damage inflicted by consumption of tobacco on the protective antiprotease mechanisms [41]. Thus, in smokers, aneurysm, like herniation, has to be considered the result of a systemic protease–antiprotease imbalance. This conclusion is supported by a reported eightfold increase in the incidence of cerebral aneurysm in patients with α_1-antitrypsin deficiency correlated with a similar change in plasma elastase [42].

4.8 Congenital and Genetic Influences

Smoking does not always lead to death from lung cancer or a heart attack. Similarly, not all smokers develop aneurysms or hernias. Further, these latter may arise in patients who have never used tobacco. Thus many hernias occur soon after birth, especially if premature. Such congenital defects have been ascribed to a delay in normal development, i.e., closure of the processus vaginalis. However, herniation may be multiple, familial, or part of various connective tissue disorders, including osteogenesis imperfecta, Marfan's or Ehlers-Danlos syndromes, congenital elastolysis (cutis laxae), or, more commonly, hip dislocation in childhood. Some of these conditions are known to arise from genetic mutations.

In 1992, Deak et al. [43] demonstrated abnormal synthesis (collagen gene expression) in cultured skin fibroblasts taken from two patients with multiple aneurysms, suggesting sporadic mutation. However, a number of individuals with single aneurysm showed no such change despite a positive family history. The following year, this group studied nine men, 17–67 years of age, with either indirect or direct inguinal herniation. Few smoked, some had a familial history, and a third demonstrated joint hypermobility. Isotopically labeled skin fibroblasts secreted twice as much type III collagen (one of the two common forms among the 29 different ones) as controls. The altered ratio with predominant type I collagen led to a decrease in insoluble (polymeric) fibrils, confirming our original observations. The collagen type proportions also regulate fibrillogenesis, fibril diameter, and bundle architecture. It was commented that "an increase in type III collagen (a metabolic abnormality of production) may predispose certain individuals to the development of inguinal herniation and recurrence after corrective surgery" [44].

Genitourinary prolapse in women was shown in 1990 [45] to be similarly associated with hypermobility, suggesting an underlying connective tissue disorder. In 1996, collagen deficiency with increased cross-linking and decreased solubility associated with collagenolysis was identified [46] in this condition. The role of smoking in herniogenesis was emphasized in 1998 by Scott [47], who found that the use of tobacco was twice as common in 130 patients operated upon for recurrence, compared to those treated for primary herniation. At the same meeting, Pans et al. [48, 49] used biomechanics and immunohistochemistry to confirm the changes in collagen that we had previously described. They concluded that

The collagen framework of the transversalis fascia was modified, mainly in the direct hernia group, associated with increased vascularity and cellularity. Similar changes were observed on the non-herniated sides, suggesting that a connective tissue pathology plays a role in the genesis of groin hernias.

4.9 Conclusion

In infancy, herniation is known to relate to prematurity or known connective tissue disorders. In adults, cigarette smoking has now been shown repeatedly to damage connective tissue, causing attenuation of the fascia transversalis, thus leading to inguinal and incisional herniation (metastatic emphysema). Genetic mutation can also interfere with collagen type I and III synthesis, thereby playing a role in herniogenesis. Thus, 75 years later, Keith's suggestion that a pathological change in connective tissue could cause herniation has been confirmed by a number of investigators.

4.10 Summary

Modern herniology began with the underlying assumption that the tissues lining the various abdominal defects were normal and would remain so. Even though Harrison, Keith, and Andrews questioned this dictum in the 1920s, it was not until 1964 that the possibility of connective tissue abnormalities was suggested. Thirty years ago, I noticed attenuation of the rectus sheath and therefore of the fascia transversalis in veterans undergoing preperitoneal repair. Evidence was accumulated suggesting leakage of proteases from the lungs of these heavy smokers as the mechanism (metastatic emphysema). A similar phenomenon was cited to explain the development of aortic aneurysm in this population. The evidence to support these concepts is reviewed and the mechanism has been extended to include incisional herniation. Recently, studies primarily in nonsmokers have shown that the genetic expression of collagen type I and III synthesis can be influenced by mutation. These data indicate that more than one factor can cause a systemic metabolic disease of collagen leading to abdominal herniation.

4.11 Discussion

Filipi: I enjoyed your presentation. How would you evaluate an individual who you suspect has a collagen disorder? How would you work them up? What tests would you do in somebody that has had five or six incisional hernia repairs and has a dehisced thoracotomy incision, for example?

Read: What I think you should do nowadays is get a biopsy of their tissue if you can; I think you can suspect a collagen disorder if you take a blood sample and have evidence of increased circulating (elastolytic) activity, but from the point of view of genetic expression, you have to have a biopsy of the rectus sheath, which is made of collagen. You have to have the biopsy analyzed to see what proportion of the various types of collagen are present. These are early days and this is not being done at the moment, but the main purpose of my talk today was to point out that we must face the fact that abnormality of the tissue itself may play a role apart from any anatomical variation where there is abnormal thickening or an abnormal anatomical mass.

Filipi: Where is this done in the United States? If a type III collagen defect is discovered on collagen analysis, how would it influence you when performing an abdominal operation?

Read: That is a very good point. Collagen analysis is being done in various collagen laboratories and various universities have them; I am sure you could get it done if you could find a biochemist that would do it for you and you set it up. An important lesson I have found has been that we need to use more reinforcement of the abdominal wall with an artificial Marlex mesh or some other mesh than we thought we needed in the past. We cannot rely on the tissues themselves to accept sutures, as they are liable to tear out and are not as strong in some people as they should be.

Kingsnorth: The message is that you cannot refashion defective tissue; you have to reinforce it with prosthetic material.

Read: You have to keep this tissue factor in mind.

Wantz: I agree that there is something wrong with the fascia and that you never get a hernia where a fascia is covered by intact muscle. The first defect to occur is absence of muscle before hernia. So which comes first, the chicken or the egg? Actually, the most important point is that muscle disappears in the groin before hernia occurs.

Read: We have always said that, and that has been the dogma, that hernia is due to muscular failure. The evidence has been that the muscle is frequently normal; in other words, a child can be born with abnormal tissue, for instance, and can have a defect in the tissue with associated connective tissue disease regardless of muscle.

Wantz: I agree with that, but you never see direct hernias in children because the floor of the canal is always covered in muscle. It is in adults that muscle disappears.

Hartel: Is it not possible that there might be an additional cause of hernia in chronic smokers, i.e., chronic bronchitis, because coughing increases the intra-abdominal pressure ten times more than just the standing position. Could this be an additional cause of hernia?

Read: It may be. People who develop hernias in later life tend to have abnormal lung function. We have always assumed that it was coughing which stressed the abdominal cavity, but the evidence is that the abdominal cavity is remarkably resistant to stress. A paper was published in the Lancet a number of years ago that said that hernias were unusual in weight lifters. If you lift 50 t or whatever they do, you do not get a hernia just by increasing intra-abdominal pressure.

Ferguson: You may know that elastase has actually become a very interesting enzyme for wound healing defects in the skin. A series of studies show that with normal ageing the level of active elastase increases partly because elastase goes up and the inhibitor goes down, which is partly why you get wrinkles in your skin. It is exacerbated by UV damage and by smoking, so there is a parallel in the skin for what you are describing. The result is that some people, including ourselves, have developed elastase inhibitors which are undergoing clinical trials for chronic ulcers such as chronic venous ulcers of the skin, where they show some promise. My suggestion would therefore be that perhaps some of these elastase inhibitors may be of interest in hernia surgery, because you could dampen down some of the proliferative activity. Do you have any comments on that?

Read: I made that suggestion in a paper in 1982, but I think at the time we did not have very good elastase–antielastase. Now, with the AIDS epidemic, we have good antiproteases and it may well be that your suggestion could be adopted. In the skin, we have similar changes to what I think we have seen in the fascia of the groin.

Scott: Have any similar collagen studies been done on patients with incisional hernias?

Read: Our original work was done on the rectus sheath, and that is a very important point. I am going to comment on that tomorrow or the next day, so if you come to that you can learn what work has been done on incisional hernias. I will present what seems to be known in the literature.

Schumpelick: You mentioned the paper by Dr. Scott showing the difference between smokers and nonsmokers after a laparoscopic approach for inguinal hernia. Does it really matter, because I think smokers have different habits in coughing, etc.?

Read: Experience with the smoking habit seems to be that there will more frequently be a recurrence with smokers than with primary hernia.

Schumpelick: How do you explain the difference?

Scott: We just looked at epidemiological data on our recurrent hernias versus our primary hernias. We found that our recurrent hernia patients had a much higher rate of significant smoking history than our primary hernia patients.

Schumpelick: But you do not make any conclusion about elastase level?

Scott: No.

Simmermacher: Does that mean that any kind of increase in abdominal pressure will create a hernia?

Read: An increase in intra-abdominal pressure certainly causes a hernia with ascites – we know that ascites are a major cause of hernia formation – but it is remarkable how few hernias we see in people who have been exposed to high abdominal pressure. In the narrowing of the belly, the muscle, as Dr. Watts pointed out, is so strong that it is difficult to produce a hernia even with massive trauma.

Devlin: Patients on chronic ambulatory peritoneal dialysis get hernias because of raised intra-abdominal pressure.

Read: Yes, I agree that does occur, but other factors may be involved. The point is that we do not generally carry a lot of fluid in the belly. I agree with you that ascites are not the only mechanism that increases intra-abdominal pressure. It used to be said that hernias were related to cancer of the colon because of increased obstruction, because of the distended colon increasing intra-abdominal pressure, but I think that the idea of an association between hernia and cancer of the colon has not stood up.

Klinge: We are still measuring the contents of different collagens in patients with incisional hernia or primary hernia, and up to know it appears that there is an increase in collagen I in patients with incisional hernia but not in patients with a primary hernia but particularly in the patients with a scar hernia or recurrent hernia. I think that underlines the importance of metabolic changes, particularly for incisional hernia.

Read: That is an important point, and I think I will comment on that in the next couple of days.

Bendavid: I agree on the fact that increased intra-abdominal pressure may not be a factor. You are right, and I still have the published paper proving that carcinomas of the colon and chronic constipation are not a factor; we are now also showing that benign prostatic hypertrophy is not a factor. Certainly, it is very rare to see hernias associated with pregnancy, and you cannot get a better example of increase intra-abdominal pressure.

Devlin: Did you comment on polycystic kidneys in hernias?

Read: No, I did not.

Devlin: Because there is a lot of evidence of a defect in the collagen.

Read: I think there may be a point there. It may be renal disease with peritoneal irritation. With renal disease there may be an abnormality with an effect on the connective tissue of the renal disease itself.

Devlin: There has been some very good work coming from Oxford recently, showing that 10% of polycystic kidneys with renal disease have hernias; they are quite different from the ordinary polycystic kidney disease and have a collagen defect.

Kingsnorth: There are two studies that connect hernia with genetic abnormalities; the first is study of the Eskimos in Greenland, who have a high incidence of connective tissue disorders such as rheumatoid arthritis, and there is a high incidence of hernias in these populations. The second is an epidemiological study from China, in which young people under the age of 15 years with hernias have been studied and the family histories carefully analyzed. The results show a high incidence of hernia in relatives due to dominant inheritance with limited penetrance and paternal transmission. The causes are multifactorial, and there are genetic factors that probably affect collagen synthesis.

Bendavid: I was very impressed with the original work you and also Earl Peacock have done. It is a shame that we have almost abandoned it, and in the last 30 years very little has been added. We are fortunate at the University of Toronto to have a collagen laboratory, and we are starting some work there; in particular, there is the idea that we may be dealing with a genetic disease. You very rarely see hernias in women; look at the chromosomal distribution in XX versus men's XY and the fact that direct inguinal hernia, for example, is rare in women – as a matter of fact, they account for only 0.2% of all the abdominal wall hernias. Why do women have that sort of anatomy? I also think that hernia patients are a very particular type of patient; I think we do a lot more operations than most people, and I have seen normal muscular floor of the canal. If you look at the textbooks, they all describe natural and abnormal anatomy, and that is not true. I think most textbooks describe the conjoined tendon, for example. We all know that a conjoined tendon exists in about 3% up to about 11% of people, so we are emphasizing an anatomy which is not exact and which also promotes this belief of herniation resulting from anatomical misrepresentation. As a matter of fact, with my new way of thinking about genetic defects, I even wonder whether McVay's description of perhaps 12–16 varieties of insertions of the internal oblique muscle are not in fact various stages of degeneration of the muscle that may eventually lead to a hernia formation.

Schumpelick: Raymond, do you have an explanation for why there is spontaneous healing of umbilical hernia in infants or newborns and never inguinal hernia? Is it a question of metabolism or a question of anatomy?

Read: I rather assumed it was the size of the defect and the fact that the umbilicus is a normal defect which is supposed to heal. We are all born with an umbilicus, and there are mechanisms which allow for healing in the umbilicus which are not available in the groin.

Devlin: All males are born with testicles and therefore must have a processus vaginalis. Why do some of them persist as hernias, indirect hernias, and some do not? A total of 40% of premature babies under 1000 g have hernias.

Read: Again, I think that the fact that a patient has an open processus vaginalis does not mean that he has a hernia.

Devlin: No, but was it not said many years ago that if you look at all adult men and you put pressure in their peritoneal cavity, they would develop hernias.

Read: Yes.

Devlin: So there may be something persisting there.

Read: Yes, I agree that there is a normal mechanism whereby there is a closure of the peritoneum in most people. But a significant proportion never close, and they may never get a hernia, so there are other factors involved besides the presence of a sac.

Devlin: This was pointed out by Sir Cecil Wakely of your old medical school many years ago.

Bendavid: I am running at loggerheads with Professor Devlin again, if that is true. When you look at a series of thousands of patients, your indirect hernias are really not much more frequent than direct inguinal hernias. In our series, they account for roughly 50%, so the presence of a processus vaginalis and the fact you have a defect at the internal ring should really promote hernias and possibly give an incidence of 90%–95% of indirect as opposed to direct hernias; yet we do not see that. However, especially when you see the highest incidence of hernias closer to the age of 55 or perhaps a little older, I feel that this sort of statistics perhaps supports some genetic theory rather than an anatomical malfunction or a dysfunction or abnormality.

Read: I do not think that everything is necessarily related to genes. The genetic theory alone does not necessarily cover everybody.

Skandalakis: If we take all the so-called congenital abnormalities (since I am a physician and South-American embryologist), I would say that in 50% of cases we do not know how to explain the crime or how to reconstruct the crime, so I do not know if it is true. We believe that in 77% of cases the posterior inguinal wall is normal, and in 23% of cases the posterior inguinal wall is not normal; we therefore still have a lot of open questions.

References

1. Cooper, A.P.: The anatomy and surgical treatment of inguinal and congenital hernia. London: Longman 1804.
2. Cloquet, J.: Recherches sur les causes et l Anatomie des Hernies Abdominales. Paris: Mequignon-Marvis, 1819
3. Russel, R.H.: The saccular theory of hernia and the radical operation. Lancet 1906; 3:1197–1203.
4. Harrison, P.W.: Inguinal hernia: A study of the principles involved in the surgical treatmet. Arch Surg 1922; 4:680–689.
5. Keith, A.: On the origin and nature of hernia. British J Surg 1924; 11:455–475.
6. Andrews, E.: A method of herniotomy utilizing only white fascia. Ann Surg, 1924;80:225–238.
7. Wirtschafter, Z.T., and Bentley, J.P.: Hernias as a collagen maturation defect. Ann Surg. 1964; 160:852.
8. Zimmermann, Leo M., and Anson, Barry J.: Anatomy and Surgery of Hernia. Second Edidion. Baltimore: Williams and Wilkins Co., 1967.
9. Read, R.C.: Preperitoneal exposure of inguinal herniation. Am J Surg, 1968; 116:653–658.
10. Read, R.C.: Attenuation of the rectus sheath in inguinal herniation. Am J Surg, 1970; 120:610–614.
11. Wagh, P.V., and Read, R.C.: Collagen deficiency in rectus sheath of patients with inguinal herniation. Proc Soc Exper Biol Med, 1971; 37:382–384.
12. Wagh, P.V., and Read, R.C.: Defective collagen synthesis in inguinal herniation . Am J Surg, 1972; 124:819–822.
13. Wagh,P.V., Leverich, A.P., Sun, C.N., White, H.J., Read, R.C.: Direct inguinal herniation in men: A disease of collagen. J Surg Res 1974; 17:425–433.
14. Sun, C.N., White, H.J., Wagh, P.V., Read, R.C.: Alteration of collagen fibrils in direct inguinal herniation in men. Eighth International Congress on Electro Microscopy, Canbera, 1974. II; 482–483.
15. McVay, C.B.: Hernia: The pathological anatomy of the more common hernias and their repair. Springfield, III., Charles C. Thomas 1954.
16. Read, R.C.: Presidential address: Systemic effects of smoking. Am J Surg 1984; 148:706–711.
17. Laurell, C.B., Eriksson, S.: The electrophoretic alpha-1-globulin pattern of serum alpha-1-antitrypsin deficiency. Scand J. Clin Lab Invest 1963; 15:132–140.
18. Gross, P.E., Pfizer, E.A., Tokler, E., et al.: Experimental emphysema and it's production with papain in normal and silicotic rats. Arch Environ Health 1965; 11:50–58.
19. Wewers, M.D., Gadek, J.E.: The protease theory of emphysema (editiorial) Ann Intern Med 1987; 107:761–763.
20. Cannon, D.J., Read, R.C.: Metastatic emphysema: A mechanism for acquiring inguinal herniation: Ann Surg 1981; 194:270–278.
21. Lee, P.C., Howard, J.M.: Fat necrosis. Surg Gynecol Obstet 1979; 148:785–789.
22. Cannon, D.J., Casteel, L., Read, R.C.: Abdominal aortic aneurysm, Leriche syndrome, inguinal herniation and smoking. Arch Surg 1984; 119:387–389.

23. Kadunce, D.P., Burr, R., Gress, R., et al: Cigarette smoking: Risk factor for premature facial wrinkling. Ann intern Med 1991; 114:840–844.
24. Peacock, Erle E., Jr.: Biology of Hernia. Chapter 3, Hernia. Second Edition, edited by Lloyd M. Nyhus and Robert E. Condon. Philadelphia: J.B. Lippincott Company, 1978.
25. Bielecki, K., Puawski, R.: Is cigarette smoking a causative factor in the development of inguinal hernia. Pol Tyg Lek 1988; 43:974–976.
26. Weitz, J.L., Crowley, K.A., Landman, S.L., et al: Increased neutrophil elastase activity in cigarette smokers. Ann Intern Med 1987; 107:680–682.
27. Hammond, E., Garfinkel, L.: Coronary heart disease, stroke and aortic aneurysm. Arch Environ Health 1969; 19:167–182.
28. Auerbach, O., Garfinkel, L.: Atherosclerosis and aneurysm of the aorta in relation to smoking habits and age. Chest 1980: 78:805–809.
29. Cronenwett, J., Murphy, T., Zelnock, G., et al: Actuarial analysis of variables associated with rupture of small abdominal aortic aneurysms. Surgery 1985; 98:472–483.
30. Swanson, R. J., Littooy, F.N., Hunt, T.K. Stoney, R.J.L Laparotomy as a precipitating factor in the rupture of intra-abdominal aneurysms. Arch Surg 1980; 115:299–304.
31. Busuttil, R.W., Abou-Zamzam, A. M., Machleder, H.I.: Collagenase activity of the human aorta. A comparison of patients with and without abdominal aortic aneurysms. Arch Surg 1980; 115:1373–1378.
32. Cannon, D. J. Read, R.C.: Blood elastolytic activitiy in patients with aortic aneurysm. Ann Thoracic Surg 1982; 34:10–15.
33. Cohen, J. R., Faust, G., Tenenbaum, N., Sarfati, I., Rogowsky, P., Wise, L.: The calcium messenger system and the kinetics of elastase release from human neutrophils in patients with abdominal aortic aneurysms. Annals of Vascular Surgery 1990; 4(6) 570–574.
34. Cohen, J. R., Sarfati, I. and Wise, L.: The effect of cigarette smoking on rabbit aortic elastase activity. J Vasc Surg, 1989; 4:580–584.
35. Stevick, C. A., Long, J. B., Jamasbi, B., Nash, M.: Ventral hernia following aortic reconstruction. Am Surg, 1988; 51:287.
36. Hall, K. A., Peters, B., Smyth, St. H., et al: Abdominal wall hernias in patients with abdominal aortic aneurysmal versus aortoiliac occlusive disease. Am J Surg 1995; 170:572.
37. Holland, A.J., et al: Incisional hernias are more common in aneurysmal aterial disease. Eur J Vasc Endovasc Surg 1996; 12:196–200.
38. Brown, S.L., Buckstrom, B., Busuttil, R.W.: A new serum proteolytic enzyme in aneurysm pathogenesis. J Vasc Surg 1985; 2:293–399.
39. Rizzo, R.J., McCarthy, W.J., Dixit, S. N., et al: Collagen types and matrix protein content in human abdominal aortic aneurysms.. J Vasc Surg 1989; 10:365–373.
40. Misra, B.K., Whittle, I.R., Steers, A. J., Sellar, R. J.: De novo saccular aneurysms. Neurosurg 1988; 23:10–15.
41. Dubick,M. A., Hunter, G.C., Perez-Lizano, E., et al: Assessment of the role of pancreatic proteases in human abdominal aortic aneurysms and occlusive disease. Clin. Chim. Acta 1988; 177:1–10.
42. Baker, C. J., Flore, A., Connoly, E. S., Jr., et al: Serum elastase and alpha-1-antitrypsin levels in patients with ruptured and unruptured cerebral aneurysms. Neurosurg 1995; 37(1):56–61.
43. Deak, S. B., Ricotta, J.J., Mariani, Th. J., et al: Abnormalities in the Biosynthesis of Type III Procollagen in Cultured Skin Fibroblasts from Two Patients with Mulitple Aneurysms. Matrix Vol. 12, Gustav Fischer Verlag: Stuttgart, 1992; 92–100.
44. Friedmann, D. W., Boyd, Ch. D., Norton, P., et al: Increases in Type III Collagen Gene Expression and Protein Synthesis in Patients with Inguinal Hernias. Ann Surg: 1993, 6, 218:754–760.
45. Baker, N. P., Baker, J., Sharp, H., et al: Genitourinary prolapse: relationship with joint mobility. Neurourol Urodynam 19990; 9:321–22.
46. Jackson, S. R., Avery, N.C., Tarlton, J. F., et al: Changes in metabolism of collagen in genitourinary prolapse. Lancet June 15, 1996; 347:1658–1661.
47. Scott, J. St.: Causes of groin hernia recurrence following open repair. Presented at the 1st Annual Scientific Meeting of the American Hernia Society, Miami Beach, Florida: Feb., 1998.
48. Pans, A., Pierard, G. E., Albert, A., et al: Adult groin hernias: new insight into their biomechanical characteristics. Eur J of Clin Invest, 1997; 27:1–6
49. Pans, A. and Pierard, G.E.: Immunohistochemical study of the rectus sheath and transversalis fascia in adult groin hernias. Presented at the 1st Annual Scientific Meeting of the American Hernia Society, Miami Beach, Florida: Feb., 1998.

CHAPTER 5

Growth Factors and Hernia

A.N. Kingsnorth

Wound healing is a complex programmed sequence of cellular and molecular processes which includes inflammation, cell migration, angiogenesis, provisional matrix synthesis, collagen deposition and re-epithelisation. Hernia repair is achieved by correction of the defect in the fascia transversalis. The specific events in wound healing that could be utilised to augment the defect in the fascia transversalis, matrix synthesis and collagen deposition can be specifically identified [1].

5.1 Function

Growth factors are part of a large number of polypeptides that transmit signals affecting cellular activities and modulate cell function [2]. The term "growth factor" does not ideally describe their function, because they stimulate and inhibit cell division, differentiation, migration or gene expression, depending on the cell involved. Hundreds of growth factors have been described and have been grouped 20 families or superfamilies, but only a few have been fully researched to identify their specific role in wound healing.

The specific qualities that identify growth factors as potential therapies to enhance repair can be identified as the following [3]:

- They are synthesised and stimulated by tissue repair cells such as platelets, macrophages, endothelial cells and fibroblasts
- They are deficient in chronic wounds (and since collagen synthesis is deficient in the fascia transversalis of patients with hernia, they may also be deficient in this condition).
- They enhance normal and reverse deficient tissue repair.

5.2 Availability

Due to progress in recombinant DNA technology, growth factors are now being produced in sufficient quantity for clinical use [4]. Over 100 companies are involved in the recombinant growth factor research and development for soft tissue repair (Table 1), and at least one third of these are conducting pre-clinical or clinical trials (Table 2). However, to date the outcomes of clinical trials have been confused by conflicting

Table 1. Growth factor-based products under development for the acceleration of wound healing

Growth factor	Company	Method of production	Source
EGF	Amgen	Recombinant	*E. coli*
EGF	Chiron	Recombinant	Yeast
EGF	Creative Biomolecules	Recombinant	*E. coli*
EGF	Ethicon	Recombinant	Licensed from Chiron (yeast)
aFGF	Merck Sharp & Dohme	Extracted	Bovine brain
bFGF	Amgen	Recombinant	*E. coli*
bFGF	Scios Nova	Recombinant	*E. coli*
bFGF	Progen	Recombinant	*E. coli*
bFGF	ZymoGenetics	Recombinant	-[a]
IGF-1	Amgen	Recombinant	Bacterial cells
IGF-1	Chiron	Recombinant	Yeast
IGF-1	Kabi	Recombinant	Yeast
IGF-1	Merck Sharp & Dohme	Recombinant	Mammalian cells
PDGF	Amgen	Recombinant	Mammalian cells
PDGF	Beirsdorf AG	Recombinant	Mammalian cells
PDGF	Chiron	Recombinant	Yeast
PDGF	Creative Biomolecules	Recombinant	*E. coli*
PDGF	Ethicon	Recombinant	Licensed from Chiron (yeast)
PDGF	ZymoGenetics	Recombinant	Yeast
PDWHF	Curative Technologies	Extracted	Platelets
TGF-b1	Genentech	Recombinant	Mammalian cells
TGF-b2	Oncogen	Recombinant	Mammalian cells
TGF-b2	Celtrix Pharmaceuticals	Extracted	Bovine source
		Recombinant	Mammalian cells

EGF, epithelial growth factor; FGF, fibroblast growth factor; aFGF, acidic FGF; bFGF, basic FGF; IGF, insulin-like growth factor; PDGF, platelet-derived growth factor; PDWHF, platelet-derived wound-healing formula; TGF, transforming growth factor; *E. coli*, *Escherichia coli.*
[a] Source not revealed by the company.

Table 2. Growth factors in clinical trials

Growth factor	Company	Indication
EGF	Chiron/Ethicon	Skin ulcers, venous-stasis ulcers
bFGF	Scios Nova	Chronic soft tissue ulcers, pressure sores
PDGF	Amgen	Chronic dermal ulcers, pressure sores
PDGF	Chiron/Ethicon	Skin ulcers
PDGF	ZymoGenetics	Diabetic ulcers
TGF-β2	Celtrix Pharmaceuticals	Venous-stasis ulcers

EGF, epithelial growth factor; bFGF, basis fibroblast growth factor; PDGF, platelet-derived growth factor; TGF, transforming growth factor.

results utilising the same growth factor in the same chronic wound, and questionable controls are used in many studies, few of which were blinded [1, 5].

5.3 Experimental Findings

For a specific review of the properties of growth factors which have been investigated to date, the reader is referred to Pierce and Mustoe [1]. The best characterised growth factors involved in wound healing and their major properties in the wound healing process are as follows:

- Platelet-derived growth factor (PDGF) is the most potent stimulator of fibroblast proliferation, thereby enhancing matrix synthesis and wound remodelling.
- Transforming growth factor beta (TGF-b) is a powerful chemotactic agent for wound-healing cells and significantly enhances pro-collagen type I synthesis and fibronectin and collagen deposition.
- Fibroblast growth factors (FGF) are powerful angiogenic factors.

A summary of some of the clinical trials carried out with these agents is shown in Table 3. Current knowledge indicates that PDGF or TGF-b would be the most likely agents to be successful in enhancing wound healing in hernia because of their effects on matrix synthesis and collagen deposition.

The free polypeptide growth factors, however, are vulnerable to digestion by tissue proteases and are rapidly degraded in the wound environment; in addition, they have a short biological half-life in serum of a few minutes. Growth factors should therefore be administered with a vulnerary agent such as an ointment, gel or collagen sponge [5]. This has added considerably to the complexity of clinical research in order to identify a vulnerary agent which can slowly release active growth factor over a period of time in a healing wound. To ensure the highest quality of clinical trials, the Food and Drug Administration (FDA) of the United States requires that a dressing or device marketed as a wound-healing agent should augment optimal repair [1]. Moreover, the International Committee on Wound Management consensus statement in 1993 stated that the means of healing must be conducted by scientifically based procedures and materials [5].

Table 3. Growth factors and cytokines in clinical development

Growth factor/cytokine	Preclinical effect	Clinical trial results
PDGF-BB	⇑ Neovessels	⇑ Healing in pressure and diabetic ulcers; phase III trials in progress
	⇑ Reepithelialization ⇑ Granulation tissue	
TGF-β2	⇑ Collagen-containing granulation tissue not successful	⇑ Healing in venous-stasis ulcers; repair of macular holes
TGF-β3	⇑ Healing ⇓ Scarring	Chronic ulcers, in progress
bFGF	⇑ Neovessels in a provisional matix	Pressure ulcers – biological effect; diabetic and veno stasis ulcers, no effect
	⇑ Reepithelialization	
IL-1β	⇑ Healing in infected open wounds	Pressure ulcers, phase I study in progress
GM-CSF	⇑ Healing in incisions	Chronic ulcers, in progress
aFGF	⇑ Neovessels	Diabetic and venous stasis
	⇑ Matrix ulcers, in progress	
EGF	⇑ Reepithelialization	
ulcers, minimal effects	Donor graft sites, chronic	

PDGF-BB, platelet-derived growth factor-BB; TGF, transforming growth factor; FGF, fibroblast growth factor; bFGF, basic FGF; aFGF, acidic FGF; GM-CSF, granulocyte-macrophage colony-stimulating factor; EGF, epithelial growth factor.

Topical agents for wound healing fall into five categories [5], with the following properties:

1. Removing the cause of tissue breakdown such as infection/inflammation
2. Reducing pain (local anaesthetics)
3. Removing necrotic tissue
4. Assisting wound closure, such as tissue glues manufactured from fibrin or cyandarcrylate
5. Augmenting the healing process, such as growth factors

In hernia repair, local anaesthetics are widely used, and the ability to return to immediate gentle physical activity may in itself enhance wound healing in its early phases. Tissue glues have been utilised for the fixation of mesh. Targeting growth factors in order to achieve improved tissue formation and function involves the process of tissue engineering [6]. Tissue engineering involves the use of synthetic materials, xenograft replacement, cells in diffusion chambers or growth factors. Synthetic materials are already widely used in hernia surgery, and the challenge will be to augment these materials with growth factors.

Orthopaedic surgeons have begun to use targeted delivery systems to achieve tissue engineering [6]. For instance, TGF-b adsorbed onto resorbable microcrystals of hydroxyappetite or 3% methocellulose with cross-linked type I collagen can be used in bone fractures. In addition, ethylene vinyl acetate copolymer with bovine serum albumin and PDGF can be coated onto a Kirschner wire to achieve accelerated fracture healing. PDGF has also been used by incorporation into a rapidly dissolving collagen type I film, wrapped around fracture sites.

In soft tissues that are a potential site of hernia, FGF has been used bind to heparin sepharose beads. Biomaterials have been used pre-coated with fibronectin, type IV collagen or gelatin, which immobilises growth factors for local delivery. Alginate (a cellulose-like polysaccharide), beads and microcrystalline collagen have also been utilised to concentrate the delivery of growth factors at wound-healing sites. Any of these systems have potential for use in hernia surgery.

5.4 Outlook

Looking to the future, targeted delivery systems could be used for gene therapy [7]. Gene therapy involves the delivery of DNA sequences (sense or antisense) into cells for transgene expression by liposome-mediated transfection. These DNA sequences could conceivably be growth factors or structural matrix molecules. These therapies have travelled beyond the conception stage for sports injuries, with a possibility of targeting mechanical ligament weaknesses. Such concepts could be extended to include disorders of mechanical weaknesses in ligaments or indeed in the fascia transversalis in hernia (Fig. 1).

Biomaterials alone have not solved the problem of recurrence or wound failure in hernia surgery. Tissue engineering is a powerful modality which could be used in the future.

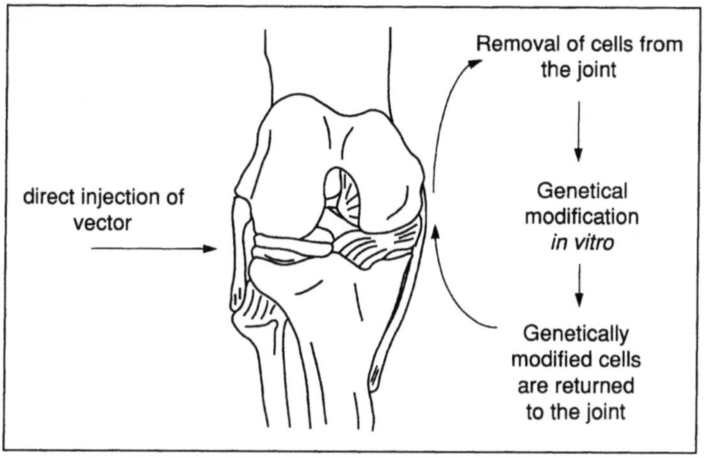

Fig. 1. A potential method of gene therapy for the repair of intra-articular injuries

5.5 Discussion

Schippers: Professor Kingsnorth, you presented excellent data concerning how to introduce growth factors, but do you know whether there is a need for growth factor in wound healing? In particular, are there patients who have a lack of growth factor who might develop such hernias?

Kingsnorth: There are no data connecting growth factor deficiency to hernia development, so this might be an area for research. Apart from growth factor deficiencies, there are numerous other defects which cause hernias.

Schumpelick: How do you explain the fact that, those with the greatest amount of growth factors, newborns, there is such a high rate of hernia?

Kingsnorth: We do not have enough data to answer that question. The experiments carried out by Peacock were very interesting; he did not merely look at defective tissue in the groin, but took samples of connective tissue from elsewhere, examining the opposite groin and the rectus sheath. He found that the metabolic disorder of collagen synthesis was universal in the connective tissues examined, so if we are going to continue these studies we are going to have to look at the presence of growth factor or some finger printing growth factor activity not only in the groin where the hernia exists, but also in the midline of the abdomen, for example. We need to look at the connective tissues and growth factor synthesis in many anatomical areas.

Klosterhalfen: I am not so optimistic, because you say you are working to modify biomaterials. I think this is a complicated field. You say that the implantation of biomaterials may produce recurrent hernias; if you look at the inflammatory infiltrate of these biomaterials such as polypropylene (studies are being carried out in Aachen), there is always an increase in TGF, tumor necrosis factor (TNF) and other growth factors over weeks.

Kingsnorth: In acute wound healing, the sequence of events is fairly well characterised. What is not well characterised are existing metabolic abnormalities in patients with hernia, i.e. growth factor abnormalities and collagen disorders that exist before the hernia repair. Even with biomaterials we have not solved the problem of recurrent hernias.

References

1. Pierce GF, Mustoe TA. Pharmacologic enhancement of wound healing. Annu Rev Med 1995; 46: 467–81
2. Greenhalgh DG The role of growth factors in wound healing. J Trauma 1996; 41: 159–167
3. Van de Kerkhof PC, Van Bergen B, Spruijt K, Kuiper JP Age-related changes in wound healing. Clin Exp Dermatol 1994; 19: 369–74
4. Meyer-Ingold W Wound therapy: growth factors as agents to promote healing. Trends of Biotechnology 1993; 11: 387–92
5. Bolton L, Fattu AJ Topical agents and wound healing. Clinics Dermatol 1994; 12: 95–120
6. Nimni ME Polypeptide growth factors: targeted delivery systems. Biomaterials 1997; 18: 1201–25
7. Gerich TG, Fu FH, Robbins PD, Evans CH Prospects for gene therapy in sports medicine. Knee Surg, Sports Traumatol, Arthroscopy 1996; 4: 180–7

Part III Abdominal Wall Defects

CHAPTER 6

Primary Hernia

D. Bennett

A hernia may be defined as a protrusion of a sac of peritoneum together with preperitoneal fat or an organ through a congenital or acquired defect in the muscles of the abdominal wall through which they do not normally pass (Ljungdahl). The anatomic feature common to all external hernias is a defect in the aponeurotic/fascial layer that lines the abdominal cavity. Hernias occupy a good deal of surgical time and account for about 10%–15% of all surgical procedures. The majority occur in the region of the umbilicus (80%), with incisional and femoral hernias accounting for only 7% and 5%, respectively. Rarer forms of hernias represent only a tiny proportion of the surgical problem.

6.1 Epigastric Hernia

Hernias of the anterior abdominal wall aponeurosis that are located in the midline are referred to collectively as hernias of the linea alba. With the exception of umbilical hernias, the most common location of a midline fascial defect is between the xiphoid process and the umbilicus. These fascial defects are termed epigastric hernias. The first epigastric hernia was described in 1285 by Arnauld de Villeneuve, but it was not until 1812 that the term epigastric hernia was introduced by Leveille. It is difficult to determine the incidence of epigastric hernia, but autopsy studies have suggested a prevalence of 0.5%–10% in the general population. There is a male predominance with a male to female ratio of at least 3: 1. Infant and child epigastric hernias are very rare, the diagnosis usually being made in the third to fifth decades.

6.2 Anatomy

The linea alba is the midline raphe formed by the junction of the rectus sheaths. It extends from the xiphoid process to the symphysis pubis. Superficial to the linea alba lie only skin and subcutaneous adipose tissue. Deep to the linea alba and the epigastric region, the fascia transversalis, preperitoneal fat, fat of the falciform ligament and peritoneum are found. The rectus muscles diverge as they proceed superiorly to insert on the fifth, sixth and seventh ribs and on the costal cartilage. Although the linea alba is narrow below the umbilicus, it may be as much as 2.5 cm wider above it. This anatomic feature may account for the rarity of midline hernias below the umbilicus.

The anterior abdominal wall aponeurosis consists of fine tendinous fibres invested in loose areolar tissue and arranged as interwoven sheets. This arrangement results in a triple-layer criss-cross pattern in the anterior and posterior rectus sheaths and contributes to the anatomic functional linkage of the muscles of the anterior abdominal wall, allowing them to work in concert. Askar reported a detailed anatomic study of the anterior abdominal wall and demonstrated that these tendinous fibres do not stop in the midline but decussate, creating an intricate interwoven pattern which links all layers of the abdominal wall with those of the other side. Decussation above the umbilicus may appear as a single line in the midline (30%) or, more commonly (70%), as a triple decussation pattern. Below the umbilicus, decussation has always been described in a single line.

Defects in the fascia may vary in diameter from several centimetres to only a few millimetres. The larger ones are usually readily reducible, whereas the smaller ones often become incarcerated. Epigastric hernias may either be a true hernia with a peritoneal sac, the incidence of which varies between 12% and 60%, or may simply contain a pre-peritoneal mass of fat attached to the peritoneum by a pedicle. Multiple fascial defects are present in between 20% and 25% of individuals.

It was originally postulated that epigastric hernias had a congenital origin (Pollack 1936). An alternative hypothesis (Moschowitz) stressed the importance of blood vessels perforating the linea alba and the prolongation of the fascia transversalis at these points. Both these theories have been criticised, as epigastric hernias are rare in childhood and isolated vessels are only rarely seen accompanying the hernial mass.

A far more attractive hypothesis was that proposed by Askar, who observed that epigastric hernias occurred exclusively in patients who had a single midline pattern of decussation. An alternative explanation relates to the structural/functional relations of the anterior abdominal wall. As noted earlier, the anterior abdominal wall aponeurosis consists of tendinous fibres which are situated obliquely in aponeurotic sheets, allowing for changes in the shape of the abdominal wall, e.g. during respiration. However, the midline can change only in length and breadth, with an increase in one necessitating a decrease in the other. During abdominal distension, the linea alba must increase in both dimensions, and the resultant tearing of fibres may play a role in the development of epigastric hernias.

Clinically, the majority of epigastric hernias (75%) are asymptomatic. Vague upper abdominal pain and nausea associated with epigastric tenderness may be present. The symptoms tend to be more severe when the patient is lying down, said to be due to traction on the hernial contents. Pain on exertion localised to the epigastrium is typical of an epigastric hernia. A subcutaneous lump, which may be tender, if incarcerated, can often cause more symptoms than larger ones. Incarceration is common, especially in smaller hernias, but strangulation is unusual.

The presence of a midline mass on physical examination usually confirms the diagnosis. In obese patients, palpation of the mass may occasionally be difficult but a local area of tenderness in the linea alba is usually present, even if the hernia is not incarcerated. Confirmation of the diagnosis can be made either by ultrasound or computed tomography (CT), both of which reveal the characteristic findings of abdominal wall hernias. These modalities may prove useful in the occasional hernia which escapes clinical diagnosis. Symptomatic hernias and those greater than 2 cm in diameter are best treated surgically.

6.3 Umbilical Hernia

There are three distinct types of hernia which occur around the umbilicus: congenital (omphalocele), infantile umbilical hernia and adult para-umbilical hernias. The term omphalocele refers to herniation of the abdominal viscera into the tissues of the umbilical cord. The hernia sac, therefore, has an internal lining of peritoneum and an external covering of thinned amnion that makes up the covering of the umbilical vessels within the cord. At 10 weeks' gestation, the gut normally returns to the abdominal cavity. When this fails to occur, normal rotation and fixation of the intestine is prevented. The umbilicus is absent and a funnel-shaped defect in the abdominal wall is present through which viscera protrude into the umbilical cord. The resulting abdominal wall defect varies considerably in size from no larger than an umbilical stump to a defect that appears to involve the entire ventral abdominal wall. Defects less than 5 cm in diameter usually contain gut only, whereas defects greater than 5 cm usually contain liver and other viscera. This condition occurs in 1 in 5000 births and is associated with other serious congenital abnormalities in 60% of cases (cryptorchidism and brain malformations are known to join omphalocele in a triad.)

Clinically, omphalocele may be diagnosed in utero or at birth . Fetal abdominal wall defects usually are not subtle and may be visualised as early as 15 weeks' gestation. On ultrasound examination, an omphalocele appears as fluid-filled loops of intestine anterior to the normal fetal abdominal wall well contained in the smooth sac. The umbilical vessels run between the layers of the sac to the abdominal wall. In large defects, the liver, spleen, stomach, pancreas or bladder may also be seen through the membrane. The management is surgical and is considered later.

6.4 Infantile Umbilical Hernia

At birth, following division of the umbilical cord, the stump heals by granulation and scarring diffuses with the umbilical ring of the abdominal wall. The obliterated umbilical vein (round ligament) is usually attached to the inferior border of the umbilical ring along with remnants of the urachus and the two obliterated umbilical arteries. The round ligament, by crossing and partially covering the umbilical ring, may protect against herniation. Non-fusion allows the peritoneal sac to protrude, usually at the superior margin of the ring. The infantile hernia, as opposed to the congenital type, is always covered with skin. In children, umbilical hernias may be the third most common surgical disorder after hydroceles and inguinal hernias. This hernia is present in about one in every five births, the incidence in black infants being up to eight times higher than in white infants.

It is most common in premature babies, and low birth weight predisposes to the umbilical hernias. There also appears to be a 9%–12% familial predisposition to umbilical hernias, but no genetic pattern of inheritance has been identified. In sets of identical twins, both children are invariably affected.

Most children with umbilical hernia present with the obvious cosmetic defect, although there may be a history of vague intermittent abdominal pain. The hernia results in a cone-like protrusion of the umbilicus that bulges every time the child cries or strains. The most important differential diagnosis is from a hernia of the umbilical cord, i.e. omphalocele. It is particularly important to identify this lesion at birth and to avoid clamping or dividing the wide base of the cord, which subsequently results in an inadvertent enterectomy. Alternative and less common differential diagnoses include an omphalomesenteric duct or a urachus. Remnants of the omphalomesenteric duct and urachus can also produce cystic masses within the umbilicus.

Infantile umbilical hernias rarely enlarge over time and will disappear in 90% of children by the age of 2 years. The majority of authors state that umbilical hernias persisting after the age of 5 or 6 years are unlikely to close spontaneously. Unfortunately, no prospective chronological studies of a stable population followed up from infancy to adulthood are available to provide clear guidelines.

Spontaneous resolution of umbilical hernias appears to be directly influenced by the size of the umbilical ring. If, at the age of 3 months, the hernia has a fascial ring of less than 0.5 cm, 96% heal spontaneously within 2 years. Defects that have a ring larger than 1.5 cm are unlikely to resolve spontaneously. Coupled with a natural tendency to closure of the fascial ring is the fact that complications of infantile umbilical hernias are extremely uncommon and probably occur in approximately 4% of cases. Reported complications include strangulation of the omentum, strangulation of the intestine and evisceration. Surgical repair is indicated if a complication occurs or if the hernia persists beyond the age of 2 years.

6.5 Acquired Umbilical Hernia

The umbilicus may become partially unfolded in patients with acute abdominal distension. Persistent elevation of the intra-abdominal pressure results in the umbilical cicatrix giving way and the development of an acquired umbilical hernia. Although uncommon, causes of acquired umbilical hernias include ascites from cirrhosis, congestive heart failure or nephrosis. Patients undergoing peritoneal dialysis also have a high incidence of these hernias. Management should be conservative, as the majority of patients have serious underlying problems and operative repair is not indicated unless the hernia incarcerates or becomes extremely large and the overlying skin is thinned down to such an extent that spontaneous rupture is possible.

6.6 Para-umbilical Hernia

Para-umbilical hernias are acquired hernias and occur in all age-groups. They are the result of disruption of the linea alba and generally occur above the umbilical cicatrix. They may occur in association with umbilical hernias and can be multiple when associated with diastasis recti. Aetiological factors include stretching of the abdominal wall due to obesity, multiple pregnancy, ascites and fat deposition in the abdominal wall. This condition is more common over the age of 35 and is five times more common in females.

Clinically, gastrointestinal symptoms are common, possibly caused by dragging on the fat and peritoneum of the falciform ligament. When the hernial sac contains bowel, colic due to intermittent intestinal obstruction is common. The hernia tends to progress over time and intertrigo and necrosis of the skin may occur in patients with larger hernias.

It is important to distinguish para-umbilical hernias from umbilical hernias, as the latter may close spontaneously in the young, whereas the former, which usually have a small neck, require surgical correction. In the para-umbilical hernia, about half the fundus of the sac is covered by the umbilicus and the remainder is covered by the skin of the abdomen immediately above or below the umbilicus. This is in contrast to the umbilical hernia, where the protrusion is directly under the umbilicus with a circumferentially symmetric bulge. Because para-umbilical hernias do not resolve spontaneously and have a high incidence of incarceration and strangulation, surgical repair is always indicated.

6.7 Umbilical Hernia in Adults

Umbilical hernias in adults do not represent persistence of infantile hernias. In contrast to the infantile hernia, umbilical hernias in adults are indirect herniations through an umbilical canal which is bordered by umbilical fascia posteriorly, the linea alba anteriorly and the medial edges of the two rectus sheaths on each side. These hernias therefore tend to incarcerate and strangulate and do not resolve spontaneously. It has been argued that they are actually para-umbilical hernias that occur just above and to the left of the umbilicus. Umbilical hernias in adults have a high associated morbidity and mortality. More than 90% of these patients are women, and almost all are obese and multiparous. In this population, umbilical hernias incarcerate half as often as inguinal hernias and three times more often than femoral hernias.

Clinically, the diagnosis of umbilical hernia in adults is usually obvious. A complete reduction is often not successful, because omentum becomes adherent to the sac. The hernia is usually painful because, as the hernia enlarges, it has a tendency to sag downward and causes traction on the stomach or transverse colon. Attacks of intermittent colicky pain may be caused by subacute intestinal obstruction. Treatment should be conservative for as long as possible, but these patients often have incarcerated hernias and prolonged preoperative therapy is not possible.

6.8 Spigelian Hernia

Spigelian hernias are rare hernias which are generally difficult to diagnose because of their frequent intramural location and vague and non-specific symptoms. A spontaneous rupture along the semilunar line was first described by Henry-Francois Lu Dran in 1742, the term "spigelian hernia" being coined after the Belgian anatomist, Adriaan van den Spieghel (the semilunar line also being known as the linea semilunaris spigeli).

There are approximately 1000 cases of spigelian hernias reported in the literature. The majority of spigelian hernias were diagnosed in patients between 40–70 years of age, with a female to male ratio of 4:3. The majority of hernias (95%) are located below the umbilicus. They occur with equal frequency on the left and right side of the body and are rarely bilateral (bilateral, 10%).

The linea semilunaris marks the transition from muscle to aponeurosis in the transversus abdominis muscle of the abdomen. The part of the aponeurosis that lies between the semilunar line and the lateral edge of the rectus muscle is known as the spigelian aponeurosis. A spigelian hernia is a protrusion of a peritoneal sac or preperitoneal fat through a congenital or acquired defect within the spigelian aponeurosis. Hernias that penetrate the aponeurosis more medially and protrude into the rectus sheath are referred to as intravaginal hernias. The spigelian hernia belt, where the spigelian aponeurosis is wider (on average approximately 2 cm), is a transverse belt lying 0–6 cm cranial to the interspinal plane (i.e. the horizontal plane through both anterior superior iliac spines).

The topographic anatomy of the abdominal wall varies above and below the umbilicus. Spigelian hernias are rare in the cranialmost part of the abdomen above the umbilicus. The muscle belly of the transverse abdominis muscle here reaches to and behind the lateral edge of the rectus muscle. The linea semilunaris lies dorsal to the rectus muscle, and there is thus no spigelian aponeurosis in this area. As a result, herniation through the transverse aponeurosis at this level is intravaginal.

Below the umbilicus, there are considerable structural variations in both muscle and aponeurotic tissue within both the internal oblique and transversus abdominis muscle. The fibres of the two muscles run almost parallel here, so that the gaps in the muscles may coincide. In such a situation, the fibres can be separated more easily, creating a risk of herniation. Above the semicircular line (the line of Douglas), the aponeurosis of the transversus abdominis muscle divides into two layers, which blend with the anterior and posterior lamellae of the rectus sheath (McVay and Anson 1940). This division occurs within the spigelian aponeurosis, which therefore consists of two lamellae. The dorsal lamella becomes thinner as it approaches the semicircular line. The medial part of the spigelian aponeurosis is weakest within the last few centimetres above the line of Douglas, and this probably is one of the most important reasons why most spigelian hernias are located in the vicinity of this line. Caudal to the line, all fibres from the transverse aponeurosis run to the anterior lamella of the rectus sheath, and the spigelian aponeurosis consists of a single layer again.

The external oblique muscle, which is the most stable structure in the anterior lateral part of the abdominal wall, is aponeurotic ventral to the spigelian aponeurosis throughout its length and prevents the hernia from entering the subcutaneous tissue. This probably accounts for the fact that the hernial sac is located subcutaneously in less than 1% of reported cases.

The aetiology of the spigelian hernia is generally considered to be related to the muscular aponeurotic structure within and ventral to the spigelian aponeurosis. The spigelian aponeurosis is one of the congenital weak areas in the ventral abdominal wall. Other predisposing factors are the same as for all other types of abdominal wall hernias (e.g. resulting in increased intra-abdominal pressure).

The diagnosis of a spigelian hernia is difficult. The symptoms vary considerably, probably because so many different organs have been reported within the hernia, resulting in diagnostic confusion. A peritoneal sac is found in most cases and usually contains the greater omentum, small intestine or part of the colon. Other organs which have been reported within the sac include stomach, gallbladder, appendix, ovary and macrodiverticulum. The usual symptoms at presentation are abdominal pain, a mass in the anterior abdominal wall or signs of incarceration with or without intestinal obstruction. The pain varies with type, severity and location, depending on the content of the hernia. Abdominal pain of uncharacteristic type, not typical of a hernia, is common, and a useful diagnostic characteristic is the provocation or aggravation of pain by manoeuvres that increase intra-abdominal pressure and the relief of pain by rest. The findings on physical examination are variable, depending on the position of the hernial sac and whether or not it is reducible. A lump may be present at the time of examination but, frequently, subjects complain of pain in the absence of a visible or palpable lump. The most useful screening test is tenderness over the spigelian aponeurosis when the abdominal muscles are tensed. This finding is not pathognomonic of a spigelian hernia, but obviously is a useful method when screening.

The most useful investigation methods for spigelian hernias are abdominal wall ultrasound and CT. Ultrasound is a rapid, accurate, non-invasive investigation which is easy to perform and which delineates the abdominal wall clearly. The diagnosis is based on demonstration of a hernial orifice in the spigelian aponeurosis and on demonstration of a hernial sac. With ultrasound scans, a congenic strip can be seen below the subcutaneous fat of the abdominal wall and the hernial orifice is visualised as a defect in the echo strip from the aponeurosis. CT provides a good alternative method for evaluating the anterior abdominal wall and provides information about the hernial orifice, the sac and the contents of the sac. If using a CT to examine the abdominal wall, it is important that the distance between slices and cross-sectional scans is very short to avoid missing the hernial orifice.

Once a spigelian hernia has been demonstrated, either by clinical techniques or by radiological investigation, the treatment is surgical.

6.9 Obturator Hernia

The obturator hernia was first described by Roland Arnaud de Ronsil in 1722. It is never externally visible and is rarely palpable, passing through the obturator canal. An obturator hernia begins with the entrance of pre-peritoneal collective tissue and fat into the pelvic orifice of the obturator canal. Subsequently, a dimple appears in the peritoneum over the internal opening of the obturator canal and progresses to the invagination of a peritoneal sac, which may remain empty at first. The sac may follow the anterior division of the obturator nerve. The symptoms usually commence when the ileum passes into the sac. Initially, this may be transitory and may reduce spontaneously, but eventually the herniated muscle of the ileum fails to reduce spontaneously. Symptoms arise due to partial (Richter type) or complete obstruction.

Obturator hernias are rare, with no clinic reporting an incidence of more than 0.073% of all hernias repaired. The male to female ratio is 1:6, and elderly individuals are most commonly affected.

The symptoms of an obturator hernia are acute, becoming progressively severe, and are only relieved by reduction of the hernia. The first signs of an obturator hernia are, in order of frequency, intestinal obstruction, the Howship-Romberg sign (pain extending down the inner surface of the thigh to the knee relieved by flexion of the thigh), a history of previous attacks and a palpable mass. The investigation of choice is herniography or ultrasonography, while laparoscopy and CT may also be useful. The treatment is surgery. Approximately 50% of obturator hernias are diagnosed intra-operatively when patients present with an acute obstruction.

6.10 Lumbar Hernia

Lumbar hernias are rare, with only around 300 cases having been reported in the literature. It has not proved possibly to provide a simple classification for these hernias. The most commonly used criterion is that of ascites or protrusion. There are three anatomic types of protrusion: the superior lumbar triangle hernia, the inferior lumbar triangle hernia and the profuse lumbar hernia. The profuse lumbar hernia is one that has become enlarged to such a degree that it encompasses most of the lumbar space and is not confined to either the superior or inferior triangle areas. These hernias are usually post-traumatic or incisional hernias. Herniation through the superior lumbar triangle, described independently by Grymseltt and Lusshast, occurs more commonly than hernias through the inferior lumbar triangle, described by Petit.

The most common finding suggesting a lumbar hernia is a flank protrusion usually discovered by the patient. The shape and size of the hernias are variable, depending on the posture of the patient. When the patient is standing, the hernia tends to become tense and larger. Coughing produces an impulse and, on percussion, the hernia is typically tympanic. Strangulation of the lumbar hernia is rare due to the large size of the lumbar defect and broad neck of the sac, and in one report strangulation was present in only 8% of 186 cases (Watson 1948). The contents of a lumbar hernia may include small and large intestine, mesentery, omentum, appendix, caecum, stomach, ovary, spleen and occasionally the kidneys. Symptoms are most severe when intestinal obstruction occurs. The diagnosis of an incarcerated lumbar hernia is suggested by cramping abdominal pains, vomiting and distension associated with a tender, irreducible mass in the lumbar area. The superior triangle of Grymseltt and Lusshast is an inverted triangle with its base formed by the inferior margin of the 12th rib along with the inferior border of the serratus posterior inferior muscle; the medial border of the triangle is the lateral edge of the quadratus lumborum muscle; the left margin is the posterior free border of the internal oblique muscle; and the whole area is referred to as the lumbocostal abdominal space. The roof of this area is formed by the latissimus dorsi muscle, while the floor is formed by the fascia transversalis along with the aponeurosis of the transversus abdominis muscle. The size and shape of the superior triangle are extremely variable, and the degree of the weakness and potential for a superior lumbar hernia depends on its size and shape. A tall, slim person with acute angulated lower ribs has a smaller superior lumbar space than a short, round-chested person with horizontal ribs, in whom the superior triangle becomes broad and larger.

The inferior lumbar triangle described by Petit is an upright triangle. The crest of the iliac bone forms the base of the triangle; the lateral border is the posterior free margin of the external oblique muscle; the medial border is the lateral free border of the latissimus dorsi muscle. The floor of the inferior lumbar triangle is composed of lumbodorsal fascia, which is contiguous with the aponeurosis of the internal oblique and transversus abdominis muscles. It is generally agreed that the weakest point is the apex of the inferior lumbar triangle.

Lumbar hernias rarely result in strangulation, and the prognosis is therefore good for most patients. The hernias do however increase in size and become symptomatic as well as being cosmetically displeasing to patients. As the hernias increase in size, a corrective surgical procedure becomes increasingly more difficult and complicated, and most patients with lumbar hernias should therefore undergo operative repair at the time of discovery. In infants, surgical repair should be delayed until the child is at least 6 months of age, unless the intensity of symptoms or physical findings suggest a danger of incarceration or strangulation, in which case corrective surgery should be performed immediately.

6.11 Discussion

Read: How many spigelian hernias do you operate on in your hospital each year?

Bennett: Very few indeed. I am not aware of any spigelian hernias having been operated on in the last 5 years.

Read: We operate on about half a dozen a year in our hospital. It seems to me that it is more common than we have realized. You compared a thousand cases of spigelian hernias with 300 cases of lumbar hernia. We very rarely see lumbar hernias, but we do see spigelian hernias as an unusual type of hernia.

Schumpelick: You mentioned the low spigelian hernia. I think that is a real entity, because in female patients after hysterectomy with a Pfannenstiel incision we see some spigelian hernias down in the Hesselbach triangle. That is not so uncommon.

Bennett: There is a difficulty perhaps in identifying them. I suspect a lot of people describe them as direct inguinal hernias, which might be occurring slightly higher up in the inguinal canal than is otherwise recognized. The incidence might be a lot higher than we realize. It just fails to be recognized that it is a low spigelian as supposed to a high direct hernia.

Schumpelick: Why do we not see low epigastric hernias below the level of the umbilicus? The pressure is higher in the lower abdomen.

Bennett: Askar suggests that it may be related to the way that the function of the abdominal wall above the umbilicus is organized. It can expand in either volume or length, but not both at the same time. If you stress it in both volume and length, you cause a defect to occur, whereas below the umbilicus the abdominal wall can expand both in volume and length and is therefore not exposed to the same stress. This shearing sensation, which may produce an epigastric hernia, does not occur below the umbilicus.

Amid: Perhaps the reason that your review of literature showed 1000 spigelian hernias but only 300 lumbar hernias is the fact that lumbar hernias are not really that uncommon. Therefore people do not report them.

I think I have an answer for Professor Schumpelick. Epigastric or midline incision hernia below the umbilicus is less common because of the fact that the rectus muscles below the umbilicus are really together. As they go up, they diverge and leave a defect between the two rectus muscles above the umbilicus. The stage is more set for an epigastric hernia above the umbilicus than below.

Bendavid: We see lumbar hernias extremely rarely. However, spigelian hernias are more common than you suspect. We see them regularly. If you examine the hernias that you call interstitial hernias at the level of the internal ring really closely, you will often see that they go through transverse and internal oblique muscle just medial to the internal ring itself. Careful dissection sometimes reveals the spigelian fascia, and these are actually spigelian hernias rather than true interstitial hernias, which come through the internal ring itself.

Bennett: There is probably a large gray area in our dissections. Many of us are perhaps not so precise in our descriptions when we are carrying out repairs. There is a very high incidence of incisional lumbar hernias. We see a lot of lumbar hernia repairs which are secondary. However, my review of the literature has revealed 300 primary cases not related to trauma or any other events which might predispose a patient to developing a flank hernia.

Filipi: We perform an open technique for laparoscopic cholecystectomy. This involves a small vertical incision below the umbilicus. Especially in males, we find a second layer of fascia below the midline in 30% of patients. This makes it impossible to use the technique that I like to use, i.e. the blunt finger entry technique. That might be one of the reasons why these midline hernias do not occur below the umbilicus.

Schumpelick: What is a para-umbilical hernia? Is it an old umbilical one, a degenerated one or an entity in its own right?

Bennett: If you look through the literature, the description given is of a hernia which is asymptomatic to the umbilicus. Some people actually say that an umbilical hernia is simply a sliding para-umbilical hernia which originates through a defect in the linea alba represented through the umbilicus. I suspect the para-umbilical hernia actually originates through the linea alba defect and combines part of the umbilical hernia to form the so-called para-umbilical hernia. It is therefore a primary defect in the linea alba.

Bendavid: I would also like to point out the high incidence of incarceration of umbilical hernia in patients with liver disease and ascites. I do not think that it has ever been explained, but it is a real entity. You mentioned in one of your slides that the umbilical hernia in adults does not represent the persistence of an infantile hernia. How can you tell the difference?

Bennett: There have been a couple of case reports of presentations in the literature which have actually followed people through from infancy to adulthood, and it has been shown that the patients did not have an infantile lump and that the lump appeared during adulthood. It is on that basis that we believe the acquired umbilical hernia in adults is different to the infantile hernia, which is of a congenital origin.

CHAPTER 7

Nonhernial Defects

C. Peiper

Surgeons, themselves are the most common cause of abdominal wall defects. These occur mostly as the result of tumor resection, harvesting of muscle in reconstructive breast surgery, or open abdomen management due to traumatic or infectious disorders. The latter situation, in particular, has caused a significant increase in the number of full-thickness defects due to a more aggressive therapeutic approach in recent decades. Congenital abnormalities only lead to reconstructive procedures in adults in rare cases such as in prune belly syndrome patients.

The deficiency may be limited to the fascial layer or may involve the full thickness of the abdominal wall. In general, these defects may lead to disturbances in the integrity, strength, and contour of the muscular and fascial layers of the anterior and lateral abdominal wall. Primary or secondary closure of the defect therefore has to be carried out using native tissue, local or distal flaps, prosthetic reinforcement, or replacement.

Abdominal wall defects can be classified according to the severity of the trauma and the biology of the wound (Table 1). Here, hernial defects are classified as either grade I or II. The main focus, however, will be on the severe defects classified as grade III or IV.

7.1 Tumor Resection

Many malignant tumors may cause infiltration of the abdominal wall and require full-thickness resection for potential cure or good palliation for the patient. They range

Table 1. Abdominal wall defect classification [20]

Grade	Definition	Example
I	Limited trauma to native tissue, no infection	Recurrent inguinal hernia
II	Defects – Have required multiple reoperations – Are associated with high-stress areas of the abdominal wall – Involve poor-quality soft tissue	Recurrent ventral hernia
III	Infected Contaminated	Enteric fistula Infected mesh material
IV	Full-thickness abdominal wall loss	Tumor, traumatic or infectious process

from primary sarcoma of the abdominal wall such as rhabdomyosarcoma or liposarcoma [19] to invasion by intra-abdominal tumors such as colonic or the cervical cancer [19] to metastases of distant malignancies [12]. Exotic entities such as carcinoid of the umbilicus [11] have also been described. Malignancies possibly causing abdominal wall resection include the following:

- Rhabdomyosarcoma
- Bladder carcinoma
- Desmoid tumor
- Chondrosarcoma
- Myxosarcoma
- Malignant fibrous histiocytoma
- Basal cell carcinoma
- Cervical cancer
- Endometrial cancer
- Metastases
- Leiomyosarcoma
- Urachus carcinoma
- Osteosarcoma of the rib
- Fibrosarcoma
- Liposarcoma
- Dermatofibrosarcoma protuberans
- Infiltrating colonic carcinoma
- Squamous cell carcinoma
- Carcinoid of the umbilicus

When present, abdominal wall tumors may ulcerate, become infected, or bleed, causing unsightly painful lesions with a foul-smelling discharge. The main suggestion for all these cases is to perform adequate debridement and complete excision of tumors without any fear of the resulting size and complexity of the defect, as the radicality of the resection is the most important factor determining the patient's life expectancy. Margins should cover at least 4–6 cm of the adjacent healthy tissue. Any reoperation for tumor recurrence entails an elevated perioperative risk due to infiltration or adhesion to the parietal peritoneum, the underlying intestine, or the greater omentum. Furthermore, in most cases, the treatment of choice is surgical extirpation. Ample local excision of the tumor therefore remains of primary importance [1].

7.2 Trauma

Post-traumatic defects are due either to intra-abdominal injuries with septic complications or to direct disruption. This happens in about one per thousand of all blunt traumas, mostly after high-speed motor vehicle crashes. The so-called seat belt syndrome includes bowel injury, lumbar spine fracture, and direct abdominal wall trauma. These traumata are most common in the flank and the anterior inferior region of the abdominal wall [2]. The defects result either from direct trauma, e.g. after contact with bicycle, motorcycle, or snowmobile handlebars, or are the result of indirect injuries. Here, an acute increase in intra-abdominal pressure associated with tangential shearing stress may lead to muscular disruption [21]. These injuries are rare in the supraumbilical position, probably due to the added strength of the posterior rectus sheath, which is present only above the arcuate line [7].The findings range from bruising to ecchymosis to a full-thickness defect, occasionally with evisceration. This diagnosis leads to laparotomy. Concomitant injuries are involved in more than 50% of cases. Intestinal reconstruction should be performed separate from and before any attempt at delayed abdominal wall repair is made [2]. Less violent injuries may lead to defects of the musculo-aponeurotic layers with intact skin, resulting in an acute traumatic hernia. These cases, however, are very rare. Up to 1994, less than 30 cases were reported in the literature [3, 7].

Other causes of abdominal wall injuries include electrical burn trauma [9] and close-range shotgun blasts, which have a high mortality rate of 85%–90% due to hemorrhage from solid viscus injury or multiple hollow viscus perforations [10]. Both injury patterns can also lead to full-thickness wall loss. Destructive abdominal wall trauma patients have an overall mortality rate of 38% due to an average of 3.3 associated organ injuries [18].

After excluding or treating intra-abdominal associated injuries and adequate debridement of the abdominal wall margins, primary closure is only advisable if possible without any tension. As these wounds are typically associated with massive soft tissue injury requiring extensive debridement, primary closure is not feasible. The use of tissue whose viability is questionable for closure under "minimal" tension will fail. In addition, many of these patients develop a post-traumatic visceral edema in their intra- or postoperative course. This is the effect of the total amount of the fluid volume necessary for the stabilization of the patient's circulation. The same situation may arise during ongoing intraoperative volume resuscitation in ruptured abdominal aortic aneurysm repair, after intraoperative visceral ischemia and reperfusion, and in mesenteric venous obstruction caused by traction on the mesentery or temporary occlusion of the portal vein. Resulting tension during abdominal closure will lead to tissue necrosis, wound sepsis, and fascial dehiscence as well as evisceration. If bleeding has been controlled, necrotic tissue debrided, and tissue oxygenation restored, visceral edema should be resorbed in the early postoperative period and secondary reconstruction can be performed [17].

7.3 Necrotizing Fasciitis

Postoperative necrotizing fasciitis of the abdominal wall is often fatal. Failure to recognize the potential severity of these infections, with resultant delays in treatment, is responsible for the attendant morbidity and mortality. The necrotizing fasciitis in the classical sense is due to clostridial organism infection. More frequently, however, a synergism between multiple organisms is the cause, especially after bowel injury. The treatment follows an aggressive schedule including surgical debridement and broad-spectrum antibiotics, as well as repeated abdominal reexplorations and an open abdomen management. The early debridement of the infected regions, however, often leads to full-thickness defects of the abdominal wall. Areas of small bowel necrosis are often noted during subsequent operations and are apparently due to contact with necrotic abdominal wall tissue [8]. Definitive reconstruction of the abdominal wall is carried out after complete stabilization of the infectious process. Despite this modern form of management, the mortality rate remains at about 25% [18].

7.4 Laparostomy

All the above-mentioned situations may lead to open abdomen management, so-called laparostomy. The most common cause, however, for the initiation of laparostomy is peritonitis. This may be caused by perforation or bacterial transmigration of an infected organ. Other causes are ascending infection and iatrogenic complications. These may occur after operative or interventional procedures or following diagnostic examination. Maintenance of a chronic ambulatory peritoneal dialysis (CAPD) is also a risk factor for the development of peritonitis. Severe diffuse intra-abdominal infection is often associated with multiple organ failure and has a very high mortality rate of up to 46% [15].

The current therapeutic approach to peritonitis includes repeated operative explorations and the use of laparostomy. Laparostomy treats the peritoneal cavity as a whole abscess. This leads to better pulmonary function due to improved diaphragmatic excursions. The decreased intra-abdominal pressure also improves the microperfusion of the organs, especially the kidney, the liver, and the bowel. Necrosis of the abdominal wall closed forcefully and repeatedly is avoided [5].

Laparostomy can be performed leaving the abdominal cavity completely open or using a synthetic mesh for temporary closure. This includes the advantage of covering the abdominal cavity. The mesh has to be safe and biologically inert. After implantation, it has to be well tolerated in the organism. The main advantage of using a mesh is the prevention of organ evisceration. The risk of enteric fistulas appearing spontaneously or after minimal trauma is reduced, while the free drainage of fluids is ensured [5]. The exact methodology for this temporary closure may vary (i.e., abdominal zipper, absorbable or nonabsorbable mesh), but the basic principle of open management and easy intra-abdominal access for local care and debridement remains the same.

After the sepsis has been brought under control, reexploration of the peritoneal cavity is no longer necessary, and organ support has been discontinued, the defect is then ready for reconstruction. The current concept of open abdomen management includes local wound care to enable rapid growth of granulation tissue through and over the synthetic mesh and early skin grafting to close the wound. This prevents fistulization and fluid and protein loss through the stitches of the mesh. The intra-abdominal organs are protected against exogenous infection, and the catabolic state of the organism can thus be controlled. After the patient has fully recovered, the definitive reconstruction of the abdominal wall is carried out [13].

7.5 Radiotherapy

Defects of the abdominal wall related to iatrogenic procedures may also occur after the end of percutaneous radiotherapy, especially following radical or palliative surgical treatment. The list of relevant malignancies is long and has already been mentioned (see Sect. 7.1). Due to the kind of damage to the abdominal wall, there are some peculiarities in the postradiation situation. The radiated part of the abdominal wall does not mobilize easily, and the different layers are fixed together. Furthermore, the radiated skin cannot tolerate any tension whatsoever. Both facts are due to a decreased blood supply, secondary to obliterative endarteriitis and vasculitis caused by the radiation. This chronic ischemia has a significant effect on wound healing and has to be taken into consideration during reconstruction [19].

7.6 Donor Defect After a Transverse Rectus Abdominis Musculocutaneous Flap

A further iatrogenic defect might occur after harvesting a part of the rectus abdominis muscle for a transverse rectus abdominis musculocutaneous (TRAM) flap in reconstructive breast surgery after radical mastectomy. Investigations show that, even after preserving the caudal and lateral part of the muscle, more than 60% of patients show denervation of the residual strip of rectus [6]. This is probably due to the fact that the motor branches of the lower intercostal nerves, which innervate the rectus muscle, enter the deep surface of the muscular belly approximately 3 cm from the lateral edge. A nerve injury is possible here even during selective harvesting of muscle. Additional strangulation of muscular fibers and operative reduction of the blood supply may lead to fibrosis and degeneration of the muscle and to a functional defect of the abdominal wall [4].

7.7 Prune Belly Syndrome

Prune belly syndrome is also relevant in surgery in adults. In addition to anomalies of the urogenital and gastrointestinal tract, luxation of the hip, spina bifida, and hydrocephalus, hypoplasia or aplasia of the muscles of the abdominal wall is one of its pathognomonic symptoms. If the patient's condition allows him to reach adolescence, the competence of the abdominal wall may be restored. In the Monfort operation, the overstretched floppy fascial parts of the abdominal wall are excised and the oblique muscles refixed to the rectus muscle [14].

7.8 Congenital Abdominal Wall Necrosis

One unusual report describes so-called congenital soft tissue necrosis in infants, which is described in two cases. In one case, full-thickness necrosis was caused by the subcutaneous injection of radiopaque contrast material into the fetus during an improperly performed fetal amniography. In the other case, neither a traumatic nor an iatrogenic episode could be ascertained from the maternal gestational history. The etiology of the defect was therefore presumed to be spontaneous. It closed within 8 weeks with conservative management [16].

7.9 Discussion

Scott: In the literature, there is a discussion of difficult abdominal wall closures with patients who have a large edema. Surgeons use parachute material and bring that together over time. Have you found any of that in the literature or have you ever used that technique?

Peiper: There are many suggestions for these indications. There is also the idea of putting sutures into the wound; by pulling the sutures, the margins will be joined together over time. However, I do not think this is a common concept which can be recommended for all cases. The better idea is not to perform the primary closure if there is any doubt whether the tension might be too high. It is better to implant synthetic mesh for the early postoperative phase until the patient is stable and the edema is resorbed. The definitive reconstruction can then follow within a few days.

Bruch: What kind of mesh do you use to reconstruct the abdominal wall in the initial postoperative phase? Do you use a resorbable mesh or do you use xenoplastic mesh?

Peiper: For the acute situation, we use resorbable mesh as we do not know how the situation of the patient will develop. It might be necessary to perform reoperations and it might not be advisable to perform a definitive reconstruction too soon. Many patients need several weeks or months to stabilize, and if you use an absorbable mesh you can leave it in situ. If you have a nonabsorbable mesh in an infective situation, I do not think it is advisable to leave it in situ for a longer period.

Greenburg: We have been closing complicated wounds following major surgery or after trauma and have used the bladder pressure. We measure the pressure using a Foley catheter as means of assessing increased intra-abdominal pressure as we try to pull tension-free walls together. I wonder whether you have any experience of that?

Peiper: We do not have any experience of that, but there are reports in the literature about measurement of the intra-abdominal pressure using a balloon catheter in the bladder or the rectum. You can also measure the tension of the abdominal wall directly during closure if you use a device which tells you the tension via strain gauge tension transducers. While closing the abdominal wall, you can measure the tension, which might be directly on the suture line.

Greenburg: There may be a real difference in the tension in the suture because it is probably related as much to the physical characteristics of the suture material as to the actual tension of the abdominal wall. I think we should consider looking at intra-abdominal pressure as measured primarily in the bladder or the rectum.

Peiper: I wonder whether it is advisable to take a definite parameter and to say up to 20 mmHg we should close it and above that we should not. If you are in any doubt, you should not perform a primary closure.

Greenburg: I have no problem with that concept. However, I think the pressure by itself is not sufficient. The other thing that has to be looked at is the ventilator compliance at the same time, because what you are doing when you increase intra-abdominal pressure of course is to raise the diaphragm and make it more difficult for the ventilator to work. Three weeks ago, when we saw a 20-mmHg increase in bladder pressure, we had a 50% decrease in compliance and had to make more adjustments to lower the intra-abdominal pressure.

Kingsnorth: I wonder whether classifying the defects of the anterior abdominal wall can give us any indication of the severity. I would imagine that it is far more serious to have a defect which is lateral to the rectus muscle, because there are only the flat muscles of the abdominal wall. Once they become disrupted, necrotic, or defective, you have a much more serious problem than if you have only got a defect that is in some way related to the rectus muscle itself and the sheath anteriorly and posteriorly.

Peiper: Any full-thickness wall defect is classified as a severe situation. The anterior wall defects might be easier to close, because the fascial landmarks are closer than they are in the flank. Defects in the flank are more difficult to repair. Another point is the loss of the motoric nerves, which is more prominent if the defect is in the flank. Then the whole area might be denervated.

Read: It is interesting that the tensor fascia lata flap was first used by Dr. Wallenstein of Minnesota in 1942. He did not use that flap as a composite flap, but used it for cancers of the colon that extended to the abdominal wall. He also used it for ulcers which were anaerobic combined infections of the abdominal wall in the preantibiotic era. It is interesting that this flap is a very good flap for the lower abdominal wall.

Devlin: Is there any coincidence between metabolic diseases such as diabetes and the development of ventral defects?

Peiper: Diabetes will not cause a nonhernial defect of the abdominal wall. Another exogenic factor must be present for a full abdominal wall defect to develop. Metabolic diseases probably predispose to a hernial defect.

Kingsnorth: Measuring the intra-abdominal pressure in the bladder is very dependent on the type of anesthesia that you are using. I would not have thought it very reliable, unless you have very consistent anesthesia in terms of muscle relaxation, which is related to the patient's body weight.

References

1. Blom WF, Schraffordt Koops H, Vermey A, Oldhoff J: Abdominal wall resection and reconstruction with the aid of Marlex mesh. Br J Surg 1982;69:353–355
2. Brenneman FD, Boulanger BR, Antonyshyn O: Surgical management of abdominal wall disruption after blunt trauma. J Trauma 1995;39:539–544
3. Damschen DD, Landercasper J, Cogbill TH: Acute traumatic abdominal hernia: Case reports. J Trauma 1994;36:273
4. Duchateau J, Declety A, Lejour M: Innervation of the rectus abdominis muscle: implica-tions for rectus flaps. Plast Reconstr Surg 1988;82:223–227
5. Fayman MS, Schein M, Saadia R: Abdominal wall reconstruction after open manage-ment of the septic abdomen. S Afr J Surg 1990;28:62–65

6. Galli A, Adami M, Berrino P, Leone S, Santi P: Long-term evaluation of the abdominal wall competence after total and selective harvesting of the rectus abdominis muscle. Ann Plast Surg 1992;28:409–413
7. Gill IS, Toursarkissian B, Johnson SB: Traumatic ventral abdominal hernia associated with small bowel gangrene. Case report. J Trauma 1993;35:145
8. Howard CA, Turner WW Jr: Successful treatment of early, postoperative, necrotizing infection of the abdominal wall. Crit Care Med 1989;17:586–587
9. Kumar P, Varma R: Immediate reconstruction of chest and abdominal wall defect follow-ing high voltage electrical injury. Burns 1994;20:557–559
10. Ledgerwood AM, Lucas CE: Management of massive abdominal wall defects: role of porcine skin grafts. J Trauma 1976;16:85–88
11. Nanni G, Gangeri G, Magalini SC, Grieco A, Piantelli M: Primary carcinoid of the umbilicus. Description of the 1st case. Minerva Chir 1994;49:1165–1170
12. Neven P, Shepherd JH, Tham KF, Fisher C, Breach N: Reconstruction of the abdominal wall with a latissimus dorsi musculocutaneous flap: a case of a massive abdominal wall metastasis from a cervical cancer requiring palliative resection. Gynecol Oncol 1993;49:403–406
13. Okunski WJ, Sonntag BV, Murphy RX Jr: Staged reconstruction of abdominal wall defects after intra-abdominal catastrophes. Ann Plast Surg 1996;36:475–478
14. Parrott TS, Woodard JR: The Monfort operation for abdominal wall reconstruction in the prune belly syndrome. J Urol 1992;148:688–690
15. Schein M, Decker GAG: Gastrointestinal fistulas associated with large abdominal wall defects: experience with 43 patients. Br J Surg 1990;77:97–100
16. Shija JK: Congenital soft tissue necrosis of the right anterior abdominal wall. J Pediatr Surg 1987;22:1003–1004
17. Smith PC, Tweddell JS, Bessey PQ: Alternative approaches to abdominal wound closure in severely injured patients with massive visceral edema. J Trauma 1992;32:16–20
18. Stone HH, Fabian TC, Turkleson ML, Jurkiewicz MJ: Management of acute full-thick-ness losses of the abdominal wall. Ann Surg 1981;193:612–618
19. Weinstein LP, Kovachev D, Chaglassian T: Abdominal wall reconstruction. Scand J Plast Reconstr Surg 1986;20:109–113
20. Williams JK, Carlson GW, Howell RL, Wagner JD, Nahai F, Coleman JJ: The tensor fascia lata free flap in abdominal-wall reconstruction. J Reconstr Microsurg 1997;13:83–90
21. Wood RJ, Ney AL, Bubrick MP: Traumatic abdominal hernia: A case report and review of the literature. Am Surg 1988;54:648

CHAPTER 8

Acute Wound Failure

M.A. Carlson

8.1 Incidence

The incidence of acute wound failure (also known as wound dehiscence, wound disruption, burst abdomen, evisceration, or eventration) has remained relatively constant during this century. If data from retrospective studies of large numbers of surgical patients are combined, rates of 0.4% (representing 71,000 incisions), 0.59% (320,000 incisions), and 1.2% (18,000 incisions) are obtained for the time periods 1900–1940, 1950–1984, and 1985 to the present, respectively [7, 13, 54]. The incidence of dehiscence is higher in prospective studies (failure rates ranging from 1% to 3%) compared to retrospective studies [54].

8.2 Pertinent Aspects of Fascial Healing

Fascial incisions have no inherent strength during the first week of healing, so the early integrity of a fascial wound depends entirely on the suture. In the second week of healing, there is a rapid increase in tensile strength; animal data has been variable, but in general a fascial incision regains 50% of the tensile strength of unwounded fascia after 4–6 weeks and plateaus at about 60%–80% after 1 year [2, 19, 24, 47, 51]. Rarely has it been documented that a healed fascial wound reaches 100% or more of the strength of unwounded fascia. The general belief is that wounded fascia never regains its full tensile strength.

The healing zone of a noninfected fascial wound is defined as the area within about 5 mm of each wound edge in which collagen deposition, degradation, and reorganization occurs [1]. An incision closed with sutures placed within this zone is more prone to dehiscence, as the suture can easily tear through the tissue of this biochemically active region. The healing zone may be avoided by placing fascial sutures 10 mm or more from the wound edge.

The presence of a mild degree of inflammation is important for timely gain of fascial strength after wounding. Wounds that have been sutured, allowed to heal for several days, forcefully disruptured, and then resutured regain strength faster than a primarily sutured wound [33, 56, 59, 62]. The explanation for this is that the inflammatory process healing is further along in the disruptured/resutured wounds, shortening the lag time to wound strength development. The injury from the scalpel blade usually results in adequate inflammation to ensure timely healing of a typical wound [50]. Use of coagulation current from a cautery device, however, may be too destructive, as there is evidence in animals that making an incision with this technique results in slower gain of wound strength compared to use of the scalpel [55]. Inflammation from a mild wound infection may speed gain of tensile strength, as has been shown in animals [6, 65]. There is no data, however, to support the administration of a routine bacterial inoculum to the human wound as a healing aid.

8.3 Choice of Incision

There is considerable retrospective data which supports the superiority of the transverse incision over the vertical midline with respect to dehiscence prevention [16, 29, 30, 41, 43, 61]. A partial explanation for the lower rate of wound failure with the transverse incision is that it cuts the abdominal wall parallel to the aponeurotic fibers, so that contraction of the abdominal wall musculature will tend to pull the incision together. This is opposite to the situation with the vertical midline incision, which has been called "nonanatomic." Study of wound-bursting strength in cadavers has demonstrated that transverse wounds are slightly stronger than midline wounds when 0.5- to 1-cm bites of fascia are taken with the suture needle [27, 68]. However, if a midline incision is closed with wide fascial bites (such that the needle goes through and through the rectus sheath), the bursting strength is 1.5 times greater than the above transverse incision [68]. The available randomized prospective patient data comparing transverse and midline incisions do not show a difference in the dehiscence rates [21, 27]. Two English groups have enjoyed vanishingly low dehiscence and hernia rates with the lateral paramedian incision [15, 18], but confirmatory trials have not appeared yet. A strong declaration regarding the choice of incision to prevent acute wound failure cannot be made.

8.4 Mechanisms

There are four main causes of acute wound failure: a suture break, a slipped suture knot, a loose or excessive stitch interval which allows protrusion of viscera, and suture tearing through the fascia. A wound may fail secondary to a necrotizing infection, but this is rare. Suture tearing through the fascia is by far the most common cause (70%–95%) of acute wound failure, as noted in numerous prospective and retrospective reports and in animal and cadaver wound-bursting experiments [3, 26, 28, 48, 52, 53, 58, 60]. There may be a select few patients in which poor fascia may be blamed for tearing, but the predominance of evidence indicates that an inadequate bite of fascia with the suture needle is responsible for suture tearing through the fascia.

8.5 Choice of Closure

The technique of suturing the incision is the area where an individual surgeon can make the biggest impact in reducing acute wound failure. Taking a large (>1 cm) bite of fascia with each turn of the needle while maintaining a short (about 1 cm) stitch interval seems to produce the strongest closure [42]. This has been quantified as the suture to length ratio [25, 36, 37, 40, 44, 49]. The minimum ratio which has been advocated to optimize wound strength is 4:1, i.e., the length of the suture used to close the wound should be at least four times longer than the length of the wound. Groups which have followed this precept obtain wound failure rates approaching zero. Recently, however, there has been some concern that employment of a ratio greater than 5 will result in an increased chance of wound infection in the obese individual [38, 39].

Much has been written regarding the choice of suture material for abdominal incision closure. The two basic choices are absorbable versus nonabsorbable; another less important characteristic is monofilament versus multifilament. No clear favorite (in terms of dehiscence prevention) for fascial suture has emerged from randomized trials [8, 10–12, 44, 46, 70]. Suture choice, therefore, seems relatively unimportant as long as a rapidly absorbing material (e.g., chromic catgut) is not used for fascial closure [26, 28].

Excessive tension on the suture during wound closure can result in ischemic necrosis of the entrapped fascia, and tightly tied sutures will cut through fascia earlier than loose sutures during wound-bursting experiments [31, 45, 57]. Ideal suture tension should approximate the fascia, yet allow perfusion of the healing wound edges. This translates into a relatively loose closure; the risk of a knuckle of bowel protruding through such a closure can be eliminated by using a short (about 1 cm) stitch interval [40].

There are other aspects of wound closure which, though less important, deserve mention. There is no benefit to closing the peritoneum as a separate layer [22, 35]. There is no benefit to layered closure over mass closure [4]; the latter may be preferable simply because it is quicker. There is no advantage of interrupted closure over running closure [8, 14, 23]; the latter may also be preferable because it is quicker. Knot security is improved by using more throws overall, more double throws in particular, and using all square knots [17, 66, 67, 69]. Routine placement of prophylactic retention sutures is controversial and has not been of benefit in the one prospective trial that has been done [34].

8.6 Risk Factors

The implication from the preceding paragraphs is that an inadequate surgical technique is responsible for the vast majority of burst abdomens, and this is generally true. There are some conditions, however, which have been associated with dehiscence, including male sex, advanced age, emergency operation, operator inexperience, obesity, diabetes, renal failure, jaundice, hemorrhagic shock, protein malnutrition, vitamin C deficiency, zinc deficiency, steroids, and chemoradiation [13]. The significance of the association between these factors and acute wound failure has been given mostly in small retrospective studies, so the amount that any one of these factors adds to the dehiscence risk of a given patient is difficult to quantify. Intuitively, it would seem that the presence of multiple risk factors forebodes worse for the patient than the presence of zero or one factor, but this has not been shown conclusively.

8.7 Role of Infection

Wound infection is a frequently cited risk factor for dehiscence, but again data are lacking to support a causative role. The cause of fascial disruption is obvious in the rare patient whose fascia has disintegrated from a necrotizing infection, but dehiscence usually occurs before most wound infections have an opportunity to become established. The animal data on the role of wound infection is conflicting; both salutary and detrimental effects of a bacterial inoculum on healing have been observed [5, 6, 9, 63, 65].

8.8 Postoperative Increases in Intra-abdominal Pressure

A common observation is that dehiscence is precipitated by a patient coughing or straining; elevated intra-abdominal pressure is often cited as a cause of burst abdomen. It has been demonstrated that a healthy awake man (during inguinal herniorrhaphy) can raise his intra-abdominal pressure to 60–80 mmHg with a Valsalva maneuver [32]. Continuous monitoring of intra-abominal pressure with an intraperitoneal balloon has shown that resting pressure is 8 cm H_2O (1 mmHg=1.36 cm H_2O), pressure during defecation may rise to 35 cm, and it may go up to 60–80 cm with vomiting or coughing [20]. Wound-bursting experiments on cadavers required intra-abdominal pressure in the 200-mmHg range to rupture a midline or transverse incision [31]. One might conclude that, based on the cadaver wound-burst data, a properly sutured incision should withstand the stress of intra-abdominal pressure generated by the average individual.

8.9 Summary

The incidence of acute wound failure in abdominal incisions has remained around 0.5%–1% during this century. There is little inherent strength in a fascial wound during the first postoperative week, but during the next month or so there is a rapid climb to 50% of baseline strength, and this increases to 60%–80% by 1 year. The predominant mechanism of acute wound failure is suture tearing through the fascia. The technique of wide fascial bites with a short stitch interval is the most important step an individual surgeon can take to prevent dehiscence. The rational behind this technique lies within what we know about fascial strength and healing. The soundness of this technique has been demonstrated both retrospectively and prospectively.

8.10 Discussion

Filipi: Are there any studies to suggest that retention sutures impair wound healing?

Carlson: Strictly speaking, no. Two studies were published back in the 1930s. One was by Dr. Kennedy, who claimed that, in 56 years of abdominal surgery by himself and his mentor Josef Price in Detroit, they did not have one dehiscence with evisceration. He attributed this to his closure technique, which was a fascial closure with catgut reinforced with retention sutures. His technique of retention sutures was three to an inch, and an inch away from the incision.

Kingsnorth: You said less significant factors were interrupted versus running for closure of an abdominal wound. My concept of this is that, if you put interrupted stitches in, some are going to be tight and some are going to be loose. If there is any problem with the wound, the tightest one is going to give first, and then there will be a domino effect. If you have a running stitch of a monofilament suture, the tension will be spread equally across the whole wound. I wonder where you got this information from concerning interrupted versus continuous sutures for closing wounds.

Carlson: There has been one very good study from France in which 3000 patients were enrolled – a number large enough to prove the point – comparing interrupted versus running closure.

Kingsnorth: I think you have to define what you mean by absorbable. We have all decided that absorbable in terms of catgut is out. Gynecologists prove that to us time and time again. Many of us here in this room have had to reoperate gynecological wounds that were closed with catgut. Could you be a little more accurate in defining what you mean by absorbable?

Carlson: I did not mention catgut, but I should have. Generally, if you close a wound with chromic catgut, you can expect a dehiscence rate of 10% or more. That was shown by a number of investigators in the United Kingdom 30 years ago. Catgut is bad. On a scale of absorbability, Vicryl and Dexon would be intermediate. They have a half-life of 2–3 weeks of tensile strength. In prospective randomized trials, no one has been able to show that using those two sutures – Dexon, Vicryl – has resulted in greater dehiscence rates compared to nonabsorbable sutures.

Kingsnorth: Have they shown any difference in the late wound failure rate?

Carlson: The hernia rate is going to be affected by that type of choice.

Treutner: You told us that a certain degree of wound infection may enhance the tensile strength of the wound in the later course. From my recollection, patients who experience wound infection after hernia surgery are more prone to recurrence than those have had an uneventful course. How could you explain this fact?

Carlson: That would relate more to late wound failure. The effect of wound infection on late wound failure is probably more an issue than it is in acute wound failure.

Bendavid: To answer your question, I am not so sure any more either that wound infection is necessarily a prognostic factor in recurrence. You also have to distinguish in wound infection between a superficial and a deep wound infection. I find that most of the infections we see are superficial. What you often have to do is open the wound and drain it. I have never seen a deep wound infection that went right through to the peritoneal cavity. Such infections might be associated with increased incidence of recurrence. It is very important to distinguish the two.

Klaiber: Is there any data comparing fascial incisions with the scalpel and electrocautery? It is becoming increasingly fashionable to work with electrocautery.

Carlson: There are some animal data suggesting that using a coagulation current produces a slower course of healing than using a cutting current or scalpel. If you use a coagulating current, it causes more tissue destruction. I use the scalpel.

Israelsson: At our clinic, we have a dehiscence rate of 0.4%. We have collected eight patients with wound dehiscence during the last 7 years. We measure the suture length to wound length ratio in all patients. Of these eight patients, one was sutured with a suture to wound length ratio greater than 4. In this patient, dehiscence occurred 10 days after the laparotomy. He suffered from a deep wound infection and showed necrotizing infection with complete disintegration of the entire abdominal wall. No suture in the world could have saved this patient from wound dehiscence. In one patient, the suture broke at the middle. That was clearly a surgical mistake, because modern suture material does not break unless you do not handle it properly. It was probably the grasp with a needleholder. In the other six patients, the suture length to wound length ratio was less than 4, and in three patients less than 2. In our experience, wound dehiscence is almost invariably due to a bad surgical technique. I would also like to mention a rather nasty way of establishing this. When you reoperate on a person with wound dehiscence, you can measure the length of the skin incision, and the suture is still in the wound. Just take the suture out, measure it, calculate the suture to wound length ratio, and you will find that it is very low. It is probably below 3.

Gislason: I carried out a study of the English literature and looked at all the prospective studies. I found that the continuous method is safer than the interrupted method. There are significantly fewer cases of burst abdomen using the continuous suture method. Regarding the effect of wound infection on burst abdomen, I found that late burst abdomen is associated with high wound infection rates. If you get a burst abdomen after the eighth or tenth day, you have a high incidence of wound infection. The early burst abdomen is probably due to a failure in surgical technique.

Carlson: I would suggest that one of the reasons why wound infection is greater with late dehiscence is probably that the tissue is being strangulated. That is just a hypothesis.

Schumpelick: If the surgeon and the tension of the knotting are really the risk factors, is there any device in the world available to measure it?

Carlson: That was actually done in one prospective study and it contradicts what I have been saying. There was a group in England that took a spring, put 5 kg of tension on each loop as they closed the wound, and found that their burst abdomen rate was lower in the wounds that had the tight closure than the loose closure. Unfortunately, they had a large number of wound infections in the patients that had a tight closure.

Schumpelick: A lot of surgeons are trained without this device. We do not know how to knot. We do it as best we can, but perhaps a lot of our incisional hernias, which are a late result of wound rupture, are caused by knotting in the wrong way. We do not have easily available devices to control our knotting strength. What about bed rest, coughing, weight-lifting, and all these things that are predominantly discussed by practitioners that the patient should avoid.

Carlson: You have to figure out when it is safe for patients to exert themselves, and therefore you have to know how quickly incisions are going to heal. There is a very wide variety from patient to patient. It may not even reflect what is the case in the animals, which is what a lot of these estimates are based on. But in the animals you reach a 50% point at about 4–6 weeks. That might be a safe point, but what exactly is a safe point, I really do not know. And I do not know how you really can determine it. To be safe, I would generally keep patients from exerting themselves for at least 2 months, and if they had a lot of risk factors it should be longer than that.

Kingsnorth: We are talking about acute wound failure. We have a clear distinction between later wound failure and acute wound failure, and I would completely agree with your conclusion about the incidence of acute wound failure being a surgeon-dependent variable. One additional point is the work of T.P.M. Jenkins. In his experimental studies, he found the figure 4. But he also looked at the figure 5. If you have too much suture material, you then begin to have failing wounds. You actually have to get it right. This highlights your point about pulling up the suture tight.

You did mention the spring balance man, who was actually a Pole. He did another very interesting study, in which he put clips along the wound edge in midline wounds. He then X-rayed the patients that day and at intervals up to 1 year. He found that his incidence of acute wound failure was also quite low. The late wound failures were the patients in which the clips separated on day 1. In other words, the surgeon is still an important factor.

Skandalakis: Do you use any gastrointestinal intubation postoperatively?

Carlson: Generally not. Not unless patients have a gastric distension or any reason to have gastrointestinal contents far back enough in the stomach.

References

1. Adamsons RJ, Musco F, Enquist IF: The chemical dimensions of a healing incision. Surg Gynecol Obstet 123:515, 1966
2. Adamsons RF, Kahan SA: The rate of healing of incised wounds of different tissues in rabbits. Surg Gynecol Obstet 130:837, 1970
3. Alexander HC, Prudden JF: The causes of abdominal wound disruption. Surg Gynecol Obstet 122:1223, 1966
4. Ausobsky JR, Evans M, Pollock AV: Does mass closure of midline laparotomies stand the test of time? A random control clinical trial. Ann Roy Coll Surg Engl 67:159, 1985
5. Bierens de Haan B, Ellis H, Wilks M: The role of infection on wound healing. Surg Gynecol Obstet 138:693, 1974
6. Botsford TW: The tensile strength of sutured skin wound during healing. Surg Gynecol Obstet 72:690, 1941
7. Bowen A: Postoperative wound disruption and evisceration: an analysis of thirty-four cases with a review of the literature. Am J Surg 47:3, 1940

8. Brolin RE: Prospective, randomized evaluation of midline fascial closure in gastric bariatric operations. Am J Surg 172:328, 1996
9. Bucknall TE: The effect of local infection upon wound healing: an experimental study. Br J Surg 67:851, 1980
10. Bucknall TE, Ellis H: Abdominal wound closure--A comparison of monofilament nylon and polyglycolic acid. Surgery 89:672, 1981
11. Cameron AEP, Gray RCF, Talbot RW et al.: Abdominal wound closure: a trial of Prolene and Dexon. Br J Surg 67:487, 1980
12. Carlson MA, Condon RE: Polyglyconate (Maxon) versus nylon suture in midline abdominal incision closure: a prospective randomized trial. Am Surg 61:980, 1995
13. Carlson MA: Acute Wound Failure. Surg Clin N Am 77:607, 1997
14. Colombo M, Maggioni A, Parma G et al.: A randomized comparision of continuous versus interrupted mass closure of midline incisions in patients with gynecologic cancer. Obstet Gynecol 89:684, 1997
15. Cox PJ, Ausobsky JR, Ellis H et al.: Towards no incisional hernias: lateral paramedian versus midline incisions. J Roy Soc Med 79:711, 1986
16. Del Junco T, Lange HJ: Abdominal wound disruption with eventration: report of forty cases. Am J Surg 92:271, 1956
17. Dinsmore RC: Understanding surgical knot security: a proposal to standardize the literature. J Am Coll Surg 180:689, 1995
18. Donaldson DR, Hegarty JH, Brennan TG et al.: The lateral paramedian incision--experience with 850 cases. Br J Surg 69:630, 1982
19. Douglas DM: The healing of aponeurotic incisions. Br J Surg 40:79, 1952
20. Drye JC: Intraperitoneal pressure in the human. Surg Gynecol Obstet 87:472, 1948
21. Ellis H, Coleridge-Smith PD, Joyce AD: Abdominal incisions--vertical or transverse? Postgrad Med J 60:407, 1984
22. Ellis H, Heddle R: Does the peritoneum need to be closed at laparotomy? Br J Surg 64:733, 1977
23. Fagniez PL, Hay JM, Lacaine F et al.: Abdominal midline incision closure: a multicentric randomized prospective trial of 3,135 patients, comparing continuous vs interrupted polyglycolic acid sutures. Arch Surg 120:1351, 1985
24. Fast J, Nelson C, Dennis C: Rate of gain in strength in sutured abdominal wall wounds. Surg Gynecol Obstet 84:685, 1947
25. Gallup DG, Nolan TE, Smith RP: Primary mass closure of midline incisions with a continuous polyglyconate monofilament absorbable suture. Obstet Gynecol 76:872, 1990
26. Gislason H, Gronbech JE, Soreide O: Burst abdomen and incisional hernia after major gastrointestinal operations--comparison of three closure techniques. Eur J Surg 161:349, 1995
27. Greenall MJ, Evans M, Pollock AV: Midline or transverse laparotomy? A random controlled clinical trial. Part I: influence on healing. Br J Surg 67:188, 1980
28. Greenburg AG, Saik RP, Peskin GW: Wound dehiscence: pathophysiology and prevention. Arch Surg 114:143, 1979
29. Halasz NA: Dehiscence of laparotomy wounds. Am J Surg 116:210, 1968
30. Hampton JR: The burst abdomen. Br Med J 2:1032, 1963
31. Haxton H: The influence of suture materials and methods on the healing of abdominal wounds. Br J Surg 52:372, 1965
32. Haxton HA: Intra-abdominal and intrauterine pressures (letter). Br Med J 1:856, 1948
33. Hinshaw DB, Hughes LD, Stafford CE: Effects of cortisone on the healing of disrupted abdominal wounds Am J Surg 101:189, 1961
34. Hubbard TB Jr, Rever WB Jr: Retention sutures in the closure of abdominal incisions. Am J Surg 124:378, 1972
35. Hugh TB, Nankivell C, Meagher AP et al.: Is closure of the peritoneal layer necessary in the repair of midline surgical abdominal wounds? World J Surg 14:231, 1990
36. Israelsson LA, Jonsson T: Suture length to wound length ratio and healing of midline laparotomy incisions. Br J Surg 80:1284, 1993
37 Israelsson LA, Jonsson T: Closure of midline laparotomy incisions with polydioxanone and nylon: the importance of suture technique. Br J Surg 81:1606, 1994
38. Israelsson LA, Jonsson T, Knutsson A: Suture technique and wound healing in midline laparotomy incisions. Eur J Surg 162:605, 1996
39. Israelsson LA, Jonsson T: Overweight and healing of midline incisions: the importance of suture technique. Eur J Surg 163:175, 1997
40. Jenkins TPN: The burst abdominal wound: a mechanical approach. Br J Surg 63:873, 1976
41. Keill RH, Keitzer WF, Nichols WK et al.: Abdominal wound dehiscence. Arch Surg 106:573, 1973
42. Kennedy JW: Tragedies of the abdominal incision. Am J Surg 25:512, 1934

43. Kimberly RC, Coxe WS, Koontz AR: Abdominal wound disruption. Trans South Surg Assn 74:300, 1962
44. Krukowski ZH, Cusick EL, Engeset J et al.: Polydioxanone or polypropylene for closure of midline abdominal incisions: a prospective comparative clinical trial. Br J Surg 74:828, 1987
45. Leaper DJ: Angiography as an index of healing in experimental laparotomy wounds and colonic anastomoses. Ann Roy Coll Surg Engl 65:20, 1983
46. Lewis RT, Wiegand FM: Natural history of vertical abdominal parietal closure: Prolene versus Dexon. Can J Surg 32:196, 1989
47. Lichtenstein IL, Herzikoff S, Shore JM et al: The dynamics of wound healing. Surg Gynecol Obstet 130:685, 1970
48. Lythgoe JP: Burst abdomen. Postgrad Med J 36:388, 1960
49. Martyak SN, Curtis LE: Abdominal incision and closure: a systems approach. Am J Surg 131:476, 1976
50. Miro D, Julia MV, Sitges-Serra A: Wound breaking strength and healing after suturing noninjured tissues. J Am Coll Surg 180:659, 1995
51. Nelson CA, Dennis C: Wound healing: technical factors in the gain of strength in sutured abdominal wall wounds in rabbits. Surg Gynecol Obstet 93:461, 1951
52. Niggebrugge AHP, Hansen BE, Trimbos JB et al.: Mechanical factors influencing the incidence of burst abdomen. Eur J Surg 161:655, 1995
53. Poole GV Jr, Meredith JW, Kon ND et al.: Suture technique and wound-bursting strength. Am Surg 50:569, 1984
54. Poole GV Jr: Mechanical factors in abdominal wound closure: the prevention of fascial dehiscence. Surgery 97:631, 1985
55. Rappaport WD, Hunter GC, Allen R et al.: Effect of electrocautery on wound healing in midline laparotomy incisions. Am J Surg 160:618, 1990
56. Sandblom P: The tensile strength of healing wounds: an experimental study. Acta Chir Scand 90 (Suppl 89):1, 1944
57. Sanders RJ, DiClementi D, Ireland K: Principles of abdominal wound closure: I. Animal studies. Arch Surg 112:1184, 1977
58. Sanders RJ, DiClementi D: Principles of abdominal wound closure: II. Prevention of wound dehiscence. Arch Surg 112:1188, 1977
59. Savlov ED, Dunphy JE: The healing of the disrupted and resutured wound. Surgery 36:362, 1954
60. Seid MH, McDaniel-Owens M, Poole GV Jr et al.: A randomized trial of abdominal incision suture technique and wound strength in rats. Arch Surg 130:394, 1995
61. Singleton AO, Blocker TG Jr: The problem of disruption of abdominal wounds and postoperative hernia. JAMA 112:122, 1939
62. Sisson R, Lang S, Serkes K et al.: Comparison of wound healing in various nutritional deficiency states. Surgery 44:613, 1958
63. Smith M, Enquist IF: A quantitative study of impaired healing resulting from infection. Surg Gynecol Obstet 125:965, 1967
64. Standeven A: Rupture of laparotomy wounds. Lancet 1:533, 1955
65. Tenorio A, Jindrak K, Weiner M et al.: Accelerated healing in infected wounds. Surg Gynecol Obstet 142:537, 1976
66. Tera H, Aberg C: The strength of suture knots after one week in vivo. Acta Chir Scand 142:301, 1976
67. Tera H, Aberg C: Tensile strengths of twelve types of knot employed in surgery, using different suture materials. Acta Chir Scand 142:1, 1976
68. Tera H, Aberg C: Tissue strength of structures involved in musculo-aponeurotic layer sutures in laparotomy incisions. Acta Chir Scand 142:349, 1976
69. Tera H, Aberg C: Strength of knots in surgery in relation to type of knot, type of suture material and dimension of suture thread. Acta Chir Scand 143:75, 1977
70. Wissing J, van Vroonhoven TJMV, Schattenkerk ME et al.: Fascia closure after midline laparotomy: results of a randomized trial. Br J Surg 74:738, 1987

CHAPTER 9

Natural History and Patient-Related Factors

W. Hartel, H.P. Becker

9.1 Introduction

In studies with sufficient follow-up evaluation, the incidence of primary incisional hernia is about 11% of laparotomies [4, 12]. Documented recurrence rates after repair range from 30% to 49% [1, 6, 7, 16, 19]. The present article analyzes the natural history and the patient-related risk factors for developing an incisional hernia of the abdominal wall.

9.2 Natural History of Wound Healing

Any factor which impairs normal wound healing may contribute to the development of incisional hernias. Normal wound healing is divided into several phases. Consequently, different pathological mechanisms disturbing the tissue reparation can be discussed.

The exudative phase (days 1–3) is characterized by hemostasis, aggregation of thrombocytes, and release of fibrin. Tissue defects are filled by coagulated blood and fibronectin. Any tension on the tissue leads to early disruption and destabilization of the fibronectin network. Exudation begins again, and deshiscence of the wound edges is promoted.

The resorptive phase (days 4–7) is characterized by degradation of blood products and fibrin. It comprises the immigration of neutrophil granulocytes and fibroblasts. Thereafter, capillary multiplication begins granulation and synthesis of collagen.

In the phase of reparation (days 8–12), new fibers of collagen are produced by fibroblasts. This phase is often affected by drugs (Fig. 1).

The transformation of the granulation tissue into a scar takes a long time (a period of months). It includes the decrease of capillaries, the resorption of exudate, and the definitive contraction of collagen fibers. The collagen network is responsible for the stability of the scar.

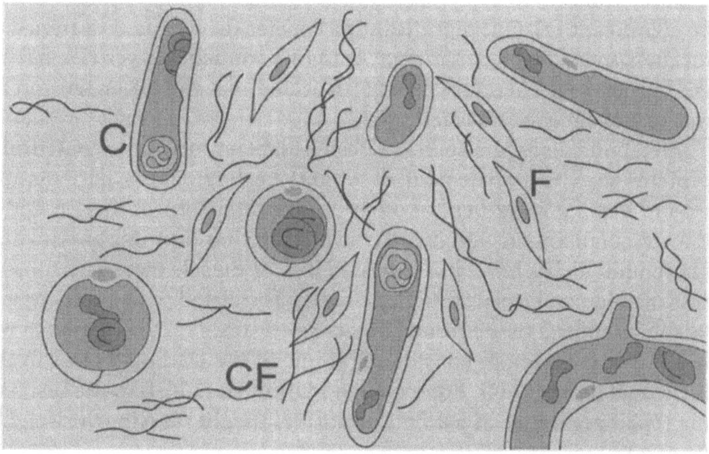

Fig. 1. Reparative phase of wound healing with synthesis of collagen fibers. Possible interference with various drugs. C, capillary with erythrocyte; *CF*, collagen fiber; F, fibroblast. (Modified from [3])

9.3 Wound Infection

Postoperative wound infection after primary surgery is probably the most important event contributing to the development of incisional hernia. Several authors have been able to implicate wound infection as a significant risk factor [2, 4, 6, 11, 13, 19]. Houck et al. found that a proven wound infection from the previous operation was the strongest predictor for the development of reinfection [9]. The repair of incisional hernias has a significantly higher risk of infection than do other clean surgical procedures [9]. Hesselink et al. showed an increase in recurrence rate after the repair of incisional hernias with wound infection, but this was not significant because the number of cases was too small in this study [7].

9.4 Patient-Related Risk Factors

Several patient-related factors may predispose to the development of incisional hernias. Tissue perfusion is the ultimate determinant of wound oxygenation and nutrition. Sufficient blood supply is essential for normal wound healing. The activity and growth of the fibroblasts depend on a partial oxygen pressure of at least 15 mmHg. Therefore, arteriosclerosis and diabetes mellitus, with their reduced blood supply, predispose to prolonged wound healing in old age. Hesselink et al. did not find age to be of significance [7]. Gender was not significant either, but it was found that 50% of the incisional hernias in females derived from gynecological and obstetrical operations [7].

In the study carried out by Hesselink et al., obesity, diabetes mellitus, and lower midline incision led to a higher recurrence rate, but these factors were not shown to be significant [7]. One significant parameter for hernia recurrence was the size of the incision. Incisional hernias smaller than 4 cm had a lower risk of recurrence than larger hernias [7]. Therefore, it was suspected that the lower tension in smaller wounds was responsible for this fact.

Metabolic disorders such as obesity, diabetes mellitus, renal insufficiency, or lack of proteins lead to impairment of wound healing. Obese patients often have difficult wound healing regardless of other risk factors. Poor perfusion and necrotic debris in the subcutaneous tissue usually favor infection and impaired wound healing. Many obese individuals have an associated loss of muscle mass and tone and therefore possess inadequate fascial strength. Obesity associated with a fatty omentum and excessive subcutaneous tissue results in increased strain on the operative wound during early healing. It is therefore considered as one of the leading factors in the development of incisional hernias [15]. According to Manninen et al. [11], the results of incisional hernia repair are better in patients of normal weight than in overweight individuals (88% vs. 61%).

Diabetes mellitus makes glucose unavailable for normal cell metabolism and leads to a decrease in amino acids and proteins. Secondarily, fibroblasts and leukocytes become dysfunctional because of the lack of glucose to meet their energy requirements. Finally, hyperglycemia interferes with ascorbate transfer, which is important for the synthesis of collagen [15]. Any hepatopathy predisposes to incisional hernias because of ascites, decreased albumin level, and insufficient formation of coagulation factors.

Renal insufficiency is characterized by hemorrhagic diathesis, renal anemia, toxic damage of thrombocytes, and hypoproteinemia. All these risk factors interfere with normal wound healing. In patients with vitamin C deficiency, wound healing is arrested during the proliferative phase. With vitamin C lacking, the enzymes responsible for the hydroxylation of the amino acids are not activated. Thus the synthesis of collagen cannot be completed. Further negative factors affecting wound healing include granulocytopenia and congenital defects of leukocyte chemotaxis and phagocytosis.

9.5 Increased Intra-abdominal Pressure

According to Klinge et al., intra-abdominal pressure varies from 0.2 kPa at rest to up to 20 kPa while standing [10]. Increased intra-abdominal pressure and tension on the suture line seems to be important for the development of wound deshiscence. Permanent traction on the adapted wound edges and instability of the wound destroy the early fibrin network. In an experimental study, Högström et al. demonstrated that tension on the wound margins led to increased neutrophil accumulation and decreased laparotomy wound strength [8]. The tensile strength and energy-to-failure studies carried out by Stone et al. showed loosely approximated wounds to be far stronger, because they had proper alignment of the wound edges and greater proliferative activity in the clefts [17] (Fig. 2). It was suspected that the quality of the collagen network was reduced in tight suture lines.

In two clinical studies, the majority of patients with burst abdomen had postoperative distention, coughing, retching, and vomiting [14, 18]. Chevrel found that burst

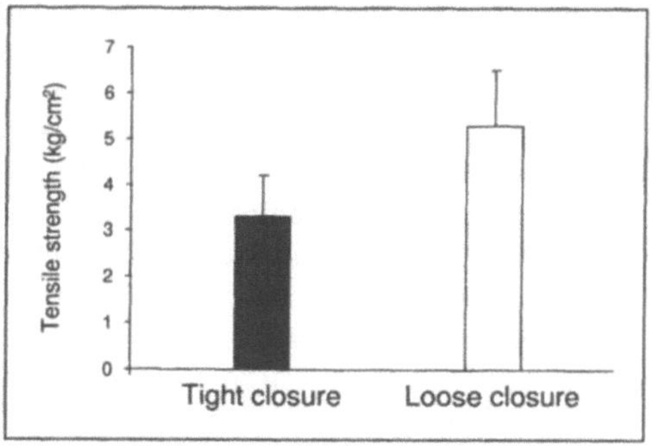

Fig. 2. Tensile strength of loosely and tightly approximated wounds. (Modified from [17])

abdomen was often the origin of an incisional hernia [5]. It occurred in 40% after emergency surgery associated with increased intra-abdominal pressure or with chronic protein depletion. Although chronic cough, constipation, prostatism, and postoperative bowel distention had no significance on the incidence in the study carried out by Hesselink [7], it can be assumed that postoperative intra-abdominal pressure plays an important role in the genesis of incisional hernia.

Postoperative disorders with increased intra-abdominal pressure include respiratory failure and bowel distention by gas and fluid, which may have negative effects on the blood supply of the bowel wall, transition time, and defecation. The bacterial contamination of the peritoneal cavity by anastomosis leakage or perforation of the gastrointestinal tract predisposes to incisional hernias. Splenomegaly may lead to anemia, leukopenia, and thrombopenia with wound healing interference.

9.6 Drugs

Certain medications have been demonstrated to lead to poor wound healing, especially when given in the first 3 days after surgery (Table 1). Steroids and chemotherapeutic

Table 1. Effects of drugs on wound healing

Medication	Phase	Mechanisms
Antacids	Exudation, reparation	Inhibition of vitamin C resorption, impairment of collagen synthesis
Antihistamines	Reparation	Inhibition of histamine effect
Anticoagulants	Exudation	Activation of antithrombin and plasmin, breakdown of fibrin network
Glucocorticosteroids	Exudation, reparation	Suppression of fibroblasts and formation of collagen
Immunosuppressants	Exudation, reparation	Suppression of hematopoietic system and of fibroblasts
Platelet aggregation inhibitors	Exudation	Inhibition of platelet aggregation, disturbance of coagulation
Vitamin K antagonists	Exudation	Disturbance of coagulation
Zytostatic agents	Exudation, reparation	Slowing of wound healing by suppression of dividing cells

agents are two of the more commonly used drug regimen that have been implicated in the development of incisional hernias [15]. Most of the drugs shown in Table 1 may blunt normal inflammatory responses and impair the usual healing process. Both radiation and chemotherapy have their greatest effects on dividing cells such as endothelial cells, fibroblasts, and keratinocytes.

The present article demonstrates that there are relevant patient-related risk factors for the development of an incisional hernia in abdominal surgery. Consequently, these permanent risk factors have to be taken into careful consideration by the surgeon during the primary closure of incisions. The timing of the surgical repair of an incisional hernia must be determined individually. Whenever possible, the repair should be carried out when the patient's underlying medical condition has stabilized, the nutritional status has been optimized, and no further contraindications impair the success of surgery.

9.7 Discussion

Schumpelick: I have a question on the natural course of incisional hernias. When do they start, and does their volume increase, or does it stop increasing over time?

Hartel: Incisional hernias very often develop after 1–2 years. Most of them develop in the first year, but some may appear after 1–2 years. If you examine long enough, you will find incisional hernias in up to 10% or 11%. The figure usually quoted in the literature is about 2%–5%.

Kingsnorth: There are two very good longitudinal studies by Ellis and Hughes, one from London and the other from Cardiff, which illustrate that point. You can examine large numbers of patients 1 year after their incision has been closed and find a perfectly intact wound. If you then examine them at 5 years, you will find a lot of incisional hernias. The hernias that occur up to about 5 years double the incidence. In other words, half of all incisional hernias will be found before 1 year, and these are probably technical failures, and after 1–5 years the other half occur, and these are probably due to defects in the wound. The collagen tissue gives way for some reason. I am sure that this is an area in which improved wound healing substances, tissues, or biomaterials can be targeted. It is something that surgeons cannot tackle alone with only their suture techniques.

Hartel: The publication by Ellis is entitled *Incisional Hernias;* when do they occur?

Devlin: I was going to make the same point that Dr. Kingsnorth made, particularly looking at the work of Hughes and Mudge in Cardiff, where they followed the patients for 20 years and found an increasing incidence of incisional hernia. So it happens later on in the healing of the wound.

Simmermacher: Returning to the natural history, how many incisional hernias are diagnosed later. How many people walk around with an incisional hernia after 5 years and never present to a physician? How many incisional hernias cause pain to patients, and how many should be operated upon due to problems later? What is the natural history of that?

Hartel: That is what we do not know. A few patients probably hesitate to go to a surgeon so as not to be operated on again, and that might be the next topic: Diagnosis of incisional hernia may show us how to detect them. I am sure that many patients are not willing to see a doctor or to have an operation unless they are in pain.

Read: With regard to fairly late herniation, Dr. Hughes indicated in his presentation that most of these cases were fairly small. What interested me is the paper by Krukowski and Matheson, who presented their work on paramedian herniation, buttonhole herniation, in 1987. In the two cases that they wrote their original paper on, it was also late. We have seen some of these buttonhole herniations earlier as well.

Devlin: If you examine a whole lot of incisions with ultrasound, you find quite a lot of these buttonhole hernias perhaps 6 months to 1 year after the operation. They have been closed with thick, nonabsorbable material such as thick polypropylene or thick nylon, but whether they cause symptoms I do not know. The paper by Krukowski concerned symptomatic hernias.

Hartel: I think that is right. I do remember patients in whom we did a reoperation and found a small incisional hernia without the patient knowing about it beforehand.

Schumpelick: We all agree that, in acute wound failure, the surgeon is the most predominant risk factor. How big is the responsibility of the surgeon in incisional hernia? Is it less than 10%? Is it more than 80%? Can it be calculated? Some say it is only the surgeon.

Hartel: I would suppose that the surgeon can be a risk factor too, especially if he or she is not experienced. About 20%–25% may be caused by technique.

Simmermacher: I disagree with your opinion that an inexperienced surgeon is a greater danger to the patient than an experienced one to some extent. Several studies have been done on different topics in surgery, indicating that, when you are doing your first operation or when residents do their first operations, they are very keen to do it very well. They are dangerous when they think that they are experienced. The greatest problems therefore develop when they think that they are good surgeons, which is after some experience. It is not only residents at the start of their career, but mainly those who think that they are already surgeons.

Hartel: I am aware of these papers, but we have to ask the following question: What was the grade of difficulty in each case? You cannot compare the cases. A doctor who deals with the worst cases might have more recurrences. But in my experience, in the last 5 years before my retirement, I had very few complications. My learning curve always rose throughout my whole life.

Bendavid: I would like to come back to importance of the surgeon's ability. I am getting to find hernias now associated with mesh and prosthetic materials. Mesh is usually inserted 5–6 cm beyond the main defect. It is supposed to protrude into good area and no one finds herniation lateral to the mesh itself. I doubt whether the surgeon's ability is really a factor here, and it cannot be explained logically.

Read: The surgeon should have put it 10 cm away. That might be the surgeon's task. If we use a bigger mesh, it might not have happened.

Skandalakis: What has happened to the gastrostomy that we did in the past? What about the Prostigmin (neostigmine) injection that we gave for better intestinal peristaltics? What about the rectal tube, which we sometimes put it in just above our anastomosis?

Hartel: I am sure that it helps to decrease intra-abdominal pressure and that might help to avoid an incisional hernia.

References

1. Amgwerd M, Decurtins M, Largiadèr F (1992) Die Narbenhernie – Prädisposition oder insuffiziente Nahttechnik. Helv Chir Acta 59: 345–349
2. Blomstedt B, Welin-Berger T (1972) Incisional hernias. Acta Chir Scand 138: 275–278
3. Böcker W, Denk H, Heitz PU (1997) Pathologie. Urban & Schwarzenberg, Munich, Vienna, Baltimore
4. Bucknall TE, Cox PJ, Ellis H (1982) Burst abdomen and incisional hernia. BMJ 284: 931–934
5. Chevrel JP (1997) Hernias and surgery of the abdominal wall. Springer, Berlin Heidelberg New York, 1997
6. George CD, Ellis H (1986) The results of incisional hernia repair: a twelve-year review. Ann R Coll Surg Engl 68: 185–187
7. Hesselink VJ, Luijendijk RW, DeWilt JHW, Heide R, J. J (1993) An evaluation of risk factors in incisional hernia recurrence. Surg Gynecol Obstet 176: 228–234
8. Högström H, Haglund U, Zederfeldt B (1990) Tension leads to increased neutrophil accumulation and decreased laparotomy wound strength. Surgery 107: 215–219
9. Houck JP, Rypins EB, Sarfreh J, Juler GL, Shimoda KJ (1989) Repair of incisional hernia. Surg Gynecol Obstet 169: 397–399
10. Klinge U, Conze Z, Limberg W, Brücker C, Öttinger AP, Schumpelick V (1996) Pathophysiologie der Bauchdecken. Chirurg 67: 229–233
11. Manninen MJ, Lavonius M, Perhoniemi VJ (1990) Results of incisional hernia repair: A retrospective study of 172 unselected hernioplasties. Eur J Surg 157: 29–31
12. Mudge M, Hughes LE (1985) Incisional hernia: a 10 year prospective study of incidence and attitudes. Br J Surg 72: 70–71
13. Pollock AV, Evans M (1989) Early prediction of incisional hernia. Br J Surg 76: 953–954
14. Reitamo J, Möller G (1972) Abdominal wound deshiscence. Acta Chir Scand 138: 170–175
15. Sabiston DC (1997) Textbook of surgery. W.B. Saunders, Philadelphia 1997
16. Schumpelick V, Arlt G, Klinge U (1997) Versorgung von Nabelhernie und Narbenhernie. Dt Ärztebl 94: A-3471–3476
17. Stone IK, Fraunhofer JA, Masterson BJ (1986) The biomechanical effects of tight suture closure upon fascia. Surg Gynecol Obstet 163: 448–452
18. Tweedie FJ, Long RC (1954) Abdominal wound disruption. Surg Gynecol Obstet 99: 41–47
19. vanderLinden F, vanVroonhoven TJ (1988) Long-term results after surgical correction of incisional hernia. Neth J Surg 40: 127–129

CHAPTER 10

Diagnosis of Abdominal Wall Defects

S.N. Truong, M. Müller

In general, pathological findings of the abdominal wall and inguinal region are easily accessible due to their superficial location. In most cases, the correct diagnosis can be reached on the basis of history, symptoms and clinical examination. Although ultrasound investigations are part of our standard routine and in the majority of our patients merely confirm the clinical findings, there are, however, two groups of patients whose complaints are difficult to classify:

- Patients, especially obese people, with palpable masses within deep layers of the abdominal wall
- Patients with pain and complaints located within the abdominal wall or the inguinal region but without any causative clinical findings

For these patients, various diagnostic tools can be used to help us to detect pathology and to treat them adequately. In most cases, ultrasound is the method of choice, but in some cases computed tomography (CT) or magnetic resonance imaging (MRI) may be helpful.

Diagnostic procedures for pathology of the abdominal wall include the following:

- Anamnesis (clinical history)
- Clinical examination
- Sonography
- CT
- MRI
- Herniography

10.1 Sonography

For sonographic examination of the abdominal wall or inguinal region, real-time ultrasound equipment with a 7.5-MHz linear scanner is preferable. Vessels are verified by a colour coded duplex scan.

Sonography is performed with the patient in a supine and standing position. The examination is carried out in two planes, vertical and horizontal. Dynamic studies while the patient performs the Vasalva manoeuvre, coughing or straining are useful.

10.1.1
Sonographic Anatomy of the Abdominal Wall

Although the echographic representation of the anatomy of the abdominal wall and inguinal region is highly variable, depending on the amount of fatty tissue and muscle, there are typical sonographic structures that should be identified in all patients (Figs. 1, 2).

The epidermis and dermis are represented by a superficial homogenous echoic layer. Underlying subcutaneous fatty tissue varies considerably between thin and obese patients. It is generally a hypoechoic and heterogeneous layer above the muscles of the abdominal wall muscles.

Two kinds of abdominal wall muscles can be identified, the rectus muscle at both sides of the midline and the three flat lateral abdominal muscles. The longitudinally running rectus muscle appears as a hypoechoic and homogenous structure with fine internal, parallel lines of greater echo reflection. It is enveloped by the rectus sheath as a surrounding echogenic line. The anterior lamina of the rectus sheath is formed by fibres of the oblique muscles, while the posterior lamina derives from the aponeurosis of the transverse muscle. In the midline, both rectus sheathes unite to form a thick echogenic aponeurotic layer, the linea alba, extending from the xiphoid to the symphysis pubis.

Below the arcuate line, the semilunar line can be identified; this is the boundary between the body of the rectus muscles and the transverse aponeurosis. This zone is of special interest because it represents a weak area, and the rare spigelian hernia can occur here.

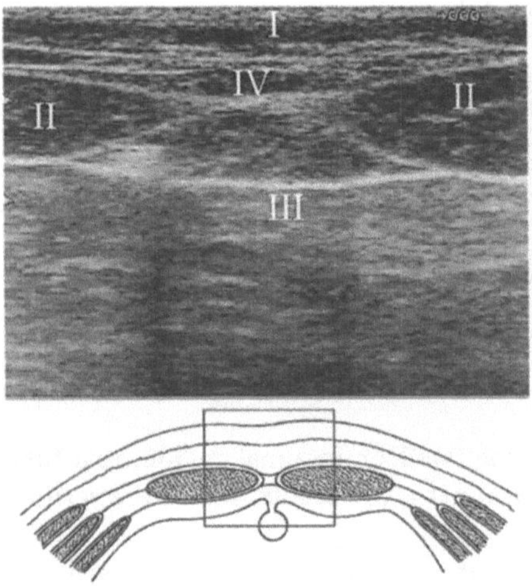

Fig. 1. Normal sonographic anatomy of the abdominal wall above the umbilicus in the midline. *I*, subcutaneous fat; *II*, rectus muscle; *III*, peritoneum; *IV*, linea alba

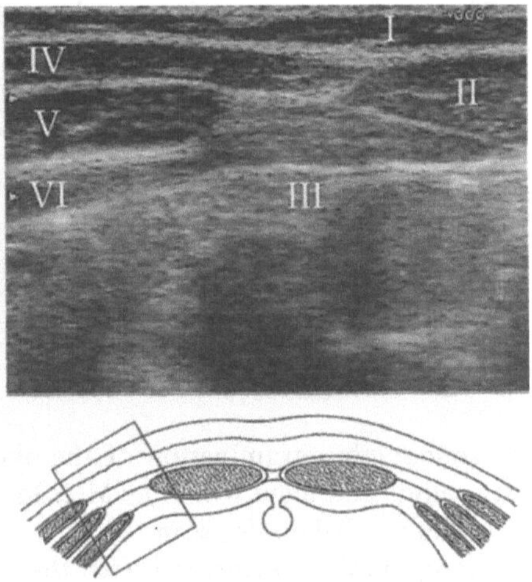

Fig. 2. Normal sonographic anatomy of the abdominal wall above the umbilicus between rectus muscle and lateral abdominal muscles. *I*, subcutaneous fat; *II*, rectus muscle; *III*, peritoneum; *IV*, oblique external muscle; *V*, oblique internal muscle; *VI*, transverse muscle

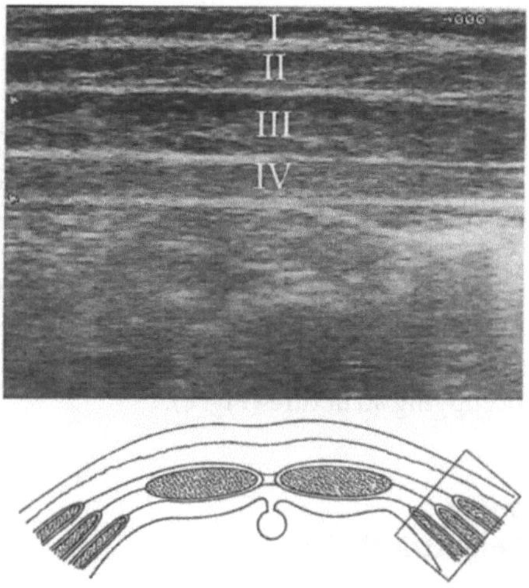

Fig. 3. Normal sonographic anatomy of the abdominal wall above the umbilicus above the lateral abdominal muscles. *I*, subcutaneous fat; *II*, oblique external muscle; *III*, oblique internal muscle; *IV*, transverse muscle

The three flat abdominal muscles in the flanks – the oblique external, oblique internal and transverse muscles – can be distinguished as three different layers, separated by their thin, highly echogenic aponeuroses (Fig. 3). In the inguinal region, the oblique external muscle disappears and only its aponeurosis can be identified above the oblique internal muscle.

The very thin echogenic line of the peritoneum separates the abdominal wall from the abdominal viscera. It is sometimes difficult to identify this line as a single layer beneath the muscles, especially in young, athletic patients. In obese patients, a hypoechoic heterogeneous zone can often be found between the muscle layers and peritoneum, representing aureolar preperitoneal fat tissue.

10.1.2 Sonographic Differential Diagnosis of Pathological Findings

Pre- and postoperative sonographic investigations help us to identify surgical diseases of the abdominal wall and inguinal region. Indications are mainly obesity and complaints without clinical findings in preoperative and postoperative investigations for fluid collection.

10.1.3 Preoperative Investigations

Diagnosis of hernia and differential diagnosis are important to lead the surgeon to the correct surgical treatment. It is therefore important to know the sonographic criteria and patterns of the different types of hernia as well as other undetermined palpable masses of the abdominal wall.

10.2 Sonographic Criteria for Hernias

The sonographic image of a hernia is a fascial gap with protruding hernial contents. The hernial sac or hernial contents should be reducible into the peritoneal cavity. The hernial sac should generally reveal an increase in size or a change of location when the patient coughs or presses. In minor hernias, only a small fascial gap or a hillock is found during dynamic examination. In addition, the hernial contents can be identified by sonography. Intestinal structures are characterized by peristaltic movements and air bubbles, while the omentum appears as a stationary, highly reflective, space-occupying structure (Fig. 4).

10.2.1 Epigastric Hernia

For diagnosis of epigastric hernias, the transducer is placed in the epigastric region over the linea alba. The reference structures are the rectus sheath and the linea alba , and the hernia is visualised by a characteristic midline fascial defect (Fig. 5).

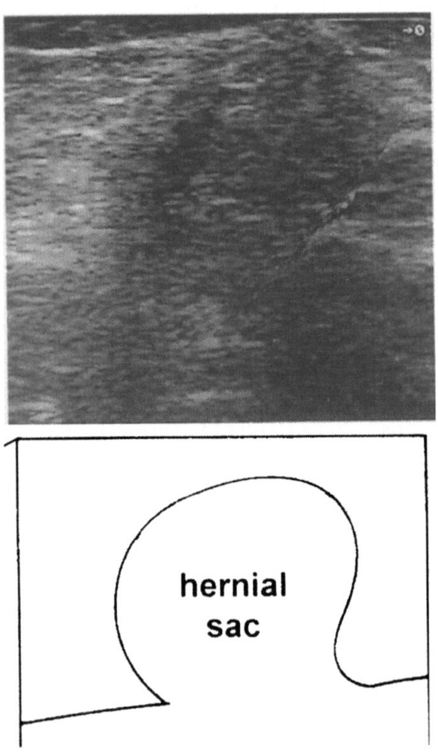

Fig. 4. Typical sonographic findings of an umbilical hernia

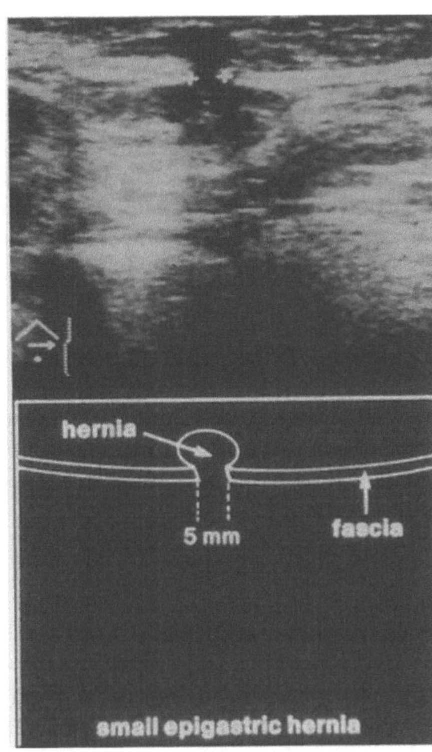

Fig. 5. Typical sonographic findings of a small epigastric hernia

10.2.2
Inguinal Hernia

Inguinal hernias are found by placing the transducer over the inguinal ligament. The reference structures are the rectus sheath medially and the internal oblique and transverse abdominal muscle laterally. Epigastric vessels are identified by a colour coded duplex scan. Although it is difficult to distinguish between direct and indirect hernia, the location of the epigastric vessels might be of help; thus direct hernias lie medial and indirect hernias lateral to the epigastric vessels (Fig. 6).

10.2.3
Femoral Hernia

For femoral hernias, the transducer is placed caudal to the inguinal ligament over the oval fossa. The reference structures are the femoral artery with a constantly filled and pulsating lumen laterally and the femoral vein with a variable volume medial to the artery; this vein expands during the Vasalva manoeuvre. Between these vessels and the symphysis pubis, femoral hernias demonstrate a low-echo area that bulges caudally during pressing or coughing (Fig. 7).

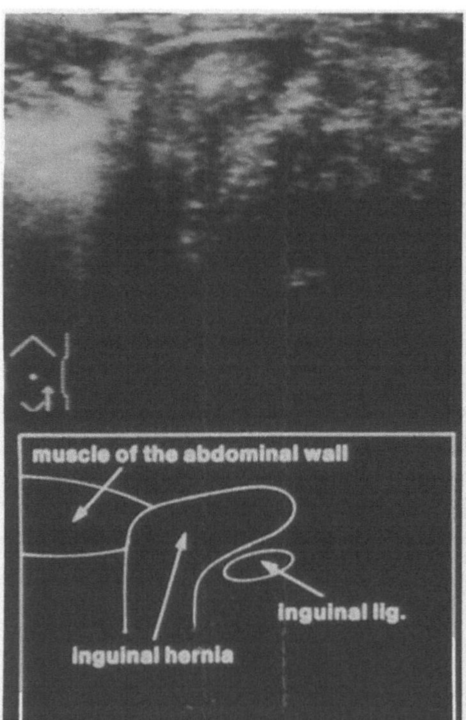

Fig. 6. Typical sonographic findings of an inguinal hernia

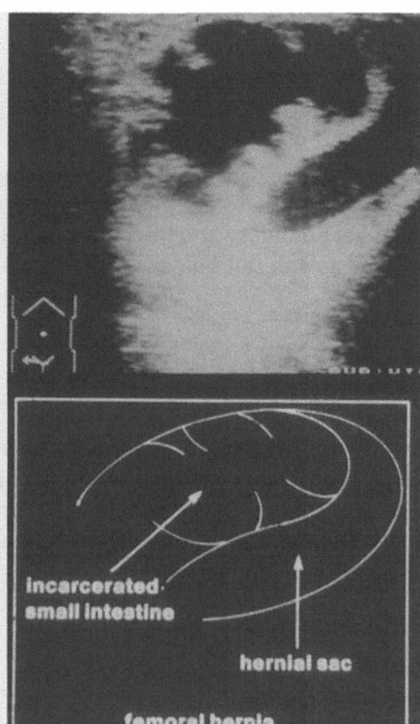

Fig. 7. Sonographic findings of a incarcerated femoral hernia with dilated small bowels

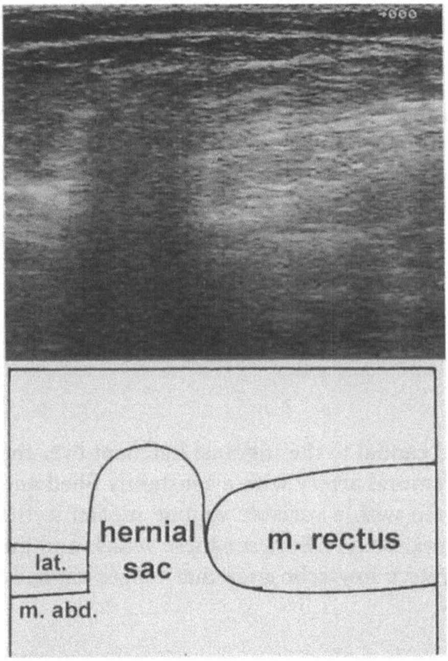

Fig. 8. Typical sonographic findings of a spigelian hernia

10.2.4
Spigelian Hernia

A spigelian hernia is identified by placing the transducer over the semilunar line. The reference structures are the semilunar line, with the lateral abdominal wall muscles as its lateral boundary and the rectus muscle as its medial boundary. A defect in the outline and an anterior bulging of the rectus margin confirms the hernia (Fig. 8).

10.2.5
Lumbar Hernia

For lumbar hernias, the transducer is placed over the lumbar and costolumbar triangle. The reference structures are the iliac crest caudally and the inferior costal arch cranially. A hernial orifice below the latissimus dorsi plane is evident to a superior lumbar hernia. Lateral bulging at the lower insertion of the latissimus muscle indicates an inferior lumbar hernia.

10.2.6
Incisional Hernia

Incisional hernias can occur at nearly any point in the abdominal wall following surgery. They show the typical hernial pattern with a fascial gap and protruding hernial

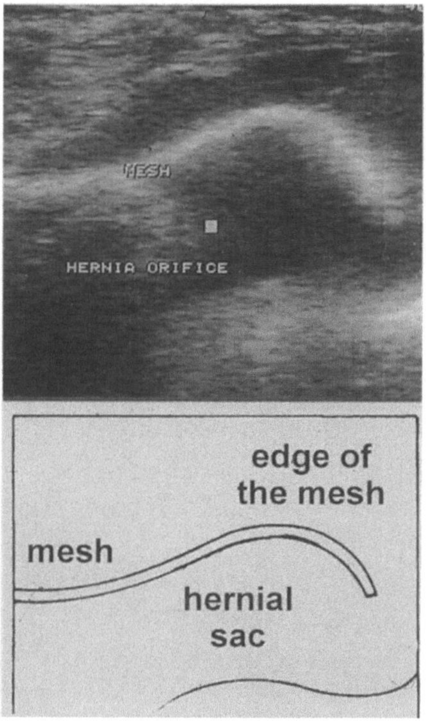

Fig. 9. Sonographic findings of a recurrent incisional hernia at the edge of the mesh

sac. In addition, after mesh repair for hernia, a recurrence can occur at the edge of the mesh (Fig. 9).

10.2.7
Umbilical Hernia

Umbilical hernias occur at the umbilicus due to a persistent omphalenteric duct. The transducer is placed over the umbilicus, and the sonographic image shows the fascial gap and the protruding hernial sac (Fig. 4).

10.3
Further Anomalies

10.3.1
Metastasis

Metastases present sonographically as homogenous, solid, space-occupying structures with plump or polycyclic outlines. Processes in the abdominal wall that are close to the peritoneum can be distinguished from intra-abdominal tumours by observing them during inspiration and expiration (Figs. 10, 11).

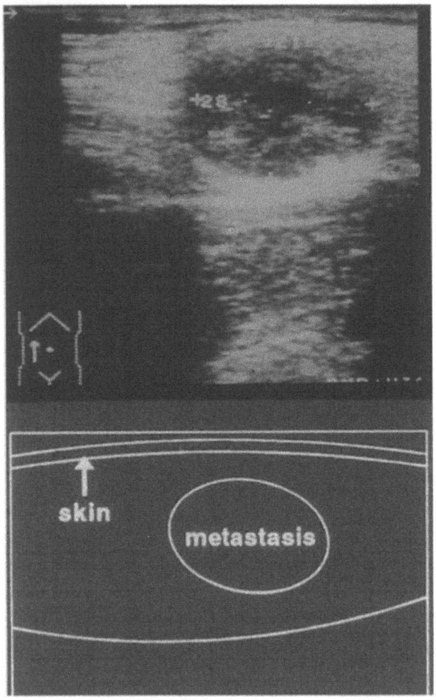

Fig. 10. Sonographic findings of a metastasis within the abdominal wall

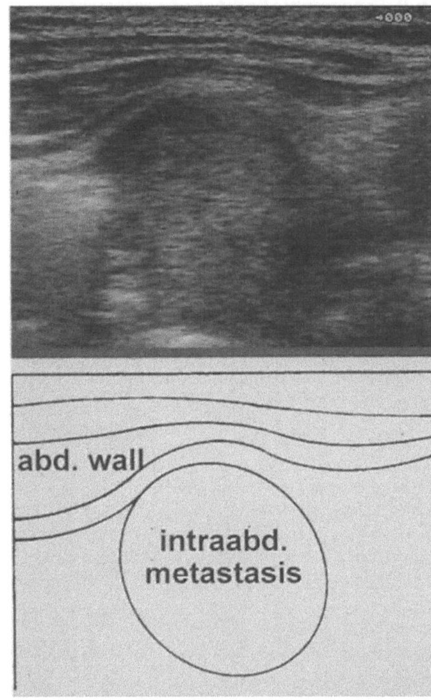

Fig. 11. Sonographic findings of an intra-abdominal metastasis without infiltration of the abdominal wall. In real-time ultrasound, visceral slide can be observed

10.3.2 Lipoma

Lipomas present as hypoechoic structures, often with a sharp margin and constant location during dynamic examination (Fig. 12).

10.3.3 Lymphoma

Lymphomas are located along the anatomical lymphatic drainage routes. They are homogenous hypoechoic or central hyperechoic space-occupying structures. Lymphomas do not show any connection to deeper structures or the peritoneal cavity. During dynamic examination, they remain constant (Fig. 13).

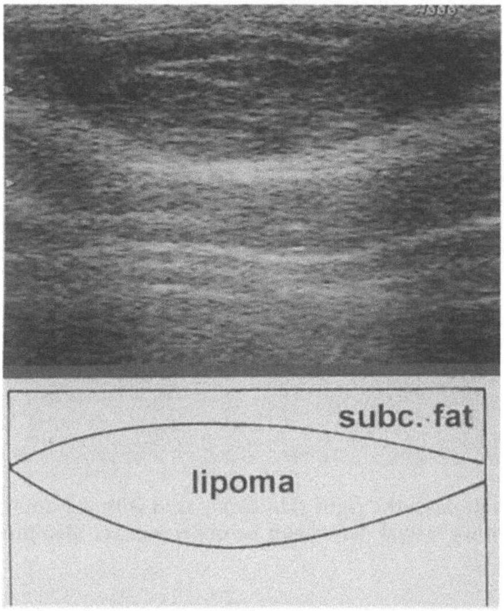

Fig. 12. Typical sonographic findings of a subcutaneous lipoma

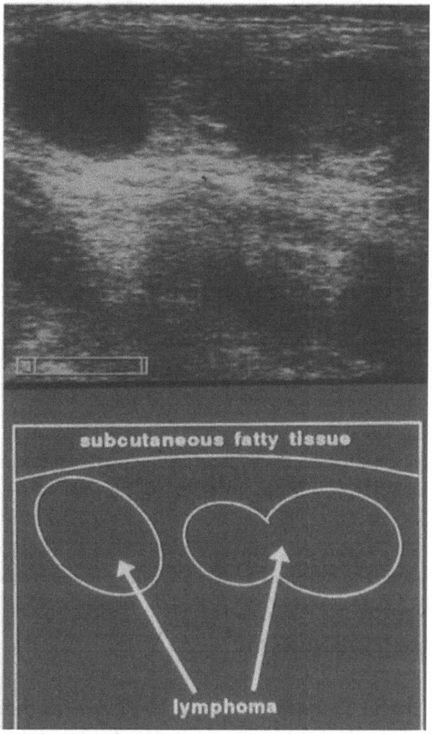

Fig. 13. Typical sonographic findings of a lymphoma

10.3.4 Endometriosis

Endometriosis shows a hypoechoic structure with irregular margins. The sonographic findings are accompanied by a typical history of complaints and pain during menstruation.

10.3.5 Abdominal Wall Relaxation

Abdominal wall relaxation following surgery, mainly after retroperitoneal approaches to the kidney [1], can clinically mimic an incisional hernia. Sonographically, there is no discontinuity of the aponeurosis or fascial gap. All muscle layers of the abdominal wall may be present, but they appear thinner in comparison with the unaffected side (Fig. 14).

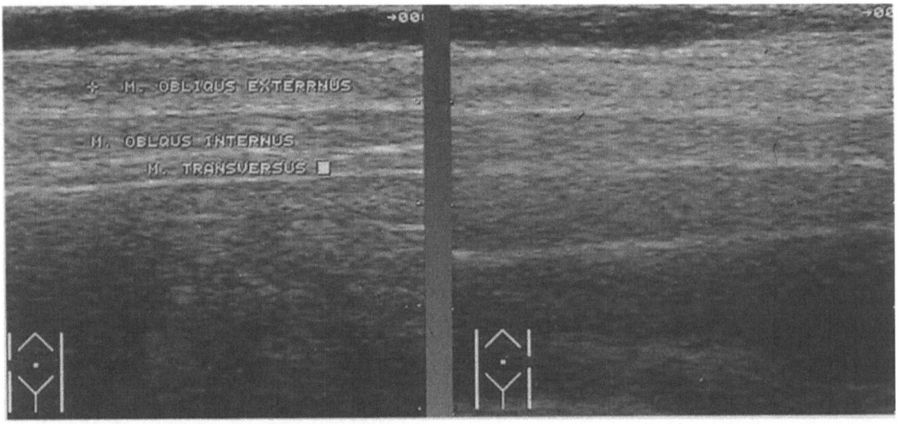

Fig. 14. Sonographic findings of abdominal wall relaxation on the right side. Compared with the unaffected left side, the typical thinner muscle layers without fascial defect can be observed. See also the magnetic resonance imaging (MRI) scan (Fig. 22)

10.3.6 Varicose Nodules

In the transverse plane, varicose nodules of the saphenous vein appear as round, hypoechoic structures in the femoral region. The longitudinal plane reveals a tubular structure with a connection to the femoral vein. Colour coded duplex sonography shows blood flow inside the structure.

10.3.7 Postoperative Investigations

Fluid collection is one of the main indications for sonography, because it presents one of the most common postoperative complications after hernia repair. The indication for fluid aspiration depends on the estimated volume.

Although it is not easy to determine the type of fluid sonographically, there are sonographic criteria that help us to distinguish between different fluid collections.

10.3.8 Hematoma

Fresh hematomas show a hypoechoic, space-occupying structure with a fine and regular inner echo and distinct margins. Organised hematomas appear as more echogenic structures (Fig. 15).

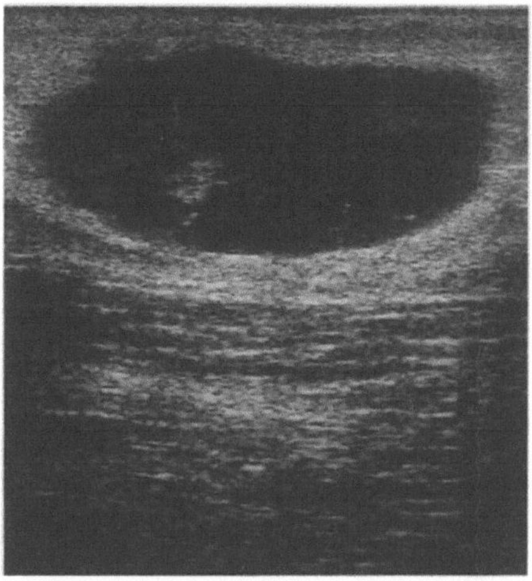

Fig. 15. Typical sonographic findings of a fresh hematoma

10.3.9
Seroma

Seromas present as anechoic structures without inner reflections or sharp margins (Fig. 16).

10.3.10
Abscess

An abscess is seen as a hypoechoic process with a heterogeneous structure caused by cell debris and small, plump hyperechoic reflections caused by gas bubbles (Fig. 17).

10.3.11
Hematoma of the Rectus Sheath

Further postoperative complications include hematoma of the rectus sheath and wound rupture. Sonography of a hematoma of the rectus sheath shows an increase in the volume of the rectus muscles. The hematoma is situated between the anterior and posterior layer of the rectus sheath (Fig. 18).

10.3.12
Wound Rupture (Burst Abdomen)

Postoperative wound rupture or burst abdomen occur in 0.05%–3% of patients [2]. Three types of lesions can be distinguished:

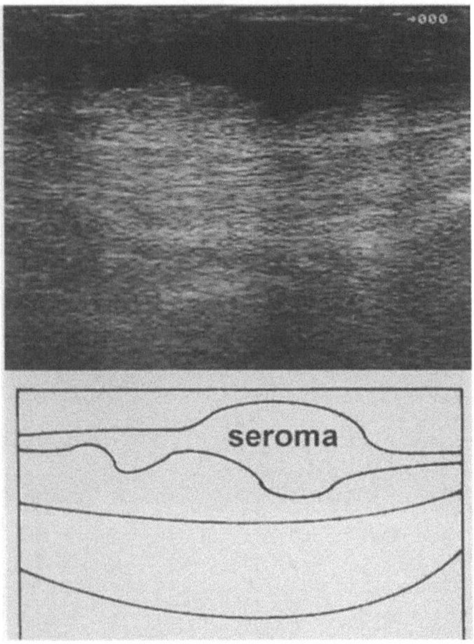

Fig. 16. Typical sonographic findings of a seroma

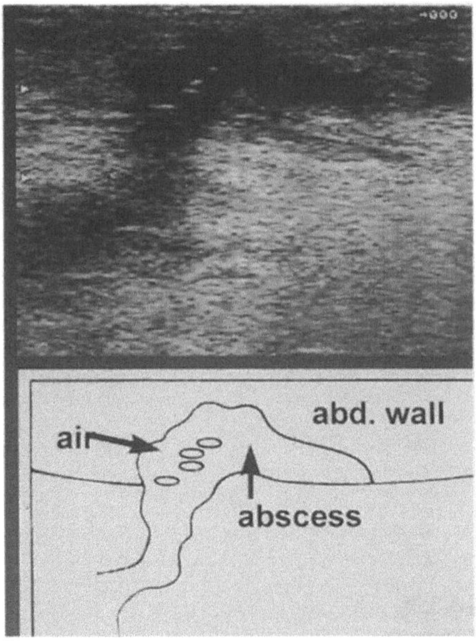

Fig. 17. Typical sonographic findings of an abscess with gas bubbles

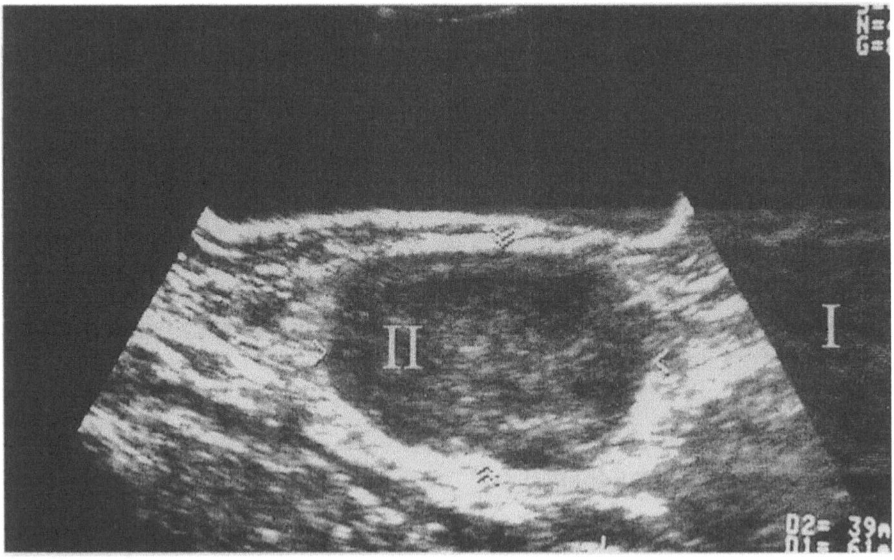

Fig. 18. Sonographic findings of a hematoma of the rectus sheath. *I*, rectus musle; *II*, hematoma

- Free, with complete rupture of all layers and protruding viscera out of the abdominal cavity
- Fixed, with complete rupture of all layers, but fixed viscera that remain in the abdominal cavity
- Covered, with rupture of the deeper layers while the cutaneous suture remains intact

The covered burst abdomen is an indication for sonography. The discontinuity of the sutured fascia or aponeurosis is revealed. Seroma or abscess may also be observed (Fig. 19).

10.4 Results

We studied the specificity and sensitivity of sonography for undetermined pain and palpable masses of unknown origin in 105 patients [3]. Altogether, the correct diagnosis was made sonographically in 89 of 105 patients (84.8%). Sonography showed a sensitivity and specificity of 100% for epigastric hernias. Inguinal hernias were found sonographically with a sensitivity of 82.3% and a specificity of 98.9%. Poor results were found for femoral hernias, with a sensitivity of 72.7% and a specificity of 97.8%, especially due to confusion with lymphoma (Table 1).

10.4.1 Sonography

In a prospective study for unknown pain and swelling of the abdominal wall or inguinal region, sonography showed a sensitivity of 87.5% and specificity of 97.8% for recognition of hematoma. Sonographic diagnosis of seroma had a sensitivity of 100% and

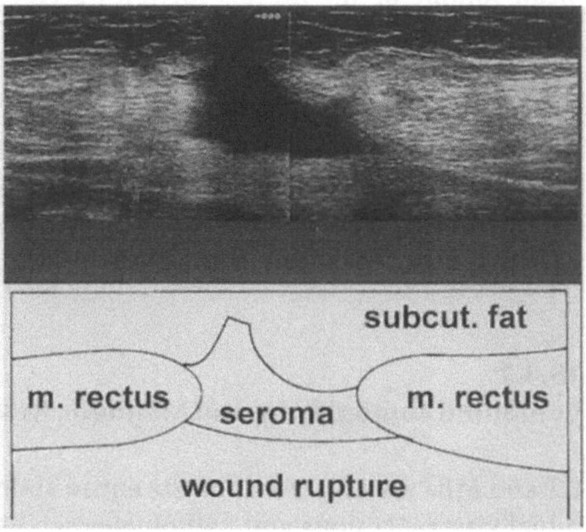

Fig. 19. Sonographic findings of a covered wound rupture (burst abdomen type 3) with fascial defect and seroma

Table 1. Sensitivity and specificity of abdominal wall sonography

	Sensitivity (%)	Specificity (%)
Epigastric hernia	100	100
Inguinal hernia	82.3	98.9
Femoral hernia	72.7	97.8
Seroma	100	97.8
Hematoma	87.5	97.8
Abscess	66.6	100
Metastasis	85.7	98
Total	85	93.8

Table 2. Postoperative sonographic examination after mesh implantation

Period	Patients (n)	Seroma (>10 ml)					Hematoma		Revision		Infection		Mesh removal (n)
		(n)	(%)	Aspiration (n)	Volume on day 6 (ml)		(n)	(%)	(n)	(%)	(n)	(%)	
					Mean	SD							
1989–1996	50	20	40	13	33.9	32.6	6	12	1	17	2	4	0
1996–1998	18	5	28	5	16.4	13.2	4	22.2	0	0	0	0	0
1997–1998	17	6	35.3	5	31.2	16.3	5	29.4	0	0	0	0	0

a specificity of 97.8%. Less good results were found for abscess, with a sensitivity of 66.6% and a specificity of 100% (Table 1).

With postoperative sonography after mesh repair, we were able to study typical wound complications and compare different mesh types (Table 2).

As the most frequent wound complication, we detected seroma (>10 ml) in 40% of cases in which Marlex mesh was used (n=50); the mean volume was 33.9 ml (SD 32.6) at the sixth postoperative day. Of these, 65% were confirmed by aspiration. In 35.3% of cases in which Atrium mesh was used (n=18), seroma (>10 ml) developed, with a mean volume of 31.2 ml (SD 16.3); it developed in 28% of cases in which Soft Hernia Mesh was used (n=19), with a mean volume of 16.4 ml (SD 13.3). All seroma in these two groups were aspirated. The difference in volume between Marlex mesh and Soft Hernia Mesh was significant (p<0.05, t test).

A total of 12% of the patients with Marlex mesh, 29.4% with Atrium mesh and 22.2% with Soft Hernia Mesh developed hematomas. One hematoma had to be released operatively. We detected wound infections in 4% of the Marlex group. We did not have to remove the mesh in any of the patients.

10.4.2 Computed Tomography and Magnetic Resonance Imaging

CT and MRI are ideal to show the entire abdominal wall and its relations to the abdominal viscera. Lesions and pathologies can be identified easily. Indication are big her-

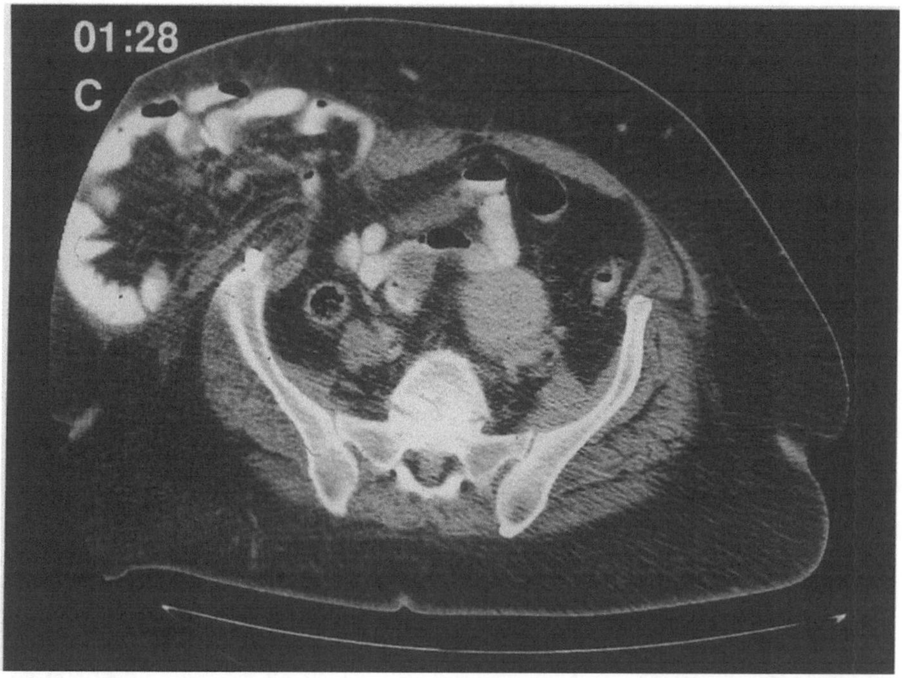

Fig. 20. Computed tomography (CT) scan of a giant incisional hernia with protruding bowels

nias, abdominal wall tumours, sonographically uncertain results and obturator hernias. The images allow the volume of giant hernias and the corresponding abdominal cavity to be estimated, and the surgeon therefore discovers whether the hernial contents will fit into the abdominal cavity and primary closure of the fascial defect is possible.

CT allows evaluation of suspicious and clinically occult hernias and the complete extension of giant hernias. The fascial defect can be identified on the axial cuts, as can the protruding hernial sac and its contents. Volume estimation is possible (Fig. 20).

The different soft tissue layers of the abdominal wall can be demonstrated by MRI scan. The fascial lesion and extension of hernial contents are easily identified (Fig. 21). In addition, abdominal wall relaxation can be diagnosed by direct comparison with the unaffected side (Fig. 22).

10.5 Conclusion

Ultrasound is an excellent tool for the preoperative evaluation of hernias and other pathological findings of the abdominal wall. The examination is easy to carry out with the aid of a 7.5-MHz scanner. Early detection and evaluation of postoperative complications such as seroma, hematoma and abscess is also possible.

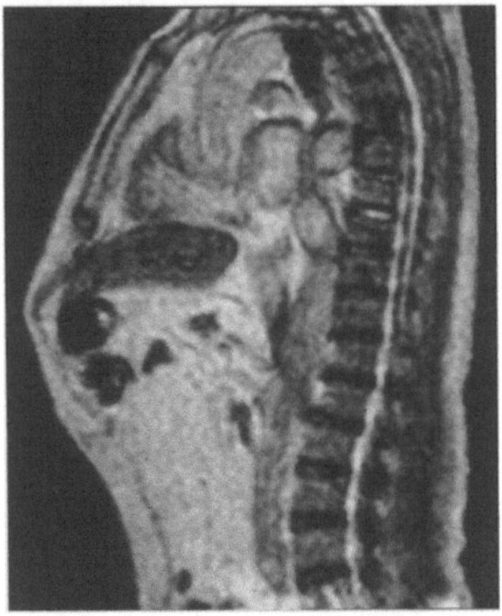

Fig. 21. Magnetic resonance imaging (MRI) scan of an incisional hernia

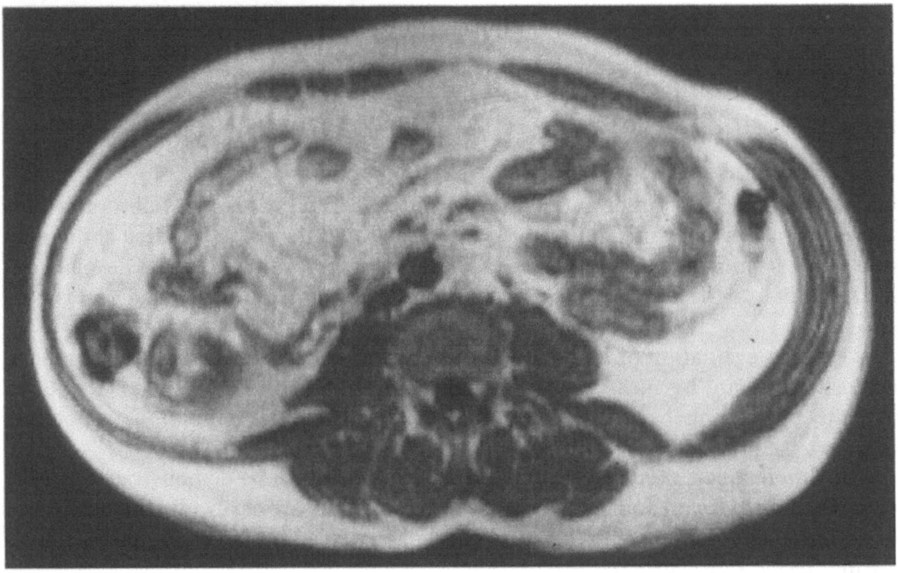

Fig. 22. Magnetic resonance imaging (MRI) scan of abdominal wall relaxation on the right side. There is no fascial defect, and all three muscle layers can be identified, with a thinner muscle layer on the right side. See also the sonographic findings in Fig. 14

In comparison with CT or herniography, ultrasonographic examination saves both time and money and does not entail the risks of invasive methods or contrast medium allergy.

Sonography can be used repeatedly by all examiners at any time in the diagnosis of small hernias or in obese patients with barely palpable findings.

Sonographic differentiation between seroma, hematoma and abscess is sometimes difficult. In this case, aspiration is required.

CT and MRI allow clear identification of abdominal wall pathologies. They play an important role in the diagnosis of uncertain clinical or sonographic findings and in preoperative planning for giant hernia repair. Malignant tumours can also be clearly demonstrated, showing their exact location in deeper layers and their spread in the abdominal wall. In the case of abdominal wall relaxation, MRI scan allows direct comparison of the affected and unaffected side. The disadvantages include higher costs, limited availability and the danger of contrast medium allergy when contrast medium is necessary.

Using postoperative sonography, we were able to demonstrate the rate of wound complication after mesh repair. Although only the seroma volume between Marlex and Soft Hernia Mesh at the sixth postoperative day showed statistical significance, we were able to demonstrate a lower seroma rate and volume after Soft Hernia Mesh repair compared to the other meshes. Further investigations are required to show that Soft Hernia Mesh lead to fewer seroma, reflecting lower alloplastic material reaction.

10.6 Discussion

Carlson: Does obesity have an effect on the accuracy of your ultrasound investigations?

Truong: Obesity does have a big influence on ultrasound, but for the diagnosis of the abdominal wall we can use a 5-MHz scanner and can see about 7 cm deep. That is not a problem.

Simmermacher: I was wondering whether you can measure the defect with ultrasound. Can you say that it is 10x4 cm or 20x25 cm?

Truong: The measurements of the defect can be determined by ultrasound quite exactly if the patient is examined in the supine position, not in the standing position.

Schumpelick: Who should do the ultrasound, because it is not a very reproducible method?

Truong: Surgeon should carry out the ultrasound themselves for greater diagnostic value. Furthermore, they are able to look for postoperative complications, which may lead to early treatment.

Schumpelick: Are they sufficiently trained to do that?

Truong: Yes, training takes 6 months.

Kingsnorth: My questions relates to the previous talk about incisional hernias and their importance. Do we need to know what the size of the problem is, in other words the late wound failure rate? We imagine that there are a lot of patients out there with late wound failure. Are these just small defects – are they bulges that are insignificant? Can your investigation tell us what is in the sac of an incisional hernia, because a patient who has bowel in it has a risk of strangulation in an incisional hernia. If we knew that and if a patient was not particularly keen on surgery, we could tell them that there is a bit of omentum or preperitoneal fat or something like that in the defect, and they might be persuaded to have an operation.

Truong: The hernial contents can be determined in over 90% of cases. We can see small intestine, omentum, and a direct finding of ileus is the dilatation of the bowel. We can see all that with ultrasound. In the burst abdomen, everything is covered. In open burst abdomen, we do not need ultrasound. However, in covered burst abdomen, the skin is intact. Ultrasound shows the disruption, the discontinuity of the aponeurosis.

Bendavid: Another application I have found for ultrasound, especially for colour-coded Doppler ultrasound, is in determining the future of the testicle. We often see patients with a very swollen testicle in whom we used to predict testicular atrophy. We are now able to determine that in fact only 50% of patients with marked swelling and very woody, hard testicles will go on to atrophy, and we have been able to demonstrate the circulation at that time. That is very important. The other thing we were hoping to do but have not been successful in doing is to determine whether arterial or venous circulation was in fact affected during that period postoperatively.

Truong: Two factors cause orchitis: the arterial and the venous flow. We have two patients with reduced arterial flow, but no orchitis was observed in these patients. Venous flow is very difficult to diagnose with colour-coded ultrasound.

Filipi: I may be a little presumptuous in saying this, as there are so many European and especially German surgeons here. It has been clearly demonstrated that surgeons can perform ultrasound accurately with the highest specificity and sensitivity not only for examination of the common bile duct, but also in patients with intraperitoneal hematomas after trauma. Prospective studies have actually been done that show that surgical residents can carry it out as well and even better than radiologic residents. One of the questions that I have is what the technical problems were that created the lack of sensitivity for the detection of inguinal hernias with ultrasound.

Truong: I have a high sensitivity and specificity for the diagnosis of inguinal hernia, but very low sensitivity for femoral hernia. Small hernias are very difficult to diagnose by ultrasound. If you do not see the hernial contents, you cannot see the hernial orifice and you see only a hypoechoic structure in this region with an increase in the volume by pressing or coughing. That is the only criteria. It is very difficult in small hernias.

Schumpelick: What is the sensitivity and specificity in clinical examination?

Truong: In the literature, the sensitivity of the clinical examination of inguinal hernias is about 85%. In 15% we have unclear findings of the abdominal wall.

Simmermacher: Are you able to distinguish between a direct and an indirect inguinal hernia with the same sensitivity and specificity?

Truong: We have a low specificity of about 70%. If we see the epigastric inferior artery, we can distinguish between direct and indirect, but it is only seen in 20% of patients.

References

Honig MP, Mason RA, Giron F. Wound complications of the retroperitoneal approach to the aorta and iliac vessels. J Vasc Surg 1992;15: p 28–34.

Chevrel JP. Hernias and surgery of the abdominal wall. Springer, Berlin Heidelberg New York, 1997: p 118.

Truong SN, Pfingsten F, Dreuw B, Schumpelick V. Value of ultrasound in the diagnosis of undetermined findings in the abdominal wall and inguinal region. in Inguinal Hernia Repair, Expert Meeting on Hernia Surgery, St. Moritz, 1994. Schumpelick V, Wantz GE (eds), Basel, Karger, 1995: 29–41

Part IV Principles of Repair

CHAPTER 11

Preparation of Patients for Hernia Surgery

S. Willis

11.1 General Aspects

A thorough preparation of patients is a mandatory prerequisite for successful hernia surgery with low complication rates. It must not be neglected even if only minor surgical procedures are planned. The initial consultation starts with carefully history-taking of the patients' complaints, previous operations and concomitant diseases. Special emphasis should be placed on cerebrovascular, coronary artery, cardiac or pulmonary diseases. Patients should be asked whether they have had any previous allergic reactions, especially to disinfectants or local anaesthetics, in order to avoid complications. Psychiatric disorders must be ruled out, since in general they require in-patient treatment. The social situation must also be assessed to determine whether the patient should receive treatment on an in- or outpatient basis. It is important to list current medications completely. This may sometimes reveal disorders that have not been asked for the physician or mentioned by the patient.

With this information in mind, a complete physical examination is then performed. An electrocardiogram and a chest X-ray are indicated in patients older than 40 years or in those with a special history or abnormal clinical findings. An additional pulmonary function test and a blood gas analysis should be carried out in patients with a history of severe pulmonary disease, in those with clinical signs of respiratory insufficiency and in those with giant hernias (see below). All patients should undergo standard laboratory tests (i.e. blood count, electrolytic levels, coagulation analysis, glucose, transaminases, urea and creatinine).

In addition to the patient's general condition, the examination should focus on the site of the hernia to be repaired. Location and diameter of the hernial orifice should be assessed. It must be evaluated whether the hernia is reducible or not. The condition of the skin in the region of the planned operation has to be thoroughly examined. For better validation and in order to exclude asymptomatic hernias, an ultrasound of the abdomen and the abdominal wall is performed in all patients in our clinic (see Chap. 10).

This information should be borne in mind when planning the operative procedure. The choice between outpatient and in-patient treatment is based on various aspects:

1. The hernia has to be reducible and treated by an elective procedure. If there are any signs of incarceration, an operation should be performed immediately under emergency conditions.

2. The technique of repair has to be considered. While primary repair is ideal for ambulatory surgery, patients undergoing a giant prosthetic reinforcement have to be admitted to hospital.
3. The general condition of patients and their personal attitude must support the decision. Only patients classified as ASA class 1 or 2 are good candidates for ambulatory surgery.

Local anaesthesia usually can be considered for all patients suitable for outpatient treatment. Patients with large hernias in which extended preparation can be expected should be given general anaesthesia. Patients with primary or recurrent inguinal hernias or small incisional hernias can usually be operated on under local anaesthesia. The majority of patients can be scheduled for an elective procedure. If there is any way of improving the patient's condition, every effort must be made and surgery should be postponed.

The preparation is concluded by informing the patient about the perioperative management and the operative procedure and its risks. Patient have to give formal consent to the operation and receive instructions on how to behave on the day of the surgery. They should also receive printed information [1–3].

11.2 Progressive Pneumoperitoneum

Preoperative progressive pneumoperitoneum is a sporadically used preoperative procedure for patients with giant inguinal or incisional hernias. In 1940, the Argentine surgeon Goni Moreno was the first to use intraperitoneal injections of oxygen to reduce an incarcerated epigastric eventration and to prepare the patient for repair under local anaesthesia [4].

11.3 Pathophysiology

The underlying problem during repair of giant hernias is how to make room to accommodate herniated viscera if they have "forfeited their right of domicile" in the abdominal cavity (Fig. 1) [5]. The principle of the progressive pneumoperitoneum consists of gradual stretching of the abdominal wall by intermittent insufflation of air into the abdominal cavity. This facilitates the operative reduction of hernial contents and allows fascial repair under minimal tension. The skin and hernial sac have a limited capacity even when they are stretched, and additional air stretches the abdomen. Although the immediate result is distension of the hernial sac and the overlying skin, a gradual increase in the size of the abdominal cavity becomes apparent over time. Experimental studies in our department showed that progressive pneumoperitoneum leads to dilatation of all structures of the abdominal wall, including muscles, fasciae, and aponeuroses without hyperplasia [6].

An elevation of the diaphragm also contributes to the increase in the abdominal cavity. Due to eventration, patients with giant hernias have a decreased intra-abdomi-

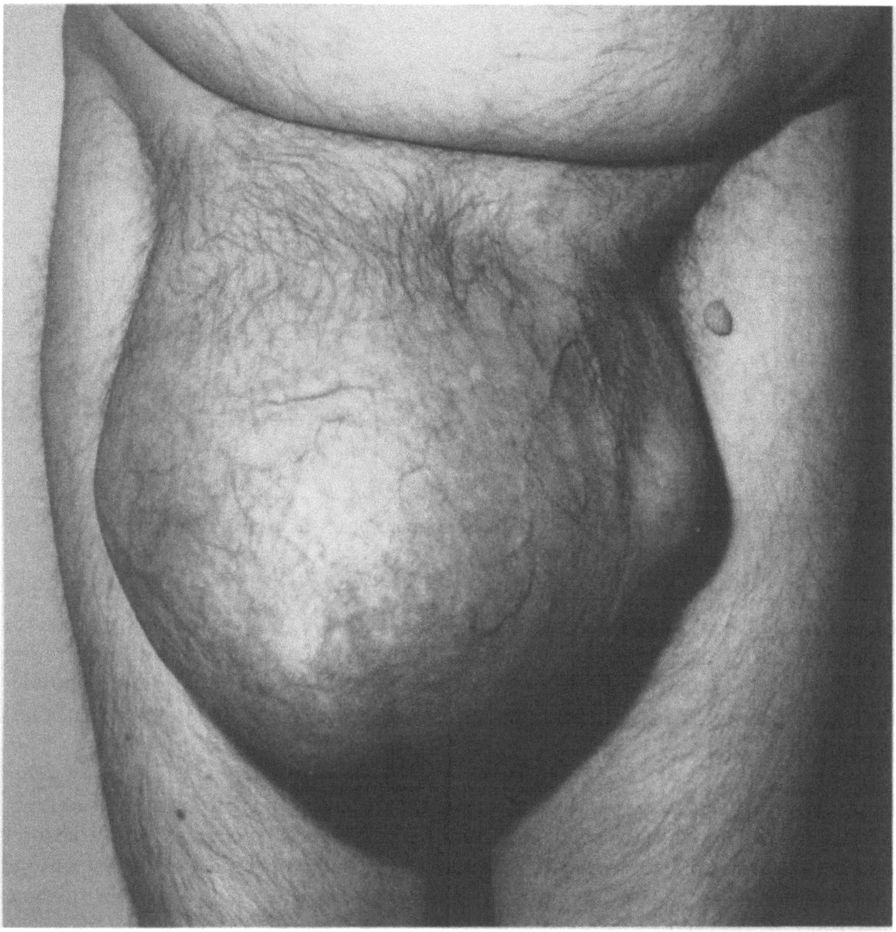

Fig. 1. Patient with giant scrotal hernia with "loss of domicile" in the abdominal cavity

nal pressure with a disequilibrium between intra-abdominal and intrathoracic pressure. As a result, the diaphragm is weak and relaxed, leading to a deterioration in respiratory function. Pneumoperitoneum leads to an increase in the intra-abdominal pressure, thereby leading to the elevation of the diaphragm with restitution of its physiological tension and function [7, 8]. The patient can thus gradually adapt to the postoperative situation. As Fig. 2 shows, there is only a slight decrease in the vital capacity during the treatment. Pulmonary function tests in the immediate postoperative period reveal a constant vital capacity. Patients who cannot tolerate the gradual insufflation of air should not be accepted for surgical treatment. Pneumoperitoneum can therefore be considered to be both a diagnostic and a therapeutic treatment. The air allows the surgeon to increase the abdominal volume gradually while observing the reaction of the awake and alert patient. Contraindications to the use of pneumope-

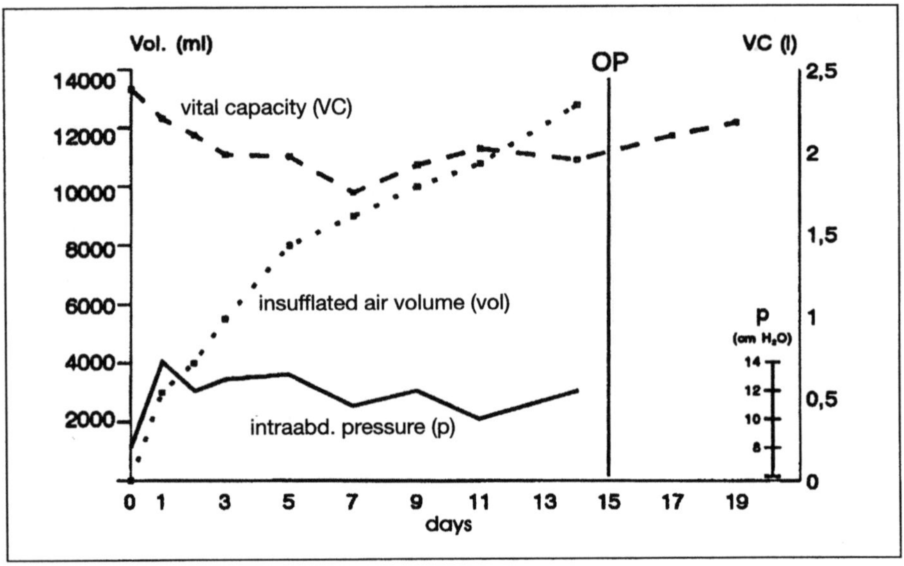

Fig. 2. Respiratory function and abdominal pressure during progressive pneumoperitoneum

ritoneum are those that would also make the patient a poor candidate for hernia repair even after completion of pneumoperitoneum, such as cardiac and respiratory insufficiency. The insufflation of 500 ml air may be the best way to determine candidates for such treatment and to exclude patients with limited cardiac pulmonary reserves [9, 10].

Other advantages of pneumoperitoneum are the gradual preoperative lysis of adhesions between the intestine and hernial ring, the discovery of additional areas of fascial weakness and potential sites of recurrent herniations and a decrease in the chronic edema of the mesentery. Furthermore, the stretching of the hernial sac has been found to be helpful in skin cleansing before the operation and potentially decreases the incidence of infection [11].

11.4 Technique

Originally, intermittent percutaneous puncture of the abdominal wall was used for the frequent insufflation of air into the abdominal cavity. CO_2 is absorbed four times more readily in the peritoneal space than air and should therefore not be used [10]. In 1965, Steichen described the placement of an indwelling catheter for daily injections of air [12]. We adapted this technique by using an indwelling standard urinary catheter, which is placed in the upper left abdominal quadrant under local anaesthesia. The site of the placement of the catheter should be at a distance from the hernia and from previous incisions. The correct placement of the catheter should be checked by the outflow of air. Insufflation of air may be started at once. Injections of 500 ml to 2 l air are performed every 1–3 days. Pain in the shoulder signifying diaphragmatic irritation indicates the end-point of daily injections. In addition, the intra-abdominal pressure should be measured by manometry. It must not exceed a maximum of 15 mmHg in order to avoid renal or circulatory complications. To reduce the risk of vomiting and aspiration, we request the patient to remain upright and not to eat for several hours before and after the procedure. This facilitates weight reduction in patients, who are usually obese.

If respiratory or cardiac compromise or severe discomfort is noted, air may be withdrawn through the catheter. Complications of the technique are often associated with the puncture of the abdominal wall. Nevertheless, perforation of viscera, peritonitis and air embolism are rare complications [9, 10, 13, 14]. The use of an indwelling catheter rather than intermittent puncture to induce pneumoperitoneum should reduce the likelihood of these complications. In a series of 587 patients, Moreno described 11 local infections of the catheter, nine cases of pneumonia, four cases of lung embolism due to deep vein thromboses and three heart infarctions. Six of his patients died because of complications from the pneumoperitoneum [11].

11.5 Results

The results of preoperative progressive pneumoperitoneum are impressive (Table 1). Controlled randomised studies do not exist because patients with giant hernias are rare and often exhibit unique features caused by their disease. Recurrence rates in different studies are between 0% and 43%, with a medium of 3.6%. Compared with recurrence rates for conventional repair (20%–49%) or alloplastic repair (7%–15%), these results are impressive [16].

In our department, preoperative progressive pneumoperitoneum was performed in three patients with incisional hernias and in two patients with inguinal hernias. Two patients with incisional hernias received mesh repair without complications, while preoperative pneumoperitoneum had to be withdrawn in one patient because of local infection of the catheter. Of the two patients with inguinal hernias, one refused further treatment during the treatment, while the other patient had a Shouldice repair without complications (Fig. 3).

Table 1. Recurrence rates following incisional hernia repair using progressive pneumoperitoneum

Reference	Patients (*n*)	Recurrences (*n*)	(%)
[5]	8	1	12.5
[14]	10	0	0
[11]	487	14	2.9
[15]	7	3	42.9
[13]	40	2	5
Total	552	20	3.6

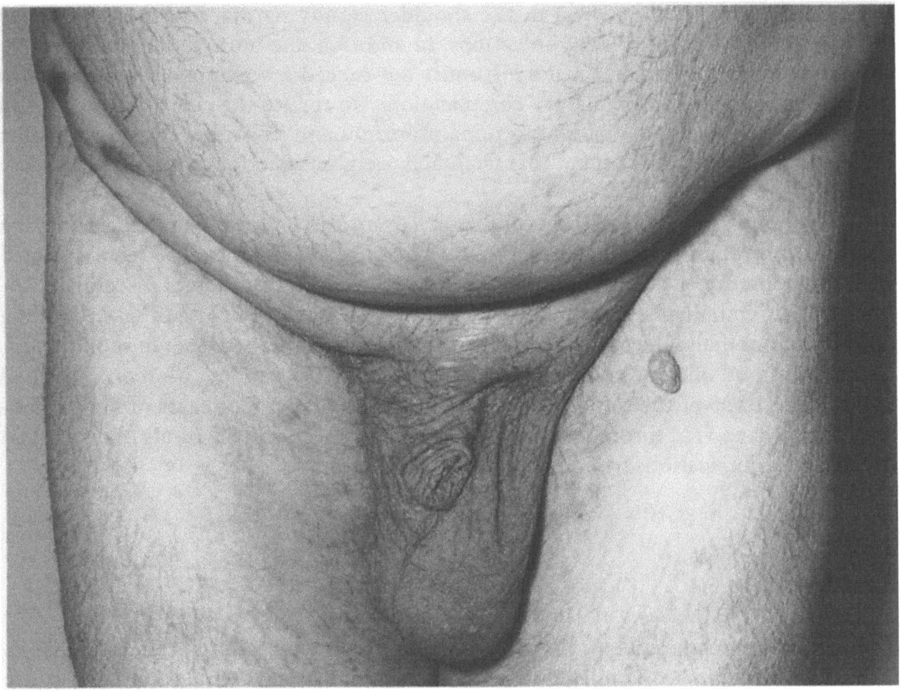

Fig. 3. Patient with previous giant scrotal hernia after pneumoperitoneum and Shouldice repair

11.6 Conclusion

Preoperative progressive pneumoperitoneum is a useful adjunct in the treatment of giant inguinal or incisional hernias with "loss of domicile" in the abdominal cavity. The advantages of pneumoperitoneum include the expansion of the abdomen, allowing reduction of herniated viscera, and the possibility of carrying out tension-free repair of the defect. The restoration of the physiological intra-abdominal pressure improves the patient's respiratory function by elevation of the diaphragm. The use of preoperative pneumoperitoneum cannot be substitute for fascial integrity. Alloplastic reinforcement with meshes should therefore be additionally used to improve fascial tightness. On the other hand, mesh alone does not solve the problem of creating room for the reduction of the herniated viscera. Therefore, in giant hernias with a large hernial orifice and fascial weakness, the combination of preoperative progressive pneumoperitoneum and mesh repair seems to be useful.

11.7 Discussion

Flament: The question everyone asks in this kind of meeting is how you choose a patient for pneumoperitoneum. Do you use a CT scan? We usually do pneumoperitoneum in about 25% of patients with huge incisional hernias; we choose to it if, when we see the CT scans, more than 25% of the bowel is outside the abdominal cavity. Do you do that?

Willis: No, we do not do that. We decide by estimation. If you look at the patient and you feel it would be absolutely impossible and that there is no chance of reducing the herniated viscera, then pneumoperitoneum should of course be performed. We do it in all patients where we have doubts, where we are not absolutely sure. Mason described it as "better air than err(or)". You can see from the five patients we have had so far that we handle it restrictively. So I think it is a good method, but only a good method if the indication is right.

Amid: My comment applies to incisional hernia. With large incisional hernia, the effect of pneumoperitoneum is to expand the abdominal wall to make room for the intestine, and this is crucial for tissue repair. However, the same thing can be achieved with mesh repaid by using a larger piece of mesh and bypassing the cumbersome process of pneumoperitoneum. I understand that when you do pneumoperitoneum you preserve some of the respiratory function of the broad abdominal wall and as you expand the abdominal cavity with mesh you do not have this advantage, but I wonder whether it would be a viable alternative to use a larger piece of mesh instead of going through a pneumoperitoneum.

Willis: I have two points about your comments, Dr. Amid. The first is that all these patients with giant hernias normally have a poor respiratory function. I refer to a study by Dr. Flament, who also showed that obese patients have a kind of protective effect for their ventilation system if they have a hernia. If you carry out forced or immediate repair by mesh, you do not have this advantage, and it is not only the stretching of the abdominal wall muscle, it is also the elevation of the diaphragm; you do not have this using mesh. The second point is that pneumoperitoneum offers the chance of the patient returning to the physiological state. Mesh repair is not physiological; you put the viscera into the abdomen with a mesh. However, with pneumoperitoneum you have the chance of reaching the physiological state.

Schumpelick: What happens to the abdominal wall in these cases of pneumoperitoneum; is it a reversible dilatation?

Willis: If there is a giant hernia, the retraction of the abdominal muscle will of course be fixed after a certain time. We have done some animal experiments showing that there is also a tearing of the fascia and muscle. We know from the other patient who had an abdominal wall infection that if you stop or have to stop pneumoperitoneum and wait for some time, all the air will be resorbed within 5 days and all the effect will be gone.

Schumpelick: Do you think that happens by gravity?

Willis: Yes, I think it does.

Kingsnorth: The results that you have presented are very heavily different from Morino's results. You say that he treated about 700 patients, so his indications for the threshold for which he uses pneumoperitoneum must be very much lower than in your clinic, where you only treated five patients. Also in terms of the recurrent rates: you calculated an overall recurrence rate of 3.6%, but Morino had recurrence rates of 2.9%, so I suspect he must be treating rather small hernias with pneumoperitoneum in cases in which most of us would feel it not indicated. I think it is important that we agree on some way of deciding which patients need pneumoperitoneum rather than saying that this looks like a massive hernia so let's put a couple of catheters into the peritoneal cavity for a few days.

Willis: I almost completely agree with you. I also think that 700 patients is a hard figure to believe, but there are other data, e.g. from Reno or Calderoni, who have a recurrence rate of 20%–30% without prosthetic repair, and that is not too bad either. I think their indications are correct. As I said before, in our clinic, where we certainly see a lot of huge hernias, there have still only been five patients where we decided to do pneumoperitoneum. So in our opinion, the indication for pneumoperitoneum should be set very strictly. We do not have 25% as you do, Prof. Flament. Another problem is probably that, in Western Europe, people do not develop such giant hernias any more; they go to the doctor earlier, and then there is no necessity for it.

Klaiber: I have experience with five patients. I had one patient with renal failure during pneumoperitoneum; we saw it and then stopped, and the renal function returned to normal. However, this patient was not operated on, because we could not operate on him. I saw another patient die because he did not have pneumoperitoneum. The patient asked the surgeon to open his wounds because he could not stand the pressure. Five hours later the patient was dead. I think this pneumoperitoneum is a very good method.

Willis: Did you monitor the intra-abdominal pressure?

Klaiber: No, we just asked the patients how much they can tolerate, and we had about the same amount of air, about 10–12 l.

Willis: I know from my own limited experience that these patients with such a giant hernia are rather indolent, and they stand pressures of up to 40 mmHg; we also know of animal experiments in which urine flow is completely stopped at 30 mmHg. That is why we always monitor the intra-abdominal pressure, although many authors say that it is not necessary; I think it is necessary and your example shows that.

Klaiber: It is very easy with laparoscopy, and monitoring can be done very easily, but I do not think it is obligatory.

Willis: But there is always a normal manometer on the ward and you can just connect it to the catheter to see the pressure; even without laparoscopy it is no problem.

Schumpelick: I would like to put a question to Dr. Herszage, who is following in the tradition of Morino in Argentina: What is the role of progressive pneumoperitoneum now?

Herszage: In my series, for socio-economic reasons, we do not use pneumoperitoneum. We only use it in extreme cases. We prefer relaxing incisions, because they are easier for us and cheaper, and the social costs are lower.

Schumpelick: How can we calculate the work of Moreno? Is it true, as Dr. Kingsnorth said, that he operated on small hernias as well. Are there only huge ones – 700 cases is a lot – and why did he obtain such good results? Is it because he operated on small hernias?

Herszage: No, only huge hernias, not small ones. I was invited to work in a city far from Buenos Aires on the coast. They did not show me the patient previously; I went directly from the airport to the operating theatre and found a big incision from the xiphoid to the suprapubis, but they did pneumoperitoneum for 3 months, and it was easy for me to make an anatomical repair. This case showed that it is an advantage to use pneumoperitoneum, but it is not an innocuous method.

Flament: Just one point that we have missed so far: I know that Morino mentioned in his paper that insufflation facilitates dissection, and there is a kind of pneumodissection exactly like there is in laparoscopic procedures, so that the adhesions of the bowel are very easy to free after insufflation.

Filipi: How do you decide how much air you have to insufflate? Is it adapted to the patient's tolerance plus monitoring the pressure, or do you have a protocol that you use?

Willis: We perform it until the patients complains about pain in the shoulder; that is normally due to the supplementary ligaments of the liver being stretched, and then we stop. We always stop at that point and then check the pressure afterwards. It must not exceed 20 cm water column.

Wantz: How may times have you had to stop because of mediastinal emphysema?

Willis: We only occasionally see mediastinal emphysema; we do see it, of course, but it is not a problem. We have never had to stop because of it.

Bendavid: We do not do pneumoperitoneum, but we do have to encourage weight loss. We have had patients who have lost up to 50 kg, over 100 pounds; has this been forgotten as a technique, or should we forsake the technique of having the patient lose weight?

Willis: The patient should of course lose weight, because we know or at least presume that obesity is one of the factors involved in recurrences; therefore Mason performed laparoscopic gastric banding additionally. When we perform pneumoperitoneum for 2 weeks, patients are always nauseous because they do not eat during that time, and they always lose weight. When these patients see the chance to be operated on, they are very motivated; they try to lose weight, and they come back weighing less. Pneumoperitoneum supports this effect. So they all lose weight preoperatively. The question is what happens after the operation; do they eat again and gain weight? I am afraid they do.

Skandalakis: The last time I used pneumoperitoneum was 30 years ago, and of course I did not know how to do it, so I asked a pneumologist to come who used pneumothorax, and he did it. In the Atlanta area, we do not use pneumoperitoneum anymore.

References

1. Schumpelick V, Treutner KH., Arlt G. (1994) Inguinal hernia repair in adults. Lancet 344: 375
2. Chevrel JP (ed) Hernias and surgery of the abdominal wall, Springer, Paris, 1997
3. Treutner K (1995) Preparation of patients for hernia surgery. In: Schumpelick V, Wantz GE (eds) Inguinal Hernia Repair, Karger, Basel, p. 79
4. Moreno IG (1947) Chronic eventrations and large hernias. Surgery 22: 945
5. Koontz A (1958) Hernias that have forfeited the right of domicile: Use of pneumoperitoneum as aid in their operative cure. South Med J 51: 165
6. Willis S, Conze J, Müller S, Klosterhalfen B, Schumpelick V (1996) Progressives Pneumoperitoneum in der Behandlung von Leisten- und Narbenhernien. Tierexperimentelle Ergebnisse und klinische Anwendung. Langenbecks Archiv Chir. 381: 132
7. Champetier J, Laborde Y, Letoublan Ch, Durand A (1978) Traitement des eventrations abdominales postoperatoires: bases biomechanique elementaires. J Chir (Paris) 115:585
8. Rives J, Lardennois B, Pire J, Hibon J (1973) Les grandes eventrations: importance du "volet abdominal" et troubles respiratoires qui lui sont secondaires. Chirurgie 99: 547
9. Raynor RR, Del Guerico L (1989) The place for pneumoperitoneum in the repair of massive hernia. World J Surg 13: 581
10. Mason EE (1995) Pneumoperitoneum in giant hernia. In: Nyhus LM, Condon RE (eds) Hernia. 4th ed., JB Lippincott, Philadelphia, p. 515
11. Moreno IG (1978) The rational treatment of hernias and voluminous chronic eventrations: Preparation with progressive pneumoperitoneum. In: Nyhus LM, Condon RE (eds) Hernia. 2nd ed., JB Lippincott, Philadelphia, p. 536
12. Steichen FM (1965) A simple method for establishing, maintaining, and regulating surgically induced pneumoperitoneum in preparation for large hernias repair. Surgery 58: 1031
13. Caldironi MW, Romano M, Bozza F (1990) Progressive pneumoperitoneum in the management of giant incisional hernias: a study of 41 patients. Br J Surg. 77: 306
14. Hamer DB, Duthie HL (1972) Pneumoperitoneum in the management of abdominal incisional hernia. Br J Surg 59: 372
15. Raynor RW, Del Guerico L (1985) Update on the use of pneumoperitoneum prior to the repair of large hernias of the abdominal wall. Surg Gyn Obstet 161: 367
16. Schumpelick V, Conze J, Klinge U (1996) Die präperitoneale Netzplastik in der Reparation der Narbenhernie. Eine vergleichende retrospektive Studie. Chirurg 67: 1028

CHAPTER 12

Augmentation with Autologous Material

H.P. Bruch, U.J. Roblick, H. Schimmelpenning

12.1 Introduction

Abdominal wall hernias are frequent findings after abdominal operations. The incidence has increased with each increment of abdominal surgical interventions. In the postoperative course, 5%–10% of the patients develop an incisional hernia [1, 2]; this rate increases up to 14% in patients undergoing a re-laparotomy [5]. The occurrence rate of such hernias is influenced by complications in wound healing or metabolic disorders such as diabetes, protein deficiency or renal insufficiency. Long-term respirator therapy or chronic-obstructive pulmonary disease are among the aetiological factors involved in the development of an abdominal hernia. In addition, there are a considerable number of large umbilical, inborn and acquired midline hernias. All these abdominal wall defects present a great individual and economical problem which should be overcome with appropriate surgical methods, including repair techniques with biological material.

Prosthetic materials for hernia surgery were established early on; the use of fascia, cutis and corium as augmentation materials was described in 1910 by Kirschner, in 1913 by Loewe and in 1914 by Rehn [6–8]. Gallie et al. [9] used autologous fascial strips in 1923. Wangensteen introduced “the repair of recurrent and difficult hernias and other large defects of the abdominal wall with the iliotibial tract” in 1934 [10]. Since that time, tendons, cutis and whole skin grafts, both homo- and heterografts, have been advocated and found to have different problems.

12.2 Technical Aspects

The aims of hernia reparation are the sufficient closure of the abdominal wall defect and the prevention of a hernia recurrence. Nowadays, hernia repair is usually performed using synthetic materials such as Marlex (polypropylene) or Gore-Tex (polytetrafluoroethylene, PTFE). The only real substantial disadvantages of these materials become obvious if the mesh is directly attached to the intestine. Infections and cutaneous or intestinal fistula formations are described in up to 10% of these cases [11, 12]. The infections can be treated conservatively in most cases (approximately 70%). Surgical removal of the alloplastic graft is necessary in 30% [13]. In the case of giant wall defects where a large mesh had to be implanted, a syndrome that may be referred to as

Table 1. Recurrence rates following incisional hernia repair using synthetic mesh

Author	Year	Patients (n)	Follow-up (months)	Recurrences (%)
Molloy et al.	1991	50	6–120	8
Liakakos et al.	1994	49	12–156	8
Condon et al.	1995	62	1–82	13

the "knight-in-armour syndrome" may develop. This means that stooping to tie shoe lashes or secure boot straps may be impossible for the patient. In contrast, there are a number of advantages to these non-biological prosthetics. The tension resistance and the stability of these materials are 1000-fold higher than that of biological grafts. If the mesh is fixed properly, hernia recurrence is seldom seen (8%–13%; Table 1). The number of allergic and hyperergic reactions is low. Taking all these factors into account, it remains to be shown whether there is any indication left for biological materials in abdominal hernia repair.

12.2.1 Cutisplasty

Cutisplasty was originally introduced by Loewe [7] and Rehn [8] under different conditions. It is a full-thickness skin graft from which the epidermis is dissected.

This repair technique using autologous material has several striking advantages compared to synthetic materials:
- Smooth wound healing
- High resistance to infection
- High elasticity
- Availability at low costs (it could be removed from the redundant hernia sac)

The indications for cutisplasty are as follows:
- Large abdominal wall and incisional hernias
- Recurrent hernias
- Abdominal muscle deficiency syndrome
- Retraction of the hernia rims based on scar contraction
- Hernia repair under high tension
- Associated diseases causing high intra-abdominal pressure

12.2.1.1 Operation Technique

The cutis flap is removed from the hernia sac. This should be followed by ablation of the tegumentary epidermal epithelium to avoid epithelial cysts [14, 15]. The flap has to be perforated with a puncture needle to prevent seroma formation [15]. After that, the skin graft should be sewn under tension in overlapping technique (overlapping zone, 2–3 cm) to the rims of the hernia [15, 18] using non-absorbable suture material. A drainage tube should be positioned. To ensure tension-free closure of the abdomen, the pre-

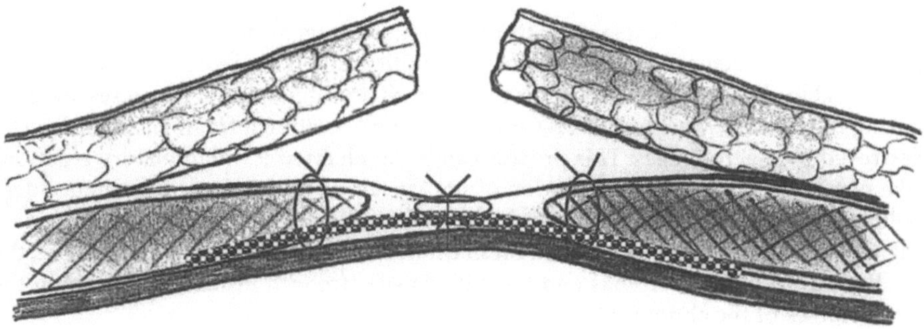

Fig. 1. Cutisplasty positioned used a sublay technique

peritoneal fascia should be reconstructed. This can be achieved by using the anterior part of the rectus sheath, which is therefore longitudinally incised and rotated like a door wing. The closure of the abdomen is accomplished using continuous non-absorbable suture. In our experience, using a modified onlay technique gives the best results (Fig. 1).

12.2.1.2
Histomorphological Aspects

The implanted cutis graft undergoes considerable structural changes. Experimental data was obtained in rats by Wilker et al. and Reith et al., who investigated morphology and wound healing following cutisplasty [16, 17]. Under the tension of the abdominal muscles, the transverse diameter of the cutis transplant increases considerably within the first 80 days [17]. The longitudinal diameter decreases at first, approaching its original length within the same period of time [16]. Two different mechanisms are responsible for these functional adaptations which lead to remodelling of the fascia structures of the abdomen. The skin plasty is initially covered by fibrin fibres. The cellular reaction shows a lympho-plasmacellular infiltration and an ingrowth of capillary bundles. Revascularisation is completed after 2 weeks. This is followed by a displacement of the grafts collagen fibres by giant cells and macrophages. The histological aspect of the transplant resembles that of a fresh scar. Under the polarisation microscope, the collagen fibres of the fresh transplant show a random pattern. Due to the tension of the abdominal wall, the collagen fibres are brought into line during the remodelling process appropriate to the mechanical stress. They show a parallel structure after 8 weeks, thus mimicking the structure of the fascia skeleton of the abdominal wall. The entire transplant has transformed into a strong, fibrous "juvenile" tissue.

As in normal wound healing, the long-term stability of such a reconstruction and the operative success in terms of prevention of recurrent herniation depend on physiological processes such as the following:

- Genesis of high quality collagen
- The metabolic state of the patient (obesity, diabetes, renal insufficiency)
- A sufficient blood supply to the graft
- Inflammatory reactions caused by local infection

Augmentation of the cutisplasty with reabsorbable polyglycolic acid mesh is described in order to achieve a higher primary stability [14]. This repair technique has a considerable disadvantage. Tension resistance of the cutisplasty decreases by 80% during the first few weeks. After 4–5 weeks, the mesh is almost fragmented and partly destroyed by macrophages. This process can be accelerated if inflammatory reactions take place and the local concentration of non-specific esterases increases, hence degrading polyester macromolecules such as polyglycolic acid. From this point of view, augmentation with polyglycolic acid mesh cannot be recommended. Furthermore, the mesh tends to induce seromas and loses its tensile strength instead of absorbing the tensile forces of the abdominal wall.

12.2.1.3
Results

These biological arguments might explain contradictory results concerning the long-term stability of augmented cutisplasties. Nevertheless, the overall results obtained by cutisplasty are good, with recurrence rates of between 0% and 14% being reported (Table 2). This seems, therefore, to be an appropriate graft for the repair of primary and recurrent hernias of the abdominal wall.

12.2.2
Tensor Fasciae Latae Transposition Flap

A second possibility to repair large defects of the abdominal wall with autologous materials may be achieved using a uni- or bilateral tensor fasciae latae flap (TFL). The use of muscle together with the overlying skin as a compound flap was first described by Owens for the reconstruction of facial defects in 1955 [23]. Based on its vascular anatomy, the TFL flap can easily be transposed in all directions and ensures a dynamic stabilisation of defects in the groin and insufficient abdominal wall (Fig. 2). This being only an accessory muscle of thigh flexion and rotation, it is unlikely that any major disability will ensue following the use of an TFL flap [24–26].

Table 2. Recurrence rates after cutisplasty

Author	Year	Operations (*n*)	Recurrences (%)
Schildberg et al.	1983	17 (PO)	4
		9 (RO)	0
Reith et al.	1989	97 (PO)	3
		33 (RO)	6
Schütter et al.	1994	14 (PO)	7
		14 (RO)	14
Results in Lubeck	1990–1998	21 (PO)	5
		11 (RO)	1

PO, primary operations; RO, recurrences operated on.

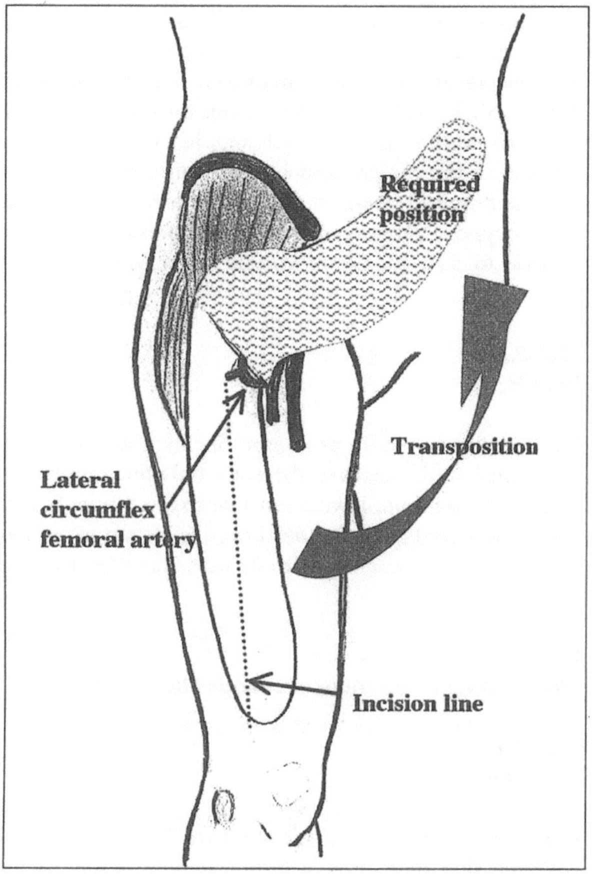

Fig. 2. Tensor fasciae latae (TFL) transposition flap

12.2.2.1 Indication

The indications for a TFL flap are seen in abdominal wall defects after trauma or infection, especially when combined with a contaminated bowel injury or a sepsis. Other indications are congenital defects and abdominal wall hernias after tumour resection [25–27].

12.2.2.2 Operation Technique

The incision of the skin starts 5 cm distal to the iliac crest and extends distally 10 cm above the fibular caput (Fig. 2). The tensor muscle and the fascia lata are freed from the adjacent tissues. The vascular pedicle enters the muscle about 4–6 cm distal to the anterior iliac crest. Two venae comitantes and one artery originating from the lateral circumflex femoral artery are usually observed. This bundle has to be preserved by all means during surgery. The flap is prosected and elevated in the disto-proximal direction. Special attention must be paid to a layer of loose connective tissue under the tendon sheath, because this layer carries the blood supply. It is advisable to cut the branch of the circumflex artery, which supplies the gluteous medious muscle. This facilitates rotation of the muscle and fascia around the iliac crest. The flap is then transposed into the required position. If all these precautions are followed, it can be extended up to the xiphoid process and most abdominal wall defects can be closed. It is usually possible to close the donor area by primary suture [26–28].

12.2.2.3 Results

The TFL flap seems to be an appropriate transplant for a dynamic stabilisation of the abdominal wall. However, there are only few reports on the method and only a small number of patients have been investigated over a short follow-up period [29]. One major disadvantage is the defect in the elevation zone of the lower extremity, particularly in younger patients, with its subsequent cosmetic deficit.

12.2.3 Free Transplanted Myocutaneous Flap – Latissimus Dorsi Free Flap

12.2.3.1 Indication

A freely transplanted myocutaneous flap consisting of the latissimus muscle and covering skin may be an appropriate alternative repair for giant abdominal wall defects that have developed after tumor surgery or severe trauma, for example. This technique offers a combination of good functional and highly aesthetic reconstruction of abdominal wall defects.

12.2.3.2 Operation Technique

The free flap is elevated in a patient positioned on the side (Fig. 3). The size of the flap is fitted to the defect. After the dissection of the myocutaneous flap and the preparation of the vascular/nerve bundle (thoracodorsal artery and vein, thoracodorsal nerve), the latter is dissected. This is followed by the anastomosis of the flap with the receiving vessels (e.g. inferior epigastric artery) [29, 30]. The thoracodorsal nerve is co-adapted to an intercostal nerve. This leads to a synergistic innervation to the abdominal muscles. The flap is then exactly adapted to the defect and sutured. The operation is completed with a direct closure of the withdrawal area. The regeneration of the co-adapted nerve and the reinnervation of the flap is completed after 2 years.

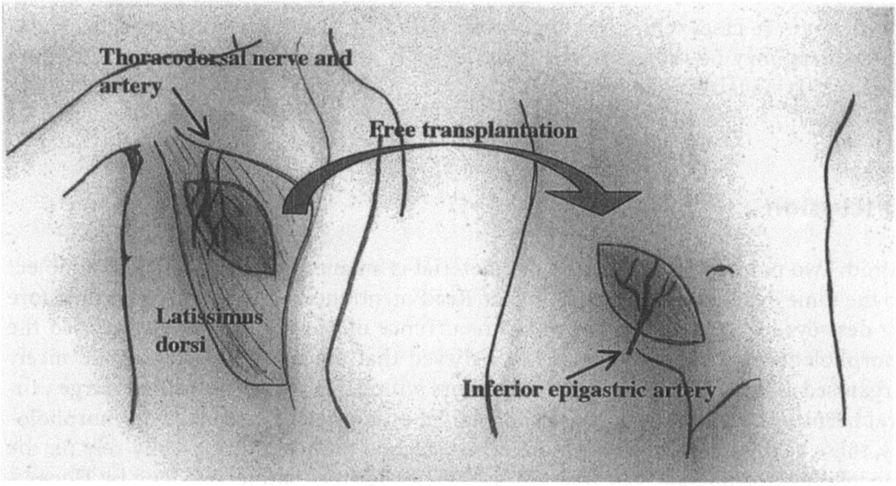

Fig. 3. Latissimus dorsi free flap

12.2.3.3
Results

There are only a few case reports in the literature reporting fairly good results [29, 30]. Such results can only be obtained if the operation is performed in centres with facilities and experience for micro-surgical interventions. Otherwise, insufficiencies of the graft's arterial or venous anastomosis or the lack of regeneration of the transplanted nerve will be the consequences.

12.3
Summary

The cutisplasty skin graft is always available and easy to handle. If a single-shot antibiotic prophylaxis is administered, infectious complications are rare. The long-term results seem comparable to those of synthetic mesh. It has not yet been established whether augmentation with reabsorbable mesh has a beneficial effect on long-term results. In our opinion, cutisplasty should not be used in patients presenting with risk factors.

The tensor fasciae latae seems to be an appropriate pedicled transplant for abdominal hernia repair. However, there are only a few reports on the method, including a small number of patients investigated over a short follow-up period. Hence, it cannot yet be advocated that this technically mandatory procedure should be part of the standard surgical methods. There remains some reasonable doubt as to whether or not a tendon-like fascia can withstand the permanent transverse tension of the abdominal wall with its parallel fibres.

In very rare cases with giant abdominal wall defects, freely transplanted myocutaneous flaps may be indicated, but there are only a few case reports in the literature demonstrating fairly good results.

12.4 Discussion

Amid: Two points. Firstly, because the material is an autogenous material, it is subject to the same degenerative process that Dr. Read mentioned yesterday. It could therefore be destroyed over time, leading to the recurrence of the hernia. You emphasised the morphology of collagen fibers. It was believed that the collagen fibres are all nicely organised and parallel, and they are therefore strong. However, we observed large ventral hernias in rabbits, in our experimental laboratory ward; despite good morphology, these rabbits developed a hernia, which means that we cannot really rely on the morphology of the collagen fibers. The same experimentation was done by Honerd, who came to the same conclusion. Something else must be important besides morphology.

Bruch: I think if the hernia sack is very big, and the hernia itself is very large, we should not apply this material for hernia repair. We also use a xenogenic mesh.

Schumpelick: Is the Farthmann group doing biomechanical studies on cutisplasty, because I think that is very important.

Bruch: I don't think so.

Schumpelick: I think that has to be done, because strength is important.

Bruch: We are doing that at the moment. We are comparing polypropylene mesh with cutisplasty, and I think it is necessary to carry out a randomised study to have valid data about this biological material.

Klaiber: I would like to make a comment on cutisplasty. I prefer to do coriumplasty, and I will tell you why. There is still an indication for cutisplasty. For example, if you have an perforated diverticulitis and a large hernia, you have to do something. That is a good indication for augmentation by cutisplasty, an infectious environment. In coriumplasty, you take away the epidermis and open the capillaries of the transplant, and within 1 day there is already vascularisation of the transplant; that is why I prefer coriumplasty.

Bruch: That is true, but it depends on the general state of the patient,. We did experiments with corium, and we saw that revascularisation takes place within 16 hours to 3 days.

Kingsnorth: You mentioned that the tensior fasciae latae flap. Is there is a tendency for bowel to appear underneath it because you only have this very thin fascia itself? We have used this technique in one giant inguinal-scrotal hernia in which we actually augmented the TFL flap with polypropylene mesh, so we actually filled the gap, first of all with the mesh, but then we still had a very big tissue gap that we were unable to fill, so we swung around the tensior fasciae latae flap on top of it, and it worked very well indeed. Do you think that it might overcome the shortcoming of the TFL flap if it is augmented with a polypropylene mesh?

Bruch: I think that is an interesting method, and I think it will work. We can ask Professor Berger about this problem with the TFL flap. He can tell us something about the possibilities and problems, I think.

Berger: From the anatomical and mechanical point of view, the flap is very good for the lower abdominal part, but not for the middle part of the abdomen, which you have mentioned before. However, when you bring it up to the thorax aperture, it is of course possible. But because of the anatomical design of this flap, it is better for the lower part. You have to fix it on both sides, not in a very good tension. In all these flaps and all these materials, as you have shown in the dermis graft, you lose tension if it is in a good direction, and in a normal direction the collagen rearranges itself as it should be. If you put it in a lose situation, you immediately lose tension and tensile strength of this part of the fascia. We have to remember that this flap is a combined flap: you have a muscle and you have fascia. The fascia very often heals like a free fascia graft, even if you like to have a long blood supply in the fascia. The distal part of the fascia is not very well supplied with blood when we use it for the abdominal wall. We are dealing with material that should be innovated, and this is possible using microsurgical methods. You will be aware of the pedicle, that you have a neurovascular pedical for your flap. It is very easy if you use a rectus femoris with innervation, and this type of material is the best type of material what we can use.

Peiper: If I understood you correctly, you just take away the epithelial coverage of the cutis during transplantation.

Bruch: It is not necessary if you implant it top down. There are many groups that do not remove the epithelium.

Peiper: So you leave all the structures of the cutis in place. How much of a problem is the formation of retention cysts within the cutis transplant?

Bruch: There is almost no problem, but nobody knows why.

Skandakakis: If you have a patient with a giant hernia, when you have a lot of peritoneal sac, is it possible to use the sac to cover the viscera, perhaps to avoid adhesions?

Bruch: That may be possible, but we have never done that, I must confess.

Amid: We always do that; as a matter of fact, in two cases I re-implanted peritoneum. What we usually do when we have to use peritoneum as a physiological barrier is to save the sac and then rotate it. On two occasions we could not rotate, so I had to use just peritoneum as a free flap to cover the viscera. We did this in only two cases, but there was no problem.

Skandalakis: Let me say something about the omentum. Sometimes it is very short and sometimes very narrow, so we might not have enough omentum to cover all the intestinal loops: perhaps what Dr. Amid says might be a good idea.

Berger: Can I come back to the definition of cutis, dermis and corium. I think we should keep to a clear definition: it is a dermisplasty. When we talk about cutis, we still have the ceratinocytes in mind. Ceratinocytes produce epithelial cysts, and this is usually the origin of an infection.

Bendavid: There were a great number of publications on all these grafts in the 1930s, 1940s and 1950s in North America, and they have largely been abandoned for obvious reasons. Certainly, in the last 20–30 years, I have never seen it done, and I consider it as a form of regression in surgery to have to revert to this. You have excellent materials nowadays, so I cannot see how such a topic would come up in discussion. I have never heard it discussed in North America in the last 20 years.

Stoppa: I wonder about the indication for your autologous material, because I see one remark about the difficulty of realising this type of operation with microsurgery and so on. The second problem is that I wonder about the security and strength of repair edge of your autologous material for a large hernia, because I doubt whether it will be sufficiently strong.

Bruch: I do not think we should use it in large hernias because of the increase in the transverse diameter by maybe 80%; we might get a new herniation if we use it in large hernias. We use a polypropylene mesh in large hernias, as everybody does.

Filipi: That seems to be the trend this morning. Let us ask who in the audience uses cutisplasty, please raise your hand. Two people.

Bendavid: May I make one more comment. It seems to me that the incidence of recurrences is 100% for all of these.

Bruch: I do not agree with that in the long run.

Bendavid: With that form and also with the resorbable meshes, it has certainly also been established. Resorbable meshes result in a 100% incidence of recurrence.

Bruch: Yes, of course, but it is only used, if at all, as an augmentation material for a few weeks, in combination with cutisplasty.

Klaiber: You have to use it as an augmentation itself; it is not sufficient except as an augmentation to the bowel. It is insufficient in an infectious environment, for example.

Skandalakis: Do you have a special dermatome or do you use a knife?

Bruch: We use a knife, because it is easier to use than a dermatome.

Skandalakis: Are you sure that you take the subcutaneous tissue?

Bruch: We remove it with the knife.

References

1. Carlson, M.A., Ludwig, K.A., Condon, R.E.: Ventral hernia and other complications of 1.000 midline incisions. South Med J, 1995, 88: 450–54
2. Gislason, H., Gronbech, J.E., Soreide, O.: Burst abdomen and incisional hernia after major gastrointestinal operations – comparison of three closure techniques. Eur J Surg, 1995, 161: 349–53
3. Zimmermann, G., Müller, G., Haid, A.: Chirurgische Therapie der Narbenhernien. Chirurg, 1991, 62: 656–62

4. Van der Linden, F.T., van Vroonhoven, T.J.: Long-term results after surgical correction of incisional hernia. Neth J Surg, 1988, 40: 127–32
5. Fuchsig, P.: Ursachen, Vorkommen und Verhinderung der Bauchnarbenbrüche. Langenbecks Arch Chir, 1963, 304: 275–86
6. Kirschner, M.: Die praktischen Ergebnisse der freien Fascien-Transplantation. Langenbecks Arch Klin Chir 2, 1910, 888–912
7. Loewe, O. et al.: Über Hautimplantation an Stelle der freien Fascienplastik. Münch Med Wochensr, 1913, 24: 1320–21
8. Rehn, E. et al.: Das kutane und subkutane Bindegewebe als plastisches Material. Münch Med Wochenschr, 1914, 61: 118–21
9. Gallie, W.E., LeMesurier, A.B.: Living sutures in the treatment of hernia. Can Med Assoc J, 1923, 13: 469–80
10. Wangensteen, O.H. et al.: Repair of recurrent and difficult hernias and other large defects of the abdominal wall employing the iliotibial tract of fascia latae as a pedicled flap. Surg Gynecol Obstet, 1934, 59: 759–66
11. Condon, R.E., Nyhus, L.M.: Hernia. Lippincott, Philadelphia, 319
12. Liakakos, T:, Karanikas, I., Panagiotidis, H., Dendrinos, S.: Use of Marlex mesh in the repair of recurrent incisional hernia. Br J Surg, 1994, 81: 248–52
13. Eisner, L., Harder, F.: Narbenhernien. Chirurg, 1997, 68: 304–9
14. Schütter, F.W., Kiroff, P.: Die netzverstärkte Kutisplastik. Langenbecks Arch Chir, 1995, 380: 249–52
15. Kranich, H.: Behandlung großer Narben- und Bauchwandhernien mit einer Modifikation der Kutislappenplastik nach E. Rehn. Zbl Chirurgie, 1990, 115: 301–9
16. Wilker, D., Betz, A., Farthmann, E.H.: Über das Verhalten versenkter Haut zum Ersatz der vorderen Bauchwand der Ratte. Zbl Chirurgie, 1987, 109: 1505–11
17. Reith, H.B., Dittrich, H., Kozuscheck, W.: Morphologie und Einteilung der Kutisplastik bei Bauchwanddefekten – Eine tierexperimentelle Untersuchung. Langenbecks Arch Chir, 1994, 379: 13–9
18. Reith, H.B., Kozuscheck, W.: Behandlung großer Narbenhernien mit der Kutisplastik. Chir Gastroenterologie, 1993, 9: 361–65
19. Schildberg, F.W., Vatankhah, M., Nissen, R.: Chirurgische Behandlung des Narbenbruchs der Bauchdecken. Langenbecks Arch Chir, 1983, 361: 319- 23
20. Piza-Katzer, H., Meissl, G., Stacher, G.: Rekonstruktion von Bauchwanddefekten mit Corium. Chirurg, 1979, 50: 775–79
21. Feifel, G.: Tradition und Fortschritt in der Korrektur von großen Narbenbrüchen. Langenbecks Arch Chir, 1995, 380: 247–48
22. Zimmermann, G., Müller, G., Haid, A.: Chirurgische Therapie der Narbenhernien. Chirurg, 1991, 62: 656–62
23. Owens, N.: Compound neck pedicle designed for the repair of massive facial defects, formation, development and application. Plast Reconstr Surg, 1955, 15: 369–72
24. McGregor, J.C., Buchan, A.C.: Our experience with the tensor fasciae latae myocutaneous flap. B J Plast Surg, 1980, 33: 270–6
25. Papp, Ch.: Die operative Behandlung großer Bauchwandbrüche mit dem M. tensor fasciae latae. Chirurg, 1986, 57: 165–68
26. Papp, Ch., Maurer, H., Zanon, E., Kollreider, A.: Der kombinierte osteomuskuläre M. tensor fasciae latae-M. glutaeus medius-Lappen. Chirurg, 1985, 56: 809–13
27. Mathes, S.J., Buchanan, R.T.: Tensor fascia lata: Neurosensory musculo-cutaneous free flap. B J Plast Surg, 1979, 32: 184–87
28. Krupp, S., Milliet, A.C.: Why and When to delay TFL flaps. Chir Plast, 1982, 7: 23–31
29. Harpf, C., Ninkovic, P., Kronberger, P., Anderl, H.: Dynamische und funktionelle Bauchdeckenstabilisierung, Wiederherstellung von ausgedehnten Bauchwanddefekten. Chirurg, 1997, 68: 488–492
30. Greulich, M., Martin, M., Gubisch, W., Reichert, H.: Anschluß freier Lappenplastiken an die Epigastrica inferior. Handchir Mikrochir Plast Chir, 1991, 23: 28–32

CHAPTER 13

Biomaterials – Classification, Technical and Experimental Aspects

P.K. Amid

While, from the chemical point of view, all these synthetics are completely biocompatible, some physical and structural properties of the prostheses are associated with certain complications. However, these complications are entirely preventable if their causes are recognized in advance and accounted for.

Prevention of biomaterial-related complications requires in-depth knowledge and understanding of the physical properties of prostheses, of which the porosity and the pore size of the materials are of paramount importance. Classification of available biomaterials for hernia surgery is essential for the everyday practical use of prostheses. Based on their pore size, the most frequently used materials in hernia surgery can be grouped into four types [1]:

- *Type I.* Totally macroporous prostheses, such as Atrium, Composix, Marlex, Prolene, Surgipro (monofilament), and Trilex. These prostheses contain pores larger than 75 μm, which is the required pore size for admission of macrophages, fibroblasts (fibroplasia), blood vessels (angiogenesis), and collagen fibers into the pores [1–3].
- *Type II.* Totally microporous prostheses, such as expanded polytetrafluoroethylene (ePTFE; Gore-Tex), surgical membrane, and dual-mesh. These prostheses contain pores that are less than 10 μm in at least one of their three dimensions.
- *Type III.* Macroporous prosthesis with multifilamentous or microporous components, such as PTFE mesh (Teflon), braided Dacron mesh (Mersilene), braided polypropylene mesh (Surgipro), or perforated PTFE patch (MycroMesh).
- *Type IV.* Biomaterials with submicronic pore size, such as Silastic, Cellgard (polypropylene sheeting), Preclude Pricardial membrane, and Preclude Dura Substitute. These are not suitable prostheses for hernia repair per se; however, in combination with type I biomaterials, they can provide adhesion-free composites (such as Composix listed above) for intraperitoneal implantation [4].

Biomaterial-related complications frequently encountered in hernia surgery include infection, seroma formation, intestinal adhesion, bowel obstruction, erosion of the prostheses into the adjacent hollow viscus, and failure of the repair due to contraction of the prostheses.

13.1 Infection

Surgical infection promoted by implantation of biomaterials, such as sutures and prostheses, is caused by infiltration and proliferation of bacteria into and within the pores and interstices of these synthetic materials. When interstices or pores are less than 10 μm in each of their three dimensions, bacteria averaging 1 μm cannot be eliminated by macrophages and neurophilic granulocytes, which are too large to enter a 10-mm three-dimensional pore [5]. Braided sutures and prosthetic material with interstices and pores less than 10 μm provide a suitable housing for bacteria and the development of infection by admitting bacteria but excluding macrophages. By admitting both macrophages and bacteria, biomaterials with pores larger than 10 mm create a major challenge for the proliferation of bacteria and thus do not contribute to the development of surgical infection.

Type II and III prostheses are similar to braided suture materials and by harboring bacteria can promote their growth, likewise resulting in biomaterial-related infection [1, 5].

In contrast to types II and III, type I prostheses deter housing and growth of bacteria, not only by admitting macrophages, but also because they allow rapid fibroplasia and angiogenesis within their sufficiently wide pores, which also prevents infiltration and growth of bacteria.

Frequently, sinus tract formation and chronic infection following type I prosthetic repair of hernias are caused by utilization of multifilamentous suture material for the fixation of the mesh, although they are mistaken for being caused by the mesh itself.

Although the infection rate associated with type II and III prostheses is within a reasonable rate, higher rates of between 9.6% [6] and 50% [7] associated with their utilization have been reported. Such numbers have not been encountered in association with type I biomaterials.

More importantly, in connection with surgical infection from other causes, the totally macroporous prostheses (type I) do not have to be extracted; drainage of the infected area, followed by local wound care, is all that is necessary to manage the infection. By contrast, total removal of the type II prosthesis and at least partial removal of the type III prosthesis is required in order to manage infection associated with their utilization.

13.2 Seroma

Postoperative prosthesis-related seroma formation is caused by host inflammatory reaction to the prosthesis (which modern biomaterials have made negligible) and by the dead space created between the prosthesis and host tissue. Adequate pore size gives type I and III prostheses sufficient molecular permeability to allow penetration of host proteinaceous material into their pores [1]. Since this results in a rapid fibrinous fixation of the mesh to the tissue and elimination of the dead space between the prosthesis and the host tissue, the chance of seroma formation is minimized [1]. Sufficient molecular permeability also results in the formation of proper scaffolding for future host tissue incorporation [2], which – by filling up the pores of the mesh and making them inaccessible to bacteria – further decreases the chance of biomaterial-related seroma formation and infection.

The risk of seroma can be reduced to virtually zero by avoiding direct contact with the subcutaneous adipose tissue by retromuscular or subaponeurotic placement of the mesh [4], as well as closed system drainage of the surgical field whenever a large sheet of mesh is used.

Because of their inadequate pore size, type II biomaterials lack sufficient molecular permeability for the host fibrinous and proteinaceous materials, thus resulting in slow elimination of the dead space between the prosthesis and the host tissue and the formation of seroma [1].

Although the reported rate of seroma formation associated with type II prostheses is within a reasonable range, higher rates of 14.6% have been reported [6]. No such increased rates of seroma formation have been cited in the surgical literature in connection with properly implanted type I and III prostheses.

13.3 Intestinal Adhesions and Fistula Formations

The most important characteristics of ideal prostheses for abdominal wall hernia surgery are macroporosity and surface texture [1, 2]. These qualities combine to create the degree of host tissue infiltration into the prostheses which is crucial for a strong and secure hernia repair. However, an undesirable side effect of macroporosity is the adherence of macroporous meshes to the bowel, when they come in direct contact with the intestinal tract [4, 8]. This in turn leads to bowel obstruction and intestinal fistula formation [4, 8]. At the present time, all available prostheses (absorbable and nonabsorbable) adhere to the intestines [4]. Covering the mesh on its intestinal side with a layer of absorbable material such as Vicryl or with an ePTFE patch does not solve this problem [8] (Fig. 1). In order to prevent mesh-related intestinal complications, we suggest covering the visceral side of the mesh with a layer of a tissue-impervious biomaterial [4]. A variety of tissue-impervious biomaterials, such as Silastic, polypropylene sheeting, and ePTFE of submicronic pore size (Preclude Pericordial Membrane and Preclude Dura Substitute; Gore) are available for this purpose. These composites or the commercially available product (Composix; Davol) offer an excellent tissue ingrown while avoiding intestinal adhesions and their concomitant complications (Fig. 2).

13.4 Shrinkage of the Prosthesis

13.4.1 Collapse of the Prosthetic Plug (Mesh Plug)

After implantation, and depending on their looseness, mesh plugs shrink up to 75% in size, thus failing to secure the repair. A loose or soft plug which can be collapsed by pinching it between two fingers (the pinch test) loses size during the patient's own scarring process. As a result, the anchoring sutures of the plug pull through the margin of the hernia defect, leading to recurrence of the hernia. More importantly, after scarification and shrinkage, even a soft plug assumes a rock-hard consistency (Fig. 3), which can erode into the bladder [1], intestines [9], and major blood vessels [10] or migrate down to the scrotum (Fig. 3).

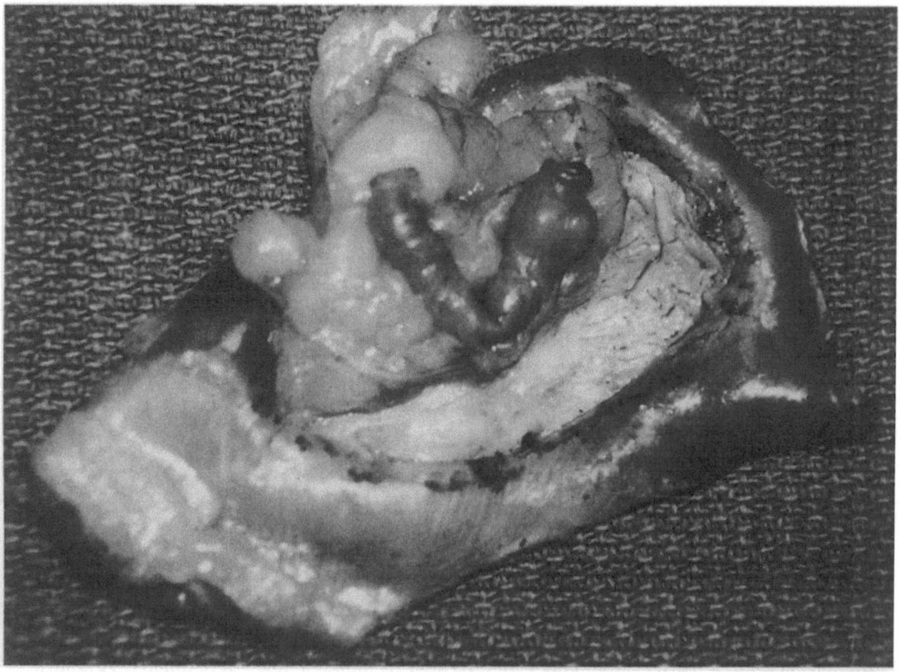

Fig. 1. Adhesion of the intestine to Marlex/Vicryl composite (rabbit model)

Fig. 2. Adhesion-free composite removed 6 months after its implantation showing no sign of adhesion (rabbit model)

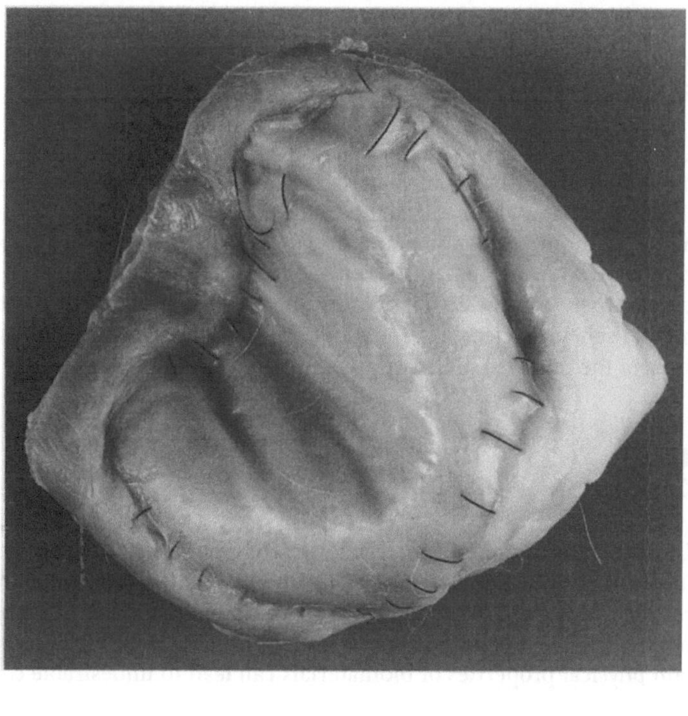

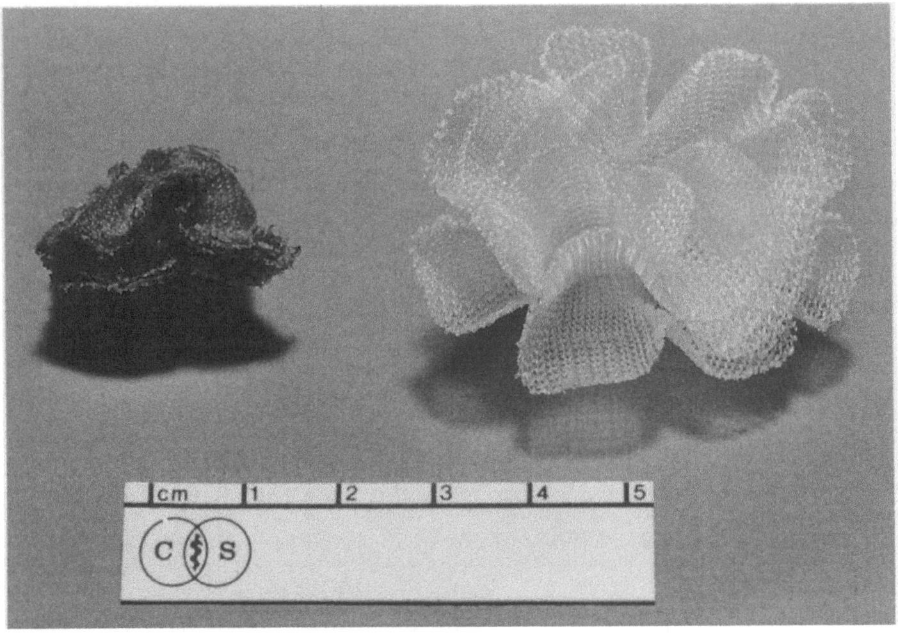

Fig. 3. Shrinkage of a "Perfix" mesh plug 4 months after its implantation. Approximately 70% shrinkage compared with an unused plug. Approximately 30% shrinkage compared with the plug after its insertion into the defect

13.4.2
Shrinkage of the Mesh Patch

Contraction of the mesh fibers during the scarring process leads to shrinkage of the mesh after implantation in vivo. Radiographic measurements of the distances between the metallic staples used for the preperitoneal mesh repair of incisional hernias [1] made 10 months after implantation reveal a contraction of approximately 20% as compared to measurements taken shortly after the procedure [1]. Furthermore, comparison between mesh removed from patients and processed through an alcohol-methyl salicylate clearing sequence with that of a control demonstrates that the pore sizes of the removed mesh are approximately 20% smaller [1].

13.5
Conclusion

Utilization of synthetic materials in abdominal wall hernia surgery has become increasingly popular. The use of synthetic mesh to achieve tension-free repair has resulted in a significant reduction in postoperative pain, the length of the recovery period, and the rate of postoperative recurrences. However, it must be noted that certain physical properties of biomaterials can lead to undesirable consequences, including increased risk of infection, seroma formation, biomaterial-related intestinal obstruction and fistula formation, and failure of the repair due to shrinkage of the mesh. If the mechanisms of these problems are understood and proper precautions are taken, prostheses can be used with minimal or no complications. These precautions include the following:

1. The risk of infection can be avoided by utilization of type I prostheses.
2. The risk of seroma formation can be virtually eliminated by subaponeurotic and retromuscular implantation of type I and III prostheses and drainage of the surgical field whenever a large sheet of mesh is used.
3. The possibility of mesh-related intestinal adhesion, bowel obstruction, and fistula formation can be eliminated by avoiding direct contact between the mesh and the intestinal tract or utilization of adhesion-free composites.
4. Finally, problems associated with contraction of the mesh can be circumvented by using a sufficiently large piece of mesh to provide adequate mesh–tissue interface beyond the boundary of the hernia defect and by maintaining adequate laxity of the mesh while it is being fixed to the abdominal wall tissue.

13.6 Discussion

Simmermacher: In your original presentation in *Hernia*, you talked about four groups of biomaterials and now you only have three. I know that the last one is probably the subporous group which you told us is not suitable for abdominal wall repair, at least not on its own. You demonstrated that the type I (macroporous) mesh is actually suitable for abdominal wall repair, but how is the pore size determined? Is it the smallest pore you can find in the three-dimensional prosthesis which determines its fate?

Amid: I did in fact have four types in *Hernia*. At that time the composite was not commercially available. So I listed those things that you can attach to a mesh yourself as a group of its own, and under that I had the surgical membrane and others. But now that this is available, I did not mention it here at all. As for the pore size: on polypropylene meshes there is no pore less than 10 mm, unless you are talking about where the two fibers are in contact with each other. I think you are probably referring to Gore-Tex, where you also see large pores. But the pore size should not be less than 1 mm in any of the two surface dimensions. If you have a pore size of 100 mm long and 3 mm wide, that can house bacteria, so even if one dimension of two surface dimensions is less than 10 mm, theoretically bacteria can be housed.

Bruch: May I ask you why the macroporous mesh shrinks by 20%–40%? Is it the effusion of softness, or is it the scar formation?

Amid: It is the scar formation – it is not like shrinking of fabrics. The shrinkage of fabrics is caused by the foreshortening of the fibers. If you have a pore size of, say, 1x1 cm, when it shrinks it contracts, and each fiber wrinkles; 1x1 cm then becomes 0.8x0.8 cm because of the shrinkage. If you leave this material for 2 weeks, its memory will come back and then you go back to the original 1x1 cm, so it is not really foreshortening, it is shrinkage. That is why the larger the original pores are, the more shrinkage you have. That can be very easily accounted for; all you have to do is use a wider mesh and leave the mesh more relaxed to allow for shrinkage.

Schumpelick: I do not think that your statement – the larger the pore size, the larger the shrinkage – is totally correct. I believe that shrinkage depends on scar formation. And there are different sizes of scar formation in relation to different type of material. Shrinkage is the result of scars around the pores, and if you have a mesh-like scar, you will not have shrinkage, but if there is a plate of scar, there will be more shrinkage. Later on, we will see a slide with whole-size polypropylene sheets in animals; within 2 years sarcomas developed in 100%, and I would therefore be very careful and would warn everyone about putting a sheet of polypropylene within the belly.

Amid: I completely agree with your first point. I am just guessing that the larger the pore, the more shrinkage there is; I have not really studied that. Your comment makes sense, because if you have less scar tissue or softer scar tissue then there is less contraction. That would be a good thing for future study – to compare two different things and see the shrinkage. I am not quite sure that I quite understand your other question. You are talking about sarcoma formation, but I have never seen anything about it in the literature. Are you talking about malignant sarcoma? That is be the first I have heard of it. I do not know whether anyone else has heard about sarcoma associated with mesh. That throws a dark shadow over mesh.

Bendavid: May I make some comments concerning any of the tumors. In a textbook on prosthesis and hernia surgery, there was an excellent chapter by Nick Stansiwick, an experienced review of all materials, and we have not yet reported a single case associated with Marlex Gore-Tex. As far as shrinkage is concerned, if you were to measure those pores after 10 years, does it mean that the shrinkage increases to 40%–50%?

Amid: I do not know. My experience is limited to about three or four patients in whom, for different reasons, I had to remove the mesh or just for the purpose of this study I removed just a little piece of mesh, and I guess the longest one was about 1 year.

Bendavid: I guess you can probably measure them regularly over the next few years. Another question, in retromuscular position, do you really need a combination of Gore-Tex and Marlex?

Amid: No, if the peritoneum is intact, there is no real need for that. But let me clarify something: although this composite is my design and I get royalties on it, it is not recommended and not necessary to use it unless you really have to, because it is expensive, so it should be used only if you do not have anything to protect the intestine from the mesh; it does not have a very wide use.

Bendavid: The staples you showed on your mesh looked pretty nasty. Have you lost any of them in the abdominal cavity?

Amid: No, this is the type of stapler that was manufactured by U.S. Surgical many years ago to close the abdominal wall. The only reason that I showed it is that I also use the articulating Endohernia stapler in some cases, and these staplers are very small and do have not enough holding power. These bigger staplers really go through; they basically do the same thing sutures do; in fact, you have to be careful if you have a skinny patient that they do not go through the skin.

Bendavid: One last comment, as a warning. As you know –we have talked about it before – I started using the combination, and approximately 1 month later Ethicon called me about a product that they had which combined Marlex and Gore-Tex; it makes sense, because Gore-Tex supposedly eliminates adhesions and Marlex allows much better incorporation within scar tissue. However, I am not so sure that the product is as good as it ought to be, because one of my objections to that mesh – and the reason why I still use the two separate sheets – is that I have had the experience on recurrent incisional hernia of finding bowel included in the Gore-Tex suture. This happened on three occasions. You actually dissect and find that you cannot remove the Gore-Tex because it is literally an integral part of the bowel; then you have to dissect it and leave it inside. If you have two sheets, separately, you can actually suture, and in certain cases continuously suture throughout the circumference of the Marlex, never picking up the Gore-Tex, which is deep to it. I think that is very important.

Amid: Are you referring to sutures that are used to suture PTFE to Marlex?

Bendavid: No, that you can do outside the patient; you can put in four sutures and actually keep the two layers together. But once you have put the combination within the peritoneum cavity, you can put interrupted sutures circumferentially, it may take 10–15 min, but once it is in place then I usually run the continuous suture to incorporate only the Marlex to the edge of the defect.

Amid: That depends on the technique you use, but for both of the things that I showed you, both the handmade and the commercially available one, the sutures that are fixing these things together are not supposed to be in the intestine.

Stoppa: A technical questions about your stitching in composite mesh; you place it intraperitoneally if I understood correctly?

Amid: No, not really, I was not referring to placement of the composite intraperitoneally. I made a vague passing remark about the way I do your procedure: it is retromuscular, it is over the peritoneum in the lower abdomen over the posterior rectum sheath, above the umbilicus or line of Douglas.

Stoppa: I am talking about composite mesh. Do you place it extraperitoneally?

Amid: Extraperitoneally, yes. So far I have not had any patient in which there was no peritoneum that I had to implant it inside. The reason why I did it in these cases was that there were holes in the peritoneum that I could not close. I made an attempt to close them, but the sutures would come through. So, although I had a layer of peritoneum, I had several holes on the peritoneum, and patients did not have omentum. I therefore used this in the retromuscular place.

Stoppa: But a composite mesh should be a simplification of the technique to cure large hernias.

Amid: That is right, it is just a matter of simplification. But only extraperitoneally.

Stoppa Do you see any neuralgia?

Amid: No, because with your technique the intercostal nerves are quite visible; if I am correct, that is the lateral border of dissection. The staplers are placed in between the neurovascular pedicals, so it is easy to avoid.

Flament: I have the same concerns as Robert; I agree with everything you told us. In France, we had a disastrous experience 20 years ago with composite mesh. It was smooth, Silastic, on one side and velvet on the other. The smooth side caused seromas, and the velvet side prevented removal of the mesh. So I agree with placing a composite mesh intraperitoneally, but I disagree with composite mesh in a closed space. One side will create seromas and then infection, and the other side will create adhesions to the muscle and prevent removal of the prosthesis if you have to.

Amid: I agree completely with you. But the reason that I used it is the fact that I had several relatively large holes on the peritoneum, so I thought any seroma would go into there. I do not recommend using it if you have a completely intact peritoneum, because (a) it is not necessary, (b) it causes the complication you mentioned, and (c) it is expensive, so there is no reason to use it.

Bendavid: Dr. Flament, you cannot compare Watergon with anything else, just like you cannot take any other two meshes we use, e.g., PTFE, which is Teflon, not ePTFE. Those results were also disastrous. What I would like to ask is, if you put it extraperitoneally, why bother with Gore-Tex?

Amid: That is exactly my point. If you are extraperitoneal and your peritoneum is intact, you do not have to use it. You see, with this procedure I try not to get into the peritoneal cavity, as Dr. Wantz has described, but we occasionally make holes in the peritoneum by accident. If the peritoneum is very thin, and you attempt to close them, the suture does not hold. Then you are left with several holes. That is the only time that I would use this in the extraperitoneal position. Otherwise it is only really good for intraperitoneal applications.

References

1. Amid PK. (1997) Classification of biomaterials and their related complications in abdominal wall hernia surgery. Hernia 1:15–21.
2. Bobyn JD, Wilson Gj, MacGregor DC, Pilliar RM, Weatherly Gc (1982) Effect of pore size on the peel strength of attachment of fibrous tissue to porous-surfaced implants, J Biomed Matér, Res 571–584.
3. White RA, Hirose FM, Sproat RW, Lawrence RS, Nelson RJ (1981) Histopathology observations after short-term implantation of two porous elastomers in dogs. Biomaterials 2:171–176.
4. Amid PK, Shulman AG, Lichtenstein IL, Sostrin S, Young J, Hakakha M.(1994) An experimental evaluation of a new composite mesh with the selective property of incorporation to the abdominal wall without adhering to the intestines. J Biomed Materials Res 28:373–75.
5. Alexander JW, Kaplan JZ, Altmeier WA (1967) Rose of suture materials in the development of wound infection. Ann Surg 165:192–1991.
6. DeBord JR, Wyffels PL, Marshall JS, Miller G, Marxhall WH (1992) Repair of large ventral incisional hernias with expanded polytetrafluoroethylene prosthetic patch. Postgrad Gen Surg 4:156–160.
7. Smith RS (1971) The use of prosthetic materials in the repair of hernias. Surg Clin North Am 51:1387–1399.
8. Soler M. Verhaeghe P, Essomba A. Sevestre H, Stoppa R (1993) Treatment of postoperative incisional hernias by a composite prosthetics (polyester-polyglactin 910). Clinical and experimental study. Ann Chir 47:598–608.
9. Danielli PG, Kurihara H, Montecamozzo G, et al (1997) Le complicanze dei plugs: Infezione e recidive. Hernia 1(1):55.
10. Cristaldi M, Pisacreta M, Elli M, et al. (1997) Femoro-poplieteal by-pass occlusion following mesh-plug for prevascular femoral hernia repair. Hernia 1:197–199.

CHAPTER 14

Biocompatibility of Biomaterials – Clinical and Mechanical Aspects

J. Conze, U. Klinge

14.1 Introduction

For good clinical results in abdominal hernia surgery, a perfect correspondence is required between the mechanical aspects of the abdominal wall and the mechanical aspects of the biomaterial used for repair. By using biomaterial for abdominal wall reinforcement or even replacement, the surgeon should try to stick as close to the original as possible in an attempt to imitate nature.

There are many mechanical aspects of the abdominal wall that have to be considered. In addition to the anatomy, which was described and discussed in Part I, it is necessary to know the different mechanical strains in the abdominal wall, and these can be measured and described in numbers. They include intra-abdominal pressure, which varies under different circumstances, tension strength, i.e., the stress within the abdominal wall resulting from intra-abdominal pressure, and tensile strength, i.e., the ability to withstand mechanical stress, a kind of holding force.

Important for clinical aspects is the mobility of the abdominal wall and its possible restriction after hernia repair.

All these different aspects of the abdominal wall should be taken into account when using biomaterials for hernia repair. This means that the tensile strength of meshes should be adapted to the physiological tensile strength of the abdominal wall. Furthermore, a mesh should show symmetric strains in all directions and should allow the same mobility as the abdominal wall.

It is mobility that is most important for patients' comfort and their ability to bend forwards and backwards and to turn around the way they did before the hernia occurred. Thus the results of hernia repair should not only be judged on the recurrence rate, but also on the mobility of the abdominal wall.

In 1995, we performed a follow-up study of all hernia patients [1]. The results in patients after repair with Marlex mesh using the sublay technique showed a very low recurrence rate. However, some patients complained of a reduction in the mobility of the abdominal wall. They had difficulties in bending forward or problems in turning round to look over their shoulder. One patient who had undergone a large mesh repair could not even tie his shoelaces by himself anymore. The personal complaints varied between the above-mentioned immobility to the sensation of a foreign body and sensitivity to the weather, all connected with the use of biomaterials.

14.2 Three-Dimensional Stereography

To investigate these complaints, we developed a method to measure and analyze the dynamics of the abdominal wall using three-dimensional stereography. This optical method to measure surface areas was first used in 1898 for planimetric examination of the back [3]. It is based on the principle of stereophotogrammetry, but uses one camera with a line projector instead of two cameras (Fig. 1).

For video documentation, a light grid is projected onto the abdominal wall in maximal abdominal wall excursion. Two video images show the surface changes at the beginning and end of movement (Fig. 2). After digitalization of the pictures, we calculate the surface deformity. We receive data on the height difference (which is calculated from the change in the highest point on inspiration and expiration), the abdominal wall curvature (which is measured over the abdominal midline as the second deviation), and a fictive adjusted radius (which is calculated as a sphere fitted into all abdominal surface coordinates) (Fig. 3).

Comparing these results with the data of a control group that did not undergo an operation, we found a highly significant reduction in all three aspects of abdominal wall mobility (Fig. 4).

With regard to the textile characteristics, the results of three-dimensional stereometry and patients' complaints led to the hypothesis that the current available meshes are oversized. Adapting the meshes to the physiological strains of the abdominal wall should improve biocompatibility.

In the following the physiological strains of the abdominal wall are described.

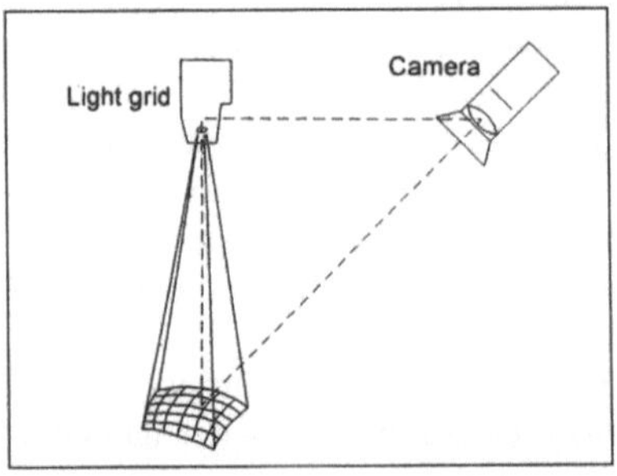

Fig. 1. Three-dimensional stereography

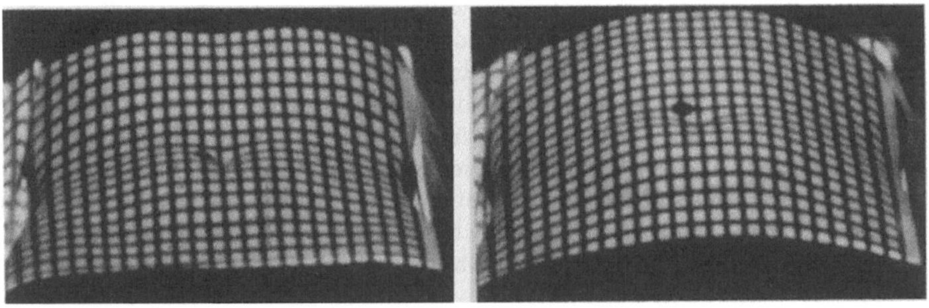

Fig. 2. Light grid projected onto the abdominal wall in maximum excursion

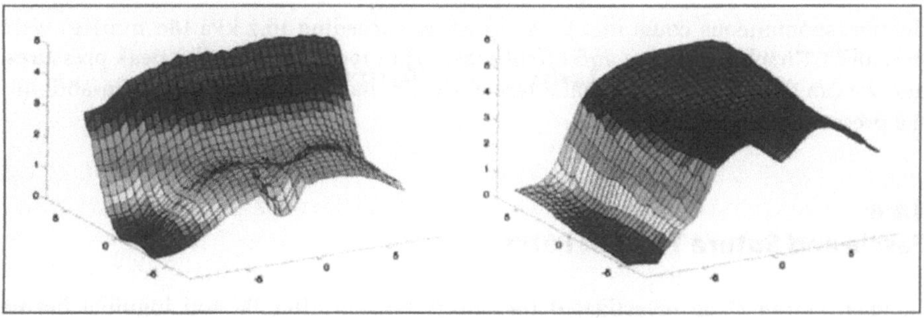

Fig. 3. Reconstruction of the abdominal surface (second deviation)

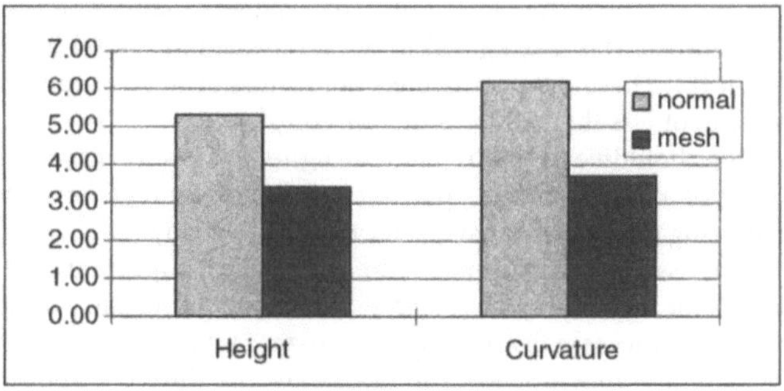

Fig. 4. Three-dimensional stereography: height and curvature after mesh repair and in control group

14.3 Intra-abdominal Pressure

Intra-abdominal pressure (Table 1) depends on the body position, standing or supine, and increases by pressing in coughing, vomiting, and defecation or in pain.

In 1870, Paul Bert [3] was the first person to describe a method to measure intra-abdominal pressure by placing a balloon in the rectum ampulla of dogs and connecting the instrument to a water manometer.

In 1948, Dyre et al. [4] investigated intra-abdominal pressure in humans and measured a mean pressure of 8 cm water column (1.45 kPa), with an increase of up to 3 cm water column on respiration. During vomiting, it could reach up to 80 cm water column (14.5 kPa).

Caix et al. [5] found a baseline pressure of about 1.07 kPa measured in humans postoperatively. In deep breathing, it increased by up to 0.5 kPa (4 mmHg), and in pro-

Table 1. Intra-abdominal pressure

Reference	Year	Baseline pressure (kPa)	Peak pressure (kPa)
[4]	1948	1.45	14.5
[6]	1973	-	19.9
[7]	1991	-	13.9
[5]	1997	1.07 kPa	10.7 kPa

ductive, spontaneous coughing, peak pressures exceeding 10.7 kPa (80 mmHg) were measured. Kirsch [6] in 1973 and Effenberger [7] in 1991 found similar peak pressures, and we can therefore assume that a fascial closure has to withstand an intra-abdominal pressure of up to 20 kPa.

14.4 Fascia and Suture Tearout Force

In 1994, Lipton et al. investigated the suture tension after Bassini inguinal hernia repair and after aponeurotic repair in humans. In the Bassini group, he measured a mean suture tension of 633±239 g; in the other group, after suturing the fascia transversalis, a suture tension of only 3.9±2.9 g was found. The tearout force of the external aponeurosis was 2–4 kg. All in all, he measured a total holding force of 1.3 kg or 1.3 *N*/cm [8]. These data confirmed the results of Read's study in 1981, in which a suture tension of less than 2 N was measured [9].

For Shouldice hernia repair, Calcagno and Wantz measured the tension required to bring tissue into precise approximation. The average tension of the imbricating layer requiring the fascia transversalis was 29±16 g [10].

Our own investigations of the mechanical aspects in the groin region confirmed values for the suture tension of less than 500 g over the wound length [11].

In postmortem examinations in 1974, Tauber and Seidel investigated the mechanical stability and resistance to tearing of the different abdominal wall structures [12, 13] (Table 2). They differentiated between longitudinal and horizontal tearing forces. The abdominal fascia of the linea alba showed the best resistance in the horizontal direction and ruptured at 82 *N*/cm; in the longitudinal direction, it ruptured at 32 *N*/cm. The ventral and posterior layer of the rectus sheath showed a tearing resistance of 74 *N*/cm and 67 *N*/cm in the horizontal direction and of only 20*N*/cm and 15 *N*/cm in the longitudinal direction, respectively. The resistance and strength of the abdominal fascia are four times as high in the horizontal direction as in the longitudinal direction.

When testing the suture tearout force, Tauber and Seidel found that the tearout force was one third to one fourth of normal tissue.

In postmortem studies Greenall investigated the force necessary to tear a thread in the transverse and longitudinal direction. Depending on the suture distance from the margin of the incisions (5 or 10 mm), he measured a suture tearout force of 1.78 or 5.75 kg in the transverse incision. In vertical incisions, rupture occurred at a force of 0.9 or 2.6 kg [14].

Table 2. Tensile strength of human fascia postmortem [12, 13]

Fascia	Horizontal (*N*/cm)	Longitudinal (*N*/cm)
Linea alba	82	32
Ventral sheet of rectus	74	20
Posterior sheet	67	15

14.5 Tension Strength

Of special interest for the mechanical aspects of the biocompatibility of biomaterials is the tension strength of the abdominal wall. This is the mechanical stress within the abdominal wall resulting from intra-abdominal pressure.

According to the law of Laplace, the tension strength of the abdominal wall is the product of the intra-abdominal pressure and the quotient of the radius and twice the wall thickness:

$$K=p^*(r/2s)$$

where K is the wall tension, p the pressure, r the radius, and s the wall thickness. By taking an abdominal circumference of 100 cm, equivalent to a radial diameter of 31.83 cm, and a thickness of the abdominal wall of 0.08 cm, we arrive at a tension strength for the abdominal wall of 20 kp/cm² or 196.2 *N*/cm².

14.6 Tensile Strength

Tensile strength is the ability of material or tissue to withstand mechanical stress, a kind of holding force.

Assuming the abdominal cavity to be a thin, hollow sphere, the total tensile strength can be calculated by multiplying the tension strength ($K=p^*r/2s$) by the area A of the abdominal wall ($A=2p^*r^*s$). A simple calculation shows that the tensile strength is not related to wall thickness:

$$F_{total}=p^*r/2s^*2\pi^*r^*s=p^*p^*r^2$$

Dividing this by the abdominal circumference of 100 cm, the total tensile strength per cm abdominal wall can be calculated by the following formula:

$$F=p^*d/4 \text{ (N/cm)}$$

where *F* is tensile strength per centimeter circumference, *d* diameter, and *p* pressure [10].

Taking into account these considerations and assuming a maximal intra-abdominal pressure of 20 kPa and a human body diameter of 32 cm, we arrive at a maximum tensile strength of 16 *N*/cm per cm abdominal wall.

The value calculated using this theoretical model shows about the same height as found by Tauber and Seidel in their postmortem examinations of human fascia, already mentioned above. This confirms the mathematical theory that tensile strength does not need to exceed 16 *N*/cm.

14.7 Mechanical Aspects of Biomaterial

A large number of different meshes are available. They differ in material, number of filaments, pore size, and various mechanical aspects (Table 3).

Amid elaborated a systematic approach, published in 1997, with four types of meshes to characterize the different mesh materials available [11]:

1. Macroporous (>75 mm): Atrium, Marlex, Prolene,Trelex, monofilament polypropylene
2. Microporus (<10 mm): expanded polytetrafluoroethylene (ePTFE)/Gore-Tex
3. Macroporus multifilament or combined with microporous components: PTFE/Teflon, perforated PTFE/MycroMesh, multifilament polypropylene/Soft Hernia Mesh (SHM) and SurgiPro, Dacron/Mersilene
4. Submicronic pore size (>1 mm): Silastic, Cellgard Sheet

Meshes are not knitted or woven materials, but hosiery. To obtain precise and comparable information, independent textile analysis according to existing rules issued by the German Standardization Institute is necessary. Mesh parameters of interest are weight (g/m^2), proportion of pores (%) or pore size, and textile surface per cm^2. Of particular interest in mechanical terms are bending stiffness ($N/100\ cm^2$), maximum tearing force ($N/5$ cm) in the vertical and horizontal direction, suture tearout force (N), tensile strength, and elongation at 16 N/cm (%).

Different tests are used to measure these parameters. A typical method to investigate the maximum tearing force in the vertical and horizontal direction is strip tensiometry. The same principle is used as for the suture tearout test.

To measure and compare tensile strength, the abdominal wall physiology is simulated by testing the strain exerted by a stamp, the so-called stamp-strain test. In comparison to strip tensiometry, a symmetric strain is achieved not only between the two ends of a mesh strip, but also of an determined area with a fixed stamp radius. A respective value can be determined using the stamp-strain test by relating the stamp pressure to the mesh perimeter.

Table 3. Alloplastic materials used for hernia repair

Material	Trade name
Polypropylene	Marlex (monofilament)
	Prolene (double monofilament)
	Surgipro (multifilament)
	Soft Hernia Mesh (multifilament)
	Atrium (monofilament)
Polytetrafluoroethylene (PTFE)	Teflon (multifilament)
	Gore-Tex (soft tissue patch)
	Dual Mesh
	MycroMesh (2-mm perforations)
Polyvinyl	Ivalon Sponge
Polyamid	Nylon
Polyester	Mersilene (multifilament)
	Dacron
Polyglactin 910	Vicryl (absorbable)
Polyglycolic acid	Dexon (absorbable)

We have tested several meshes and mesh modifications in collaboration with a textile institute. In summary, the results of strip tensiometrty and, even more so, of the stamp-strain test prove the hypothesis that meshes are oversized compared to the required physiological strains of the abdominal wall. They revealed a striking asymmetry, which is indicated by the linear rupture in the stamp-strain test.

As a consequence of this, we decided to develop a new mesh, adapted to the physiological strains.: We decided to use polypropylene because of the uncertain long-term reaction by hydrolytic degradation of polyester in vivo [17–19]. Just recently, Riepe and colleagues were able to demonstrate that hydrolytic degradation of polyester takes place with increasing time of implantation in humans. Analysis by linear regression showed a decrease in bursting strength of over 31% in 10 years and a 100% loss of bursting strength in 25–39 years [20].

We chose a multifilament polypropylene, temporarily named Soft Hernia Mesh (SHM), with a polypropylene part (PP) of less than 30% of the Marlex mesh and with an increased pore size of 5 mm (Fig. 5) (Vypro). The very low stiffness of the permanent structure requiered a combination with an absorbable polyglactin to temporarily ease its use by the surgeon and to decrease the polypropylene-related inflammatory response [21].

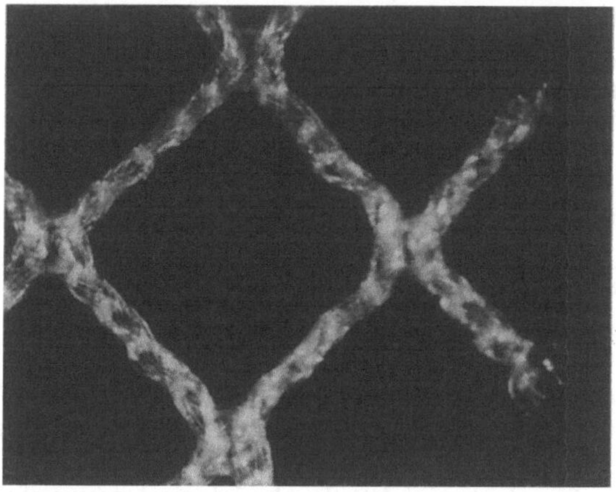

Fig. 5. Vypro® Mesh

14.8 Textile Analysis Results

Table 4 shows a textile analysis of nonabsorbable mesh materials. The most common meshes, Marlex, Prolene, and Mersilene, were compared with the new SHM. When testing SHM, we differentiated between the complete mesh and the remaining polypropylene part of the mesh.

Comparison of the mechanical aspects such as tensile strength in different directions, measured by strip tensiometry, showed not only that the meshes were oversized, as expected, but also a striking asymmetry when tearing in different directions.

By testing the meshes with the stamp-strain test, it became even more obvious that the common meshes are too strong compared with the physiological strains of the

Table 4. Textile analysis of nonabsorbable mesh materials

	Mersilene	Marlex	Prolene	SHM	PP (part of SHM)
Material	Polyester	Polypropylene	Polypropylene	Polypropylene and polyglactin	Polypropylene
Filament	Multifilament	Monofilament	Monofilament	Multifilament	Multifilament
Weight (g/m²)	39.5	95.09	108.5	56.64	26.77
Pore proportion (%)	89.78	85.26	83.2	90.77	92.86
Textile surface per cm² (mm²)	0.1	1.3	1.5	0.4–1.0	0.2
Bending stiff ness (*N*/100 cm²)					
Vertical	0.4	34.7	6.7	6.6	1.8
Horizontal	0.1	134.4	12.9	2.0	0.6
Tensile strength (*N*/5 cm)					
Vertical	205	432	597	387	132
Horizontal	101	567	767	63	55
Suture tearout test (*N*)					
Vertical	15.2	57.2	57	29.6	17.5
Horizontal	15.5	55.8	74.6	29.0	22.7
Rip continuation force (*N*)					
Vertical	6	7	<0.1	10	9
Horizontal	7	40	44	11	12
Stamp-strain test tensile strength/*r* contact (*N*/cm)	19.5	58.8	90.9	31.9	16.1
Elongation under 16 *N*/cm (%)	15.8	13.7	6.9	15.8	31.2

SHM, Soft Hernia Mesh; PP, polpropylene part.

abdominal wall. Considering a tensile strength of 16 *N*/cm as the maximum necessary, the tensile strength of Marlex and Prolene meshes far exceed this figure, with a tensile strength of 58.8 and >90 *N*/cm, respectively.

In order to simulate the physiological strains of the abdominal wall, we investigated the elongation of the meshes under a stamp pressure of 16 *N*/cm. For Prolene, we found a elongation of only 6.9%, for Marlex 13.7%, for Mersilene 15.8%, and for SHM 31.2% . This value corresponds to the elongation of the abdominal wall. Furthermore, SHM showed a circular rupture when exceeding the pressure above the tensile strength in comparison to the linear rupture of all the other meshes.

The primary aim of reducing the proportion of foreign material can be seen when comparing the different values for weight, pore proportion, and textile surface per cm2. The lightest mesh is the new SHM, with the largest pore size and proportion and a weight of 26.77 g/m². The Marlex mesh weighs more than three time as much, with a textile surface per cm² of 1.3 mm² compared to 0.2 mm² in SHM.

The textile characteristics with the mechanical aspects shown above can only give an indication of clinical suitability. They cannot show the interaction in vivo between incorporated mesh and induced scar tissue.

Until now, by reducing polypropylene and using larger pore sizes, there has been a remarkable improvement in tissue reaction and abdominal wall mobility. In the following chapter, Dr. Klinge and Dr. Klosterhalfen will present the experimental and histological results.

14.9 Discussion

For a discussion, please see Chap. 16.

References

1. Schumpelick V, Conze J, Klinge U (1996) Die praeperitoneale Netzplastik in der Reparation der Narbenhernie. Chirurg 67:1028–1035
2. Gäbel H (1993) Photogrammetrisches Verfahren zur Erfassung von menschlichen Körperoberflächen. Dissertation: Fachbereich Bauingenieur- und Vermessungswesen, Technische Universität Braunschweig
3. Bert P (1870) Lecons sur la physiologie comparee de la respiration. Bailliere,Paris,pp338–346)
4. Dyre JC (1948) Intraabdominal pressure in the human. Surg-Gynecol-Obstet87:472–475).
5. Caix et al.(1997) Functional anatomy of the muscles of the anterolateral abdominal wall: electromyography and histoenzymology. In: Hernias and surgery of the abdominal wall, JP Chevrel (ed), pp 32–42, Springer, Berlin Heidelberg New York
6. Kirsch U (1973) Zu Naht and Knoten. In Melsunger Med. Mitteilungen, Fa. Braun Melsunger, Band 47, 117:95–116
7. Effenberger T (1991) Druckparameter des abdomnellen Faszienverschlusses. Ethicon Symposium, Hamburg
8. Lipton S, Estrin J, Nathan I. (1994)A biomechanical study of the aponeurotic inguinal hernia repair. J-Am-Coo-Surg. 178:595–9.
9. Read R, McLeod C.(1981) Influence of a relaxing incision on suture tension in Bassini and McVay's repairs. Arch Surg 116:440–5.
10. Calcagno D, Wantz GE. (1985) Suture tension and the Shouldice repair. Lancet 22:1446(letter)
11. Peiper et al. In press
12. Tauber R (1975) Bedeutung mechanischer Faktoren bei der Entstehung der abdominellen Wunddehiszenz. Zentrbl Chir 19:1178–82)
13. Seidel W (1974) Messungen zur Festigkleit der Bauchdeckennaht. Chirurg 45:366.272.
14. Greenall MY, Evans M, Pollock AV.(1980) Midline or transverse laparotomy? A random controlled clinical trial. Br J Surg 64:733–736
15. Klinge U, Conze J, Limberg W, Brucker C, Oettinger AP, Schumpelick V (1996) Pathophysiologie der Bauchdecke. Chirurg 67(3):229–33.
16. Amid P. (1997) Classification of biomaterials and their related complications in abdominal wall hernia surgery. Hernia 1:5–8.
17. Smith R, Olivier C, Williams DF (1987) The enzymatic degradation of polymers in vitro.J-Biomed-MatRes,Vol.21,991–1003.
18. Schwertassek K, Dvorak J.(1972) Beitrag zum Studium des Abbaues von Polyester-Gefäßprothesen im menschlichen Organismus. Biomed Technik, 17:105–9.
19. Maarek J, Guidon R, Aubin M, et al.(1984) Molecular weight characterization of virgin and explanted polyester arterial prosthesis. J Biomed Mat Res 18:881–894.
20. Riepe G, Loos J, Imig H, et al.(1997) Long term in vivo alterations of polyester vascular grafts in humans. Eur J Vasc Endovasc Surg 13(6):540–8.
21. Klinge U, Klosterhalfen B, Conze J, et al (1998) A modified mesh for hernia repair adapted to abdominal wall physiology. Eur J Surg, in press.

CHAPTER 15

Biomaterials – Experimental Aspects

U. Klinge, B. Klosterhalfen

The abdominal wall is mainly strengthened in two ways [1]:

- By a mechanical block, e.g. as sublay or even onlay, at least as long as the fixation works (problem of implantation technique)
- By induction of scar tissue, e.g. by polyester or polypropylene, not by polytetrafluoroethylene (PTFE) (problem of tissue response)

In contrast to the only slight influence of suture material, the type of mesh material greatly affects the clinical results, as indicated by Amid [2]. Mesh is a vast amount of material implanted in a very extended area. Mesh-related complaints [3], complications such as adhesions, mesh dislocation, meshes cutting up the spermatic cord [4], fistulas to bowels and bladder, the macroscopical appearance of explanted meshes being shrunk, folded and rolled and the histological evidence of persistent inflammation over a period of years. Alltogether indicate that meshes are not always inertly incorporated. It is worth noting that up to 30% of all mesh recipients are younger than 40 years [5], meaning that the mesh has to guarantee full function for up to 50 years. Some patients are as young as 13 years old [6].

Type, quantity and structure of the implanted meshes determine the resulting tissue reactions, biocompatibility or the overall suitability. Factors to be considered when choosing meshes include textile characteristics, experience and, last but not least, experimental results.

15.1 Textile Characteristics

Since the first report by Witzel [7] in 1889 using silver meshes for hernia repair, many different materials have been introduced. Having decided to implant a mesh, a choice has to be made between a monofilament or multifilament, absorbable or non-absorbable, small or large pore-sized, polypropylene, polyester or PTFE mesh. Unfortunately, manufacturing firms rarely deliver satisfactory information. Amid elaborated a systematic approach characterizing four different types of mesh materials [2], published in 1997.

To obtain precise information on the hosieries (meshes are usually not knitted or woven materials), we initiated on independent textile analysis of meshes according to existing rules issued by the German Standardization Institute. Testing of the tensile strength and moreover of the symmetric strength by pressing through the stamp proves that meshes are inappropriate considering the physiologically required strength (Fig. 1). Furthermore, individual testing, e.g. of the subsequent tearing force or the recovery angle, reveals dissatisfactory asymmetries.

The improvement of mesh quality demands both a reduction in the amount of material, adapting the strength to 16 N/cm, as already mentioned [8], and an improvement in the hosiery structure to obtain more symmetrical properties. As polyester always degrades, entailing a loss of mechanical stability, and PTFE does not induce scar tissue formation, polypropylene appears to be the best suitable polymer of the materials available. As a result of these demands, the newly constructed mesh (originally named Soft Hernia Mesh = SHM, now Vypro) contains a reduced polypropylene fraction of less than 30% compared with Marlex and has large pores of about 5 mm. In the test pressing through the stamp, the mesh now ruptures in a circular line, indicating a more symmetrical strain. The very low stiffness of the permanent structure requires an additional supply with filaments of absorbable polyglactin. This temporarily eases its use by the surgeon and decreases the inflammatory response by covering the polypropylene surface.

The textile characteristics can only give an indication of clinical suitability, because they do not reflect the interaction between incorporated mesh and induced scar tissue. The consequences of the polypropylene reduction with regard to tissue reaction

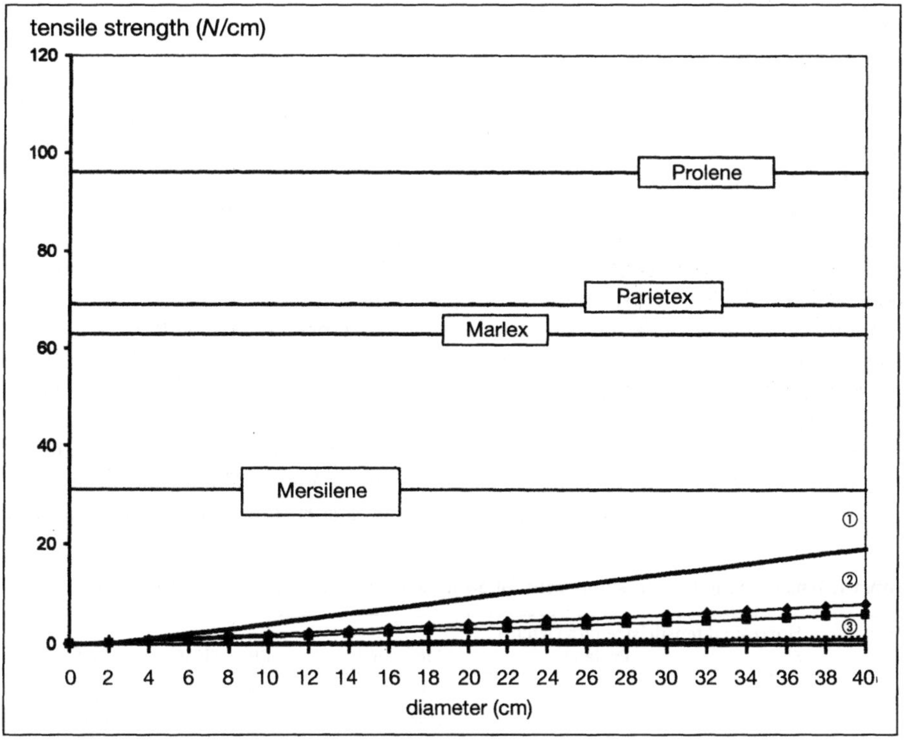

Fig. 1. Tensile strength F of meshes in relation to physiological strain. $F=Pxd/4$. Maximum ①, 150 mmHg (19.95 kPa); cough, pressing ②, 7.9 kPa; pain ③, 5.9 kPa; standing position, 1.7 kPa; reduced blood flow, 1.3 kPa; supine position, 0.8 kPa

and abdominal wall function are remarkable and have been shown both in animals and in humans [9].

15.2 Experimental Aspects

Mesh is usually implanted for a few days up to 6 months as an inlay in rats or rabbits, and only rarely in dogs or pigs, and thus does not reflect the real clinical situation in humans, making evaluation of the suitability of meshes in animal experiments questionable.

15.2.1 Mechanical Testing

The central task of meshes is to strengthen the abdominal wall. The tensile strength is therefore of particular interest.

15.2.1.1 Pulling Strength

The tensile strength of strips of usually 1–2 cm in width is 36±17 *N*/cm for the abdominal wall in dogs (muscles and fascia), 10–25 *N*/cm in rabbits [10, 11] and 11–16 *N*/cm in rats [12, 13] (12.3±3.2 *N*/cm vertically and 19.5±3.6 *N*/cm horizontally [14]). Inaccordance to the tensile strength in humans, these values reveal slight differences in the vertical direction and differences of approximately 20%–30% in the horizontal direction. In rats, the tensile strength of a simple laparotomy, closed by continuous suture, regains half of its original strength within 3 weeks and approaches normal values after 3 months [14] (Table 1). Various meshes show no differences as inlay with regard to the tensile strength of the sutured zone. Because of the extraordinary strength of meshes, it is obvious that rupture usually occurs at the suture line in accordance with Bellon's observations [15], no matter which material is used.

Repeated testing just for the isolated mesh area alone showed no significant alteration over 3 months except for the meshes consisting of Vicryl. The tensile strength of Soft Hernia Mesh decreased in proportion to the absorption of polyglactin, always

Table 1. Tensile strength of the suture zone following sham operation or mesh implantation

Day	Horizontal tensile strength (*N*/cm)				
	Sham	Prolene	Mersilene	PP of SHM	SHM
3	3.4	1.7	2.1	2.0	8.1
7	7.8	7.9	10.8	7.8	8.3
14	7.8	7.9	12.3	13.7	10.1
21	11.1	10.1	14.0	11.8	7.3
90	16.7	21.8	18.4	21.6	11.1

PP, polypropylene; SHM, Soft Hernia Mesh.

Table 2. Decreasing tensile strength of Soft Hernia Mesh (mesh alone)

Day	Tensile strength (*N*/cm)
3	62
7	44
14	38
21	48
45	30
90	24

exceeding the required 16 *N*/cm (Table 2). A pronounced increase in strength by the developed scar tissue was not able to be proven.

15.2.1.2
Bursting Pressure

Testing the bursting pressure by increasing the tension on an area until rupture occurs can be performed either in vivo, as described by Arnaud [16], or in vitro, by using an excised piece of abdominal wall, stretching it out over a cylinder.

The great strength of meshes requires a pressure of more than 100 kPa in vivo to produce a rupture within the mesh area – far beyond the physiological range. Generally, in vivo hernias occur in the inguinal or diaphragm region, increasing pressure to over 25 kPa [17–19]. In vitro, the rupture pressure exceeds 100 kPa because the specimen is usually fixed onto a special sealing film [20–22].

With regard to the very high forces, both methods seem to be inappropriate to reveal subtle differences between the meshes.

15.2.1.3
Abdominal Wall Stiffness

Measurement of the resulting abdominal wall stiffness enables a far better detection of differences than the determination of tensile strengths. We therefore developed a special, non-invasive three-dimensional stereography at the Institute of Aerodynamics in order to determine the curvature of the implant as a parameter of the resulting stiffness. The method has been described previously [14]. In general, a light pattern is projected onto the abdominal wall after filling up the abdominal cavity with water. The resulting deformation of the grid permits the calculation of the surface and of the curvature over the mesh.

As a result, after mesh implantation, the stiffness of the abdominal wall increases both in rats and, as previously described, in humans. After a sham operation in rats (Fig. 2), the curvature decreases at low intra-abdominal pressures with water flowing out through the flanks. Later on, beyond a pressure of 2–3 kPa, the curvature increases steadily to maximum values of 20–25 $^1/_{100}$ cm. This changes markedly after mesh implantation. The radius increases as a consequence of the reduced mobility of the abdominal wall 21 days after implantation at an intra-abdominal pressure of 1 kPa (Fig. 3). Compared with controls and Soft Hernia Mesh, the stiffness increases significantly with Prolene and even more so with Mersilene mesh, although the latter is considerably more flexible in the textile form.

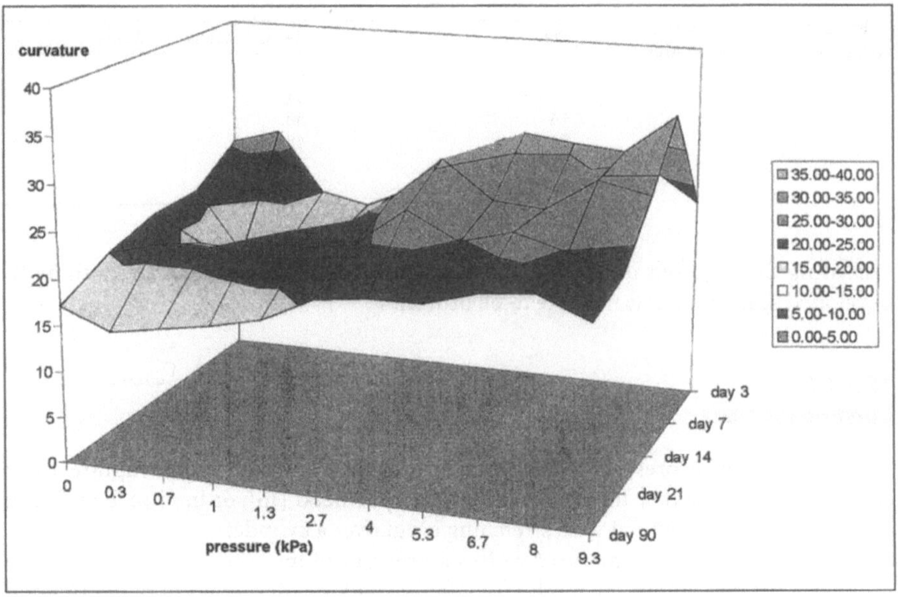

Fig. 2. Curvature following sham operation

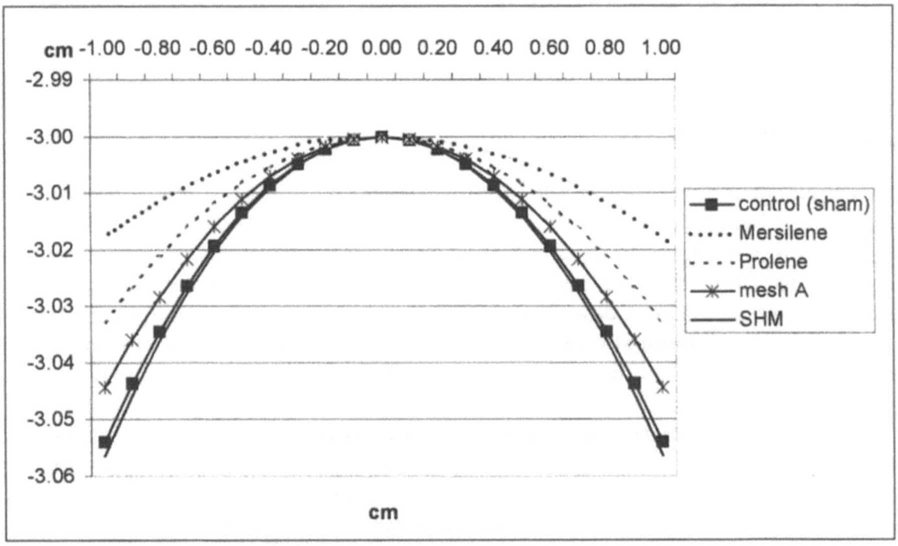

Fig. 3. Radius of the abdominal wall following mesh implantation in rats. Day 21, fitted radius at 1 kPa=7.5 mmHg. *SHM* = Soft Hernia Mesh

Analysing the course of the curvature between 0 and 9.3 kPa 90 days after implantation, both the Prolene and Mersilene meshes restricted abdominal wall mobility, whereas Soft Hernia Mesh did not show any significant restriction compared with controls (Fig. 4).

For the stiff Prolene mesh (Fig. 5) and the comparatively soft Mersilene mesh (Fig. 6), a remarkable decrease in curvature and an increase in stiffness are detectable. This process begins 3 weeks after implantation and is proportional to the development of scar tissue. In contrast to this decrease in curvature, Soft Hernia Mesh (Fig. 7) with reduced amounts of polypropylene showed no remarkable difference compared with the sham-operated rats. This applies to both pure polypropylene and to the combination of polypropylene with Vicryl.

With the aid of three-dimensional stereography, slight differences between the various materials can be detected. As expected, the mesh with the lowest amount of polypropylene and the highest elasticity reveals no detectable reduction in abdominal wall mobility (Tables 3, 4).

Comparing all tested meshes, the mesh weight and the surface of the alloplastic material seem to be strongly associated with the resulting stiffness. Heavy meshes with a large surface tend to have an increased stiffness and a reduced curvature (Figs. 8, 9).

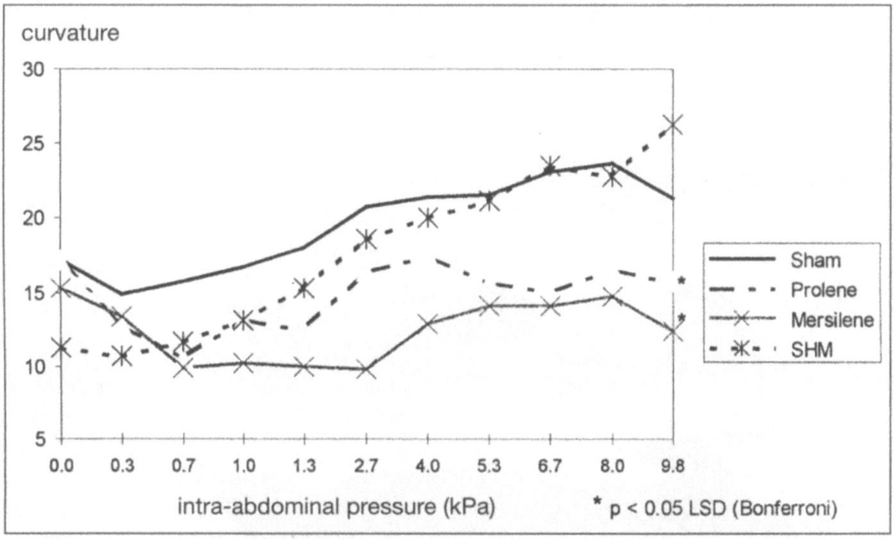

Fig. 4. Curvature following mesh implantation after 90 days. *Asterisk*, $p<0.05$ LSD (Bonferroni). *SHM*, Soft Hernia Mesh

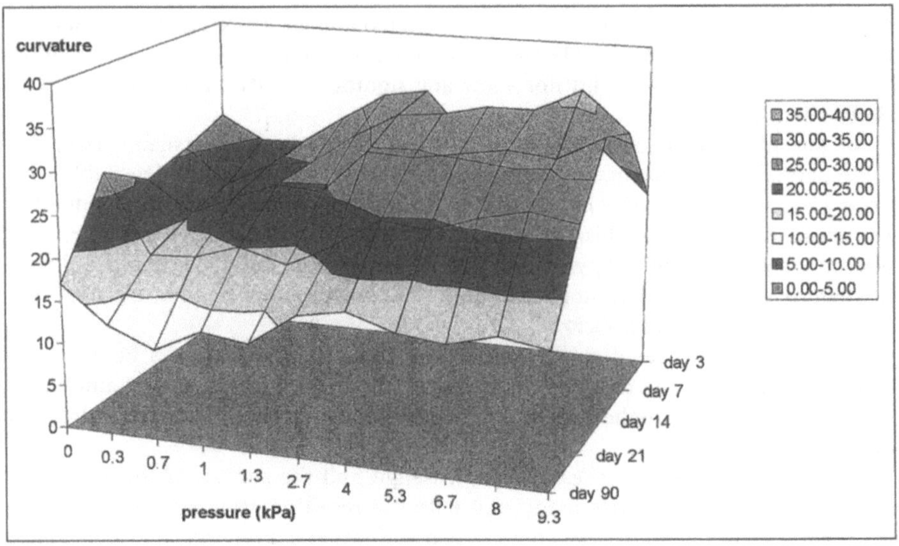

Fig. 5. Curvature following Prolene mesh implantation

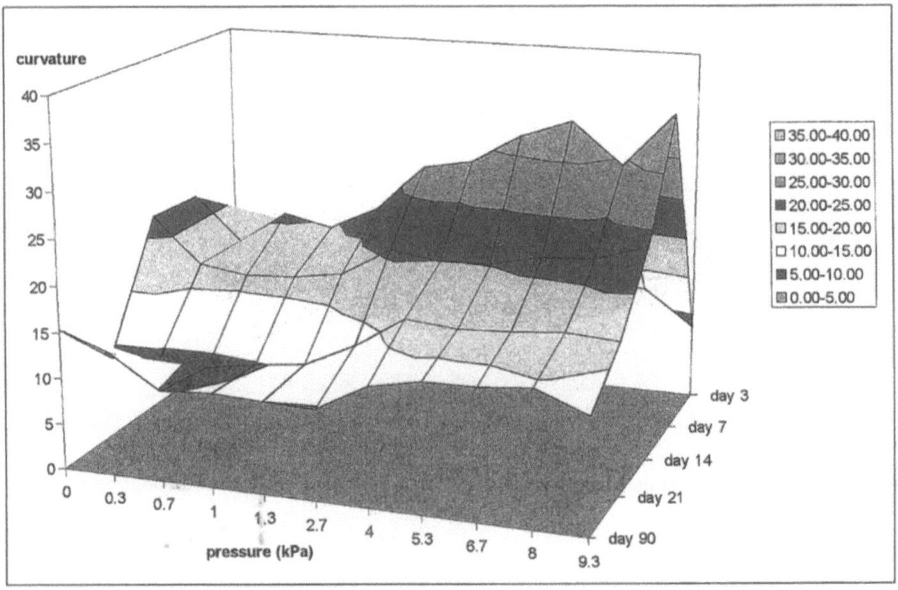

Fig. 6. Curvature following Mersilene mesh implantation

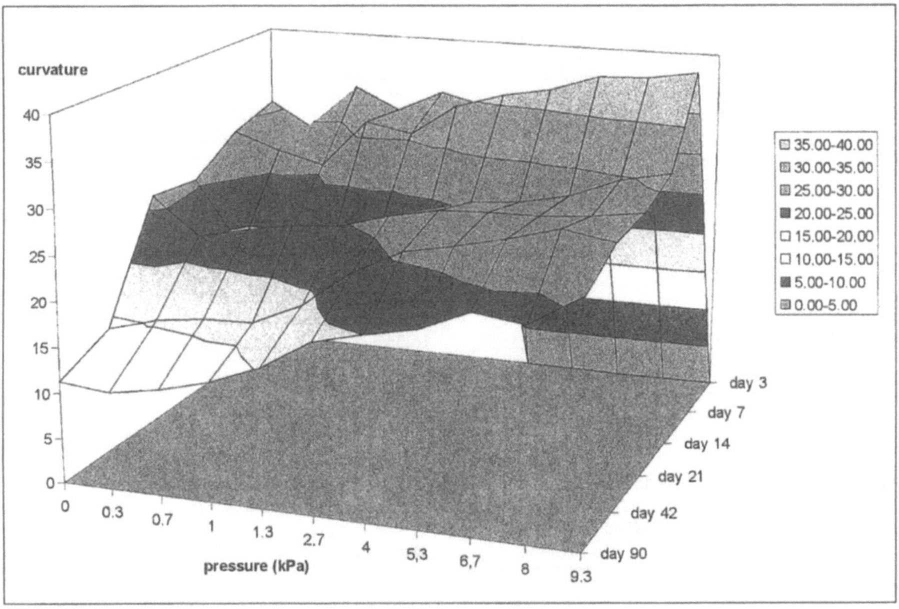

Fig. 7. Curvature following Soft Hernia Mesh (SHM) implantation

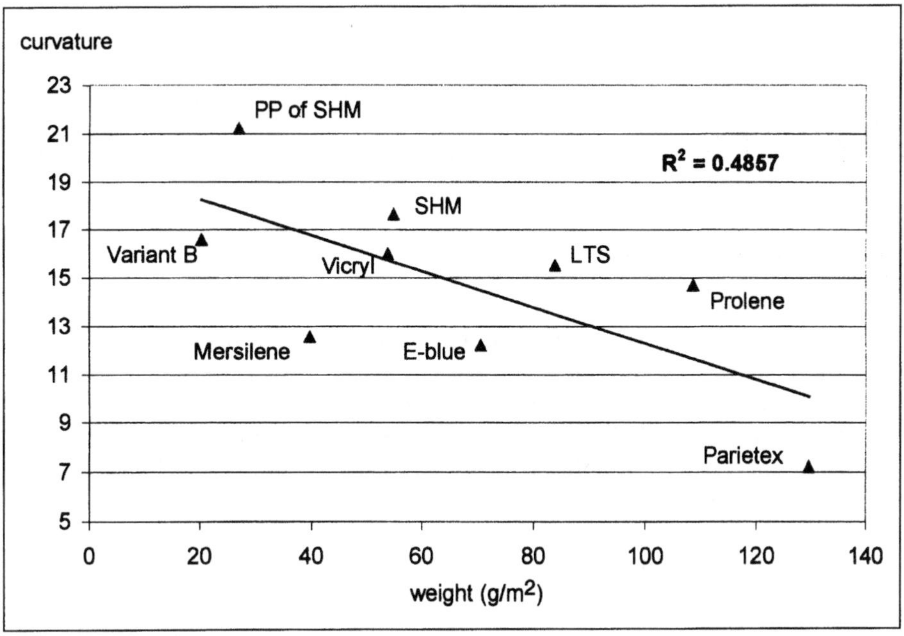

Fig. 8. Mesh weight and curvature (implantation in rats for 90 days). PP, polypropylene; *SHM*, Soft Hernia Mesh

Table 3. Curvature after 21 days in rats

Pressure	Curvature (1/100 cm) Sham	Prolene	Mersilene	PP of SHM	SHM
0	19.9±6.6	27.4±4.5	8.80±4.5	23.2±3.8	26.2±2.4
0.3	21.4±7.7	17.9±4.5	8.90±3.8	16.9±0.8	22.1±3.2
0.7	21.4±8.6	18.3±3.9	8.86±6.8	16.4±2.2	23.3±3.8
1.0	23.1±6.7	20.0±3.2	9.80±6.9	17.4±3.3	24.2±4.8
1.3	22.7±6.4	18.4±3.9	10.5±5.6	20.1±3.0	24.7±6.3
2.7	23.4±7.4	21.3±2.1	13.1±8.5	22.8±4.1	26.3±5.4
4.0	27.7±6.8	24.8±3.4	16.7±5.4	22.9±3.7	27.4±6.0
5.3	24.8±4.3	24.1±2.9	16.1±4.8	23.0±4.1	27.7±7.3
6.7	26.4±7.7	26±5.7	16.4±4.1	22.3±5.9	27.8±7.4
8.0	24.8±2.6	27.2±5.3	17±3.5	22.3±4.4	28.3±7.0
9.3	22.9±5.8	26.4±5.7	16.5±3.3	26.6±4.6	29.0±7.5

The differences between Mersilene and sham are statistically significant (LSD Bonferroni).
PP, polypropylene; SHM, Soft Hernia Mesh.

Table 4. Curvature after 90 days in rats

Pressure	Curvature (1/100 cm) Sham	Prolene	Mersilene	PP of SHM	SHM
0	17.2±6.0	17.7±4.6	16.5±3.4	12.8±0.0	11.3±3.6
0.3	14.9±3.8	12.9±8.5	13.5±6.1	14.2±8.9	10.7±2.6
0.7	15.8±4.3	10.8±7.3	11.3±3.8	15.6±8.4	11.6±3.8
1.0	16.7±4.4	13.2±7.3	14.7±9.4	16.3±8.6	13.0±3.4
1.3	16.2±6.3	13.8±6.6	18.4±10.8	17.7±9.3	15.2±2.8
2.7	20.7±4.5	17.4±9.0	20.3±12.8	22.1±11.9	18.6±3.6
4.0	22.2±4.2	16.6±10.4	20.4±11.4	24.4±14.4	20.0±4.3
5.3	19.5±5.5	19.5±13.5	18.5±9.8	27.9±14.6	21.1±4.0
6.7	19.5±6.0	15.0±17.0	16.8±6.9	27.7±9.9	23.4±5.9
8.0	20.6±9.5	15.3±17.0	19.5±10.6	29.2±5.2	22.8±5.7
9.3	21.3±2.4	–	–	–	26.3±7.9

The differences between Mersilene and Prolene versus sham are statistically significant (LSD Bonferroni).
PP, polypropylene; SHM, Soft Hernia Mesh.

15.2.2
Histology

The large pores of Soft Hernia Mesh induce a mesh scar but prevent an all-embedding scar plate, as seen with the polypropylene meshes usually implanted. The collagen is orientated circularly around the polypropylene fibres, and the pores are filled mainly with fat tissue. This missing scar plate might be responsible for the preserved and persistent elasticity of Soft Hernia Mesh. Histology reveals the absence of marked inflammation but pronounced vascularisation. Further details are presented in Chap 16.

This improved incorporation of the mesh into the surrounding tissue has even been shown in humans. In two patients, 3 and 9 months after implantation of Soft Hernia Mesh, a revision was performed not connected with the initial hernia repair. In each case, clinical examination of the mesh area revealed no palpable stiffness. Histological analysis totally confirmed the findings in the animal experiments.

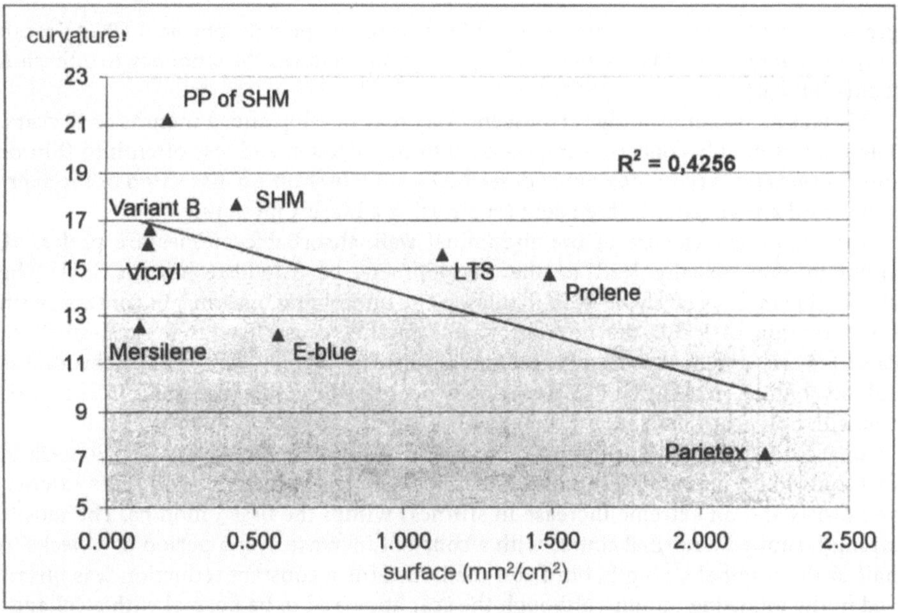

Fig. 9. Mesh surface and curvature (implantation in rats for 90 days). PP, polypropylene; *SHM*, Soft Hernia Mesh

15.2.3 Conclusion

In conclusion, all tested standard meshes are oversized compared with the physiologically required forces. Recommended stability can be obtained through reduction of the material, loading to a reduction in the resulting stiffness following mesh implantation and an improved integration of the mesh into the surrounding tissue.

The described experimental model is suitable to test further improvements, e.g. by using either long-term absorbable material or non-absorbable material with better textile properties or by coating the alloplastic material with wound-healing components.

15.3 Adhesions and Fistulas

Both meshes and surgical trauma promote the formation of adhesions or the development of fistulas if there is direct contact with the bowels. Clinical registration of adhesions is difficult. Statistically, a bowel occlusion caused by adhesions occurs with an average delay of 11 years [24]. The extent of adhesions, which usually develop in the first 48 h, varies depending on the used material. Polyester causes only small adhesions and PTFE slightly more [18, 25]. Polypropylene meshes [26–29] account for the greatest extent, even more than induced by absorbable polyglycolic acid (PGA) mesh [24]. In general, covering the mesh with peritoneum reduces the tendency to adhesion formation [30].

Fistulas are generally only rarely seen. They may develop after 3 months or 15 years. The reports mainly concern a migration into the bladder, and less often into thin or thick bowels [31–34]. In 1997, Silich described for the first time a dissection of the spermatic cord 4 years after Lichtenstein repair using a Marlex mesh [4].

For temporary closure of the abdominal wall, absorbable meshes are preferred, although they usually lead to the development of extended hernias [35]. The absorbable meshes rarely develop fistulas to the underlying intestine. In contrast, with the exception of PTFE, the non-absorbable meshes cause fistulas in 50%–100% of cases [36–41], and 60%–90% of these meshes have to be removed [35]. Bleichrodt was able to confirm in rats that PTFE markedly decreased the rate of fistulas in comparison with polypropylene [26, 27].

In accordance with expectations, the implantation of an absorbable Vicryl mesh in rats leads to hernias after 6 months. The surprising fact is that Vicryl induces extensive fibrosis and an extreme increase in stiffness within the first 3 months. The tensile strength showed a normal course with a constant increase over a period of 3 weeks to half of the original strength, but from then onwards a constant reduction was observed in the following months, although the scar appeared to be normal with a collagen fraction of more than 90%. There has not yet bee any valid explanation why the induced scar tissue loses its mechanical strength completely over time (Fig. 10).

Absorbable meshes can prevent direct contact between intestine and the non-absorbable meshes until the wound is completely covered by peritoneum. Furthermo-

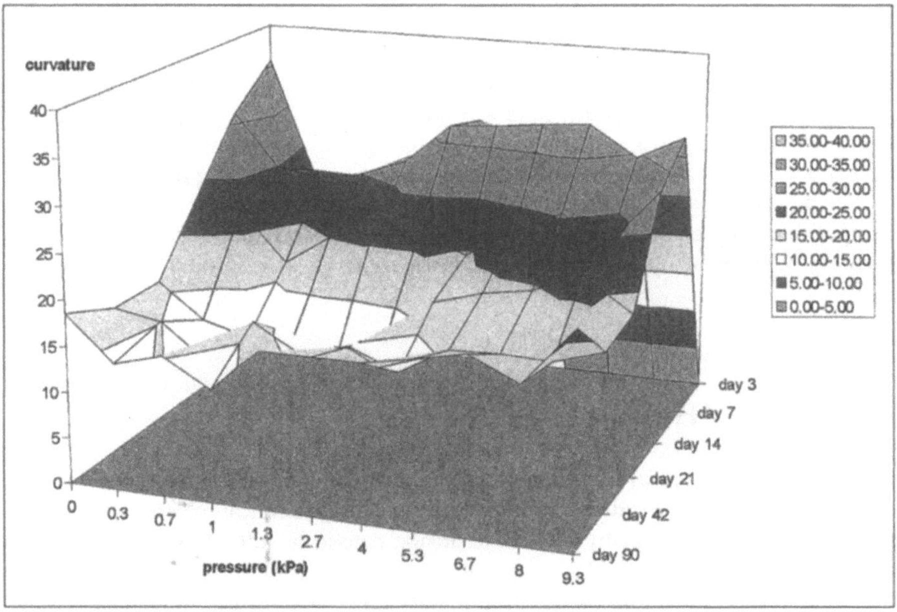

Fig. 10. Curvature following Vicryl mesh implantation

Table 5. Adhesions (mm²) in rats following Marlex or Marlex/Vicryl mesh implantation

Marlex mesh	Marlex and Vicryl mesh
351	93
309	88
247	71
191	96
153	158
237	165
157	50
213	67
171	73
226±69	96±40

p=0.0003 (t test).

re, Vicryl-induced adhesions may disappear, as was shown in rats, rabbits and even humans [18, 25, 42].

At least in rats, the underlying of a Vicryl mesh can reduce the extent of adhesions compared to the single implantation of a Marlex mesh (Table 5). In each of nine rats, the area of adhesion after 14 days was recorded by Treutner et al. [43] and showed highly significant decreases from 225±68 to 95±39 mm². Complete prevention of adhesions was not possible.

15.3.1 Clinical Prevention

To prevent adhesions or fistulas to the intestines, any direct contact between bowel and the polypropylene or polyester has to be avoided very carefully. There are several options to achieve this aim.

In 1994, Amid described that, in rabbits, combining polypropylene meshes with films of Silastic or polypropylene can prevent adhesions to the bowel [44]. For temporary closure, Losanoff [45] covered the whole intestine in a polypropylene film and did not find any fistula in 29 patients.

Alternatively, an absorbable mesh can be underlaid [46] or the much more expensive PTFE meshes can be used [47].

In any case, the most successful, simplest and by far the cheapest method is to interpose omentum tissue [48, 49] or hernial sac [50].

15.4 Infection

Even after alloarthroplastic operations, bacteria are found in the wound in more than 40% of patients. The risk of an apparent infection rises markedly, especially if the alloplastic material is not fully integrated into the surrounding tissue, e.g. in the case of haematomas or seromas.

Early experiments in the late 1950s showed a marked increase in infection rates in the presence of biomaterials, whereas fortunately this has not been seen in modern clinical studies with meshes.

In 1957, Elek and Conen found that, for silk, the number of bacteria necessary to cause an abscess decreased in the presence of biomaterials from 100,000 to 100 [51]. In 1982, Sharp saw that the infection rate in the presence of monofilaments was lower than with multifilaments [52]. This was confirmed by Blomstedt in 1977, who found the highest inflammatory activity with multifilament polyester, whereas monofilament polypropylene led only initially to a smooth inflammation [53], probably due to the increased adherence of the bacteria to the suture material [54].

A higher incidence of infections was not seen in all experiments. For example, Paterson-Brown used monofilament and multifilament sutures in pigs and did not find any pronounced differences [55]; moreover, no differences were reported by Edlich in the early 1970s either [56, 57].

The existence of small pores and caves might encourage germs to nest [58]. In 1981, Bucknall found no difference in the extent of inflammation, but showed a much longer persistence of bacteria attached to multifilaments (for over 70 days) [59]. In the presence of knots, the influence of the material decreases far more. Even if a slight difference between the materials has been found, this disappears in the presence of knots [60–62]. For the detection of bacteria in the wound, the structure of the material and their attachment to the filaments seem to be much more important than the type of filament itself.

Even if mesh infection occurs, the mesh may be left in place, except if a PTFE mesh has been used. Experimentally, these meshes seem to be more resistant to bacteria adhesion [63], but their small pores make complete destruction of microbes by macrophages impossible. Thus, if infections occur, these meshes generally have to be removed [2, 64, 65].

We tested the infection rate of a monofilament versus a multifilament mesh in rats over 7 days. Increasing concentrations of *Staphylococcus aureus* (ATCC 25923) were added. Without biomaterial, 50 million micro-organisms were required to cause an infection, whereas in the presence of biomaterial 5 million were enough to cause a wound infection in about 30% of the rats. In all animals, even after dilution down to 50,000 microbes per ml, some bacteria can be detected.

Comparing the multifilament Soft Hernia Mesh with the monofilament Marlex mesh (n=36 in each group), there was no significant difference with regard to the infection rate (Table 6), although in almost all cases bacteria were detectable.

The infection rate between monofilament and multifilament meshes did not differ after 7 days, although the multifilament meshes sometimes led to a slight increase in persisting bacteria. This confirms the reports in the literature of detectable bacteria for 30–70 days [53, 54, 59]. Germ detection does not correlate with the clinical manife-

Table 6. Bacteria contamination of infected meshes in rats (5×10^6 *Staphylococcus aureus*, n=36, 7 days)

	Monofilament (Marlex)	Multifilament (Soft Hernia Mesh)	Significance (p, χ^2 test)
Infection	4	3	0.69
Germs detectable in diluted extract (24 h)	9	13	0.31
Germs detectable in culture (48 h)	32	35	0.16

station of infections. This might explain the lack of increased infections following the use of multifilament sutures or meshes [66–68]. Regarding the non-elevated infection rate in clinical practice, the importance of experimental findings has to be questioned.

Experimentally, the adherence of bacteria to the alloplastic material can be decreased by coating the polymers [69]. The amount of bacteria can be reduced both by topical or systemic application of antibiotics [70]. Whether or not this is really necessary remains open for discussion.

15.5 Mesh Shrinkage

It is well known that the physiological wound contraction increases with the extent of inflammation. Amid reported mesh shrinkage of implanted meshes of approximately 20% of the length and 30%–40% of the mesh area [2]. Using a collagen-coated Vicryl mesh, Meddings was able to show shrinkage of the mesh area from 16 to 6.5 cm^2 (40.6%) after 2 weeks in rats, followed by a slight recovery to 10 cm^2 (62.5%) after 3 months [13].

Mesh-induced inflammation is largely determined by the material itself, especially its chemical properties, structure and the total amount of alloplastic material. The type of implanted material therefore influences the amount of shrinkage, as was proven in dogs both radiographically and histologically.

Both a Marlex mesh and the polypropylene-reduced Soft Hernia Mesh were implanted in dogs in a sublay position. The edges of the mesh were marked by clips and the clip position was examined radiographically. After 3 and 6 months, respectively, histological analysis of explanted meshes was also performed. With both methods, a shrinkage of 40% in area and of 20% in length of the implanted meshes was found. Furthermore, the mesh with the reduced inflammatory response seemed to show a decreased extent of shrinkage, appearing to recover as polyglactin was absorbed (difference not significant, t test) (Table 7; Fig. 11).

Mesh dislocation has never been seen, but a pronounced folding of the explanted Marlex meshes has been observed (Fig. 12). The folding of this relatively stiff material seems to be the consequence of the inevitable wound contraction, pushing together the textile material. The extent of the observed shrinkage highlights the fact that a sparse subduction of the meshes of less than 2–5 cm will provoke recurrence.

Table 7. Mean area (cm^2) ± SD of meshes implanted in dogs as measured on radiographs

Day	Marlex (monofilament)		SHM (multifilament)	
	n	Area	*n*	Area
0	5	139±11	5	116±18
7	5	119±13	5	110±16
14	4	71±16	5	85±9
28	4	75±8	5	78±20
56	4	45±55	5	74±23
84	1	81	2	57±98
168	1	63	2	70±97

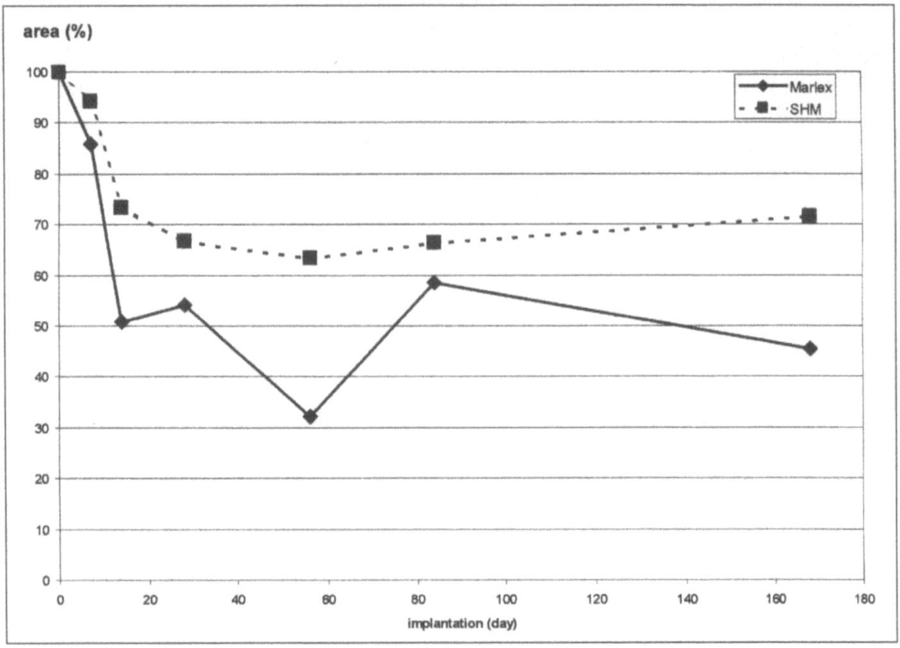

Fig. 11. Shrinkage of meshes as assessed by radiographs in dogs. *SHM*, Soft Hernia Mesh

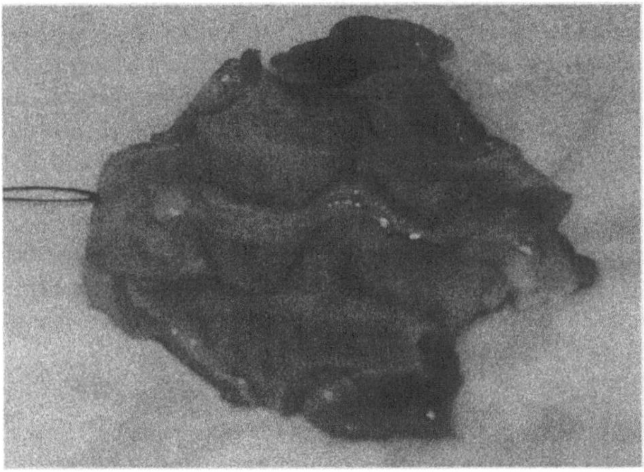

Fig. 12. Folding of Marlex mesh after 3 months in a dog

15.6 Meshes and Tumourgenesis

Since the 1960s it has been known from animal experiments, especially in rodents, that nearly all foreign bodies can induce sarcomas after implantation for more than 6 months. The incidence mainly results from the thickness of the fibrous capsule rather than from the chemical properties of the implanted material [71]. Corresponding follow-up studies in humans, i.e. for 30–50 years are not available, particularly because the survival of patients with implanted biomaterials is often limited. However, occasional reports of sarcomas following Dacron vascular grafts have been published (Table 8).

In 1980, Brand collected nearly 100 sarcomas induced by scars. A total of 50% of these appeared within 25 years [76]. In 1988, Jennings reported 40 sarcomas induced by foreign bodies. They appeared after a mean of 17.6±24.9 years, seeming to have two peaks within 5 years or after 15 years (Table 9). In the 1970s, on the basis of his experimental results in animals, Brand postulated a multiphasic appearance of induced sarcomas [77].

Chapter 16 discusses whether there really is a risk for the development of sarcomas, especially in very young patients.

Table 8. Sarcomas induced by biomaterials [71–75]

Author	Year of publication	Latency (years)	Material
Dargent	1997	–	Dacron
Caralps-Riera	1996	2.3	Dacron
Fyfe	1994	4	Dacron
Raso	1993	–	Femoral vascular graft
Weiss	1991	–	Dacron
Weinberg	1980	1.2	Dacron
Fehrenbacher	1981	12	Dacron
Moncure	1987	–	Dacron
Wallnofer	1977	3	Graft
O'Connell	1976	1	Dacron
Burns	1972	10	Dacron
Ott	1970	19	Sutures
Jennings	1988	20	Swab
Leinhardt	1988	20	Sutures, polyethylene
Levis	1980	–	Silicon injections

Table 9. Latency of foreign body-induced sarcomas [75]

Latency (years)	Sarcomas (*n*)
≤5	14
≤10	3
≤20	14
≤30	5
≤40	3
>40	1

15.7 Summary

Experimental results indicate that clinical results are largely influenced by the type of mesh chosen. In contrast to normal suture material, it is necessary to choose the material very carefully.

Amid published recommendations for meshes in 1997 [2]:

1. The risk of infection is better if meshes with large pores of monofilament material are used. The newly developed Soft Hernia Mesh reaches this aim, although it is made of multifilaments, because up to now all monofilaments that have been tested are very stiff. New materials are necessary for further improvements.
2. The increased number of seromas indicates that meshes with large pores and the smallest amount of material possible should be used. A mesh with a reduction of polypropylene to less than 30% still maintains sufficient strength. With the reduction of polypropylene to less than 30% in Soft Hernia Mesh, seromas are less frequently seen compared to other materials.
3. The risk of fistula formation and dislocation requires elastic meshes with little inflammatory reaction and large pores to prevent folding and mesh movement. With all meshes, it is essential that direct contact between the mesh and the intestines is prevented.
4. The risk of shrinkage requires prostheses which promote little or no inflammation in a sublay position with sufficient subduction of several centimetres. The newly developed Soft Hernia or Vypro Mesh also seems to be favourable in this respect.

Notwithstanding questions concerning the best approach or the best mesh position, it should not be neglected to examine whether meshes are necessary at all and whether they are specifically suitable. The newly developed Soft Hernia Mesh does not fulfil all of the above-mentioned recommendations but might be an improvement in several respects.

The issue of recurrence rates no longer seems to be the sole criterion. The method of implantation and the biocompatibility of the different materials is now also becoming important. Among other aspects, we need to discuss whether open or laparoscopic surgery, an onlay, sublay or inlay position, and polypropylene, polyester or PTFE should be used. Above all, we need to be aware of local mesh problems such as seromas, shrinkage, dislocation or restriction of abdominal wall mobility.

15.8 Discussion

For a discussion, see Chap. 16.

References

1. Klinge U, Prescher A, Klosterhalfen B, Schumpelick V. [Development and pathophysiology of abdominal wall defects]. Chirurg 1997;68(4):293–303.
2. Amid P. Classification of biomaterials and their related complications in abdominal wall hernia surgery. Hernia 1997;1:5–8.
3. Schumpelick V, Arlt G, Schlachetzki A, Klosterhalfen B. Chronic inguinal pain following TAPP. A case of mesh shrinkage. Chirurg 1997;68:1297–1300.
4. Silich RC, McSherry CK. Spermatic granuloma. An uncommon complication of the tension-free hernia repair. Surg Endosc 1996;10(5):537–9.
5. Kunath U, Lambert H. [Laparoscopic hernioplasty]. Chirurg 1995;66(4):404–8.
6. Felix EL, Michas CA, Gonzalez MH, Jr. Laparoscopic hernioplasty: why does it work? Surg-Endosc 1997;11(1):36–41.

7. Witzel O. Über den Verschluß von Bauchwunden und Bruchpforten durch versenkte Silberdrahtnetze (Einheilung von Filigranpelotten). Zbl Chirurgie 1900;10:257–60.
8. Klinge U, Conze J, Limberg W, Brucker C, Ottinger AP, Schumpelick V. [Pathophysiology of the abdominal wall]. Chirurg 1996;67(3):229–33.
9. Klinge U, Klosterhalfen B, Conze J, et al. A modified mesh for hernia repair adapted to abdominal wall physiology. Eur J Surg 1998;in press.
10. Nilsson t. Biomechanical studies of rabbit abdominal wall. Part I the mechanical properties of specimens from different anatomical positions. J Biomech 1982;15,2:123.9.
11. Neugebauer R, D Wolter, L Claes, B Bültmann. Die Bauchdeckenersatzplastik durch ein unbeschichtetes Kohlenstoffgewebe. Langenbecks Arch Chir 1979;350:83–93.
12. Bellon JM, Bujan J, Contreras LA, Carreras San Martin A, Hernando A, Jurado F. Improvement of the tissue integration of a new modified polytetrafluoroethylene prosthesis: Mycro Mesh. Biomaterials 1996;17(13):1265–71
13. Meddings RN, Carachi R, Gorham S, French DA. A new bioprosthesis in large abdominal wall defects. J Pediatr Surg 1993;28(5):660–3
14. Klinge U, Conze J, Klosterhalfen B, et al. [Changes in abdominal wall mechanics after mesh implantation. Experimental changes in mesh stability]. Langenbecks Arch Chir 1996;381(6):323–32.
15. Bellon JM, Contreras LA, Bujan J, Carrea San Martin A. Experimental assay of a Dual Mesh polytetrafluoroethylene prosthesis (non-porous on one side) in the repair of abdominal wall defects. Biomaterials 1996;17(24):2367–72
16. Arnaud JP, Eloy R, Adloff M, Grenier JF. In vivo exploration of the tensile strength of the abdominal wall after repair with different prosthetic materials. Experimental study in the rat. Eur Surg Res 1979;11(1):1–7.
17. Arnaud JP, Eloy R, Adloff M, Grenier JF. Critical evaluation of prosthetic materials in repair of abdominal wall hernias: new criteria of tolerance and resistance. Am J Surg 1977;133(3):338–45
18. Jenkins S, Klamer T, Parteka J, Condon R. A comparison of prosthetic materials used to repair abdominal wall defects. Surgery 1983;94,2:392–8.
19. Greenstein SM, Murphy TF, Rush BF, Jr., Alexander H. Evaluation of polylactic acid-carbon mesh for repair of ventral herniorrhaphy. Am J Surg 1986;151(5):635–9.
20. Cerise EJ, Busuttil RW, Craighead CC, Ogden WWD. The use of Mersilene mesh in repair of abdominal wall hernias: a clinical and experimental study. Ann Surg 1975;181(5):728–34
21. Myers B, M Rightor, W Donovan. Inguinal hernia repair. Arch Surg 1981;116:463–5.
22. Marmon L, CD Vinocour, SB Standiford, CW Wagner, JM Dunn, WH Weintraub. Evaluation of absorbable polyglycolic acid mesh as a wound support. J Ped Surg 1985;20,6:737–42.
23. Kingsnorth A, J Slavin. Peptide growth factors in wound healing. Br J Surg 1991;78:1286–90.
24. Delany HM. Intraperitoneal mesh–a word of caution [editorial; comment]. Surg Endosc 1994; 8(4):287–8
25. Pans A, Pierard GE. A comparison of intraperitoneal prostheses for the repair of abdominal muscular wall defects in rats. Eur Surg Res 1992;24(1):54–60.
26. Bleichrodt RP, Simmermacher RK, van der Lei B, Schakenraad JM. Expanded polytetrafluoroethylene patch versus polypropylene mesh for the repair of contaminated defects of the abdominal wall. Surg Gynecol Obstet 1993;176(1):18–24
27. Simmermacher RK, Schakenraad JM, Bleichrodt RP. Reherniation after repair of the abdominal wall with expanded polytetrafluoroethylene. J Am Coll Surg 1994;178(6):613–6
28. Christoforoni PM, Kim YB, Preys Z, Lay RY, Montz FJ. Adhesion formation after incisional hernia repair: a randomized porcine trial. Am Surg 1996;62(11):935–8.
29. Eller R, Bukhari R, Poulos E, McIntire D, Jenevein E. Intraperitoneal adhesions in laparoscopic and standard open herniorrhaphy. An experimental study. Surg Endosc 1997;11(1):24–8
30. Schlechter B, Marks J, Shillingstad RB, Ponsky JL. Intraabdominal mesh prosthesis in a canine model [see comments]. Surg Endosc 1994;8(2):127–9
31. Bothra R. Late onset small bowel fistula due to tantalum mesh. Am J Surg 1973;125(5):649–50
32. DeGuzman LJ, Nyhus LM, Yared G, Schlesinger PK. Colocutaneous fistula formation following polypropylene mesh placement for repair of a ventral hernia: diagnosis by colonoscopy. Endoscopy 1995;27(6):459–61.
33. Kaufman Z, Engelberg M, Zager M. Fecal fistula: a late complication of Marlex mesh repair. Dis Colon Rectum 1981;24(7):543–4
34. Soler M, Verhaeghe P, Essomba A, Sevestre H, Stoppa R. [Treatment of postoperative incisional hernias by a composite prosthesis (polyester-polyglactin 910). Clinical and experimental study]. Ann Chir 1993;47(7):598–608.
35. Greene MA, Mullins RJ, Malangoni MA, Feliciano PD, Richardson JD, Polk HC, Jr. Laparotomy wound closure with absorbable polyglycolic acid mesh. Surg Gynecol Obstet 1993;176(3):213–8
36. Dayton MT, Buchele BA, Shirazi SS, Hunt LB. Use of an absorbable mesh to repair contaminated abdominal-wall defects. Arch Surg 1986;121(8):954–60

37. Dion YM, Laplante R, Charara J, Marois M. The influence of the number of endoclips and of mesh incorporation on the strength of an experimental hernia patch repair. Surg Endosc 1994;8(11): 1324–8
38. Fansler RF, Taheri P, Cullinane C, Sabates B, Flint LM. Polypropylene mesh closure of the complicated abdominal wound. Am J Surg 1995;170(1):15–8
39. Jones JW, Jurkovich GJ. Polypropylene mesh closure of infected abdominal wounds. Am Surg 1989;55(1):73–6
40. Voyles CR, Richardson JD, Bland KI, Tobin GR, Flint LM, Polk HC, Jr. Emergency abdominal wall reconstruction with polypropylene mesh: short-term benefits versus long-term complications. Ann Surg 1981;194(2):219–23
41. Nagy KK, Fildes JJ, Mahr C, et al. Experience with three prosthetic materials in temporary abdominal wall closure. Am Surg 1996;62(5):331–5
42. Zachariou Z, R Daum. Gewebereaktivität prostethischer Materialien bei der Rekonstruktion von Defekten in der Chirurgie. Ein Vergleich zwischen Gore-Tex, Vicryl-Netz und Dura im Rattenmodell. Langenbecks Arch Chir 1995;Suppl II:1337–44.
43. Treutner K, G Winkeltau, MM Lerch, R Stadel, V Schumpelick. Postoperative intraabdominelle Adhäsionen – ein neues standardisiertes und objektiviertes Tiermodell und Testung von Substanzen zur Adhäsionsprophylaxe. Langenbecks Arch Chir 1989;374,2:99–104.
44. Amid PK, Shulman AG, Lichtenstein IL, Sostrin S, Young J, Hakakha M. Experimental evaluation of a new composite mesh with the selective property of incorporation to the abdominal wall without adhering to the intestines. J Biomed Mater Res 1994;28(3):373–5
45. Losanoff JE, Kjossev KT. Mesh-foil laparostomy. J Am Coll Surg 1997;185(1):89–92.
46. Wantz GE. Incisional hernioplasty with Mersilene. Surg-Gynecol-Obstet 1991;172(2):129–37
47. Bellon JM, Contreras LA, Sabater C, Bujan J. Pathologic and clinical aspects of repair of large incisional hernias after implant of a polytetrafluoroethylene prosthesis. World J Surg 1997;21(4):402–6.
48. Brandt CP, McHenry CR, Jacobs DG, Piotrowski JJ, Priebe PP. Polypropylene mesh closure after emergency laparotomy: morbidity and outcome. Surgery 1995;118(4):736–40; discussion 740–1
49. Saiz A, Willis I, Paul D, M S. Laparoscopic ventral hernia repair: a community hospital experience [Authors response]. Am Surg 1997;63(5):465–466.
50. Klein P, Konzen G, Schmidt O, Hohenberger W. [Reconstruction of scar hernias–intraoperative tensiometry for objective determination of procedure of choice]. Chirurg 1996;67(10):1020–7.
51. Elek S, PE Conen. The virulence of staphylococcus pyogeneus for man. Br J Exp Path 1957;38:573.
52. Sharp WV, Belden TA, King PH, Teague PC. Suture resistance to infection. Surgery 1982;91(1):61–3.
53. Blomstedt B, Österberg B. Suture materials and wound infection. Acta Chir Scand 1977;144:269–274.
54. Österberg B, Blomstedt B. Effect of suture materials on bacterial survival in infected wounds. Acta Chir Scand 1979;145:431–4.
55. Paterson-Brown S, Cheslyn-Curtis S, Biglin, J, Dye J, Easmon C, Durdley H. Suture materials in contaminated wounds: a detailed comparison of a new suture with those currently in use. Br J Surg 1987;74:734–5.
56. Edlich R, PH Panek, GT Rodeheaver, VC Turnbull, LD Kurtz, MT Edgerton. Physical and chemical configuration of sutures in the development of surgical infection. Ann Surg 1973;177,6:679–88.
57. Edlich RF, Panke PH, Rodehaver GT, Kurtz L, Edgerton M. Surgical sutures and infection: a biomaterial evaluation. J Biomed Mat Re Symposium 1974;5(1):115–126.
58. Osterberg B. Influence of capillary multifilament sutures on the antibacterial action of inflammatory cells in infected wounds. Acta Chir Scand 1983;149(8):751–7.
59. Bucknall TE. Abdominal wound closure: choice of suture. J Royal society Medicine 1981;74:580–5.
60. Scher KS, Bernstein JM, Jones CW. Infectivity of vascular sutures. Am Surg 1985;51(10):577–9.
61. Shuhaiber H, Chugh T, Burns G. In vitro adherence of bacteria to sutures in cardiac surgery. J Cardiovasc Surg Torino 1989;30(5):749–53.
62. Chu CC, Williams DF. Effects of physical configuration and chemical structure of suture materials on bacterial adhesion. A possible link to wound infection. Am J Surg 1984;147(2):197–204.
63. Smith S, Gantt N, Rowe MI, Lloyd DA. Dura versus Gore-Tex as an abdominal wall prosthesis in an open and closed infected model. J Pediatr Surg 1989;24(6):519–21.
64. Slim K, Pezet D, Le Roux S, Chipponi J. Mesh infection after laparoscopic herniorrhaphy. Eur J Surg 1996;162(3):247–8.
65. Law NW, Ellis H. A comparison of polypropylene mesh and expanded polytetrafluoroethylene patch for the repair of contaminated abdominal wall defects–an experimental study [see comments]. Surgery 1991;109(5):652–5
66. Sitzmann J, DW McFadden. The internal retention repair of massive ventral hernia. Am Surgeon 1989;55:719–23.
67. Thill RH, Hopkins WM. The use of Mersilene mesh in adult inguinal and femoral hernia repairs: a comparison with classic techniques. Am Surg 1994;60(8):553–6; discussion 556–7

68. Gilbert AI, Felton LL. Infection in inguinal hernia repair considering biomaterials and antibiotics [published erratum appears in Surg Gynecol Obstet 1993 Nov;177(5):528]. Surg Gynecol Obstet 1993;177(2):126–30
69. Farrah SR, Erdos GW. The production of antibacterial tubing, sutures, and bandages by in situ precipitation of metallic salts. Can J Microbiol 1991;37(6):445–9.
70. Troy MG, Dong QS, Dobrin PB, Hecht D. Do topical antibiotics provide improved prophylaxis against bacterial growth in the presence of polypropylene mesh? Am J Surg 1996;171(4):391–3
71. Ott G. Fremdkörpersarkome. 1st ed. Springer, Berlin Heidelberg New York, 1970.
72. Weiss WM, Riles TS, Gouge TH, Mizrachi HH. Angiosarcoma at the site of a Dacron vascular prosthesis: a case report and literature review. J Vasc Surg 1991;14(1):87–91.
73. Weinberg DS, Maini BS. Primary sarcoma of the aorta associated with a vascular prosthesis: a case report. Cancer 1980;46(2):398–402.
74. O´Connell TX, Fee HJ, Golding A. Sarcoma associated with dacron prosthetic material: case report and review of the literature. J Thorac Cardiovasc Surg 1976;72(1):94–6.
75. Jennings T, Peterson L, Axiotis C, Freidlaender G, Cooke R, Rosai J. Angiosarcoma associated with foreign body material. A report of three cases. Cancer 1988;62(11):2436–44.
76. Brand KG, Brand I. Risk assessment of carcinogenesis at implantation sites. Plast Reconstr Surg 1980;66(4):591–5.
76. Brand KG, Buoen LC, Brand I. Multiphasic incidence of foreign body-induced sarcomas. Cancer Res 1976;36(10):3681–3.

CHAPTER 16

Biocompatibility of Biomaterials – Histological Aspects

B. Klosterhalfen, U. Klinge

16.1 Current Status of Mesh Research

The history of surgical meshes is an outstanding example of the progress that has taken place in hernia surgery and the possible benefits for patients from the use of biomaterials in general. Whereas in the 1960s the introduction of polymer meshes was considered a revolutionary and unconventional step in hernia repair, modern hernia surgery would not be conceivable without the use of these special biomaterials. Finally, the era of laparoscopic surgery further increased the use of polymer meshes, representing a central prerequisite of this progressive surgical technique. Overall, hernia repair using polymer meshes achieves satisfying results in the majority of patients, with recurrence rates lower than 10% (Amid et al. 1992; Shulman et al. 1992). In particular, the repair of complicated or large incisional hernias mainly depends on the employment of meshes (Walker et al. 1976; Sugarbaker 1980; Imvrios et al. 1994). The effectiveness of the implants is based on their method of working either by mechanical closure of the defect (sublay technique) or the integration of the mesh into the artificial abdominal wall mainly by the induction of a strong scar tissue around the mesh fibres (Klosterhalfen et al. 1997).

Thus, in the literature of the last few decades, numerous clinical reports and studies prove the successful application of different mesh modification in hernia surgery (Notaras 1974; Walker and Langer 1976; Sher et al. 1980; Blom et al. 1982; Matapurkar et al. 1991; Wantz 1991). However, parallel to the spread of polymer meshes in hernia surgery, the literature shows an increasing number of reports about major and minor complications after mesh implantation. Visceral erosions after implantation of polypropylene (PP) and polyester (PE) mesh modifications with subsequent formation of fistulas are well-known clinical and experimental complications (Subramanyam et al. 1989; Bleichrodt et al. 1993; Miller et al. 1997; Leber et al. 1998). Common minor complications of these meshes are local wound disturbances, including seromas in 30%–50% (Schumpelick et al. 1996; Wantz 1996; Leber and Garb 1998), discomfort in 10%–20% (Lichtenstein et al. 1988; V Schumpelick et al. 1996; Schumpelick et al. 1997) and restriction of abdominal wall mobility in 25% of all cases (Klinge et al. 1996a,b). Reasons for the failure of the implants generally include persistent and active inflammatory processes, irregular or low formation of scar tissues and unsatisfactory integration of the mesh in the regenerative tissue area, biomechanical properties of the implant and improper surgical techniques during implantation (Lichtenstein et al. 1990, 1993; Bellon et al. 1996, 1997; Klinge et al. 1996a; Klosterhalfen et al. 1997).

Despite the clinical significance of meshes in hernia surgery, basic experimental data about the pathophysiology of hernias themselves and the artificial abdominal wall after mesh implantation are rare. Moreover, in the last few decades, specialists involved in hernia surgery have developed and optimized surgical techniques to take advantage of the therapeutic potential of mesh repair and to evaluate the use of surgical meshes in patient. Most clinical studies have primarily compared mesh-operated operations using mesh with standard procedures of hernia repair without using implants (Lichtenstein et al. 1993; Amid et al. 1994).

Whereas the operative techniques for optimization of the results are more or less defined by surgery, mesh modifications available for hernia surgery are still being produced and have been established on the market for decades. Research in the field of surgical meshes has mainly remained descriptive, although modern techniques in textile engineering, experimental surgery and histopathology now allow a deeper insight into the function of implanted meshes and the mechanisms of mesh integration into the artificial abdominal wall. An understanding of these processes and new findings about the tissue and cellular response at the interface of defined mesh modifications will accelerate the development of optimized surgical meshes.

The present chapter will add a certain spectrum of morphological parameters, giving a more detailed impression of the local tissue and cellular response after mesh implantation. Moreover, we will describe the extent to which particular material properties of surgical meshes influence the histological picture of the implant bed and to which morphology provides an interpretation of biocompatibility. In detail, the data will demonstrate that all surgical meshes, such as Marlex, Mersilene, GoreTex and others, firstly show a persisting inflammation over a period of years after implantation, secondly show a continuous cellular stress response to the presence of polymer fibres characterized by the induction of the heat shock response (HSR), thirdly show consistent tissue damage with features of apoptosis (TUNEL), DNA strand breaks and necrosis, and fourthly show persistent and compensating tissue repair, indicated by proliferating cells in the interface (Ki67). These parameters represent basic cellular reactions and patterns of adaptation to stresses of different origin and are decisive for the estimation of the inertness and biocompatibility of surgical meshes. Moreover, persistent DNA strand breaks and persistent cell proliferation indicate a chronic irritation of the recipient host tissues by the mesh. In addition, determination of the cellular response after mesh implantation represents a helpful and exact method to describe the biocompatibility of surgical meshes in situ.

Finally, the potential of polymer meshes for chronic tissue irritation and polymer-related foreign-body (FB) carcinogenesis is discussed. Both phenomena should not be dismissed irresponsibly without continuous investigation and long-term patient follow-up.

16.2 Concept of Low- and Heavy-Weight Surgical Meshes

Klinge et al. (1996b) emphasized that mechanical data of the artificial abdominal wall after mesh implantation should be adapted to physiologic values. The original stiffness and scar formation after implantation of the Marlex and Prolene meshes have been supposed to be the basis of abdominal wall restriction (Klinge et al. 1996a; Klosterhalfen et al. 1997). Moreover, the amount of the manufactured PP, the small size of the pores and the large surface areas of these particular mesh modifications support an acute or chronic inflammatory process basically affecting the integration of the mesh fibres into the recipient tissues. However, sufficient stability of the artificial abdominal wall is guaranteed by PP mesh modifications even with a reduction of the amount of PP to about 25% of the Prolene mesh (Klinge et al. 1996a). On closer inspection of the material properties and morphological data of the different PP mesh samples with different weights, pore sizes and surface areas, the activity of inflammation and, consequently, the connective tissue formation are closely related to the amount of material implanted, the type of filament (multi- or monofilament) and the proportion of pores, which define the surface or contact area between the foreign material and the recipient tissues (Klosterhalfen et al. 1998a). In particular, larger amounts of PP with a huge surface enlargement by processing multifilaments induce a strong and active inflammatory tissue reaction in which polymorphonuclear neutrophils (PMN) dominate, whereas the reduction of the material and diminishing of the area support a chronic, macrophage-controlled tissue response.

The findings of this particular study led to the concept of low- and heavy-weight meshes, based on the idea that the integration of the surgical mesh into the artificial abdominal wall mainly depends on its textile and physical properties and secondarily on its chemistry or the manufactured polymer.

To demonstrate the importance of the physical features of surgical meshes for their biocompatibility, further details on two heavy- and two low-weight meshes. The meshes consist either of PP or of PE (Table 1).

16.3 Tissue Response in Low- Versus Heavy-Weight Meshes

Parameters of the tissue response describe the composition of the interface tissues in contact with the polymer fibres. The interface in our studies is defined as an area 300–600 μm in width of the surface area of the implanted meshes. In this region of interest, morphometry is performed on histological parameters such as the partial

Table 1. Material properties of low- and heavy-weight meshes

Name	Material	Type of filament	Coated	Weight (g/m²)	Proportion of pores (%)
Prolene	PP hosiery	Monofilament, 100%PP	–	108.5	83.52
Vypro	PP+PG910 hosiery	Multifilament, 50%PP/50%PG910	–	54.65	90.77
Parietex	Polyester hosiery	Multifilament, 100%PE	Bovine collagen	129.6	79.12
Mersilene	Polyester hosiery	Multifilament, 100%PE	–	39.5	89.78

The polypropylene (PP) heavy-weight mesh Prolene is compared with the PP low-weight mesh Vypro, and the polyester (PE) heavy-weight mesh Parietex is compared with the PE low-weight mesh Mersilene. Note the weight (g/m²) and the proportion of pores (%) of each mesh modification.

volume of the inflammatory infiltrate (Fig. 1A), the volume of fat tissues, the partial volume of connective tissue (Fig. 1B) or the vessel density (Fig. 1C). Moreover, the inflammatory reaction may be specified by differentiating between PMN (Fig. 1D), macrophages (Fig. 1E), lymphocytes and eosinophils, for example. The extracellular matrix, furthermore, can be divided into fibroblasts (Fig. 1F) and fibrocysts, endothelial cells and collagen fibre deposition, for example. Histochemistry allows further subdivisions into particular types of cells, e.g. inflammatory (27E10) and anti-inflammatory (RM3/1) families of macrophages or subtypes of lymphocytes (CD4/8).

If we classify the tissue response like this, it may be remembered that each mesh type has a mesh-specific histological picture, which again allows conclusions to be made on its biocompatibility and its acceptance and integration into the artificial abdominal wall (Fig. 2). A typical heavy-weight PP mesh is Prolene. The cell infiltrate directly in contact with the meshes of the PP type mainly consists of PMN (Fig. 1D), macrophages (Fig. 1E), eosinophils and lymphocytes. Plasma cells are always rare. Moreover, the tissue reaction is characterized by a moderate, purely seromous oedema at days 3 and 7, which then constantly decreases until it has completely vanished at day 21. The synthetic filaments of PP were surrounded by a necrosis of the fibrinoid type with a dense infiltrate of granulocytes and macrophages. However, whereas PMN sho-

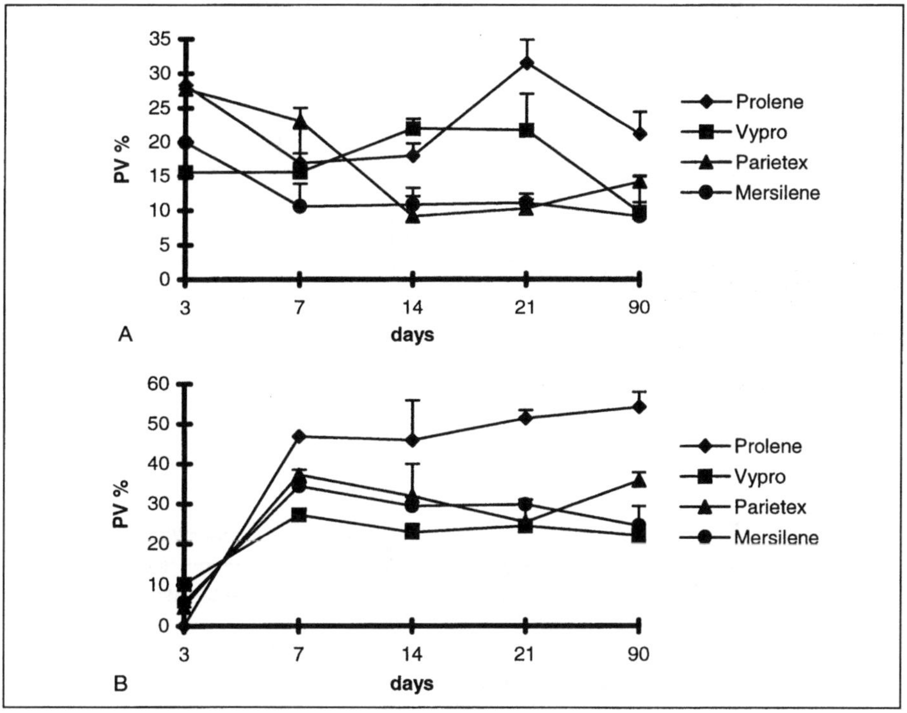

Fig. 1A–F. Tissue response. Morphometric data of the interface between polymer fibres and recipient tissues. *A* Partial volume (PV) of the inflammatory infiltrate (%). *B* PV of connective tissue formation (%). *C* PV of newly formed vessels (%). *D* Polymorphonuclear neutrophils (PMN) (%). *E* Macrophages (%). *F* Fibroblasts (%). Data are given as mean ± SD

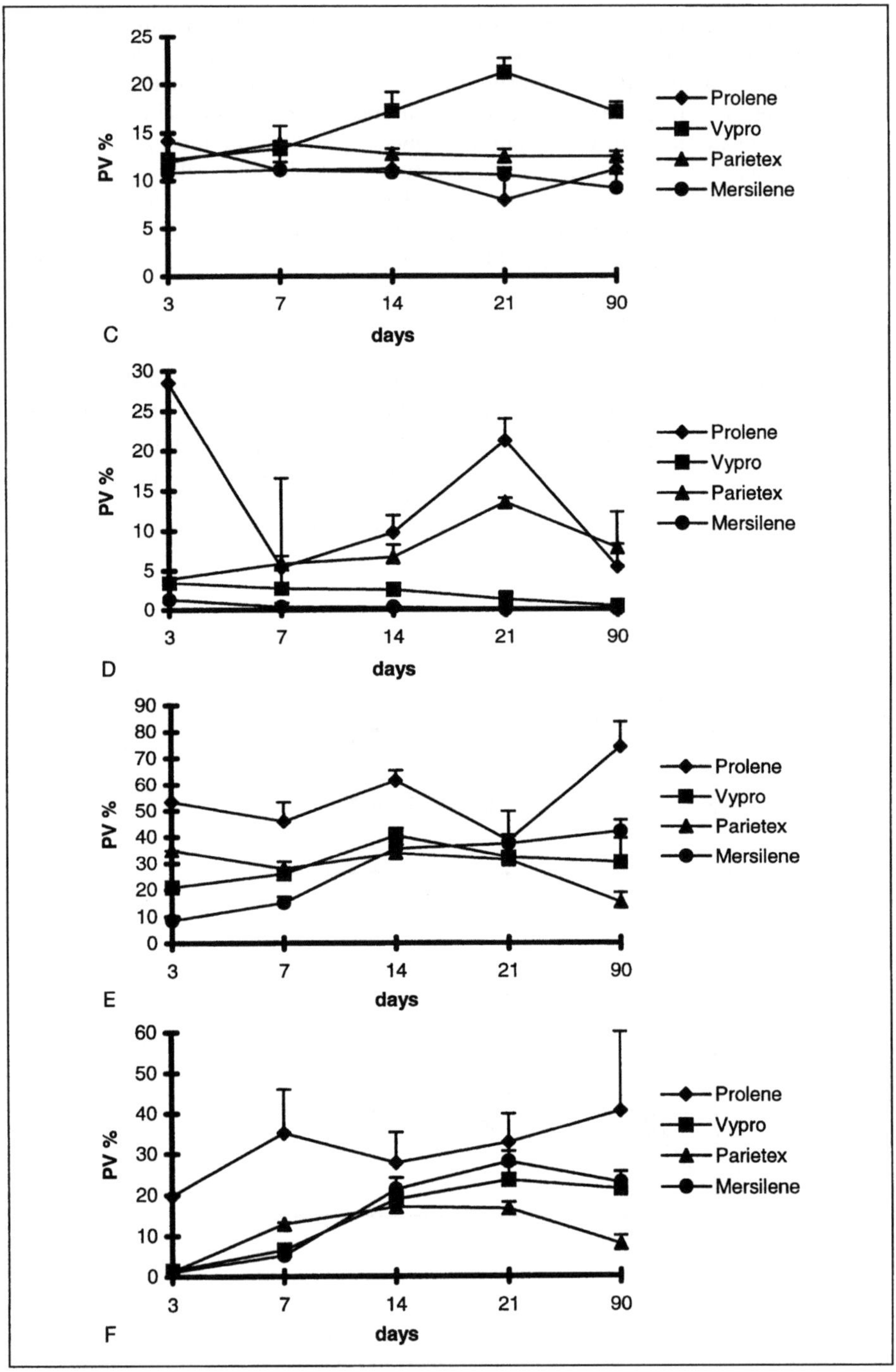

Fig. 1C–D

wed a descending density in the interface, macrophages had a rising colonization rate and were the dominating inflammatory cell type after 90 days. Moreover, macrophages were shown to transform into epitheloid-like cells from day 14 onwards, with a continuously multiplying number of multinucleated giant cells in the contact zone of the monofilament PP fibres.

Overall, at the end of the observation period of 90 days in our rat studies, a moderate persisting inflammatory interface response could be evaluated. The inflammatory reaction at day 90 should be interpreted as inflammation that is still active, with persisting PMN and a major composite, epitheloid granulomas of the FB type with a minor or moderate amount of multinucleated giant cells (Fig. 2).

Fibroblasts were found particularly from day 3 onward (Fig. 1F). The maximum number of fibroblasts were found at days 14 and 90, at the end of the observation period. Overall, Prolene showed the strongest recruitment and activation of fibroblasts. At day 14, a strong tendency of fibroblast differentiation into fibrocytes was noticed, with more spindle-shaped cell configuration and increasing amounts of collagen bundles forming the extracellular matrix.

In contrast to Prolene, the inflammatory reaction of the Vypro mesh is mainly characterized by a moderate infiltrate of macrophages and PMN at day 3. The PMN showed constantly decreasing values and finally disappeared at day 90, the end of observation. In contrast, macrophages increased until day 14, followed by a slight decrease at day 90. Compared to Prolene, the inflammatory reaction is significantly attenuated (Fig. 1A).

Parallel to the diminished inflammatory reaction in the interface of the Vypro mesh, a significantly decreased amount of fibroblasts was observed. Although the fibroblasts showed a similar maturation to fibrocytes as observed in Prolene, the overall quantity of collagen fibres deposited in the extracellular space was again significantly reduced (Fig. 1B).

The inflammatory infiltrate in the interface of the Mersilene mesh was characterized by an increasing colonization with macrophages (Fig. 1E). PMN were only observed at the beginning of the experiments at day 3 (Fig. 1D). The macrophages, however, indicated an early maturation to epitheloid cells from day 7 onwards, with a subsequent formation of numerous FB giant cells (Fig. 2). This the inflammatory infiltrate differed markedly from that of the Prolene mesh. Overall, the inflammatory response could be described as a pure, chronic FB reaction.

The recruitment of fibroblasts and the formation of connective tissue in the interface of the Mersilene mesh was low at the beginning of the experiment and later moderate (Fig. 1B,F). Collagen deposition mainly occurred in the direct surroundings of the mesh filaments, forming a circular layer of collagen tissues around each mesh fibre.

Parietex initially indicated an inflammatory reaction dominated by macrophages at days 3 and 7. However, macrophages decreased up to day 90 (Fig. 1E), whereas PMN showed constantly increasing values with a peak at day 21 (Fig. 1D). In parallel to the increase of the PMN, an enlargement of the oedema in the interstice was observed. At the end of the experimental period of 90 days, the inflammatory reaction was identified as an acute and marked inflammation.

The accumulation of fibroblasts up to day 14 of the experiment was comparable to the values recorded in Vypro and Mersilene; however, as a consequence of the enlarging oedema and acute inflammation, the fibroblast count decreased (Fig. 1F). More-

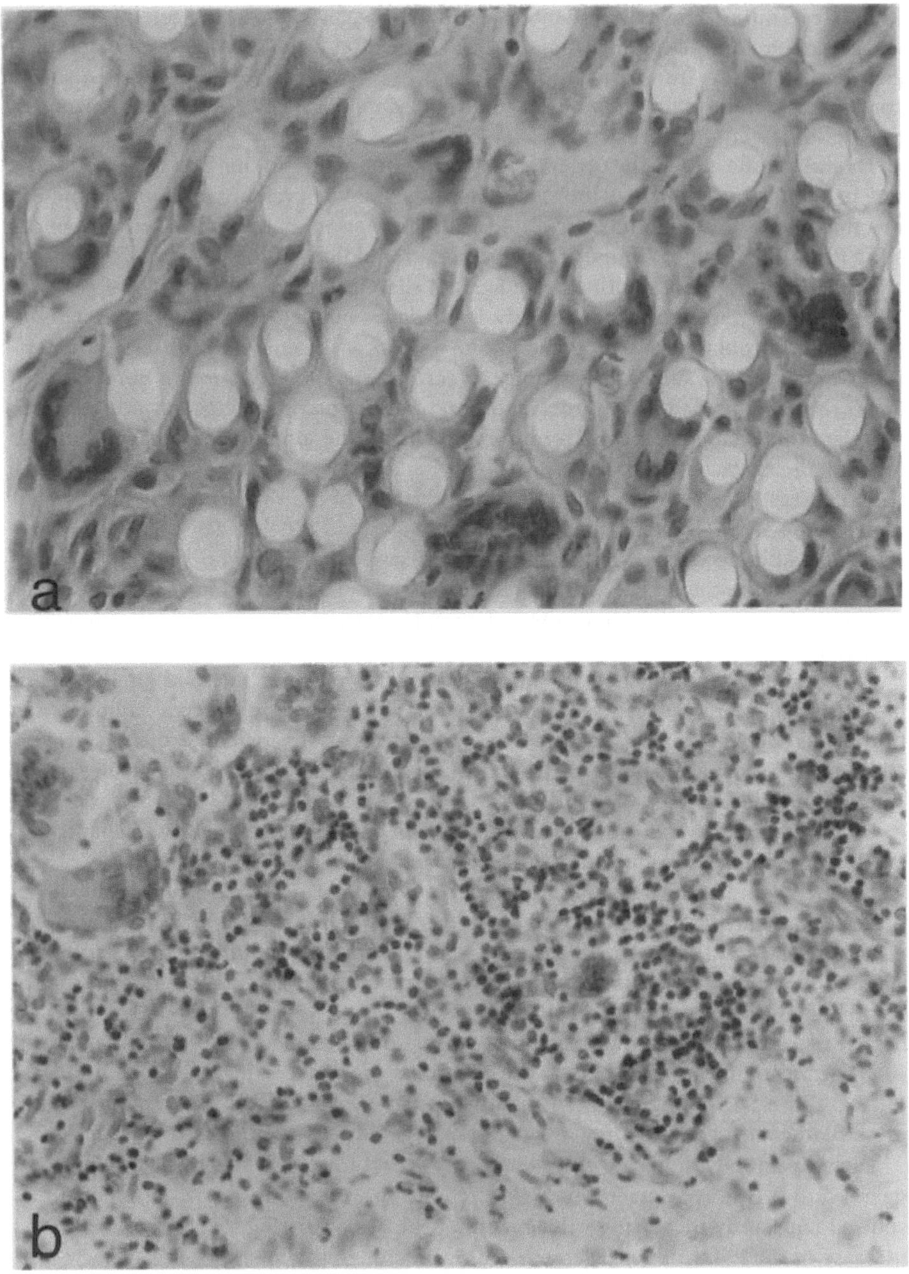

Fig. 2a, b. *a* Chronic type of inflammation with the formation of typical foreign body granulomas in the interface; note epitheloid cells and giant cells of the foreign-body type and the absence of polymorphonuclear neutrophils (PMN); this type is mainly found in the low-weight meshes Vypro and Mersilene. H&E, x250. *b* PMN-dominated acute inflammation, the main inflammatory reaction of the heavy-weight meshes Prolene and Parietex. H&E, x100. c Degradated Mersilene mesh after approximately 8 years of implantation; only particles of the mesh can be determined in the former interface. H&E, x40

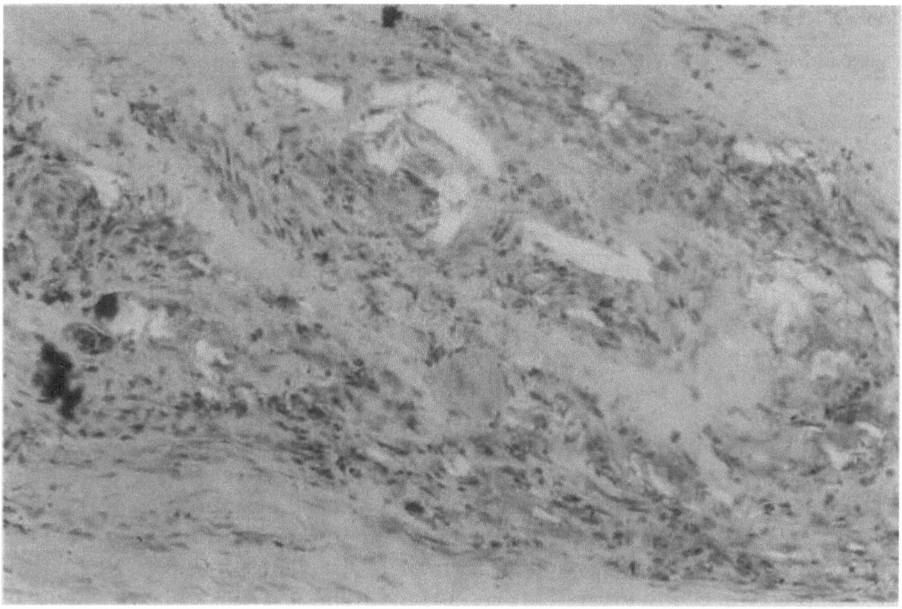

Fig. 2c

over, the maturation of the fibroblasts to fibrocytes normally observed with an onset at day 7 or 14 was markedly reduced. Consequently, collagen deposition was heavily disturbed, resulting in a diffuse fibrosis around the mesh fibres and within the mesh periphery. After 90 days, a loose collagen aggregation was found, forming a fibrosis of a scar-plate type.

Overall, the results of the tissue response clearly demonstrated that the heavy-weight meshes Prolene and Parietex induce an acute and active inflammatory reaction in the interface, whereas the low-weight meshes Vypro and Mersilene promote a more chronic inflammatory reaction. Fibrosis again directly correlates with the activity of the inflammation, as indicated by the significant increase in the partial volume of connective tissue in the interface between mesh and recipient tissues for the heavy-weight meshes Prolene and Parietex.

Another important factor influencing the activity of inflammation in the interface is the surface or contact area between mesh and recipient tissues. Our studies demonstrated that an increase in the plane area of the mesh by using multifilaments directly enhances the activity of the inflammatory reaction. Moreover, the pore size should be as large as possible in order to decrease the contact area to a minimum.

Finally, these histological observations are confirmed in part by macroscopic observations during the 90-day experiment in the rat. In particular, Mersilene and Parietex showed significant differences in the rates of local inflammations observed (Table 2). An interesting aspect remains the high rate of seromas in the Mersilene mesh, a phenomenon which was confirmed, but has yet to be explained.

Table 2. Macroscopic observations

Complications	Prolene (n)[a]	Vypro (n)[a]	Mersilene (n)[a]	Parietex (n)[a]
Seroma	2	2	25	4
Hematoma	1	3	3	5
Local inflammation	5	6	7	12
Wound edge separation	-	-	-	-
Local infection	-	-	-	-
Adhesions	Omentum	Omentum	Omentum	Omentum
Deaths	3	3	1	3

Macroscopic observations after implantation of different low- and heavy-weight polypropylene (PP) and polyester (PE) meshes and an observation period of 90 days in rats.
[a]n=45 in each group.

16.4 Cellular Response of Low- Versus Heavy-Weight Meshes

The cellular response is characterized by the cell stress and the expression of HSP70 as an inducible stress marker (Fig. 3A), the proliferation rate with Ki67 positivity (Fig. 3B) and the rate of cell damage, apoptosis and DNA strand breaks with TUNEL-positive cells (Fig. 3C). HSP70 expression (Fig. 3A) inversely correlates with the activity of the inflammatory reaction, as shown by our group in a recent study (Klosterhalfen et al. 1998b). In particular, macrophages expressing high intracellular amounts of HSP70 liberate low levels of the pro-inflammatory cytokines tumor necrosis factor (TNF)-a and possibly interleukin (IL)-1 and IL-6. This correlation may be one reason why the inflammatory reaction of the low-weight meshes Mersilene and Vypro is less active than that of the heavy-weight meshes Parietex and Prolene.

In contrast to the HSP70 expression, Ki67- (Fig. 3B) and TUNEL-positive cells (Fig. 3C) can basically be determined in the interface of the heavy-weight meshes. Here, again, the low expression of HSP70 might play a central role, because HSP70 is known to influence cell maturation and proliferation as well as to exhibit a broad spectrum of cytoprotective effects with a decrease in the rate of cell damage and apoptosis.

The results of these studies provide strong evidence for the hypothesis that all meshes are not inert and cause a chronic irritation of the artificial abdominal wall. If meshes were to be completely inert, none of the parameters HSP70, Ki67 and TUNEL would be detected in the interface. However, surgical meshes on the market and those developed for experimental studies provide at best only a marked cell stress in the interface between mesh and recipient tissues which may be tolerated by cells in contact combined with low proliferation and cell damage rates (Fig. 4). Corresponding to these results and to our best knowledge, the two low-weight meshes Mersilene and Vypro are the surgical meshes with the best short-term biocompatibility. However, Prolene and Parietex meshes show a stress level which exceeds the tolerance level of the interface tissues, leading to cell damage and subsequent tissue repair (Fig. 4).

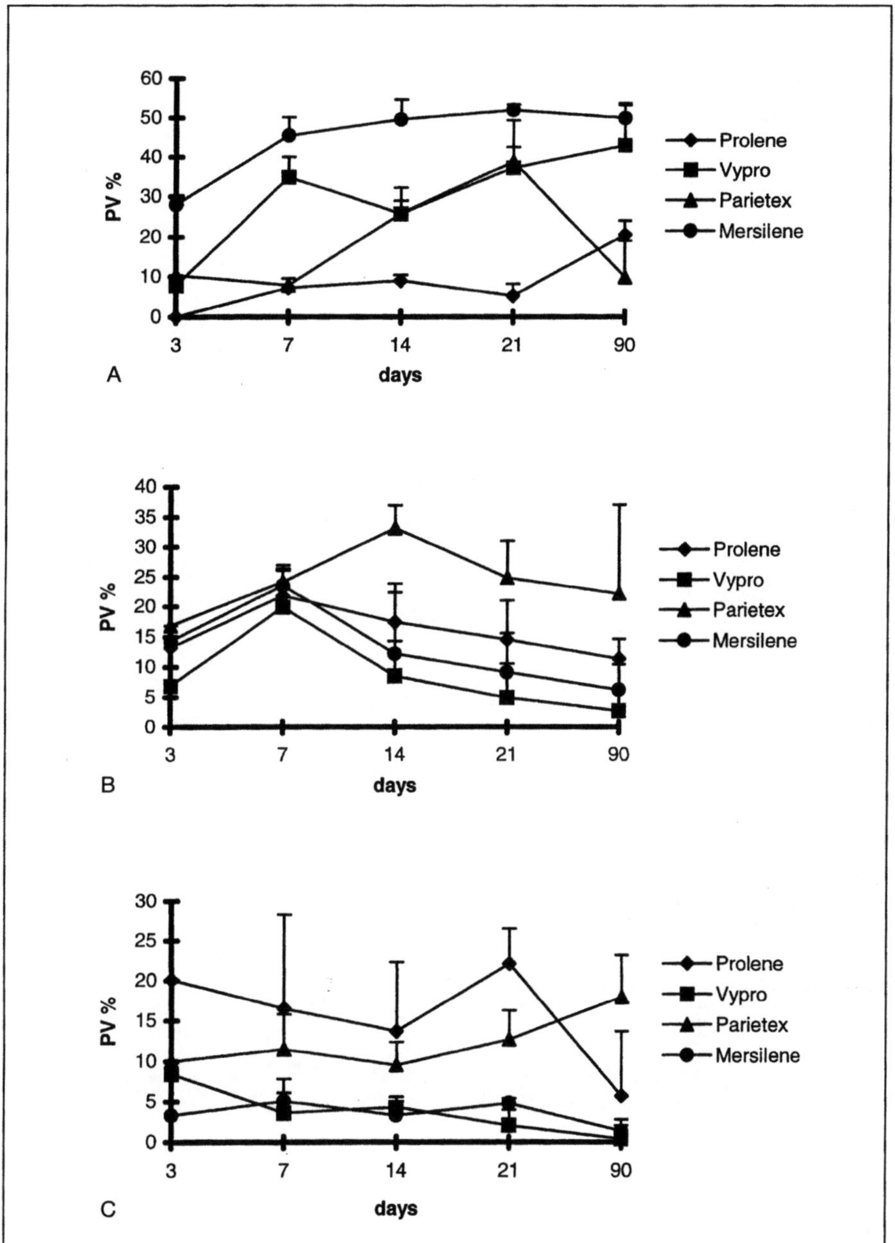

Fig. 3A–C. Cellular response. Morphometric data of the interface between polymer fibres and recipient tissues. *A* Expression of HSP70 (%) as marker of the cell stress response. *B* Ki67-positive cell fraction (%). *C* TUNEL-positive cells (%) indicating apoptosis or DNA strand breaks. PV, partial volume. Data are given as mean ± SD

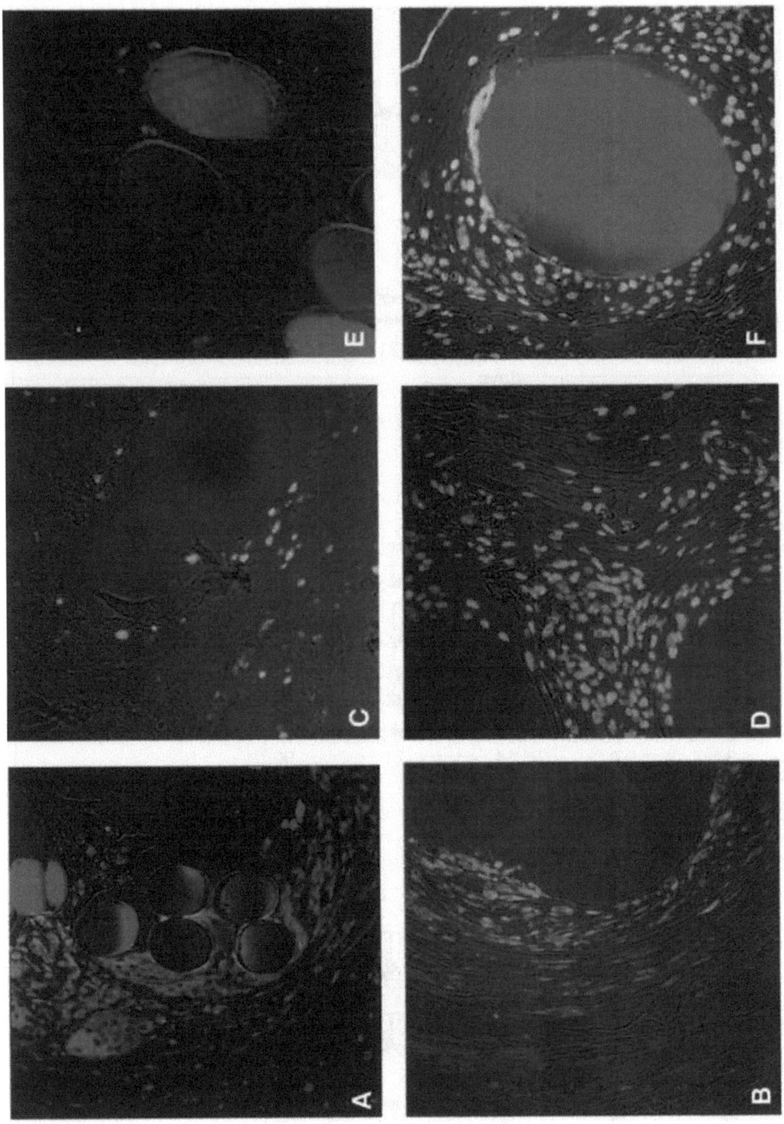

Fig. 4A–F. Confocal laser scan microscopy (CLSM) of the interface, with the Vypro mesh at the top and the Prolene mesh at the bottom. *A,B* Expression of the stress protein HSP70. *C,D* TUNEL-positive cells indicating apoptosis or DNA strand breaks. *E,F* Ki67 positivity marking proliferating cells

16.5 Short- and Long-Term Biocompatibiity of Surgical Meshes

Parallel to the studies on animals, we are very interested in investigating mesh samples explanted from patients. This is very probably the only way to obtain greater knowledge of the consequences of mesh implantation after a period of years. In mid-1998, we had 30 samples of various surgical meshes on record, and 22 mesh units have been

Table 3. Morphometric results (%) (interface, <300 mm)

Mesh	Size of group (*n*)	Time (months)	PMN (%)	Macro-phages (%)	Fibrocyts (%)	TUNEL (%)	Ki67 (%)	HSP70 (%)
Marlex	12	15.6±11.7	12.1.±6.6	44.2±11.7	19.1±7	31.8±10.6	21.3±10.1	31.3±10.5
Vypro	2	7.5±6.3	1.4±1.9	22.2±3.6	9.7±2.7	2.9±1	5.7±5.4	90.5±2.4
Mersilene	4	38±44	14.5±10.4	39.7±5.3	22.9±2.6	8.9±3.6	10.4±5.8	71.6±17.7
Gore-Tex	4	43±43	0.6±1.2	25±6.3	12.1±2.3	37.1±5.6	13.2±8.3	85.3±10.5

Study in 22 patients. Note the poor long-term results of the Mersilene mesh most probably due to the degradation of the polyester (PE) fibres. Gore-Tex is characterized by a high rate of TUNEL-positive cells in the interface. Compared to the Vypro mesh, Marlex reveals an increased rate of inflammation in the interface between mesh and recipient tissues.
PMN, polymorphonuclear neutrophils.

completely investigated (Table 3). Although the overall number of mesh samples in this study is too small to allow definitive conclusions to be made, the preliminary results indicate that surgical meshes implanted in patients reveal a tissue and cellular response comparable to the results of our rat study. Finally, the data provide an impressive report on the chronic irritation of the recipient tissues in the implant bed, even though implantation took place months or years before. Consequently, it is doubtful whether surgical meshes are inert. However, the data also show the superiority of the low-weight meshes Vypro and Mersilene. The relatively bad findings in Mersilene mesh in the patient studies compared to the animal experiments is due to the instability of the polymer PE. Implantation periods of several years are followed by a complete degradation of the mesh, and in the final histological analysis only debris or fragments can be found (Fig. 2c). It is evident that the degradation process results in an enlargement of the plane area of the mesh and an increased rate of phagocytosis, followed by activation of the inflammatory response in the interface and impaired function.

16.6 Risk of Foreign-Body Carcinogenesis

Tumour development in response to the subcutaneous implantation of plastics and other inert materials, known as FB carcinogenesis, was first observed over 40 years ago. It is a classical model of multi-stage endogenous tumourigenesis that requires one half or two thirds of the rodent life span for sarcoma or tumour development. However, unlike chemical rodent carcinogenesis, FB carcinogenesis is generally dismissed as a phenomenon unique to the rodent. The early experimental studies demonstrated unequivocally that the physical characteristics of the implant, such as size, shape and surface morphology, but not the chemical composition, were essential for FB carcinogenesis. Furthermore, a dose–response relationship was found between the implant size and tumour frequency. Materials that induce FB tumours include films of Dacron, nylon, polyethylene, polystyrene, polyvinyl chloride, saran, cellophane, polydimethylsiloxane and Teflon. It was concluded that tumour formation was directly related to cellular events during the FB reaction and formation of the fibrotic capsule surrounding the implant. Subsequent studies have extended these observations and demonstrated that subcutaneously implanted materials of any chemical composition can cause tumours in several animal species provided they possess a smooth and impermeable surface. In powdered, perforated or porous form, these materials lose their tumourigenicity, confirming a primary role for the physical characteristics of the implant rather than its chemical composition. Other studies have shown that the frequency of FB tumours varies directly with the capsule thickness. Taken together, these results suggest that FB tumour initiation and progression occur in cells within the fibrotic capsule. Tumours observed have been mainly fibrosarcomas or histiocytomas (for a review of FB carcinogenesis, see Brand et al. 1975).

In 1997, James et al. reported that the cellular response in the case of FB carcinogenesis is characterized by an accumulation of proliferating and damaged cells in the interface. Silicone foils and, as positive controls, impermeable cellulose acetate filters indicated significantly elevated TUNEL- and proliferating cell nuclear antigen (PCNA)-positive cells compared to the negative control (porous cellulose acetate filters). The results of this group show direct parallels to our findings in heavy- and low-weight meshes, which also reveal a "dose-dependent" irritation of the recipient tissues, with significantly increased cell damage and proliferating rates in the heavy-weight mesh groups compared to the low-weight mesh groups.

A legitimate question is whether FB carcinogenesis is a serious topic in the case of surgical meshes. Fortunately, no case of tumour development after mesh implantation has yet been documented in the literature. However, there are an increasing number of case reports of FB carcinogenesis after implantation of other biomaterials, particularly vascular prosthetic devices, although the mean survival time of these patients is usually less than 10 years. In this context, it has to be remembered that these vascular devices are hosieries like surgical meshes. On the basis of the results in the animal models of tumour development after polymer implantation, sarcomas should be observed in humans after 30–50 years, a period of time correlating to one half or two thirds of the rodent life span. As scientific statements such as retrospective or prospective investigations on the long-term effects of meshes in hernia surgery and other implants are not available, in general FB carcinogenesis cannot be safely dismissed without continued investigation and an appropriate patient follow-up.

Principally, the data of our studies in the rodent model and in mesh samples of patients objectify a theoretical risk in hernia patients treated with a mesh of developing FB-related tumours after decades of implantation. In particular, the tendency to operate on and treat children and young adults with surgical meshes justifies our objections; surgical meshes should not simply be considered as safe, and mesh-free techniques should be reconsidered in this group of patients. Our ethical responsibility forces hernia research to minimize the risk so that new mesh modifications should be as inert as possible. Moreover, if mesh repair is necessary, low-weight surgical meshes should be regarded as the first choice, whereas heavy-weight meshes should no longer be implanted or only in exceptional cases.

16.7 General Histological Principles for the Future Development of Surgical Meshes

The surgical biocompatibility of any biomaterial or implant is defined as the sum total of all functional and histological properties. Histology is therefore an essential procedure and of immense importance in biomaterial research. Central parameters include the tissue and cellular response, which should be determined by a professional and specialized laboratory. Simple and descriptive histology, again, should no longer be regarded as sufficient in surgical mesh research. Surgeons working with and implanting surgical meshes should demand to be informed about the surgical meshes they use in as detailed a manner as possible.

In conclusion, we would like to summarize the important points of our histological studies on surgical meshes:

1. Surgical meshes are not inert, even after years of implantation.
2. Surgical meshes lead to a chronic irritation of the recipient tissues.
3. The tissue reaction is defined in a dose-dependent manner, meaning an activation of inflammation and an increase in irritation with the increase in weight (g/m^2) and surface area (multi- or monofilaments, pore size) in contact with the mesh.
4. Biocompatibility of surgical meshes is primarily influenced by physical or material properties and only secondarily by their chemical composition.
5. Conversely, the compatibility of surgical meshes increases with low weight, large pores and monofilament mesh constructions.
6. The use of heavy-weight meshes such as Prolene or Parietex should be avoided, particularly in children and young adults.
7. Low-weight meshes are advantageous.
8. Mersilene possesses excellent short-term biocompatibility, but poor long-term qualities; PE is degraded after years in the implant bed with a subsequent loss of the mechanical stability and an activation of the inflammatory reaction; all in all, PE is not suitable for use in surgical meshes.
9. The Vypro mesh is the first of a new generation of low-weight meshes and should be regarded as the surgical mesh of choice; it has excellent short- and long-term features.
10. The risk of FB carcinogenesis should not be dismissed without long-term follow-up in patients; multi-centre, prospective studies and histological databases are urgently needed.

16.8 Discussion

Skandalakis: I would like to ask the first speaker about the strength of the aponeurosis.

Conze: Tauber and Seidel were referring to the aponeurosis of the linea alba and the posterior wall of the rectum sheath.

Skandalakis: The posterior wall is pure aponeurosis, of course. Again, we need to understand the difference between fascia and aponeurosis.

Bendavid: I think that one of the most important things we should learn at this meeting is that foreign materials are not carcinogenic. We have been using Marlex since 1956, for 42 years, millions of pieces of Gore-Tex have been used in vascular surgery, and the same applies to Mersiline and Dacron. I am not aware of cases associated with sarcomas, and even though it is theoretically possible that they exist, you cannot compare animals with humans either. Do you have any convincing evidence that this does happen? Otherwise we are going to be set back for many years. It is a fear that is not warranted. Should we leave with that fear?

Klosterhalfen: Your comment is absolutely true. The whole topic of carcinogenesis of polymers was fashionable in the 1960s and 1970s. We found a book by OTT, who was working in Freiburg and who wrote this book in 1970, and he clearly states from the literature of the 1950s, 1960s and 1970s that, at least theoretically, all polymers may induce sarcomas in rodents, dogs and especially humans; these are case reports. If you have a look in Medline, you will find an increasing number of case reports now indicating fibrosarcomas and histiosarcomas when a Gore-Tex graft is used in vascular surgery. Of course, you are right, we cannot compare rodents with human beings, but if experimental models have any sense for our science or our approaches in patients, you have to say that this might be an indication . You have to remember that rodents normally have a life span of 5 years, and if we implant these polymers, the induction time is about 2 years; if you look at a human being, we are talking about a life span of 70–80 years, so we have to consider an induction time of 30–40 years in these materials. I do not think there are any prospective or retrospective studies; most of the patients have since, and that is another very important aspect. Another important aspect is that all the studies in rodents show that foils without pores and microporous materials up to a pore size of 6–8 mm are cancerogenic. Materials with larger pores are definitely not carcinogenic, and that is why we say that the proportion of pores is the most important point here.

Ferguson: The comment you make about the carcinogenesis of these materials is also currently being discussed, e.g. in dermal wound healing, because it has been shown that by trapping pieces of hydrocolic dressing, there have been several case reports of children who subsequently – 20–30 years later – developed a tumor at the site around the pieces of hydrocolic dressing. These studies were done by a company that does not make hydrocolic dressing and therefore are not treated very seriously in the literature, but it is a consideration in the long term.

Klosterhalfen: There are a lot of other examples in medicine. If you look at asbestosis, it is just the same.

Schumpelick: I think I am right in saying that your main point is not that carcinogenesis is the sword of Damocles above mesh implantation. I believe your main point is scar formation and the condition of scar and seroma formation; I think that should be the main field of consideration, and carcinogenesis is only secondary. We have to think about it, but I do not think that it has been proven that our macroporous meshes have a risk of being carcinogenic in humans, has it?

Klosterhalfen: I think that, in macroporous meshes, the risk is definitely reduced if look at the animal studies, and my main points are very simple: Firstly, I think we have to think about whether we should implant meshes in patients aged 10–20 years, and secondly, we should simply think about our mesh construction, no more. If you want to implant a mesh in a 50-year-old patient, I do not think that it is a problem.

Schumpelick: I think that the study by Ott showed that if you use only powder of polypropylene, there is no sarcoma , but if you use a sheet of polypropylene, it might develop.

Ferguson: Can I make one closing comment relating to the very elegant study on the biomechanics of the abdominal wall. I noticed that there is a piece of equipment that you might find interesting made by a company called Dimensional Analysis; it is a way of measuring mechanical properties of skin and any other tissue or wound strength along the suture line, and basically it consists of two dots that go on the skin that are then picked up by a laser when you apply a suction pressure to the skin. The amount of deformation is measured, and if you apply enough pressure, you can actually burst the wound in vivo. That is a very interesting method to supplement the very elegant stereophotogrammetry, because it would be interesting to look at the mechanical properties of the mesh and so on; I can recommend this very elegant piece of equipment that people have used; it leaves a mark on the skin that looks like a little love bite from the suction, but people have even used it to burst wounds in humans, which I think is a bit dubious ethically.

Kingsnorth: I am very concerned about the carcinogenic potential of these meshes, and I think we and the audience would like to see these case reports; I think we need to look at them in detail to see which meshes are involved, what the implantation times are, which particular different histological types of tumors there are and what the adverse oncologies are in terms of the connection between the mesh and the tumor. It is quite a serious business, especially if we are now proposing to put hundreds of thousands of meshes in the groins of patients to repair hernia.

Klosterhalfen: That is absolutely correct. I think Dr. Klinge can easily provide these case reports. I do not have the absolute numbers here right now. If you look at the different types of sarcomas, it is very simple; you only have to look at the cells that you have in the interface, and there you have macrophages, histiocytomas, fibrocytes and fibrosarcomas.

Ferguson: But the issue here is surely to look at the risk, because there is no material or no procedure that you can say does not cause any adverse reaction. So surely people putting in the meshes have an obligation to do long-term follow-up, because if you induce sarcomas in 1%of patients below a certain age, that is rather different than if you induce it in 20% of patients over a longer period of time. A very careful longitudinal study is required, and it is about the risk, because it is not going to be 100% safe – nothing is 100% safe. The question is, what is the relative risk and how long are the times. I am commenting from another areas which say what it requires for those people putting them in to do those longitudinal studies, so if hysteria breaks out and people say that it has caused cancer in one patient, you can actually say, well yes, that is true, but this is the risk, and this is the risk of not doing it. I think that is what is required.

Bendavid: I would like to make another comment referring to the sentence I saw on Dr. Klinge's slide that biomaterial increases the risk of infection. I would like to strongly disagree with this. We have experience of over 3000 patients now, of which about 800 are my own, and I only had infection in two cases in which it was necessary to remove the mesh, despite all the measures taken. The other cases were clean throughout. Even so, we must bear in mind the fact that infection may become manifest years after surgery, and this I have seen in one or two cases which occurred 2 years after surgery. If I recall correctly, Dr. Flambert reported some cases, as did Dr. Stoppa, 8 years following surgery, but to say that this increases the risk of infection – statistically, I cannot see it.

Klinge: I have tried to explain that the meshes or biomaterials in general are accused of increasing the risk of infection but that this has never been proven in clinical studies; I therefore think we can conclude that biomaterials do not increase the infection rate, but they do prolong the persistence of bacteria in the wound. I do not think that is of any great importance for us, and that is what our experiment shows as well.

Klosterhalfen: There are some other data, if I may add to what Dr. Klinge has said; there are a lot of data in orthopaedic surgery if look at the prosthesis and bacterial infection, and one of the main risks is this famous biofilm of this bacteria and inhibition of phagocytosis by macrophages that are in this interface.

Bendavid: May I add that, originally, when we started, we used to use antibiotics with all cases of mesh. In the last 2 years, I have not used any, but the incidence has not changed. I understand that Dr. Gilbert from Florida never uses antibiotics either. It would be interesting to see by a show of hands how many people use antibiotics with prosthetic meshes here. I can see nine hands, and the rest I presume do not use antibiotics.

Amid: You have to ask what seize of mesh is used. I saw Steve raise his hand, and he is probably using them with a laparoscopic technique, which is a big piece of mesh. So the questions should be divided into two: How many people use them for a small piece of mesh? And how many people use them for a large piece of mesh?

Scott: My own personal use of antibiotics has nothing to do with medicine or science but has everything to do with the legal system in the United States. That just applies to me personally; I personally – and the various literature I have read and the people I have talked to – have not found a medical reason to use antibiotics before the implantation of a mesh in a routine primary hernia repair; however, from a legal point of view, I think that I am safer with them than without; that might seem rather cowardly of me, but I have had bad experience.

Bendavid: I would like to hear any comments, perhaps from Dr. Chevrel or Dr. Flament, on the length of surgery. I assume that the length of the surgery, as well as the size of the mesh, is probably a factor that would be worth looking into.

Flament: Yes, I agree with you; we use prophylactic antibiotics in all cases of mesh prosthesis, but I am sure that the time of exposure of the prosthesis to the outside air is very important for the rate of infection. You have to operate rapidly.

References

Amid PK, Schulman AG, Lichtenstein IL (1992) [Surgical repair of primary or recurrent inguinal hernia by prosthesis and polypropylene plug]. Chirurgie 118, 551–558

Amid PK, Shulman AG, Lichtenstein IL, Hakakha M (1994) Biomaterials for abdominal wall hernia surgery and principles of their applications. Langenbecks Arch Chir 379, 168–171

Bellon JM, Bujan J, Contreras LA, Carreras San Martin A, Hernando A, Jurado F (1996) Improvement of the tissue integration of a new modified polytetrafluoroethylene prosthesis: Mycro Mesh. Biomaterials 17, 1265–1271

Bellon JM, Contreras LA, Sabater C, Bujan J (1997) Pathologic and clinical aspects of repair of large incisional hernias after implant of a polytetrafluoroethylene prosthesis. World J Surg 21, 402–406; discussion 406–407

Bleichrodt RP, Simmermacher RK, van der Lei B, Schakenraad JM (1993) Expanded polytetrafluoroethylene patch versus polypropylene mesh for the repair of contaminated defects of the abdominal wall. Surg Gynecol Obstet 176, 18–24

Blom WF, Koops HS, Vermey A, Oldhoff J (1982) Abdominal wall resection and reconstruction with the aid of Marlex mesh. Br J Surg 69, 353–355

Brand KG, Buoen LC, Johnson KH, Brand I (1975) Etiological factors, stages, and the role of the foreign body in foreign-body tumorigenesis: a review. Cancer Res 35, 279–286

Imvrios G, Tsakiris D, Gakis D, Takoudas D, Koukoudis P, Papadimitriou M, Antoniadis AA (1994) Prosthetic mesh repair of multiple recurrent and large abdominal hernias in continuous ambulatory peritoneal dialysis patients. Perit Dial Int 14, 338–343

James SJ, Progribna M, Miller BJ, Bolon B, Muskhelishvili L (1997) Characterization of cellular response to silicone implants in rats: implications for foreign-body carcinogensis. Biomaterials 18, 667–675

Klinge U, Conze J, Klosterhalfen B, Limberg W, Obolenski B, Ottinger AP, Schumpelick V (1996a) [Changes in abdominal wall mechanics after mesh implantation. Experimental changes in mesh stability]. Langenbecks Arch Chir 381, 323–332

Klinge U, Conze J, Limberg W, Brucker C, Ottinger AP, Schumpelick V (1996b) [Pathophysiology of the abdominal wall]. Chirurg 67, 229–233

Klosterhalfen B, Klinge U, Henze U, Bhardwaj R, Conze J, Schumpelick V (1997) [Morphologic correlation of functional abdominal wall mechanics after mesh implantation]. Langenbecks Arch Chir 382, 87–94

Klosterhalfen B, Klinge U, Schumpelick V (1998a) Functional and morphological evaluation of different polypropylene mesh modifications for abdominal wall repair. Biomaterials (in press)

Klosterhalfen B, Klinge U, Tietze L, Henze U, Muys L, Mittermayer C, Bhardwaj RS (1998b) Expression of the heat shock protein 70 (HSP70) in the interface of polymer-implants in vivo. J Mat Sci Mat Med (in press)

Leber GE, Garb JL, Alexander AI, Reed WP (1998) Long-term complications associated with prosthetic repair of incisional hernias. Arch Surg 133, 378–382

Lichtenstein IL, Shulman AG, Amid PK (1990) Use of mesh to prevent recurrence of hernias. Postgrad Med 87, 155–158, 160

Lichtenstein IL, Shulman AG, Amid PK (1993) The cause, prevention, and treatment of recurrent groin hernia. Surg Clin North-Am 73, 529–544

Lichtenstein IL, Shulman AG, Amid PK, Montllor MM (1988) Cause and prevention of postherniorrhaphy neuralgia: a proposed protocol for treatment. Am J Surg 155, 786–790

Matapurkar BG, Gupta AK, Agarwal AK (1991) A new technique of "Marlex-peritoneal sandwich" in the repair of large incisional hernias [see comments]. World J Surg 15, 768–770

Miller K, Junger W (1997) Ileocutaneous fistula formation following laparoscopic polypropylene mesh hernia repair. Surg Endosc 11, 772–773

Notaras MJ (1974) Experience with mersilene mesh in abdominal wall repair. Proc R Soc Med 67, 1187–1190

Schumpelick V, Arlt G, Schlachetzki A, Klosterhalfen B (1997) [Chronic inguinal pain after transperitoneal mesh implantation. Case report of net shrinkage]. Chirurg 68, 1297–1300

Schumpelick V, Conze J, Klinge U (1996) [Preperitoneal mesh-plasty in incisional hernia repair. A comparative retrospective study of 272 operated incisional hernias]. Chirurg 67, 1028–1035

Sher W, Pollack D, Paulides CA, Matsumoto T (1980) Repair of abdominal wall defects: Gore-Tex vs. Marlex graft. Am Surg 46, 618–623

Shulman AG, Amid PK, Lichtenstein IL (1992) The safety of mesh repair for primary inguinal hernias: results of 3,019 operations from five diverse surgical sources. Am Surg 58, 255–257

Subramanyam K, Robbins HT (1989) Erosion of Marlex band and silastic ring into the stomach after gastroplasty: endoscopic recognition and management [see comments]. Am J Gastroenterol 84, 1319–1321

Sugarbaker PH (1980) Prosthetic mesh repair of large hernias at the site of colonic stomas. Surg Gynecol Obstet 150, 576–578
Walker PM, Langer B (1976) Marlex mesh for repair of abdominal wall defects. Can J Surg 19, 211–213
Wantz GE (1991) Incisional hernioplasty with Mersilene. Surg Gynecol Obstet 172, 129–137
Wantz GE (1996) Experience with the tension-free hernioplasty for primary inguinal hernias in men. J Am Coll Surg 183, 351–356

CHAPTER 17

Biomaterials – Principles of Implantation

J.B. Flament, C. Avisse, J.P. Palot, J.F. Delattre

Prosthetic implantation allows repair of complex abdominal wall herniation and can be used to treat very big or even giant lesions, often considered beyond the scope of surgical repair, especially when they are multirecurrent. The use of prosthetic material has been the subject of much controversy, but it is now widely accepted in most European countries.

17.1 Choice of the Prosthesis

The choice of an appropriate prosthesis is based on the physical and biological properties of the material to be used. The ideal material should be as light and as solid as possible, with a certain degree of elasticity and suppleness. Elasticity allows the prosthesis to conform freely to the curvatures of the visceral sac and to "accompany" the movements of the muscles into which it is incorporated, thereby avoiding undue friction leading to chronic inflammation. It is also important that the material has a fairly open mesh structure so that a rapid fibroblastic response is able to invest the prosthesis, thereby facilitating its insertion. For these several reasons, we have chosen to use Dacron (Mersuture) over the past decades, since in our opinion this is the best (or least an appropriate) material commercially available. The results of our long experience with this material in the treatment of hernia of the groin and major incisional hernia have been confirmed by experimental studies done by Petit and Stoppa in Amiens and Adloff and Arnaud in Strasbourg in 1976. They demonstrated that fibroblastic investment of the prosthesis is best when Mersilene mesh is used, i.e., the index of fibroblastic reaction is high and is much greater than the index of inflammatory reaction, which remains low. Furthermore, we have never observed intolerance to this type of prosthetic mesh, and the cases of rejection that have been seen were related to septic contamination during operation. Thus we cannot follow the conclusions of Leber et al. [19], who say that polyester mesh should no longer be used for incisional hernia repair.

Other prostheses are also available on the market.

Polypropylene meshes are thought to be very well tolerated by the organism, because they are monofilamented. Marlex (Bard) and Prolene (Ethicon) are been studied experimentally by Amid [3]. New prostheses (Vypro, which is a combination of polypropylene and polyglactin 910) has been studied in experiments by Schumpelick [18]. These new prostheses seems to be very interesting.

Polytetrafluoroethylene (PTFE), because of its poor incorporation in the connective tissue, seems to be indicated only when there is no posterior rectus sheath. It can be placed in the abdominal cavity in contact with the bowel loops.

17.2 Site of Implantation

The site of prosthetic implantation must be chosen on an anatomical basis. A prosthesis can always be positioned intraperitoneally by attaching it to the deep surface of the abdominal wall or under the skin by fixing it to the superficial part of the abdominal wall. However, insertion of the prosthesis within the wall itself obviously requires the existing anatomical conditions to be taken into account. The best planes of cleavage within the abdominal wall are found in the rectus sheath, between the lateral abdominal muscles, and in the subumbilical part of the properitoneal space, as was clearly demonstrated by Jean Rives.

17.2.1 Intraperitoneal Positioning

Intraperitoneal positioning of the prosthetic material was recommended by Bourgeon in 1972. In a study published in 1997, Arnaud [4] reported on this procedure in 220 patients. Good results (two deaths; infection in five patients, 4.5%; recurrence in eight patients, 3.6%) were obtained in the study considering the magnitude of the lesions that were seen. However, we do not believe that intraperitoneal implantation has any advantages. Although the peritoneum rapidly envelops the prosthesis and offers a good defense against infection without hematoma formation, peritoneal envelopment of the prosthesis is also accompanied by adhesions of the bowel loops, thereby hindering intestinal transit and rendering reintervention dangerous. The adhesions may be complicated by small bowel fistulization. We have seen four cases of intraluminal migration of an intraperitoneal prosthesis. When possible, interpositioning of the omentum between the viscera and the prosthesis can afford protection against these complications.

Laparoscopic placement of a prosthesis is a variant of intraperitoneal placement. We think it is ineffective, because the prosthesis cannot be placed under good tension due to the pneumoperitoneum. This technique is dangerous, because dissection of the intrasaccular adhesions is difficult and may lead to bowel fistulas. Finally, laparoscopic treatment cannot give a good cosmetic result because it does not treat the problem of an excess of skin. In many cases, paniculectomy is required to obtain a good cosmetic result.

17.2.2 Premuscular Positioning

Premuscular positioning of the prosthesis has been proposed by Chevrel [7]. Although the author's initial published report was limited to 12 cases, his personal experience has now been extended to include over 232 patients [10]. This technique consists of obtaining closure by turndown of the anterior lamina of the rectus sheath with suturing to form a mantle-like covering, as in the Welti-Eudel technique [30], followed by implantation of a large Prolene prosthesis over the sutured area. Chevrel has demonstrated the use of fibrin glue [10]. Although precautions must be taken when this procedure is used, especially in cases where cutaneous cover is less than satisfactory, its major advantage over a deeper implantation is the absence of grave complications for patients with infection (Godquin 1979).

We use only this premuscular positioning of prosthesis in cases of a septic procedure when it is not possible to place a nonabsorbable prosthesis; after a plasty according Welti and Eudel, we placed an absorbable prosthesis in the premuscular position. In our hands, the rate of recurrences with this technique was 20%.

17.2.3 Retromuscular Prefascial Prosthesis

According to our observations reported below, the prosthesis was always implanted deep to the muscles of the abdomen, i.e., in the rectus sheath or the properitoneal space whenever possible. The space for implantation may differ for the upper and lower parts of the prosthesis.

In cases of midline incisional hernia, we place the prosthesis in contact with the muscle fibers, i.e., in the interval between the rectus abdominis and the plane of contact between the peritoneum and the posterior lamina of the rectus sheath. This requires opening of the rectus sheath near the linea alba to gain entry to the retromuscular space and exposure of the posterior belly of the rectus muscle.

Described by J. Rives as early as 1973, this technique was clearly demonstrated in 1977 in the *French Encyclopaedia of Surgery* [25]. The drawings were later reproduced in the first and second edition of *Abdominal Wall Surgery* by Chevrel have also been reproduced, with minor modifications, by Wantz [29] and Stoppa et al. [27] (Fig. 1).

17.2.3.1 Closure Anterior and Posterior to the Prosthesis

The peritoneal cavity must be closed prior to implantation of the prosthesis. In most cases, apposition and suture of the posterior rectus sheath margins can be achieved if

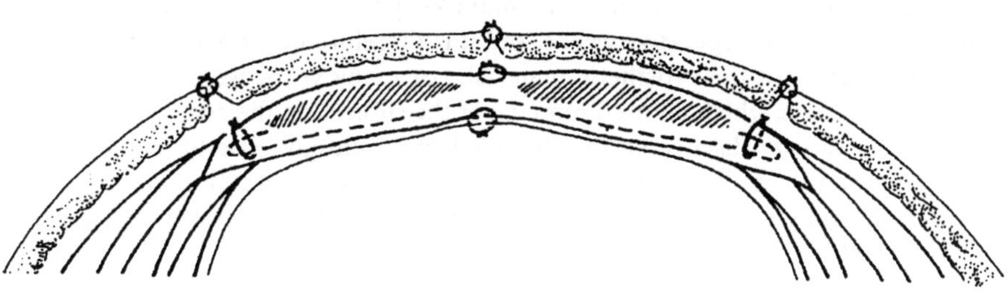

Fig. 1. Placement of the retromuscular prefascial prothesis

the peritoneum has been freed correctly and widely. In the midline, the peritoneal layer is much thicker, since it is covered by the posterior lamina of the rectus sheath in this region. If peritoneal apposition cannot be achieved, we close the defect with an absorbable prosthesis (Vicryl or Dexon sutured to the edges of the defect). Omentum, when present, can be used to protect viscera from the prosthesis. The posterior surface of the omentum allows good peritonization, while its anterior surface offers a surface of granulation tissue which invests the prosthesis. Every attempt should be made to achieve an intervening surface of cover between the prosthesis and the skin, although this is not always possible.

17.2.3.2
Placement of the Prosthesis

The upper part of the prosthesis is placed between the rectus abdominis anteriorly and the thorax and internal oblique posteriorly. The lower part of the prosthesis is fixed to Cooper's ligament and extends into the pelvic region in order to prevent its detachment; in other words, the prosthesis is implanted in the rectus sheath above the arcade line and in the properitoneal space below it.

In cases of lateral incisional hernia, the abdominal muscles may be seen only along part of the circumference of the hernial orifice. When subchondral hernia is present, it is often necessary to position the upper part of the plate beneath the diaphragm and attach it to the rib cage using transfixing costodiaphragmatic sutures. The lower part of the prosthesis then lies anterior to the peritoneum, while the upper parts are in the peritoneal envelope. In cases of inguinal incisional hernia, it is necessary to position the prosthesis so that it envelops the peritoneum and extends into the iliac fossa and pelvis. The prosthesis is sutured above to the deep surface of the muscles and below to Cooper's ligament or the iliac crest. The mesh should extend well beyond the area of the defect (in all directions) in the properitoneal space. The overlap must be at least 8 cm.

The area of insertion of the prosthesis must be as large as possible. Our experience has shown that suturing of the material to the margins of the defect (inlay prosthesis) offers no guarantee of solidity and usually results in recurrence of hernia due to lateral detachment. Accordingly, the mesh should extend well beyond the myoaponeurotic hernial orifice, with intra-abdominal pressure being used to ensure its insertion. The force of abdominal pressure holds the prosthesis against the deep surface of the muscles, thereby achieving a sort of "suture by apposition." However, this pressure-induced apposition is not sufficient to maintain the prosthesis in the correct position during the first few postoperative weeks, and it is therefore necessary to ensure solid peripheral suturing of the prosthetic material. For many years, we used pledgets to attach the prosthesis, which allowed removal of the sutures on the 20th postoperative day. However, we later discovered that the pledgets could give rise to complications and that they were not absolutely necessary. We changed our practice and now tighten each transfixing suture of the abdominal wall through a cutaneous buttonhole, which is then closed by a single stitch. In cases of midline incisional hernia, the semilunar line (Spieghel's line) is used as the site for peripheral attachment of the prosthesis.

The conditions for these surgical procedures should obey the rules of prosthetic implantation. The problems encountered are identical to those seen in orthopedic surgery. The risk of infection can be minimized by operating under conditions of scrupulous asepsis. Prosthetic surgery thus requires major precautions to be taken: perfect hemostasis, absence of direct manipulation of the prosthesis, and overnight formalin vaporization of the operating room. The overhead light should not be manipulated during the operation. Vacuum aspiration should also be proscribed during surgery to avoid the displacement of dust or other airborne particles that may be contaminated.

17.3 Fixation of the Prosthesis

Anchoring of the mesh by interrupted absorbable sutures, passed through the edge of the mesh, abdominal wall, and out through the skin through small stab incisions, is the technique we described in 1977 [25]. This technique is used by many authors [11, 21]. Staples can also be used [2]. Some have used fibrin glue to prevent slippage of the prosthesis [10].

17.4 Postoperative Care

Monitoring of body temperature may demonstrate an initial moderate rise due to inflammatory reaction. However, persistence of fever beyond the fourth postoperative day usually indicates the occurrence of late suppuration.

Aspiration drains should also be monitored. These drains, placed in contact with the prosthesis and/or beneath the skin, are used to evacuate fluid and blood in the areas of dissection, which may be very large. We remove the drains on about the sixth postoperative day.

The skin and abdominal cicatrix must be examined and should therefore be exposed as soon as possible to identify the slightest modification that may reflect the presence of local infection.

Respiratory physiotherapy should resume as soon as the patient leaves the operating room. Early ambulation is recommended in most cases, but precautions should be taken initially. It may be wise to replace early ambulation by mobilization in bed, with guidance by the physiotherapist whenever possible.

Finally, all sporting activity and physical stress are contraindicated during the period of connective tissue cicatrization, i.e., for 3–6 months after the operation.

17.4.1 Early Postoperative Infection

We obtained full cure in some cases of early postoperative infection (the last having been observed in 1987) by wide saucerization and irrigation, thereby allowing the developing granulation tissue to invest the Mersilene prosthesis. It is our impression that long-lasting wound suppuration results from overly conservative postoperative treatment (e.g., limited disunion, removal of a few stitches).

17.4.2 Late Postoperative Infection

Late postoperative complications required removal of the prosthesis.

17.5 Results

Our experience with modern procedures for repair of incisional hernia dates back to 1964. During the 1970–1997 period, we observed 1018 patients with major abdominal incisional hernias, although this figure is manifestly low since it represents those patients in which a specific procedure was done to treat the incisional hernia only, and does not take into account the numerous small incisional hernias that were identified and treated on surgical reintervention for various other reasons.

Discussed below are the results of 710 major incisional hernias (Fig. 2) treated between 1991 and 1997. These patients have been selected as they constitute a homogeneous series with respect to both the type of surgical procedure performed and the surgical team that performed the operation (four senior surgeons implanted 93.3% of the 517 prostheses in this series). Critical analysis of previous failures permitted more selective indications and resulted in a dramatic improvement of our results.

A total of 654 of our patients were elective cases, and 43 were emergencies; 499 (72.6%) required primary repair, and 211 (27.4%) had recurrent incisional hernias. The recurrence occurred after nonprosthetic repair in 112 patients (53%) and after

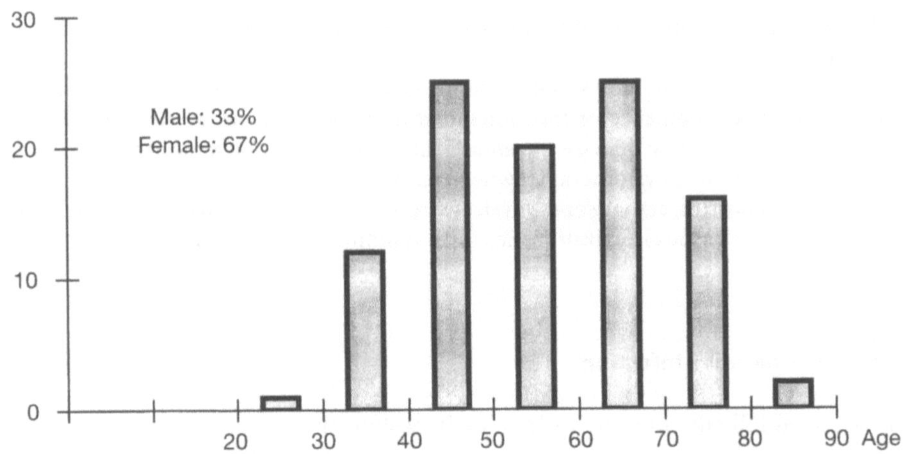

Fig. 2. Our experience with 710 patients with major incisional hernias from 1991 to 1997

prosthetic repair in 99 patients (47%). The repair was nonprosthetic in 123 patients (18%) (Tables 1, 2). The recurrence rate is about 20%. We used an absorbable mesh in 57 patients (8%) (Table 3). The recurrence rate is 54%. All the other patients (n=517) were treated with a nonabsorbable mesh – Mersuture (Ethicon) in 477 (67.2%) and Prolene in 40 (5.6%). The results are shown in Tables 4 and 5.

Table 1. Results of suture repair

	H	DCD	Follow-up (1 year)	Recurrences	
				(*n*)	(%)
Elective procedure	40	0	36	6	17
Emergency	10	2	7	2	28
Infection	26	0	24	7	20
Total	76	2	67	15	22

Table 2. Results of hernioplasty with or without absorbable prosthesis

	H	DCD	Follow-up (1 year)	Recurrences	
				(*n*)	(%)
Elective procedure	20	0	15	0	0
Emergency	4	2	2	1	50
Infection	23	1	18	6	33
Total	47	3	35	7	20

Table 3. Results of absorbable prosthetic repairs

	H	DCD	Follow-up (1 year)	Recurrences	
				(*n*)	(%)
Elective procedure	12	0	10	6	60
Emergency	29	6	19	7	53
Infection	16	3	12	9	75
Total	57	9	41	22	54

Table 4. Postoperative course of 517 prosthetic repairs

Outcome	Patients (*n*)	(%)
Uneventful course	500	96.4
Mortality[a]	3	0.6
Morbidity	16	3
Superficial wound infection	5	–
Deep wound infection[a]	5	–
Hematoma	4	–
Intestinal fistula	1	–
Bowel obstruction	1	–

[a]One patient had an infection and died.

Table 5. Long-term results of prosthetic repairs in 474 patients

Results	Patients (*n*)	(%)
Good results	446	94
Primary	438	-
After treatment of infection	8	-
Recurrences	27	5.6%
Delayed infection (2 years)	1	-
Bowel migration	1	-
Final good results[a]	466	98

[a]After reoperation for recurrence in 20 patients.

17.6 Conclusion

These results clearly show that only nonabsorbable prostheses, placed on the retromuscular prefascial space, are able to give good long-term results in patients with giant incisional hernia of the abdominal wall.

17.7 Discussion

Amid: When you told me your concerns about neuralgia, I really did not understand why you were concerned, because I put the stapler in between the intercostal neurovascular bundle and there is no way that you can catch the nerve. Now I have seen this picture of 52 staples, but there is really no need for that many staples. If you put it only between the neurovascular bundle, you need only three or four on each side. I have never stapled the upper edge or the lower edge; there are sutures to attach it under the surface of the linea alba or to Cooper's ligament.

Flament: I agree with you – we use only 12 stitches, like a clock around the abdomen, but some surgeons are like children, they trigger the stapler and go klick, klick, klick... That is why they catch the nerve, I think.

Schumpelick: Dr. Flament, do you really have to do this transcutaneous fixation? Have you tried any other method, e.g., fixing it on the fascia or at the level of the fascia? We have done it like that, and I am not quite sure whether it is sufficient, although I think it might be. Have you have any bad experience with local fixation and that is why you prefer transcutaneous fixation, or is this the way your technique has developed?

Flament: If you fix it by the posterior aspect of the rectus muscle, you put your stitches in one by one. To achieve good tension, we usually put the stitches in on one side and after that we place three, four, or five stitches. We knot them all together with the assistant pulling on the other strings, so we can achieve good tension. We feel that, for abdominal wall incisional hernias, you need good tension, unlike in inguinal hernia.

Simmermacher: Continuing the topic of transcutaneous sutures: Are they absorbable or nonabsorbable? Do you remove them and, if so, when do you remove them?

Flament: We have gone through three stages. To begin with we used pledgets, but they resulted in infection and we stopped using them in 1978. After that, we used nonabsorbable stitches, but sometimes patients complained about feeling the stitches under the skin. I do not really know exactly when we changed, but we now use absorbable sutures and patients do not feel the absorbable stitches because they are resorbed.

Bendavid: With the use of multiple layers of prosthetic material, I am always amazed that it is quite prevalent; if you take the literature on Marlex mesh, the tension under this is apparently 50 pounds per square inch, which is phenomenally strong. I always give a sheet to the patient and ask him to try to rip it, but there is no way that you can actually break it. However, with reference to Mersilene, I was interested to see that some decomposition has been reported (30%) after 10 years. I discovered a sheet of Mersilene in the Shouldice Hospital that had been sitting there for about 30 years, and when I opened it up it was powder.

Filipi: I was very impressed by your presentation. What is the mechanism of recurrence? Is it due to excessive tension at one point, or is it inadequate overlap?

Flament: We have to bear in mind different mechanisms. Firstly, tear of the mesh; this occurred once, and I know that Chevrel has had such an experience. So it is not a problem. Secondly, slipping of the prosthesis, especially in huge incisional hernias in women who have had previous gynecologic and obstetric operations. Now we fix the mesh to Cooper's ligament. And there is a problem that mainly occurs with small prostheses; these patients do not have a good abdominal wall. You put a prosthesis all over the defect, but below or above the defect the abdominal wall is very bad, and there will be recurrences around the edges of the meshes. That is why we now put huge mesh in huge incisional hernias and fix it to Cooper's ligament below and to the ribs above.

Hartel: If I understood your slides correctly, you carried out primary closures without using a prosthesis in only 18% of patients. Which patients were these, and which cases are suitable for primary closure?

Flament: None so far. The patients in which we carried out a primary closure were those where we had a small hole, but we had 30% recurrences, and these recurrences have been treated with Mersilene mesh. When we have to do a septic procedure or in emergency cases, we use relaxing incisions and closure of the midline.

Schumpelick: Dr. Flament, how often are you able to close the midline? You always try to close the midline of the linea alba? If you are not able to, what do you do then?

Flament: That is a problem. We use relaxing incisions. That is because there is a certain retraction of the lateral muscles. We use relaxing incisions on the anterior sheet of the rectus muscles and usually complete the procedure with an absorbable prosthesis as an onlay prosthesis.

Nillson: Do you always place your prosthesis in front of the peritoneum just behind the muscle layers, or do you sometimes place it in front of the posterior rectus sheath, behind the muscle itself?

Flament: That depends on the level. Above the great ligament we place the prosthesis in front of the rectus sheath or rectus muscle. So we open the posterior aspect of the rectus sheath. But below the arcuate ligament there is no more rectus sheath, so it is in the preperitonneal space. However, it is always in contact with the posterior aspect of the muscle so invasion is very quick and very fast.

References

1. Amid PK, Schulman AG, Lichtenstein IL, Sostrin 5, Young J, Hakakha M. Experimental evaluation of a new composite mesh with the selective property of incorporation to the abdominal wall without adhering to the intestines. J. of Biomedical Materials Research, 1994, 28 : 373–375
2. Amid PK, Schulman AG, Lichtenstein IL. A simple stapling technique for prosthetic repair of massive incisional hernias. The American Surgeon, 1994, 12,934–937
3. Amid PK, Classification of biomaterials and their related complications in abdominal wall hernia surgery. Hernia, 1997, 1: 14–21
4. Arnaud JP, Cervi C., Tuech JJ, Cattan F. Surgical treatment of post-operative incisional hernias by intra-peritoneal insertion of a Dacron mesh. A report of 220 cases. Hernia, 1997, 1 97–99
5. Bendavid R., Composite mesh (polypropylene - e -PTFE) in the intraperitoneal position. A report of 30 cases. Hernia, 1997, 1 5–8
6. Bendavid R. Incisional parapubic hernias. Surgery 1990; 108 898–901
7. Chevrel JP. Traitement des grandes éventrations médianes par plastie en paletot et prothése. Nouv Presse Med, 1979 ; 8: 695–696
8. Chevrel JP, Flament JB. Les éventrations de la paroi abdominale. Rapport au 92ème Congrès Francais de Chirurgie, 1990, A.F.C., Ed. Masson, Paris
9. Chevrel JP, Flament JB. Traitement des éventrations de la paroi abdominale. Editions Techniques - Encycl. Med. Chir. Techniques Chirurgicales - Appareil digestif, 40–165, 1995, l4p
10. Chevrel JP, Rath AM. The use of fibrin glues in the surgical treatment of incisional hernias. Hernia, 1997, 1 : 9–14
11. Duce AM, Muguerza JM, Villeta R, Martin J, Gutierrez A, Diez M., Noguerales F, Granell J. The Rives operation for the repair of incisional hernias. Hernia, 1997, 1 :175–177
12. Flament JB, Palot JP. Prostheses and major incisional hernias. In: Bendavid R., Prostheses and major incisional hernias, Austin Landes Biomedical publisher, 1994.
13. Flament JB, Palot JP, Burde A., Delattre J.F., Avisse C. Treatment of major incisional hernias. Problems in General Surgery, 1995; 12: 151–8
14. Flament JB, Rives, Palot JP, Burde A., Avisse C. Surgery of the abdominal wall. Major incisional hernias. Ed. by JP Chevrel, Springer, Berlin Heidelberg New York, 1995
15. Gibson CL. Operation for cure of large ventral hernias. Ann Surg, 1920;72:214
16. Goni-Moreno 1, Chronic eventrations and large hernias. Preoperative treatment by progressive pneumoperitoneum. Original procedure. Surgery, 1947; 22 : 945–53
17. Judd ES. The prevention and treatment of ventral hernia. Surg Gynecol Obstet, 1912; 15: 175–182
18. Klinge U, Klosterhalfen B, Conze J, Limberg W, Obolenski B, Ottinger AP, Schumpelick V. A modified mesh for hernia repair that is adapted to the physiology of the abdominal wall. Eur. J. Surg., 1998, 140: 1–11
19. Lardennois B., Benoist M., Hibon J., Flament JB. Résultat de l'utilisation d'une étoffe en dacron dans le traitement des grandes éventrations. A propos de 37 cas. Acta Chir. Belgica, 1971, 70, 287–290
20. Leber GE, Garb JL, Alexander AI, Reed WP. Long-term complications associated with prosthetic repair of incisional hernias. Arch Surg, 1998, 133 : 378–382
21. McLanahan D, King LT. Weems C, Novotney M, Gibson K,. Retrorectus prosthetic mesh repair of midline abdominal hernia. Am. J. Surg., 1997, 173: 445–449
22. Palot J.P., Flament JB., Avisse C., Greffier D., Burde A. Utilisation des prothèses dans les conditions de la chirurgie d'urgence. Etude rétrospective de 204 hernies de l'aine étranglées. Chirurgie, 1996, 121 : 48–50
23. Pire JC, Body C, Flament JB. La capacité vitale, un piège dans le bilan des grandes éventrations. La Nouv Presse Med 1977; 6 : 3641
24. Rives J, Lardennois B, Pire JC, Hibon J. Les grandes éventrations. Importance du "volet abdominal" et des troubles respiratoires qui lui sont secondaires. Chirurgie, 1973; 99 : 547–563
25. Rives J, Pire JC, Flament JB, Convers G. Traitement des éventrations. Encycl. Med. Chir., Paris, PARIS, 1977, 4.0.07, 40165
26. Rives J, Pire JC, Flament JB, Palot, JP, Body C. Le traitement des grandes éventrations. Nouvelles indications thérapeutiques à propos de 322 cas. Chirurgie 1985 ; 3 : 215–25.
27. Stoppa R, Moungar F, Verhaeghe P. Traitement chirurgical des éventrations médianes sus ombilicales. J Chir 1992; 129 : 335–43

28. Trivellini G, Danelli PC, Use of two prostheses in the surgical repair of recurrent hernia. Postgraduate General Surgery, Hernias, 1992, 4: 136–39
29. Wantz GE. Incisional hernioplasty with mersilene. Surgery 1991; 172: 129–37
30. Welti H, Eudel F. Un procédé de cure radicale des éventrations post-opératoires par auto-étalement des muscles grand-droits après incision du feuillet antérieur de leurs gaines. Chirurgie, 1941 ; 28: 791–798

Part V Closure of Laparotomy

CHAPTER 18

Long- Versus Short-Term Absorbable Sutures

P.J. Osther

18.1 Introduction

The cause of wound complications after laparotomy is multifactorial, conditioned by local and systemic and by pre-, peri-, and postoperative factors [1]. Several factors such as advanced age, pulmonary disease, morbid obesity, malignancy, and intra-abdominal infection are associated with impaired wound healing and predispose patients to serious wound complications such as fascial disruption (wound dehiscence), wound infection, and incisional herniation [1–4]. In patients who are at high risk for wound complications, the role of the surgical technique and suture material are especially important [3, 4].

Suture materials for fascial closure can be either absorbable or nonabsorbable, and monofilament or multifilament [2]. Although some studies have shown that the use of nonabsorbable suture materials may result in a lower incidence of incisional hernia [5–7], nonabsorbable sutures seem less ideal, as they are associated with a higher frequency of wound sinuses and wound pain [5, 6, 8–10].

The function of the suture is to maintain apposition of wound edges until the scar is strong enough to prevent displacement. In patients with impaired wound healing (high-risk patients), this process can be considerably delayed with the result that absorbable sutures may loose a significant part of their strength before there is adequate scar formation [11, 12]. Newer monofilament synthetic absorbable sutures (i.e., polyglyconate and polydioxanone sutures) have high initial and long-lasting tensile strength and a low tissue response during degradation [13]. These sutures should therefore theoretically facilitate wound healing in high-risk patients compared with multifilament sutures. Furthermore, experimental studies have shown that multifilament sutures result in a higher incidence of wound complications than monofilament sutures [14, 15]. Thus longer-lasting absorbable monofilament sutures should potentially benefit wound healing, resulting in fewer wound complications. This review was undertaken to compare absorbable multifilament sutures (short degradation time) with monofilament absorbable sutures (long degradation time) for abdominal closure with respect to wound dehiscence, wound infection and incisional herniation and with special reference to high-risk patients. For this purpose, the results of five fully randomized studies were analyzed [6, 16–19].

18.2 Wound Dehiscence

Characteristics of the five studies and incidence of wound dehiscence are presented in Table 1.

The differences in the frequencies of wound dehiscence between the five studies obviously reflect differences in the populations studied, with the highest frequency of wound dehiscence in the study that was performed in a selected group of high-risk patients [18]. However, it may be concluded that, in controlled randomized studies – regardless of the populations studied – there have been no differences in development of wound dehiscence between rapidly absorbable multifilament sutures and slowly absorbable monofilament sutures. In the "high risk" study, interrupted sutures were used [18]. The use of a continuous mass closure technique may have reduced the overall high incidence of wound dehiscence (6.4%) in these high-risk patients, since it has been shown that this technique is associated with the lowest tension in the wound compared with that of other suture techniques [20].

Table 1. Rates of wound dehiscence, wound infection, and incisional hernia

Reference	Population studied	Absorbable sutures compared	Patients (*n*)	Wound dehiscence (%)	Wound infection (%)	Incisional hernia (%)
[6]	Unselected group of patients undergoing laparotomy	Polygalactin, multifilament, interrupted	365	2.2	6.6	16.7
		Polygalactin, continuous	379	1.6	9.0	20.6
		Polydioxanone, monofilament, continuous	370	3.5*	11.6*	13.2*
[16]	Unselected group of patients undergoing laparotomy	Polyglycolic acid, multifilament, interrupted	71	1.4	0	-
		Polyglyconate, monofilament, continuous	62	4.8*	4.8*	-
[19]	Unselected group of patients undergoing laparotomy	Polygalactin, multifilament, interrupted	339	1	11	6
		Polyglyconate, monofilament, continuous	345	1*	10*	8*
[17]	Morbid obese patients undergoing gastroplasty	Polyglycolic acid, multifilament, continuous	42	0	2.4	0
		Polyglyconate, monofilament, continuous	42	0*	9.5*	9.5**
[18]	High-risk patients	Polyglycolic acid, multifilament, interrupted	100	7	16	16
		Polyglyconate, monofilament, interrupted	104	6*	7**	10*

*Not significant; **$p<0.05$.

18.3 Wound Infection

Data on wound infection in the five studies are also presented in Table 1. In the three papers studying unselected groups of patients undergoing laparotomy [6, 16, 19] and in the study of the morbid obese patients [17], there were no significant differences in frequency of wound infections between absorbable multifilament sutures and absorbable monofilament sutures. However, the monofilament polyglyconate suture was associated with a lower incidence of wound infection in the high-risk group [18], which is in agreement with experimental studies [2]. This may be related to capillary forces of the multifilament sutures, picking up bacteria into the sutures, where they subsequently escape phagocytosis [15, 21, 22]. This may have particular significance in the selected group of high-risk patients, as their overall immune response was probably already impaired because of the presence of several predisposing factors [23].

18.4 Incisional Hernia

In four of the five studies, data on the development of incisional hernia were available (Table 1). Again, the differences in frequency of incisional hernias in the different groups probably reflect differences in study populations. In three of the four studies, there were no significant differences in incidence of incisional hernia between multifilament and monofilament sutures [6, 18, 19]. In the study with morbid obese patients, the authors stated that the multifilament suture was easier to handle than the monofilament suture in very fatty tissues, which may have contributed to a higher frequency of hernias in the monofilament group [17].

18.5 Conclusion

Based on data from randomized trials, the overall impression seems to be that there are no obvious differences between absorbable multifilament sutures (with a short degradation time) and absorbable monofilament sutures (with a long degradation time) for fascial closure after laparotomy with regard to development of wound dehiscence, wound infection, and incisional hernia. The incidence of wound infection may be reduced with absorbable monofilament sutures compared with that of multifilament sutures in high-risk patients, and multifilament suture may be more appropriate in very fatty wounds. Whether a nonabsorbable or an absorbable suture should be preferred in high-risk patients still remains to be elucidated. Furthermore, it can be concluded that closure of the abdominal fascia can be performed with a continuous monofilament suture without increased risk for development of wound complications compared to that associated with absorbable interrupted multifilament sutures.

18.6 Discussion

For a discussion, please see Chap. 19.

References

1. Pennickx FM, Poelmans SV, Kerremans RP, Beckers JP Abdominal wound dehiscence in gastrointestinal surgery. Ann Surg 1979; 189: 345–52.
2. Wadström J, Gerdin B. Closure of the abdominal wall; how and why? Clinical review. Acta Chir Scand 1990; 156:75–82.
3. Israelsson LA. Wound complications in midline laparotomy incisions: the importance of the sutures technique. Thesis. Malmö, Sweden 1995, pp 1–89.
4. Haley RW, Culver DH, Morgan MW, White JW, Emori TG, Hooton TM. Identifying patients at high risk for wound infection. Am J Epidemiol 1985; 121:206–15.
5. Bucknall TE, Ellis H. Abdominal wound closure – a comparison of monofilament nylon and plyglycolic acid. Surgery 1981; 89: 672–7.
6. Wissing J, van Vroonhoven TJMV, Schattenkerk ME, Veen HF, Ponsen RJG, Jeekel J. Fascia closure after midline laparotomy: results of a randomized trial. Br J Surg 1987; 74:738–41.
7. Israelsson LA, Johnsson T. Closure of midline laparotomy incisions with polydioxanone and nylon: the importance of suture technique. Br J Surg 1994; 81: 1606–8.
8. Larsen PN, Nielsen K, Schultz A, Mejdahl S, Larsen T, Moesgaard F. Closure of the abdominal fascia after clean and clean-contaminated laparotomy. Acta Chir Scand 1989; 155:461–4.
9. Corman ML, Veidenheimer MC, Coller JA. Controlled clinical trial of three suture materials for abdominal wall closure after bowel operations. Am J Surg 1981; 141: 510–13.
10. Johnson CD, Bernhardt LW, Bentley PG. Incisional hernia after mass closure of abdominal incisions with Dexon and Prolene. Br J Surg 1982; 69: 55(Letter).
11. ABPI Data Sheet Compendium. London: Datapharm 1994
12. Hewin DF. Randomized comparison of polyglycolic acid and polyglyconate sutures for abdominal fascial closure after laparotomy in patients with suspected impaired wound healing. Br J Surg 1995; 82:1698 (letter).
13. Foresman PA, Edlich RF, Rodeheaver GT. The effect of new monofilament absorbable sutures on the healing of musculoaponeurotic incisions, gastrotomies, and colonic anastomoses. Arch Surg 1989; 124: 708–10.
14. Varma S, Ferguson HL, Breen H, Lumb WV. Comparison of seven suture materials in infected wounds – an experimental study. J Surg Res 1974; 17:165–70.
15. Chu CC, Williams DF. Effects of physical configuration and chemical structure of suture materials on bacterial adhesion. A possible link to wound infection. Am J Surg 1984; 147: 197–204.
16. Savolainen H, Ristkari S, Mokka R. Early laparotomy wound dehiscence: a randomized comparison of three suture materials and two methods of fascial closure. Annals Chirurgiae Gynaecologiae 1988; 77: 111–3.
17. Deitel M, Alhindawi R, Yamen M, To TB, Burul CJ. Dexon Plus versus Maxon fascial closure in morbid obesity: a prospective randomized comparison. Can J Surg 1990; 33: 302–4.
18. Osther PJ, Gjode P, Mortensen BB, Mortensen PB, Bartholin J, Gottrup F. Randomized comparison of polyglycolic acid and polyglyconate sutures for abdominal fascial closure after laparotomy in patients with suspected impaired wound healing. Br J Surg 1995; 82: 1080–2.
19. Sahlin S, Ahlberg J, Granström L, Ljungström KG. Monofilament versus multifilament absorbable sutures for abdominal closure. Br J Surg 1993; 80: 322–4.
20. Jenkins TPN. The burst abdominal wound: a mechanical approach. Br J Surg 1976; 63:873–6.
21. Katz S, Izhar M, Direlman D. Bacterial adherence to surgical sutures. Ann Surg 1981; 106:573–7.
22. Österberg B. Influence of capillary multifilament sutures on the antibacterial action of inflammatory cells in infected wounds. Acta Chir Scand 1983; 149:751–7.
23. MacLean LD. Significance of immunoreactivity in trauma. Acta Chir Scand 1985; Suppl 522: 151–70.

CHAPTER 19

Absorbable Versus Nonabsorbable Suture for Laparotomy Closure

M.A. Carlson

The choice of suture material is becoming increasingly complex. The multiple factors to consider when choosing a suture for closure of a fascial incision include its handling characteristics, ability to incite an inflammatory reaction, cost, knot security, and susceptibility to in vivo degradation. One of the more important factors to consider when picking a suture is the durability of tensile strength. Currently available sutures are described as rapidly absorbing, slowly absorbing, and nonabsorbable/permanent. These definitions are variable, and even some sutures described as permanent eventually degrade. Probably the most important criterion on which to judge a suture is its role in early and late wound failure (defined here as dehiscence and hernia, respectively). This review will emphasize the evaluation of suture using that criterion.

19.1 Requirements for the Ideal Suture

Seventy years ago, Moynihan wrote that the requirements for the ideal suture include adequate strength to keep tissue edges apposed and vessels ligated, no infection risk, low tissue irritability, and finally absorbability so that foreign material would not persist to cause problems [23]. The suture material which fulfilled these requirements at the time Moynihan wrote this was catgut. Unfortunately, the experience with catgut in fascial closure during the latter half of this century has been disastrous, with an average dehiscence rate of 10% or more [3a, 13]. Catgut has been condemned as a suture for fascial closure. The suture types used currently, with the possible exception of silk [18], have more than adequate strength in the fresh state to hold fascia together [15]. The issue currently of most concern is how long the suture will maintain its strength and when (if ever) will it be absorbed.

A suture used for fascial closure should maintain reasonable tensile strength for 4–6 weeks, because in animal studies this is the time required for a fascial incision to regain approximately 50% of its baseline strength [1, 10, 12, 21, 24]. The goal of 50% baseline strength is an intuition based on review of the literature; no one has ever determined the "safe" amount of healing must occur so that an abdominal incision can remain intact without the support of suture material. It would be reasonable to assume that the interval to 50% baseline strength would be longer in a patient with suspected slow healing (e.g., secondary to protein malnutrition, steroids, various metabolic diseases), which would argue for use of a more durable or permanent suture in these patients, but hard evidence for this choice is lacking.

The choice of a strong, permanent suture to close fascia would seem logical and final were it not for some long-term complications which are believed to be more common with nonabsorbable suture. "Buttonhole" hernia consists of one or more defects along the line of fascial closure and is attributed to the sawing motion of the suture on the fascia during abdominal wall motion [3]. Although the incidence of buttonhole hernia has yet to be defined, it seems to be exclusive to permanent suture. Suture sinus is a communication between the fascial suture (usually at a knot) and the skin [7, 9, 14, 16, 17]. Suture sinus has an incidence of about 1% and occurs predominately with nonabsorbable suture (although it has been seen with absorbable suture).

19.2 Current Sutures: A Sampling

The durability of suture commonly is evaluated by placing it in the subcutaneous tissue of animals for specified lengths of time, removing it, and then subjecting it to a tensiometer (ex vivo stress testing). Initial tensile strength of fresh suture is not an issue, since it has been demonstrated that fresh fascial suture will rip through the fascia during abdominal wound bursting experiments before the suture breaks [25, 26]. The tensile strength half life ($t_{1/2}$) may be estimated using several time points from ex vivo stress testing; the $t_{1/2}$ for some common absorbable sutures is given Table 1. Some "nonabsorbable" sutures are not actually so; silk has lost most of its strength at 1 year, and nylon (Ethilon, Dermalon) loses about 15%–25% of its strength per year. Polypropylene (Prolene, Surgilene), polyethylene (Ethibond, Ti-Cron, Tevdek), and polybutester (Novafil) seem to retain their strength indefinitely [22], although one study has noted some strength loss of polypropylene after 6 weeks [15].

19.3 Current Sutures: Randomized Trials

There are numerous retrospective reports (not reviewed here) in which the value of some suture is lauded based on a large experience. The use of polyglycolic acid (Dexon), which some surgeons avoid because of its relatively short $t_{1/2}$, resulted in dehiscence rates of 1.6% and 2% in a randomized trial of over 3000 patients comparing running to interrupted closure [11]. It would seem from this that using a suture which has lost half of its strength after 2 weeks (see Table 1) does not result in an inordinate incidence of wound dehiscence. The results of the eight available randomized trials which compare one suture against another do not demonstrate a difference in dehiscence rate between absorbable and nonabsorbable sutures [4–6, 8, 9, 19, 20, 27]. A

Suture	$t_{1/2}$ (weeks)
Polyglecaprone 25 (Monocryl)	1
Polyglactin 910 (Vicryl)	2
Polyglycolic acid (Dexon)	2
Polyglyconate (Maxon)	3
Polydioxanone (PDS)	6

Table 1. Ex vivo tensile strength half life ($t_{1/2}$) for some common absorbable sutures (from product insert data and [3a, 22])

Table 2. Results of prospective randomized trials comparing absorbable versus nonabsorbable suture

Location	Patients enrolled (n)	Sutures	Dehiscence (%)	Hernia (%)
Netherlands [27]	1156]	Vicryl	1.9	18.8*
		PDS	3.5	13.2
		Nylon	2.1	10.4*
Montreal [20]	200	Dexon	0	4.2
		Prolene	1.0	10.5
Aberdeen [19]	757	PDS	0.3	3.5
		Prolene	0.3	4.7
London [6]	347	Dexon	0.6	6.1
		Prolene	0.6	5.2
London [5]	210	Dexon	1.0	11.5*
		Nylon	1.0	3.8*
Burlington MA [9]	161	Vicryl	0	0
		Nurolon	0	8.9
		Prolene	1.9	4.4
New Brunswick [4]	229	PDS	0	10*
		Ethibond	1.8	18*
Milwaukee [8]	225	Maxon	0	8.7
		Nylon	2.7	4.4

PDS, polydioxanone.
*$p<0.05$.

higher ventral hernia rate with absorbable suture was found, however, in three of the eight studies (see Table 2). There does not appear to be an advantage of permanent suture over absorbable suture with respect to acute wound failure; there may be a trend for a lower hernia rate with permanent suture.

19.4 Summary

The requirements of Moynihan for the ideal suture are still applicable. The suture must have adequate strength and longevity for its job, and the suture should go away when it is no longer needed. The time required for sufficient fascial healing is not well defined and most likely is variable from patient to patient. The requirement for suture longevity, therefore, is vague. The small but real incidence of long-term complications secondary to nonabsorbable suture temper its election as the universal material for fascial closure. Conversely, the tendency to a higher ventral hernia rate may detract from the choice of absorbable suture. Knowledge of patient and suture factors should allow an intelligent choice of suture for fascial closure.

19.5 Discussion

Simmermacher: Were the techniques used in both studies comparable, or do the Dutch do something wrong compared with the rest of the world? When you used PDS, did you use the loop with a 4:1 ratio or single stitches?

Carlson: The closure technique was not constant, and therefore it is difficult to draw a conclusion.

Osther: In the Dutch study, the rate of high-risk patients is higher, and this might explain for the higher rate of recurrences.

Israelsson: Both studies lack a lot of science. For a real comparison, I think that the patient number, risk factors, closure technique, and anesthesia has to be the same in both groups.

Kingsnorth: We are probably too hung up on the small defects that the patient does not know about and which probably never become symptomatic. Therefore we have to have guidance to define what an incisional hernia is.

Israelsson: I think it is difficult to define, because in different countries the closure of symptomatic defects is a matter of social economics. We do not operate on patients with incisional hernias with the frequency that we did 10 years ago. We tend to operate on patients below the age of 65. In elderly patients, we do not operate even if they have symptoms because the economic incitement is missing.

Hartel: You mentioned that the monofilament sutures may have advantages in high-risk patients. Could you define these?

Osther: Old people, patients with a history of chronic obstructive pulmonary disease; diabetes was not included, because it was equal in both groups.

Schumpelick: How about the loop closure? Is there any experimental or clinically proven advantage?

Osther: No.

Amid: In subcuticular closures, there is less inflammatory reaction with nonabsorbable than with absorbable sutures. This is attributed to the release of substances from the absorbable suture. Is this also true of deep closure?

Carlson: I would say it is, but I have no direct support for this view.

References

1. Adamsons RF, Kahan SA: The rate of healing of incised wounds of different tissues in rabbits. Surg Gynecol Obstet 130:837, 1970.
2. Alexander HC, Prudden JF: The causes of abdominal wound disruption. Surg Gynecol Obstet 122:1223, 1966.
3. Arnaud JP, Humbert W, Eloy MR et al.: Effect of obstructive jaundice on wound healing: an experimental study in rats. Am J Surg 141:593, 1981.

3a. Bourne RB, Bitar H, Andreae PR et al: In-vivo comparison of four absorbable sutures: Vicryl, Dexon Plus, Maxon and PDS. Can J Surg 31:43, 1988.

4. Brolin RE: Prospective, randomized evaluation of midline fascial closure in gastric bariatric operations. Am J Surg 172:328, 1996.
5. Bucknall TE, Ellis H: Abdominal wound closure--A comparison of monofilament nylon and polyglycolic acid. Surgery 89:672, 1981.
6. Cameron AEP, Gray RCF, Talbot RW et al.: Abdominal wound closure: a trial of Prolene and Dexon. Br J Surg 67:487, 1980.
7. Carlson MA, Ludwig KA, Condon RE: Ventral hernia and other complications of 1,000 midline incisions. South Med J 88:450, 1995.

8. Carlson MA, Condon RE: Polyglyconate (Maxon) versus nylon suture in midline abdominal incision closure: a prospective randomized trial. Am Surg 61:980, 1995.
9. Corman ML, Veidenheimer MC, Coller JA: Controlled clinical trial of three suture materials for abdominal wall closure after bowl operations. Am J Surg 141:510, 1981.
10. Douglas DM: The healing of aponeurotic incisions. Br J Surg 40:79, 1952.
11. Fagniez PL, Hay JM, Lacaine F et al.: Abdominal midline incision closure: a multicentric randomized prospective trial of 3,135 patients, comparing continuous vs interrupted polyglycolic acid sutures. Arch Surg 120:1351, 1985.
12. Fast J, Nelson C, Dennis C: Rate of gain in strength in sutured abdominal wall wounds. Surg Gynecol Obstet 84:685, 1947.
13. Goligher JC, Irvin TT, Johnston D et al.: A controlled clinical trial of three methods of closure of laparotomy wounds. Br J Surg 62:823, 1975.
14. Greaney MG: A clinical and an experimental study of suture sinuses in abdominal wounds. Surg Gynecol Obstet 155: 712, 1982.
15. Greenwald D, Shumway S, Albear P et al.: Mechanical comparison of 10 suture materials before and after in vivo incubation. J Surg Res 56:372, 1994.
16. Israelsson LA, Jonsson T: Closure of midline laparotomy incisions with polydioxanone and nylon: the importance of suture technique. Br J Surg 81:1606, 1994.
17. Knight CD, Griffen FD: Abdominal wound closure with a continuous monofilament polypropylene suture: experience with 1,000 consecutive cases. Arch Surg 118: 1305, 1983.
18. Kronborg O: Polyglycolic acid (Dexon) versus silk for fascial closure of abdominal incisions. Acta Chir Scand 143:9, 1976.
19. Krukowski ZH, Cusick EL, Engeset J et al.: Polydioxanone or polypropylene for closure of midline abdominal incisions: a prospective comparative clinical trial. Br J Surg 74:828, 1987.
20. Lewis RT, Wiegand FM: Natural history of vertical abdominal parietal closure: Prolene versus Dexon. Can J Surg 32:196, 1989.
21. Lichtenstein IL, Herzikoff S, Shore JM et al: The dynamics of wound healing. Surg Gynecol Obstet 130:685, 1970.
22. Mathes SJ, Abouljoud M: Wound Healing. In Davis JH, Drucker WR, Foster RS Jr et al. (eds) Clinical Surgery. St Louis: CV Mosby Company, 1987, p. 493.
23. Moynihan BGA. The ritual of a surgical operation. Br J Surg 8:27, 1920.
24. Nelson CA, Dennis C: Wound healing: technical factors in the gain of strength in sutured abdominal wall wounds in rabbits. Surg Gynecol Obstet 93:461, 1951.
25. Poole GV Jr, Meredith JW, Kon ND et al.: Suture technique and wound-bursting strength. Am Surg 50:569, 1984.
26. Seid MH, McDaniel-Owens M, Poole GV Jr et al.: A randomized trial of abdominal incision suture technique and wound strength in rats. Arch Surg 130:394, 1995.
27. Wissing J, van Vroonhoven TJMV, Schattenkerk ME et al.: Fascia closure after midline laparotomy: results of a randomized trial. Br J Surg 74:738, 1987.

CHAPTER 20

Experience with Continuous Absorbable Suture for Laparotomy Closure

H. Gislason

20.1 Introduction

Suture material and suture technique may affect wound healing. Most surgeons now use a continuous or interrupted mass closure technique, and most studies performed have not shown differences in wound complication rates between these methods. Most authors favour the continuous technique because it is faster and cheaper [1–5].

Absorbable, monofilament sutures retaining their tensile strength for a long time seem to be ideal (theoretically at least) for abdominal wound closure [6, 7]. The newly introduced polyglyconate double suture with a loop (Maxon) on one needle (making the first knot unnecessary) seems to fulfil the criteria.

The patient's condition is important when evaluating the risk of developing wound complications, but the most important factor is probably the surgeon performing the operation, a factor to which too little attention is paid.

The aim of this study was to compare Maxon loop suture with the commonly used Vicryl (*p*olyglactin 910; relatively rapidly absorbed multifilament suture) using continuous mass closure and to compare the continuous suture method with the interrupted method using Vicryl. The outcome was assessed by the incidence of burst abdomen and wound infections postoperatively and by incisional hernia 1 year after the operation. Many clinical and technical factors that might be related to wound complications and the complication risk associated with the individual surgeon were examined.

20.2 Patients and Methods

A prospective trial was performed from 1990 to 1992 in which all adults (599 patients) undergoing major gastrointestinal operations were included. Urological, gynaecological and minor general surgical operations were not included. Patients who had had a laparotomy within 3 months were also excluded. All surgeons participated in the study, including residents in training. They were instructed to place the sutures a minimum of 1.5 cm from the wound edge, with a minimum of 1.5 cm between bites. Peritoneum and subcutaneous tissue were not sutured.

Patients were randomised before closure of the abdomen to have their wound closed by one of three techniques: continuous mass polyglyconate (Maxon) double suture with loop (size 0), continuous mass polyglactin 910 (Vicryl) (size 1) or interrupted polyglactin 910 (Vicryl) (size 1).

Wound infection and burst abdomen during the postoperative period were evaluated. A total of 494 patients were followed up at 1 year and examined for the presence of incisional hernia.

Statistical analysis was done using the chi-squared test or by analysis of variance (ANOVA), as appropriate.

20.3 Results

In the 599 patients, continuous Maxon was used in 203, continuous Vicryl in 199 and interrupted Vicryl in 197. There were no patient- or operation-related differences between the groups. The operations were performed by 32 surgeons with varying degree of experience, and 32% of the operations were emergency procedures. There were no differences between the groups except that the closure time was significantly longer in the group in which closure was performed with interrupted Vicryl ($p<0.001$), as shown in Table 1.

20.3.1 Early Complications

Burst abdomen was found in 14 patients (2%), eight in the Maxon loop group and three patients in each of the other two groups (Table 1). However, the difference was not statistically significant. The single most important factor related to dehiscence was postoperative wound infection, found in 11 of the 14 patients in which burst abdomen occurred ($p<0.001$). In all the patients (n=11) whose abdomen was resutured, intact sutures and knots were found.

The overall incidence of wound infection was 14% (n=84). The incidence was 20% (40 out of 199) in the Maxon group (Table 1), significantly more than in the Vicryl

Table 1. Wound complications related to suture method

Variable	Continuous				Interrupted polyglactin 910		p value (ANOVA or χ-squared)
	Polyglyconate double suture		Polyglactin 910				
	(%)	(n)	(%)	(n)	(%)	(n)	
Burst abdomen	4.1	8/197	1.5	3/194	1.6	3/192	0.13
Wound infections	20	40/197	12	23/194	11	21/192	0.015
Incisional hernia	12	19/164	6	9/163	4	7/164	0.02
Mean (±SD) closure time (min)	14±5	15±8	18±6	<0.001			

Wound infections and incisional hernia rates differ significantly between continuous polyglyconate double suture and polyglactin (continuous and interrupted); the mean closure time differs significantly between continuous and interrupted sutures.
ANOVA, analysis of various.

groups (p=0.015). Wound infections occurred in 23% (42 out of 186) of emergency operations, significantly more than in elective operations (10%; 42 out of 401; $p<0.001$). Wound infection was also highly correlated to contamination of the operation, as significantly more infections were found in operations classified as dirty ($p<0.001$). However, wound infection was not related to gender, obesity, type and length of incision or operation time.

20.3.2 Late Complications

Within 12 months of surgery, 102 patients died. Of 494 patients followed up at 1 year, 35 (7%) developed incisional hernias. Continuous closure of the abdominal wall with Maxon was associated with significantly more hernias (19 out of 164 patients; 12%) than closure with continuous (nine out of 163 patients; 6%) or interrupted Vicryl (seven out of 164 patients; 4%) (p=0.02) (Table 1). We found that herniation was strongly correlated to postoperative wound infections ($p<0.001$), as 13 (32%) of the 35 patients with incisional hernia had wound infections. Incisional hernia was also more common among older patients (66/58 years, p=0.037). We found that herniation was not related to gender, obesity, type and length of incision or emergency operation.

Wound complication rates were highly related to the surgeon performing the operation, as shown in Table 2. We did not find any difference between senior and junior surgeons (16.6% vs. 20.1%, p=0.07, in favour of the seniors). However, we found significant differences between the number of operations performed by each surgeon and the rate of wound complications (Table 2). There were also significant differences in the complication rate between individual surgeons. The three surgeons with the best results operated on 155 patients with a total of six wound failures (3.9%) (dehiscence plus incisional hernias), compared with the three surgeons with the poorest results, who operated on 50 patients resulting in ten (20%) wound failures.

20.4 Conclusion

In the present study, we examined whether wound complications were related to the closure method, i.e. continuous or interrupted, and compared two different types of suture material. We also examined the wound complication rate of the individual sur-

Table 2. Wound complications related to number of operations performed by each surgeon

Surgeons (n)	Operations (n)	Wound failure		Wound infection	
		(n)	(%)	(n)	(%)
12	<5	4/26	15.4	10/31	32.2
12	6–30	19/170	11.1	30/209	14.4
7	>30	23/305	7.5	45/347	13.0

The wound failure and wound infection rates differ significantly between the first group of surgeons and the second ($p<0.05$) and third ($p<0.01$) groups of surgeons, respectively; the wound failure rate differs significantly between the second and third groups ($p<0.05$).

geons. We found a burst abdomen rate of 2%, a wound infection rate of 14% and a 7% rate of wound hernias 1 year after the operation. Our results are in line with the results of similarly performed studies [2, 8–14].

In agreement with others [2, 4, 10], we found no differences in the rate of wound dehiscence or incisional hernia when comparing continuous and interrupted closure techniques using Vicryl (Table 1). However, significantly less time was spent when the continuous method was applied (Table 1), and the cost of material for running sutures was less than half of that for interrupted sutures. We thus recommend that the continuous method be used.

We compared Vicryl (*p*olyglactin), which is an absorbable multifilament suture that loses its tensile strength relatively soon (essentially absent by 30 days), to Maxon loop (*p*olyglyconate), which is a monofilament material that is slowly absorbed. Theoretically, one would expect Maxon to be superior to Vicryl. Surprisingly, when continuous Maxon (double suture with loop) was used, 20% of the patients developed wound infection compared to 12% when continuous Vicryl was used (p=0.015) (Table 1). Furthermore, we found more incisional hernias (12%, 40 out of 164) using continuous Maxon loop compared to continuous Vicryl (6%, nine out of 163; p=0.02). This difference is difficult to explain. A possible explanation is more tension placed on the loop sutures, resulting in reduced local blood flow and tissue necrosis and infection. Another explanation might be deposition of more suture material predisposing to infection. As demonstrated by others [6, 8, 10], we found that postoperative wound infection predisposes to the later development of incisional hernia, and in ten of 13 patients who had postoperative wound infections and developed incisional hernias, closure was carried out with Maxon loop. In a recent study. Salin et al. [2] found no difference in wound complications comparing continuous Maxon (single suture) with interrupted Vicryl, so the difference found in our study is probably related to the double suture of Maxon we used.

When comparing the results of experienced surgeons performing the same type of procedures, we found that they obtained highly different wound failure rates, ranging from 3.9% to 20%. Other authors have also noted that the skill of the surgeon is a strong predictor of wound complications [15, 16]. Other trials comparable to ours [2, 8–14] with a large number of surgeons of all levels of experience involved have demonstrated strikingly similar complication rates to the ones we found in the present study. However, studies that are similar in all aspects except that they are performed or supervised by experts (surgeons with interests in the field of abdominal wall closure) show much lower complication rates, with a burst abdomen rate of less than 0.5%, an incisional hernia rate of about 3% and a wound infection rate of 3%–4% [7, 17, 18].

Prevention of abdominal wound dehiscence and incisional hernia may be an unrealistic goal. Our findings suggest that the most important factor related to wound complications is the closure technique and the infection risk related to the specific surgeon. The incidence of wound complications could be significantly reduced by preventing abdominal wound infections. The single most important factor in reducing wound infection is to minimise contamination of the operating field. The final preparation of a stoma should therefore be carried out after closure and dressing of the wound.

We conclude that the continuous and interrupted closure methods for closure of the abdominal wall result in similar wound complication rates, but the continuous method is quicker and cheaper and should be preferred. Maxon double suture with loop is inferior to Vicryl and should not be used for abdominal wall closure.

20.5 Summary

This study present results from a prospective randomised study on abdominal wall closure involving 599 major abdominal operations. Two different closure techniques, i.e. continuous and interrupted, were compared, and the newly introduced polyglyconate double suture with loop (Maxon) was compared to polyglactin 910 (Vicryl). Wound complications, burst abdomen, wound infection and incisional hernia 1 year after the operation were examined. The wound complication rates of individual surgeons were also examined. We found a burst abdomen rate of 2%, a wound infection rate of 14% and an incisional hernia rate of 7% 1 year after the operation. We found no differences in the wound complication rates between the continuous and interrupted closure technique, but the continuous method is quicker and cheaper and should be preferred. Polyglyconate double suture with loop (Maxon) was associated with more wound infection and a higher incisional hernia rate than polyglactin 910 (Vicryl), and we conclude that the Maxon loop suture should not be used. We found great individual differences in wound complications rates between individual surgeons.

20.6 Discussion

For a discussion, please see Chap. 22.

References

1. Gislason H, Grønbech JE, Søreide O. Burst abdomen and incisional hernia after major gastrointestinal operations – Comparison of three closure techniques. Eur J Surg 1995;161: 349–354.
2. Sahlin S, Ahlberg J, Granström L, Ljungström KG. Monofilament versus multifilament absorbable sutures for abdominal closure. Br J Surg 1993;80:322–324.
3. Fagniez PL, Hay JM, Lacàine F, Thomsen C. Abdominal midline incision closure. Arch Surg 1985;120:1351–1353.
4. Richards PC, Balch CM, Aldrete JS. Abdominal wound closure. Ann Surg 1983;197:238–243.
5. Trimbos JB, Smit IB, Holm JP, Hermans J. A randomized clinical trial comparing two methods of fascia closure following midline laparotomy. Arch Surg 1992;127:1232–1234.
6. Santora TA, Roslyn JJ. Incisional hernia. Surg Clin North Am 1993;73:557–570.
7. Schoetz DJ, Coller JA, Veidenheimer MC. Closure of abdominal wounds with polydioxanone. Arch Surg 1988;123:72–74.
8. Bucknall TE, Ellis H. Abdominal wound closure- A comparison of monofilament nylon and polyglycolic acid. Surgery 1981;89:672–677.
9. Leaper DJ, Pollock AV, Evans M. Abdominal wound closure: a trial of nylon, polyglycolic acid and steel sutures. Br J Surg 1977;64:603–606.
10. Wissing J, Th JMV van Vroonhoven, ME Schattenkerk, HF Veen, RJG Ponsen, Jeekel J. Fascia closure after midline laparotomy: results of a randomized trial. Br J Surg 1987;74:738–741.
11. Osther PJ, Gjøde P, Mortensen BB, Bartholin J, Gottrup F. Randomized comparison of polyglycolic acid and polyglyconate sutures for abdominal fascial closure after laparotomy in patients with suspected impaired wound healing. Br J Surg 1995;82:1080–1082.

12. Israelsson LA, Jonsson T. Closure of midline laparotomy incisions with polydioxanone and nylon: the importance of suture technique. Br J Surg 1994;81:1606–1608.
13. Kendall SWH, Brennan TG, Guillou PJ. Suture length to wound length ratio and the integrity of midline and lateral paramedian incisions. Br J Surg 1991;78:705–707.
14. Krukowski ZH, Cusick EL, Engeset J, Matheson NA. Polydioxanone or polypropylene for closure of midline abdominal incisions: a prospective comparative clinical trial. Br J Surg 1987;74:828–830.
15. Bucknall TE, Cox PJ, Ellis H. Burst abdomen and incisional hernia: a prospective study of 1129 major laparotomies. BMJ 1982;27:931–933.
16. Medina M, Sillero M, Martinez-Gallego G, Delgado-Rodriguez M. Risk factors of surgical wound infection in patients undergoing herniorrhaphy. Eur J Surg 1997;163:191–198.
17. Corman ML, Veidenheimer MC, Coller JA: Controlled clinical trial of three suture materials for abdominal wall closure after bowel operations. Am J Surg 1981; 141:510–513.
18. Jenkins TPN. The burst abdominal wound: a mechanical approach. Br J Surg 1976;63:873–876.

CHAPTER 21

Continuous Closure of Laparotomy Incisions: Aspects on Suture Technique

L.A. Israelsson

21.1 Introduction

Wound complications such as early wound dehiscence, incisional hernia and wound infection continue to be a major source of morbidity and mortality after laparotomies.

Early wound dehiscence with evisceration, which always requires immediate reoperation, is reported to occur in 1%–3% of midline incisions [25, 63, 80]. Such reoperations are associated with considerable morbidity, and the mortality rate may be as high as 10%–40% [4, 18]. Wound dehiscence usually occurs during the first postoperative week, when the holding together of the wound is entirely dependent on the suture and the suture-holding capacity of the fascia [60]. Dehiscence may then occur if the suture breaks, knots slip or the suture cuts completely through the fascia. The latter is probably the predominant cause [18].

When incisional hernia develops, the defect in the fascia may cause the patient discomfort and pain, or strangulation of abdominal contents may be induced in the protrusion in the wound, requiring emergent surgical intervention. In midline incisions, the hernia rate 12 months after laparotomy ranges from 9% to more than 20% [3, 6, 16, 48, 56, 61, 62, 69, 81]. The regenerative powers of fascia are very limited, and a discontinuity heals by collagen bridging, which may be complicated if the fascia edges are separated [60]. They may be separated after an incomplete early wound dehiscence, after an infection with necrosis of fascia or due to factors that increase the tension on the suture line, such as overweight or abdominal distension [6, 12, 13, 23, 25, 29, 33, 34, 49, 62].

Wound infection with purulent discharge from the wound may require surgical intervention with drainage and can cause general symptoms that prolong the hospital stay. Bacterial contamination causes infection, especially if there is necrotic tissue or foreign material in the wound [60]. Gastrointestinal surgery and long duration of operation, which may increase the degree of bacterial contamination, and high tension on the suture line, which may cause tissue necrosis, have thus been associated with an increased risk of wound infection [8, 10, 20–22, 30, 43, 45, 54, 64].

Closure of midline laparotomy incisions with a continuous mass closure technique using a monofilament non-absorbable suture material is a well-established and well-documented method that produces good clinical results.

A continuous suture technique is less time consuming but equally safe as an interrupted one, and with a continuous technique less foreign material and fewer knots are deposited in the wound [1, 2, 26, 56, 65, 69, 72, 76, 79]. With a mass closure technique, the tensile strength of the wound is higher during the early postoperative period and the rate of wound dehiscence has been lower than with a layered technique [12, 18, 24, 25, 58, 57].

Monofilaments are associated with a lower rate of wound infection than multifilaments, in which bacteria may be enclosed within the interstices and be protected from phagocytosis [2, 14, 25, 55, 59, 83]. A low hernia rate with non-absorbable monofilament suture materials is well documented in several clinical studies comparing them with other materials [2, 3, 12, 15, 50]. With absorbable suture materials that retain an acceptable strength for at least 6 weeks, the rate of incisional hernia has been similar to that observed with non-absorbable sutures [5, 16, 36, 48, 52, 71, 73]. A higher hernia rate has been reported with materials absorbed within a shorter time [2, 11, 13, 19, 27, 44].

Many of the factors identified as important for the rate of wound complications are not possible to correct preoperatively or cannot be influenced by the surgeon. The suture technique, however, is totally in the hands of the surgeon and is likely to be important for the development of wound complications. The ultimate purpose of the continuing search for the optimal surgical technique is that adherence to principles found may be a way of reducing the rate of wound complications.

21.2 Suture Length to Wound Length Ratio

In a continuously closed laparotomy incision, the suture technique can be monitored through the suture length to wound length (SL:WL) ratio. This ratio depends on the stitch interval, the amount of tissue included in the stitches and the tension on the suture. An SL:WL ratio of 4 or more means that the length of the suture used is at least four times the length of the wound. The length of the suture material consumed is calculated by subtracting the length of suture remnants from the original suture length, and the wound length is defined as the length of the skin incision.

A strong correlation between the SL:WL ratio and the development of incisional hernia has been found. With an SL:WL ratio of at least 4, the wound tension seems to be distributed to the suture line in such a way that the suture-holding capacity of the tissues is not exceeded. Thus the hernia rate is lower if the SL:WL ratio is 4 or more, and suturing with a lower ratio is associated with a threefold increase in the rate of incisional hernia (Table 1) [35, 36, 38–41]. In overweight patients, the SL:WL ratio

Table 1. Suture length to wound length ratio related to incisional hernia in 802 patients at 12-month follow-up

Suture length to wound length ratio	Patients (*n*)	Incisional hernia (%)	(*n*)
<3.5	242	23	55
3.5–3.9	98	18	18
4.0–4.4	137	7	9
4.5–4.9	84	7	6
3 5.0	241	12	28

$p<0.01$ (χ-squared test).

should not be higher than 5, since this has been associated with a higher rate of both wound infection and incisional hernia, probably because a large amount of tissue other than fascia is then included in the suture [41]. If wounds are sutured with an SL:WL ratio of 4.0–4.9, the rates of wound infection and incisional hernia in overweight patients may actually be similar to those in patients who are not overweight [41].

21.3 Stitch Length

The stitch length reflects the size of tissue bites and is calculated as the ratio of the suture length and the number of stitches. If the stitch length is too long, indicating large tissue bites probably also including tissue other than fascia, the rate of wound infection is high, and an optimal stitch length should be less than 5 cm [40]. Poor circulation in tissue grasped in a suture may explain the correlation between infection and the amount of tissue included in the stitch. The suture pullout force increases with the distance from the fascia edge up to 9 mm and then reaches a plateau [17]. Thus, if the stitch length is too short, with small tissue bites close to the fascia edges, the risk of developing wound dehiscence may be increased [3, 17, 18, 51].

21.4 Tension

Excessive tension should not be placed on the suture, since this may reduce local blood flow and has been associated with an increased rate of wound infection [51]. Further, higher wound strength is achieved with a loose suture with just enough tension to approximate fascia edges than with a very tight suture [31, 70].

The causes of wound dehiscence are almost always local in the wound and seldom the result of systemic abnormalities [18, 60]. If the wound tension is distributed to the suture line in such a way that the suture-holding capacity of the tissues is exceeded during the early postoperative period, wound dehiscence follows. In accordance, a correlation has been found between suturing with a low SL:WL ratio and the development of dehiscence [35, 38, 42]. To avoid wound dehiscence, sutures should thus not be placed too close to the fascia edges and the SL:WL ratio should be 4 or more [18].

21.5 Modifying Surgical Technique

Studies on wound healing and wound complications essentially aim to reduce the risk of patients developing wound complications. To this end, surgeons not only have to be aware of a possible correlation between the surgical technique and the development of complications, but they must also be able to change their technique. This seems to be possible on a large scale and within a short time if surgeons are given proper instructions and are supplied with adequate feedback concerning their adherence to the instructions given. In one prospective study, midline incisions were found to be sutured with a mean SL:WL ratio of 3.6 [39]. Surgeons were informed about the low ratio and its correlation with a high hernia rate and were urged to suture all wounds with an SL:WL ratio of at least 4. These instructions were followed and the mean ratio was increased to 4.9; the hernia rate was thereby reduced from 19% to 11%. The rate of incisional hernias that required surgical repair within 18 months of the initial laparotomy was also decreased from 4% to 2% [38]. Thus simple adjustments in technique can considerably improve late operative results.

21.6 Knots

If an anchor knot slips totally during the early postoperative period, the wound will dehisce. The knot is always the weakest point of a suture, and a single hitch at the midpoint of a suture reduces suture strength by 30%–35% [7]. With a continuous suture technique, the anchor knots that start and finish the suture must be reliable, and – particularly with monofilament suture materials – large, complex conventional surgical knots are required [9, 28, 32, 46, 47, 53, 66–68, 74, 75, 77, 78, 82]. The suture loop has been designed and used in an attempt to overcome these difficulties. However, using the loop, twice as much suture material is deposited in the wound than is needed, and although the starting knot is safe, the finishing knot is still a bulky conventional knot. Bulky knots may cause the patient discomfort and increase the risk of a suture sinus, and self-locking knots have therefore been suggested as alternatives for continuous suturing.

With self-locking knots, the suture loses less of its strength than with conventional knots. With the large monofilament suture materials used for laparotomy closure, self-locking knots diminish the strength of the suture by less than 10% [37]. A self-locking knot cannot slip either partially or totally, whereas conventional anchor knots often slip [37]. A self-locking knot is always smaller than a conventional anchor knot, and this may be beneficial in certain situations [37]. Self-locking knots have been used in large clinical series with excellent results, and they are easy to learn to tie [38].

21.7 Recommendations

Wound complications continue to be a major source of morbidity and mortality after laparotomies. There is considerable experimental and clinical data available that allow an opinion on which methods seem best to avoid these complications.

It is recommended that midline laparotomy incisions are closed by a continuous suture technique in one layer using a non-absorbable monofilament suture material or an absorbable material that contributes to the strength of the wound for at least 6 weeks.

An optimal surgical technique includes the following:

- Suturing with an SL:WL ratio of at least 4, preferably between 4 and 5

- Suturing with a stitch length of less than 5 cm
- Not placing stitches closer than 10 mm to the fascia edges
- Not placing excessive tension on the suture
- Using self-locking knots as anchor knots

21.8 Discussion

For a discussion, please see Chap. 22.

References

1. Archie JP, Feldtman RW. Primary abdominal wound closure with permanent, continuous running monofilament sutures. Surg Gynecol Obstet 1981;153:721–722
2. Askew AR. A comparison of upper abdominal wound closure with monofilament nylon and polyglycolic acid. Aust NZ J Surg 1983;53:353–356
3. Ausobsky JR, Evans M, Pollock AV. Does mass closure of midline laparotomies stand the test of time? A random control clinical trial. Ann R Coll Surg Engl 1985;67:159–161
4. Baggish MS, Lee FWK. Abdominal wound disruption. Obstetrics & Gynecology 1975;46:530–534
5. Binnie NR, Bainbridge CL, Macintyre MC. Abdominal wound closure with polydioxanone (PDS). JR Coll Surg Edinburgh 1986;31:147–150
6. Blomstedt B, Welin-Berger T. Incisional hernias. A comparison between midline, oblique and transrectal incisions. Acta Chir Scand 1972;138:275–278
7. Bourne RB, Bitar H, Andreae PR, et al. In-vivo comparison of four absorbable sutures: Vicryl, Dexon Plus, Maxon and PDS. Can J Surg 1988;31:43–45
8. Bremmelgaard A, Raahave D, Beier-Holgersen R, Pedersen JV, Andersen S, Sørensen AI. Computer-aided surveillance of surgical infections and identification of risk factors. J Hosp Infect 1989;13:1–18
9. Brown JP. Knotting technique and suture materials. Br J Surg 1992;79:399–400
10. Bröte L, Gillquist J, Tärnvik A. Wound infections in general surgery. Acta Chir Scand 1976; 142:99–106
11. Bucknall TE. Factors influencing wound complications: a clinical and experimental study. Ann R C Surg Eng 1983;65:71–77
12. Bucknall TE, Cox PJ, Ellis H. Burst abdomen and incisional hernia: a prospective study of 1129 major laparotomies. BMJ 1982;284:931–933
13. Bucknall T, Ellis H. Abdominal wound closure- A comparison of monofilament nylon and polyglycolic acid. Surgery 1981;89:672–677
14. Bucknall TE, Teare L, Ellis H. The choice of a suture to close abdominal incisions. Eur Surg Res 1983;15:59–66
15. Burleson RL. Double loop mass closure technique for abdominal incisions. Surg Gynecol Obstet 1978;147:414–416
16. Cameron AEP, Parker CJ, Field ES, et al. A randomised comparison of polydioxanone (PDS) and polypropylene (Prolene) for abdominal wound closure. Ann R Coll Surg Eng 1987;69:113–115
17. Campbell JA, Temple WJ, Frank CB, Huchcroft SA. A biomechanical study of suture pullout in linea alba. Surgery 1989;106:888–892
18. Carlson MA. Acute wound failure. Surg Clin North Am 1997;77:607–636
19. Carlson MA, Condon RE. Polygluconate (Maxon) versus nylon suture in midline abdominal incision closure: a prospective randomised trial. Am J Surg 1995;61:980–983
20. Christou NV, Nohr CW, Meakins JL. Assessing operative site infection in surgical patients. Arch Surg 1987;122:165–169
21. Cruse PJE, Foord R. The epidemiology of wound infection: a 10-year prospective study of 62,939 wounds. Surg Clin North Am 1980;60:27–40
22. Davidson AIG, Clark C, Smith G. Postoperative wound infection: a computer analysis. Br J Surg 1971;58:333–337
23. Deitel M, Alhindawi R, Yamen M, To TB, Burul CJ. Dexon plus versus Maxon fascial closure in morbid obesity: a prospective randomized comparison. Can J Surg 1990;33:302–304

24. Dudley HAF. Layered and mass closure of the abdominal wall. A theoretical and experimental analysis. Br J Surg 1970;57:664–667
25. Ellis H, Bucknall TE, Cox PJ. Abdominal incisions and their closure. Current problems in Surgery 1985;22:5–50
26. Fagniez P-L, Hay JM, Lacàine F et al. Abdominal midline incision closure. Arch Surg 1985; 120:1351–1353
27. Gislason H, Grønbech JE, Søreide O. Burst abdomen and incisional hernia after major gastrointestinal operations – comparison of three closure techniques. Eur J Surg 1995;161:349–354
28. Greany MG. A clinical and experimental study of suture sinuses in abdominal wounds. Surg Gynecol Obstet 1982;155:712–716
29. Gys T, Hubens A. A prospective clinical study between monofilament absorbable and non-absorbable sutures for abdominal wall closure. Acta Chir Belg 1989;89:265–270
30. Haley RW, Culver DH, Morgan MW, White JW, Emori TG, Hooton TM. Identifying patients at high risk of surgical wound infection. Am J Epidemiol 1985;121:206–215
31. Haxton H. The influence of suture materials and methods on the healing of abdominal wounds. Br J Surg 1965;52:372
32. Holmlund DE. Knot properties of surgical suture materials. Acta Chir Scand 1974;140:355–362
33. Irvin TT, Koffman CG, Duthie HL. Layer closure of laparotomy wounds with absorbable and non-absorbable suture materials. Br J Surg 1976;63:793–796
34. Irvin TT, Stoddard CJ, Greaney MG, Duthie HL. Abdominal wound healing: a prospective clinical study. Br Med J 1977:351–352
35. Israelsson LA, Jonsson T. Suture length to wound length ratio and healing of midline laparotomy incisions. Br J Surg 1993;80:1284–1286
36. Israelsson LA, Jonsson T. Closure of midline laparotomy incisions with polydioxanone and nylon: the importance of suture technique. Br J Surg 1994;81:1606–1608
37. Israelsson LA, Jonsson T. Physical properties of self locking and conventional surgical knots. Eur J Surg 1994;160:323–327
38. Israelsson LA. Wound complications in midline laparotomy incisions: the importance of suture technique. Thesis 1995; From the Department of Surgery Lund University, Malmö General Hospital
39. Israelsson LA, Jonsson T. Incisional hernia after midline laparotomy; a prospective study. Eur J Surg 1996;162:125–129
40. Israelsson LA, Jonsson T, Knutsson A. Suture technique and healing in midline laparotomy incisions. Eur J Surg 1996;162:605–609
41. Israelsson LA, Jonsson T. Overweight and healing of midline incisions: the importance of suture technique. Eur J Surg 1997;163:175–180
42. Jenkins TP. The burst abdominal wound: a mechanical approach. Br J Surg 1976;63:873–876
43. Jepsen OB, Olesen Larsen S, Frølund Thomsen V. Post-operative wound sepsis in general surgery. Acta Chir Scand 1969;396 Suppl:80–90
44. Johnson CD, Bernhardt LW, Bentley PG. Incisional hernia after mass closure of abdominal incisions with Dexon and Prolene. Br J Surg 1982;69:55
45. Jones PL, Millman A. Wound healing and the aged patient. Nursing Clinics of North America 1990;25:263–277
46. Knight CD, Griffen FD. Abdominal wound closure with a continuous monofilament polypropylene suture. Arch Surg 1983;118:1305–1308
47. Knoop M, Lünstedt B, Thiede A. Maxon und PDS – Bewertung physikalischer und biologischer Eigenschaften monfiler, absorbierbarer Nahtmaterialien. Langenbecks Arch Surg 1987;371:13–28
48. Krukowski ZH, Cusick EL, Engeset J et al. Polydioxanone or polypropylene for closure of midline abdominal incisions: a prospective comparative clinical trial. Br J Surg 1987;74:828–830
49. Lamont PM, Ellis H. Incisional hernia in re-opened abdominal incisions: an overlooked risk factor. Br J Surg 1988;75:374–376
50. Leaper DJ, Pollock AV, Evans M. Abdominal wound closure: a trial of nylon, polyglycolic acid and steel sutures. Br J Surg 1977;64:603–606
51. Leaper DJ: Angiography as an index of healing in experimental laparotomy wounds and colonic anastomosis. Ann R Coll Surg Eng 1983;65:20–23
52. Leese T, Ellis H. Abdominal wound closure- A comparison of monofilament nylon and polydioxanone. Surgery 1984;95:125–126
53. Lünstedt B, Thiede A. Polydioxanone (PDS)- ein neues monofiles synthetisches, absorbierbares Nahtmaterial. Chirurg 1983;54:103–107
54. Mayer AD, Ausobsky JR, Evans M et al. Compression suture of the abdominal wall: a controlled trial in 302 major laparotomies. Br J Surg 1981;68:632–634
55. McGeehan D, Hunt D, Chaudhuri A, Rutter P. An experimental study of the relationship between synergistic wound sepsis and suture materials. Br J Surg 1908;67:636–638

56. McNeill PM, Sugerman HJ. Continuous absorbable vs. interrupted nonabsorbable fascial closure. Arch Surg 1986;121:821–823
57. Niggebrugge AHP, Hansen BE, Trimbos JB, van de Velde CJH, Zwaveling A. Mechanical factors influencing the incidence of burst abdomen. Eur J Surg 1995;161:655–661
58. Nilsson T. Closure of the abdominal wound with single-layer and double layer technique. Acta Chir Scand 1981;147:399–403
59. Osther PJ, Gjøde P, Mortensen BB, Mortensen PB, Bartholin J, Gottrup F. Randomised comparison of polyglycolic acid and polygluconate sutures for abdominal fascial closure after laparotomy in patients with suspected impaired wound healing. Br J Surg 1995;82:1080–1082
60. Peacock EE, van Winkle W. Wound healing, 3rd ed. Philadelphia: W.B. Saunders;1984
61. Pollock AV, Evans M. Early prediction of late incisional hernias. Br J Surg 1989;76:953–954
62. Pollock AV, Greenall MJ, Evans M. Single-layer mass closure of major laparotomies by continuous suturing. JR Soc Med 1979;72:889–893
63. Poole GV. Mechanical factors in abdominal wound closure: The prevention of fascial dehiscence. Surgery 1985;97:631–639
64. Raahave D. Wound contamination and postoperative infection. Danish Medical Bulletin 1991;38:481–485
65. Richards PC, Balch CM, Aldrete J.S. A randomized prospective study of 571 patients comparing continuous vs. interrupted techniques. Ann Surg 1983;197:238–243
66. vanRijssel EJC, Trimbos JB, Booster MH. Mechanical performance of square knots and sliding knots in surgery: a comparative study. Am J Obstet Gynecol 1990;162:93–97
67. Roedeheaver GT, Powell TA, Thacker JG et al. Mechanical performance of monofilament synthetic absorbable sutures. Am J Surg 1987;154:544–547
68. Rosin E, Robinson GM. Knot security of suture materials. Vet Surg 1989;18:269–273
69. Sahlin S, Ahlberg L, Granström L, Ljungström K-G. Monofilament versus multifilament absorbable sutures for abdominal closure. Br J Surg 1993; 80:322–324
70. Sanders RJ, DiClementi D, Ireland K. Principles of abdominal wound closure. I. Animal studies. Arch Surg 1977;112:1184–1187
71. Schoetz DJ, Coller JA, Veidenheimer MC. Closure of abdominal wounds with polydioxanone. Arch Surg 1988;123:72–74
72. Stone HH, Hoefling SJ, Strom PR et al. Abdominal incisions: Transverse vs. vertical placement and continuous vs. interrupted closure. S Med J 1983;76:1106–1112
73. Taylor TV. The use of polydioxanone suture in midline incisions. JR Coll Surg Edinburgh 1985;30:191–192
74. Tera H, Åberg C. Tensile strengths of twelve types of knot employed in surgery, using different suture materials. Acta Chir Scand 1976;142:1–7
75. Tera H, Åberg C. Strength of knots in surgery in relation to type of knot, type of suture material and dimensions of suture thread. Acta Chir Scand 1977;143:75–83
76. Trimbos JB, Smit IB, Holm JP, Hermans J. A randomized clinical trial comparing two methods of fascia closure following midline laparotomy. Arch Surg 1992;127:1232–1234
77. Trimbos JB, vanRijssel EJ, Klopper PJ. Performance of sliding knots in monofilament and multifilament suture material. Obstet Gynecol 1986;68:425–430
78. Trimbos JB, Brohim R, vanRijssel EJC. Factors relating to the volume of surgical knots. Int J Gynecol Obstet 1989;30:355–359
79. Trimbos JB, vanRooij J. Amount of suture material needed for continuous or interrupted wound closure: an experimental study. Eur J Surg 1993;159:141–143
80. White H, Cook J, Ward M. Abdominal wound dehiscence. A 10-year survey from a district general hospital. Ann R Coll Surg Eng 1977;59:337–341
81. Wissing J, vanVroonhoven ThJ, Schattenkerk ME et al. Fascia closure after midline laparotomy: results of a randomized trial. Br J Surg 1987;74:738–741
82. Zimmer CA, Thacker JG, Powell DM, et al. Influence of knot configuration and tying technique on the mechanical performance of sutures. J Emerg Med 1991;9:107–113
83. Österberg B. Influence of physical properties of suture materials on wound infection: an experimental study. Thesis 1983; From the Department of Clinical Bacteriology of the Karolinska Institute at the Roslagstull Hospital, Stockholm.

CHAPTER 22

Closure of the Abdomen in Acute Wound Failure

H. Gislason

Wound complications are still a challenging problem after major gastrointestinal operations. Prospective trials performed in recent years show burst abdomen rates of 1%–3%, wound infection rates of 10%–15% and incisional hernia rates of 4%–21% [1–9]. Burst abdomen is a complication associated with mortality rates of 10%–30%, high morbidity, and increased hospital stay and cost of treatment. In an effort to reduce the rate of this complication, many prospective randomized studies have been performed comparing different closure methods and suture materials [1–9]. With the incidence of burst abdomen that low, the problem with these studies is often the small number of patients included, leading to inconclusive results.

In a retrospective study (unpublished results), we found that the rate of incisional hernia in patients operated on for burst abdomen is about 50%. This figure is surprisingly high, but the only report published on this matter showed similar results [10].

This raises two questions: (1) how to minimize the incidence of burst abdomen and (2) when burst abdomen occurs, how to deal with it in order to reduce the incisional hernia rate postoperatively.

22.1 Reducing the Incidence of Burst Abdomen

Mass sutures with large bites giving a suture to wound ratio of over 4 have clearly improved results [11, 12] and are now preferred by most surgeons. However, it is still a matter of debate whether a continuous or interrupted closure technique and absorbable or non-absorbable sutures should be used. In order to obtain sufficiently large numbers of patients to answer these questions, the literature was reviewed. Nine different studies [1–9] fulfilling the following criteria were found: (a) a prospective randomized study, (b) only major laparotomies included (i.e. appendectomies, gynaecological and minor urological procedures excluded, (c) elective and acute operations included, (d) a modern suture material used, and (e) many surgeons involved.

The results of these studies are shown in Table 1. The overall results were a burst abdomen rate of 1.7% (80 out of 4790), a wound infection rate of 10.6% (495 out of 4686) and an incisional hernia rate of 11.3% (458 out of 4068). Comparison of the continuous and interrupted mass closure technique revealed burst abdomen in 1.4% (52 out of 3690) using the continuous technique compared with 2.5% (27 out of 1100) using the interrupted technique ($p=0.03$). These results are in line with the results obtained by Fagniez et al. [13], who performed a large, multicentre randomized prospective trial of 3135 patients, comparing the continuous and interrupted closure technique using polyglycolic acid sutures. They found a dehiscence rate of 1.6% in the continuous group compared with 2% in the interrupted group. However, the difference between the groups was only significant in the stratum of contaminated wounds.

These results show that the burst abdomen rate is lower when the continuous suture technique is used.

No differences were found between different suture materials and wound dehiscence. Using rapidly absorbed multifilament sutures (Vicryl/Dexon), the burst abdomen rate was 1.8% (33 out of 1794) compared with 1.9% (34 out of 1810) when more slowly absorbed monofilament sutures (Maxon/polydioxanone, PDS) were used and 1.1% (13 out of 1186) when non-absorbable monofilament sutures were used (nylon/Prolene). The data indicate that the suture material now used is of a good quality, and further improvements in results will not depend on the suture material chosen.

The most important factor related to wound complications is the operation technique and the infection risk associated with the surgeon, a factor to which surprisingly little attention has been paid in studies published on abdominal wound closure and complications. The figures shown in Table 1 represent the results obtained by a large number of surgeons. However, similar studies in which the operations were performed or supervised by experts (surgeons with a special interest in the field of abdominal wall closure) show much better results. Corman et al. [14], Scoetz et al. [15] and Jenkins [11] operated with burst abdomen rates of 0.11%, 0% and 0.007%, respectively. These results show that, with the proper operative technique, the burst abdomen rate can almost be eliminated. In a recent study, we [2] found that wound complications differ

Table 1. Incidence of burst abdomen in studies on closure methods and suture materials

Reference	Patients (*n*)	Suture material	Method of closure	Incidence (*n*)	(%)
Multifilament, rapidly absorbed					
[1]	104	Dexon	Continuous	1	1
[2]	194	Vicryl	Continuous	3	2
[3]	121	Dexon	Continuous	1	1
[4]	379	Vicryl	Continuous	6	2
[2]	192	Vicryl	Interrupted	3	2
[5]	100	Dexon	Interrupted	7	7
[6]	339	Vicryl	Interrupted	3	1
[4]	365	Vicryl	Interrupted	8	2
Monofilament, slowly absorbed					
[2]	197	Maxon[a]	Continued	8	4
[7]	405	PDS	Continued	2	0
[8]	104	PDS	Continued	0	0
[9]	285	PDS	Continued	1	0
[6]	345	Maxon	Continued	4	1
[4]	370	PDS	Continued	13	4
[5]	104	Maxon	Interrupted	6	6
Monofilament, non-absorbable					
[1]	106	Nylon	Continued	1	1
[7]	408	Nylon	Continued	3	1
[9]	295	Prolen	Continued	1	0
[4]	377	Nylon	Continued	8	2

[a]Maxon double suture with loop.
PDS, polydioxanone.

significantly between surgeons performing the same type of operation. The three gastrointestinal surgeons in our department with the best results operated with a wound failure rate (burst abdomen plus incisional hernia) of less than 4% as compared with the three with poorest results, who had a wound failure rate of approximately 20%. In order to achieve better results, postoperative complications should be reported, giving the surgeon regularly feedback about his or her results and, if necessary, offering technical instruction.

22.2 Repairing Burst Abdomen to Reduce the Incisional Hernia Rate Postoperatively

A retrospective study was performed in the Department of Surgery at Haukeland University Hospital (unpublished results), in which all the records of patients who underwent major operations for gastrointestinal conditions and were re-operated on for burst abdomen in the 10-year period from 1986 to 1996 were examined.

The surgical technique used (continuous or interrupted), the type of suture material and the use of retention sutures was recorded. Patients were followed up for the presence of incisional hernia.

A total of 78 patients were operated on for burst abdomen during this time period (55 men and 22 women). The median age at operation was 70.5 years (range, 41–91 years). Wound disruption occurred an average of 10 days postoperatively (range, 1–30 days). We found that 34 of the patients (44%) had wound infections; 43 patients had no or only minor complications, 11 (14%) died postoperatively and the remaining 24 survived after having one or more serious complications.

A total of 25 patients (32%) were excluded from the follow-up analysis: 17 patients died during the first year (including those who died postoperatively), and in eight cases the records were insufficient or patients did not come to follow-up at the outpatient clinic.

In 53 patients followed up postoperatively for the presence of incisional hernia (median, 23 months; range, 1–8 years), we found that 43% (23 patients) had an incisional hernia. The operative methods applied in these patients are shown in Table 2. The most commonly used method for treating the burst abdomen (in 29 patients) involved interrupted wound sutures and retention sutures; 38% of these developed incisional hernia. Following closure with interrupted sutures, 34% (13 out of 38) developed incisional hernia, as compared with 60% (six out of ten) where the continuous method was used ($p=0.17$, chi-squared test).

Table 2. Incidence of incisional hernia with different surgical techniques of wound closure in 53 patients

Technique	Hernia (*n*)	No hernia (*n*)
Interrupted + retention sutures	11	18
Continuous + retention sutures	5	3
Interrupted	2	7
Continuous	1	1
Retention sutures	4	1
Total	23	30

Retention sutures (external) were used in 42 patients, and 48% (20 out of 42) of these developed incisional hernia, indicating no benefit of using retention sutures.

Absorbable sutures were used almost exclusively in this study. No difference was found in the incisional hernia rate when the slowly absorbed sutures polyglyconate (Maxon) and PDS were used as compared to the more rapidly absorbed polyglactin (Vicryl) and polyglycolic acid (Dexon).

In conclusion, these results shows that conventional surgical methods for repair of burst abdomen are associated with high incisional hernia rates. If burst abdomen occurs, the wound is often infected and the strength of tissue reduced so that the sutures easily cut through the tissue. In such cases, it might be reasonable to use interrupted sutures, taking large bites in the tissue. However, retention sutures do not improve results and should not be used. In order to improve results, a mesh should probably be used as a routine, at least if tension-free repair cannot be achieved.

22.3 Discussion

Kingsnorth: How long do the wounds need to be supported with the suture material? According to Monaham, it should disappear as soon as its work has been accomplished. When is it accomplished? We know from young animals that we get only 80% of the original strength if we have made an incision in the fascia. There is quite a lot of literature that shows that your collagen weakens as you age. We should therefore look for suture material that closes wounds indefinitely, and I do not think that absorbable sutures are the right material to close midline incisions. What are your views?

Israelsson: The only important thing in our study was the suture technique, not the material. I do not think we need support from the sutures for years to come. When we open old midline incisions again, the nylon sutures are there, but they are loose. I do not think this is good for the wound.

Schumpelick: You showed that there is a higher rate of dehiscence if the ratio is higher than 4. Is this a question of ischemia or wound length?

Israelsson: The reason is multifactorial, and I do not think that we have enough time to go into it. The mean length of our wounds was 27 cm. Half of our wounds were more than 30 cm long. Therefore the loop was not long enough using a 4:1 ratio.

Schumpelick: Which suture strength did you use?

Gislason: 1–0 in my study, but I do not think that this point is as important.

Read: How did you determine the length of the suture in each patient?

Gislason: All surgeons were instructed to use a ratio greater than 4.

Israelsson: We used 150-cm-long sutures. After the closure, the remnant is measured by the nurse and subtracted from 150.

Klinge: If you accept 16 N/cm as the maximum value physiologically required and you accept that the nod decreases the tensile strength by half for a non-absorbable monofilament suture, e.g. Prolene, I think it is sufficient to use a size of 2–0. For a multifilament which is a little bit stronger, 3–0 would be enough, and for absorbable material you need a size of 1 to guarantee 16 N for 14 days.

Schippers: You said that you had not had such good experience with Maxon. Do you have an explanation for that?

Gislason: We had more infections in that group. We can only speculate on the reasons for this. Perhaps it was the loop, where we put more tension and therefore get ischemia and infection. We do not know whether it is the material or the technique.

References

1. Bucknall TE, Ellis H. Abdominal wound closure- A comparison of monofilament nylon and polyglycolic acid. Surgery 1981;89:672–677.
2. Gislason H, Grønbech JE, Søreide O. Burst abdomen and incisional hernia after major gastrointestinal operations – Comparison of three closure techniques. Eur J Surg 1995;161: 349–354.
3. Leaper DJ, Pollock AV, Evans M. Abdominal wound closure: a trial of nylon, polyglycolic acid and steel sutures. Br J Surg 1977;64:603–606.
4. Wissing J, Th JMV van Vroonhoven, ME Schattenkerk, HF Veen, RJG Ponsen, Jeekel J. Fascia closure after midline laparotomy: results of a randomized trial. Br J Surg 1987;74:738–741.
5. Osther PJ, Gjøde P, Mortensen BB, Bartholin J, Gottrup F. Randomized comparison of polyglycolic acid and polyglyconate sutures for abdominal fascial closure after laparotomy in patients with suspected impaired wound healing. Br J Surg 1995;82:1080–1082.
6. Sahlin S, Ahlberg J, Granström L, Ljungström KG. Monofilament versus multifilament absorbable sutures for abdominal closure. Br J Surg 1993;80:322–324.
7. Israelsson LA, Jonsson T. Closure of midline laparotomy incisions with polydioxanone and nylon: the importance of suture technique. Br J Surg 1994;81:1606–1608.
8. Kendall SWH, Brennan TG, Guillou PJ. Suture length to wound length ratio and the integrity of midline and lateral paramedian incisions. Br J Surg 1991;78:705–707.
9. Krukowski ZH, Cusick EL, Engeset J, Matheson NA. Polydioxanone or polypropylene for closure of midline abdominal incisions: a prospective comparative clinical trial. Br J Surg 1987;74:828–830.
10. Grace RH, Cox S. Incidence of incisional hernia after dehiscence of the abdominal wound. Am J Surg 1976; 131:210–212.
11. Jenkins TPN. The burst abdominal wound: a mechanical approach. Br J Surg 1976;63:873–876.
12. Israelsson LA, Jonsson T. Suture length to wound length ratio and healing of midline laparotomy incisions. Br J Surg 1993;80:1284–1286.
13. Fagniez PL, Hay JM, Lacàine F, Thomsen C. Abdominal midline incision closure. Arch Surg 1985;120:1351–1353.
14. Corman ML, Veidenheimer MC, Coller JA. Controlled clinical trial of three suture materials for abdominal wall closure after bowel operations. Am J Surg 1981;141:510–513.
15. Schoetz DJ, Coller JA, Veidenheimer MC. Closure of abdominal wounds with polydioxanone. Arch Surg 1988;123:72–74.

Part VI Repair of Primary Hernia

CHAPTER 23

Surgery of Umbilical, Epigastric and Spigelian Hernia

D. Bennett

23.1 Umbilical Hernias

Umbilical hernias may be sub-classified as omphalocele, infantile, acquired, paraumbilical or adult umbilical hernias.

23.1.1 Omphalocele

Omphalocele refers to herniation of the abdominal viscera into the tissues of the umbilical cord (Fig. 1). One of the most important contributors to the morbidity and mortality of isolated abdominal wall defects is the delay between delivery and appropriate repair that may be occasioned by transfer to a suitable paediatric surgical unit.

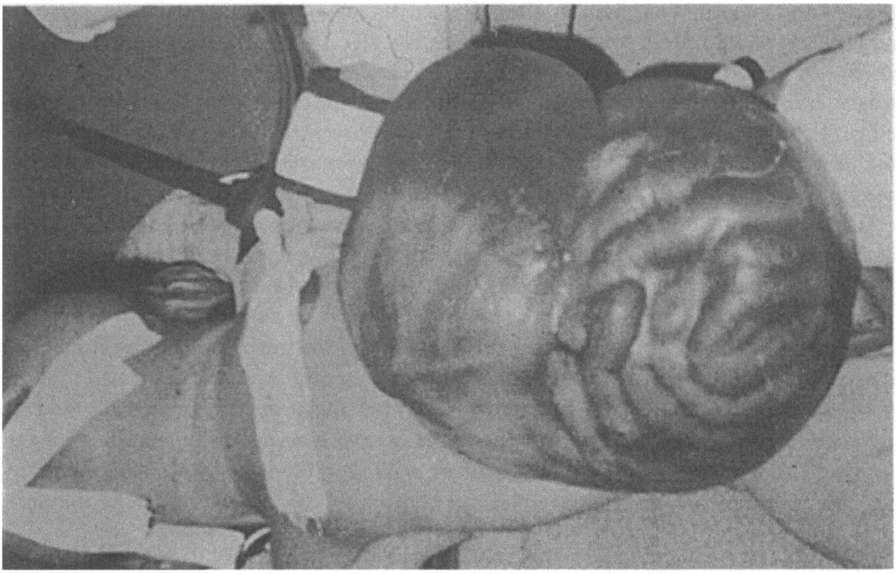

Fig. 1. Omphalocele

Antenatal knowledge of the existence of an omphalocele can allow for birth of the child at a tertiary care institution with the appropriate neonatal and paediatric surgical personnel standing by [1].

The appropriate method of delivery is still contentious. In giant omphaloceles in which dystocia or rupture may occur at the time of vaginal delivery, caesarean delivery may be advantageous. The superiority of the routine use of caesarean in smaller defects, with the attendant risks to the mother and child, has not been proven [2].

Preoperative management is directed at keeping the baby warm and hydrated and bringing him or her to theatre in a stable condition as rapidly as possible. The sac must be handled with care to avoid rupture or twisting of the sac in relation to the abdominal torso. The sac should be wrapped in moist, sterile gauze and covered with impervious plastic sheeting or aluminium foil.

Due to the high association of omphalocele with other congenital abnormalities, a thorough physical examination and chest and abdominal X-rays should be carried out preoperatively. A peripheral intravenous line is placed at the time of blood sampling, and broad-spectrum antibiotics and vitamin K are administered. A nasogastric tube is placed to decompress the gastrointestinal tract.

The surgical approach to the repair of an omphalocele has developed in parallel with the improvements in neonatal anaesthesia, intensive care, fluid management and nutritional support. The early techniques were limited by the ability to care for the infant postoperatively and a variety of skin flaps or skin escharification techniques followed by later closure of the ventral hernia emerged [3,4]. These reduced the initial mortality of these large or ruptured defects from virtually 100% to about 50%.

The initial technique of skin flap closure involved wide mobilisation of skin flaps laterally with closure over the intact omphalocele sac (Fig. 2). However, this does not allow for inspection of the intra-abdominal viscera to detect other potentially life-threatening intestinal anomalies. Alternatively the sac can be trimmed away carefully and the intra-abdominal contents inspected (Fig. 2B). The skin is freed from the fascial edges and undermined laterally (Fig. 2C,D). The umbilical vessels are ligated, or one artery is cannulated and transplanted to the lower abdomen to be used for monitoring. The skin flaps are approximated in the midline over the viscera with simple sutures (Fig. 2E). The ventral hernia is then closed primarily or by staged procedures months or even years later when it appears that the abdominal cavity has enlarged sufficiently. Unfortunately the anticipated increase in size of the abdominal cavity over time often does not occur, and the ventral hernia sac itself merely grows.

In 1967, Schuster [5] proposed using a prosthetic ventral hernia sac that could be reduced gradually in size, forcing the abdominal cavity to enlarge to allow the return of the herniated viscera (Fig. 3). This further reduced the initial mortality of the large defects to less than 50%. As experience with the technique grew, it was learned that the abdominal cavity would enlarge rapidly such that the prosthetic material could be removed within 3–7 days. The need for multiple operations and the complications of sepsis, sac dehiscence and prolonged ileus were all thereby reduced. Mortality employing this technique is now around 25%, and many surgeons believe this to be the optimal surgical technique [6].

There are many variations of the original technique using different prosthetic sheeting materials or preformed silo devices [5,8,9]. Initial trials proceeded slowly and the

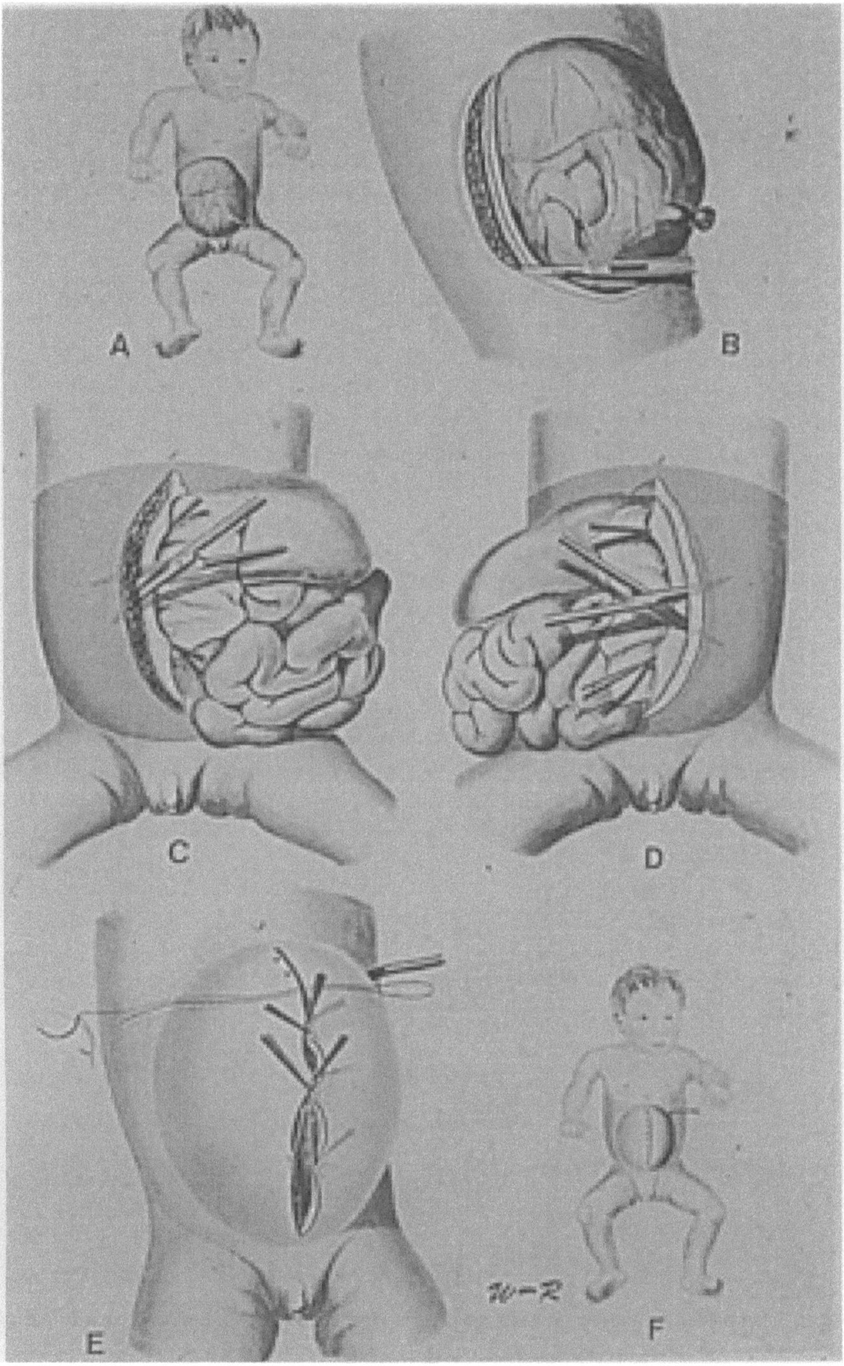

Fig. 2. Method of skin closure over an omphalocele. Reproduced with permission from [12]

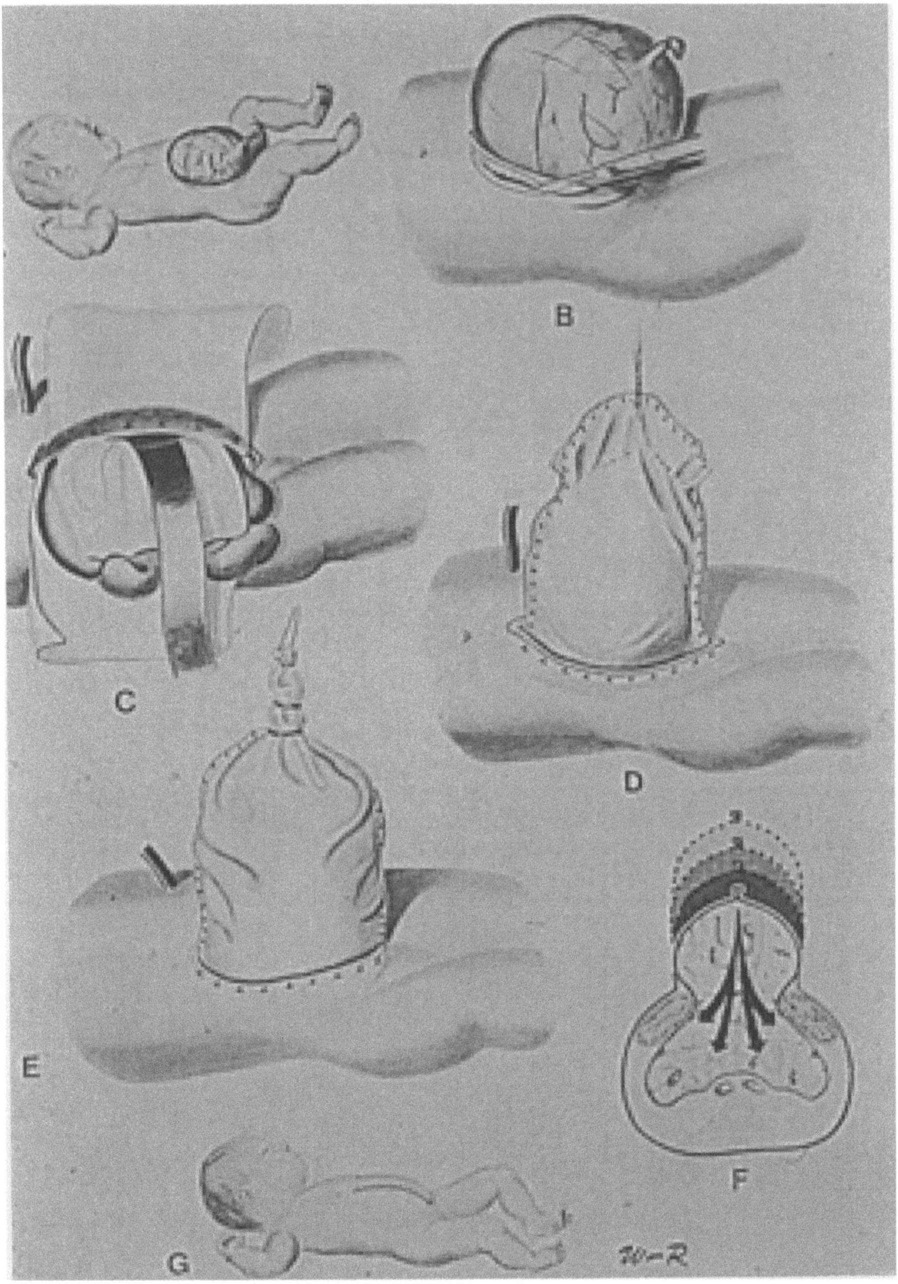

Fig. 3. Method for the staged primary repair of a large omphalocele. Reproduced with permission from [12]

process often took 3–4 weeks. With aggressive daily sac reduction, closure can usually be accomplished within 3–5 days with reduced morbidity and mortality.

The infant is taken to theatre and the entire abdomen prepared and draped. The sac is carefully trimmed from the skin edge and the skin is separated further from the fascial edge all the way around (Fig. 3B). The prosthetic material is then sewn with interrupted nonabsorbable sutures circumferentially to the full thickness of the musculofascial abdominal wall (Fig. 3C). Two sheets may be used and are joined in the midline to form a ventral pocket. When a single sheet is used, a cylinder (silo) results when the two edges of the prosthetic material are sutured together along one side. The top of the silo is closed with further sutures or simply gathered and tied with a piece of umbilical tape (Fig. 3D). The entire prosthetic pouch is wrapped with gauze soaked in antiseptic and then with a dry gauze dressing to support the pouch without kinking or tension. Attaching an umbilical tape to the apex of the sac and suspending this above the abdomen may provide further support.

The pouch is unwrapped at daily intervals, without analgesia, under aseptic conditions and inspected for signs of sepsis or dehiscence. The viscera are gently pushed into the abdomen while the infant is observed for signs of increased intra-abdominal pressure. The sac is tied or sutured at the reduced level (Fig. 3.E) and covered with an antiseptic dressing as before. When the sac is nearly flush with the abdominal wall without tension, the infant is returned to theatre and anaesthetised. The final piece of prosthetic material is removed and primary fascial closure performed with nonabsorbable interrupted sutures. Standard skin closure over the fascia completes the procedure (Fig. 3G). If dehiscence or sepsis occurs, secondary skin closure or simple covering with biological dressings may rescue the situation until the infection has subsided and a further attempt at fascial closure can be performed.

An alternative approach developed with the advent of safe muscle paralysis was primary wall closure. Abdominal enlargement was initiated in the theatre by vigorous abdominal wall stretching and the volume of the abdominal wall contents reduced by gentle evacuation of the gastrointestinal tract proximally and distally. Coupled with paralysis and ventilation after surgery, this allowed for primary closure of most omphaloceles. The initially tense abdomen softens over the ensuing 1–3 days and the infant can be weaned from the ventilator and extubated. Problems of sepsis around a foreign body, sac dehiscence and the requirement for multiple operations are virtually eliminated by this technique.

The infant is taken to theatre in a warm, sterile environment, with the intestines or intact sac covered with warm dressings and plastic sheeting. Under general anaesthesia with maximal muscle relaxant, the dressings are removed and the skin prepared with warm povidone-iodine solution. The infant is then draped.

The skin is dissected from the underlying fascia once the sac has been trimmed from the skin edge. One umbilical artery is cannulated and transplanted to the appropriate lower quadrant of the abdomen, and the other two vessels are ligated. The diaphragmatic attachments of the liver are taken down to allow increased mobility. The intestine and remainder of the abdomen are examined for additional anomalies and the intestine is evacuated proximally, via a nasogastric tube, and distally, through the anus. The abdominal wall is then stretched gradually and repeatedly by hand in quadrants. With gentleness and perseverance, the abdominal cavity can usually be more than doubled in volume. The viscera are replaced into the abdomen, usually with moderate tension. Whether vertical or horizontal closure is used depends largely on the surgeon's assessment of the best fit under least tension. Most often, vertical fascial closure is employed, especially in large defects, although there are occasions when transverse closure is obtained more easily.

After fascial closure, the abdomen is hard and tense, and the infant's haemodynamic status should be assessed for evidence of vena cava compression. Intragastric or other methods of intra-abdominal pressure monitoring may be of value. The method of skin closure attempts to provide a cosmetic umbilicus. At the completion of the fascial closure, there is an excess of skin with a ragged edge. Non-viable skin is trimmed from the edge and a nylon suture is run in and out through the edge circumferentially in a purse-string manner such that, when the purse-string is drawn tight, it brings the skin edges together in the position of a normal umbilicus. A small drain may be left in the centre of the purse-string for 1–2 days. The stitch is removed after 10 days and, in 1–2 months, this closure looks much like a normal umbilicus.

Postoperatively, the infant is nursed in the intensive care unit. Monitoring of intravenous fluid requirements includes the use of arterial blood gas determinations, urine output, blood pressure measurements and clinical assessments of overall perfusion. Nasogastric decompression is maintained with an indwelling suction catheter and broad-spectrum antibiotics are administered for at least 7 days or until the prosthetic material is removed. Parenteral nutrition is commenced on day 2 and continued until gastrointestinal function returns, the nasogastric tube is removed and oral feeding initiated. The infant is discharged from the hospital once adequate nutrition and weight gain can be maintained by oral feeding alone.

23.1.2
Infantile Umbilical Hernias

If the fascial defect is less than 1.5 cm in diameter or is asymptomatic, herniorrhaphy may be delayed until the child is 5 years old. If the hernia is tender, even if it is reduced, or if the defect is larger than 1.5 cm, repair between the ages of 2 and 3 is appropriate (Fig. 4).

Elective repair of infantile umbilical hernias is performed on an outpatient basis using general anaesthesia. The patient is placed in the supine position and the abdomen prepared. The apex of the umbilicus is elevated with a tissue holding forceps and a curvilinear incision is made within a skin fold on the inferior aspect of the hernia. The incision is carried through the subcutaneous tissue to expose the caudal aspect of the hernia sac. The sac is then dissected by blunt techniques until it is encircled. The sac should then be opened on its caudad aspect, such an incision avoiding injury to abdominal contents, which usually adhere to the fundus of the sac. Once the sac has been entered and the contents reduced, the incision is carried around to the cephalad aspect of the sac. The cut edges of the sac are held up to permit abdominal contents to fall back into the peritoneal cavity and horizontal mattress sutures are placed at the edges of the fascial defect, using absorbable material of appropriate size. It is not necessary to separate peritoneum from fascia. A tension-free repair is usually easier to obtain in a horizontal direction. If the defect is larger vertically, or there is an associated supraumbilical defect, a longitudinal closure is more appropriate. The redundant

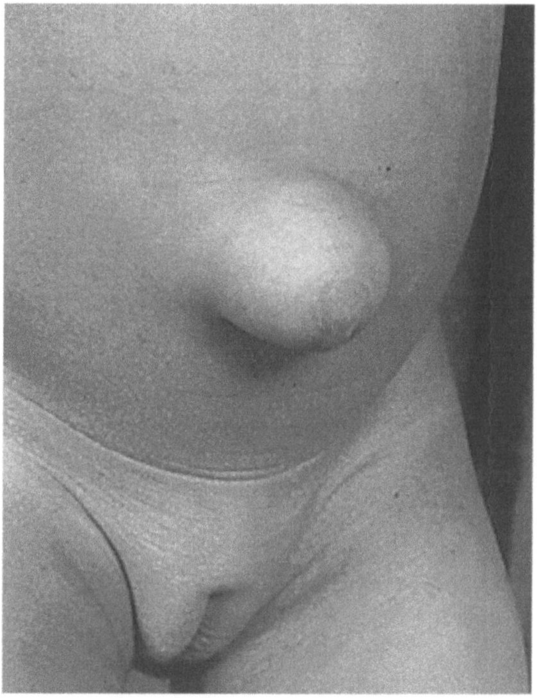

Fig. 4. Umbilical hernia

sac is excised. The umbilicus is re-fashioned by leaving a small button of the fundus of the sac attached to the inner surface of the cicatrix and tacking it down to the area of the fascial repair. Haemostasis must be meticulous. The subcutaneous tissue is closed with interrupted absorbable sutures and the skin subsequently closed with a subcuticular absorbable suture.

Alternative techniques of managing the sac include dissection of the sac intact and its subsequent inversion into the abdominal cavity without opening it (Fig. 5.A) or twisting the sac, once free, and suture-ligating it at the fascial level before excising its redundant portion.

Complications of umbilical herniorrhaphy are extremely uncommon if haemostasis is meticulous. The patient should be observed for the formation of a seroma or haematoma and the development of secondary infection. Recurrence is possible if large defects are closed under tension or if an associated paraumbilical hernia is overlooked. The undersurface of the linea alba should be palpated through the umbilical defect to identify any co-existing paraumbilical defects.

23.1.3
Paraumbilical Hernias

Paraumbilical hernias do not resolve spontaneously and have a high incidence of incarceration and strangulation, so surgical repair is always indicated. If the hernia is

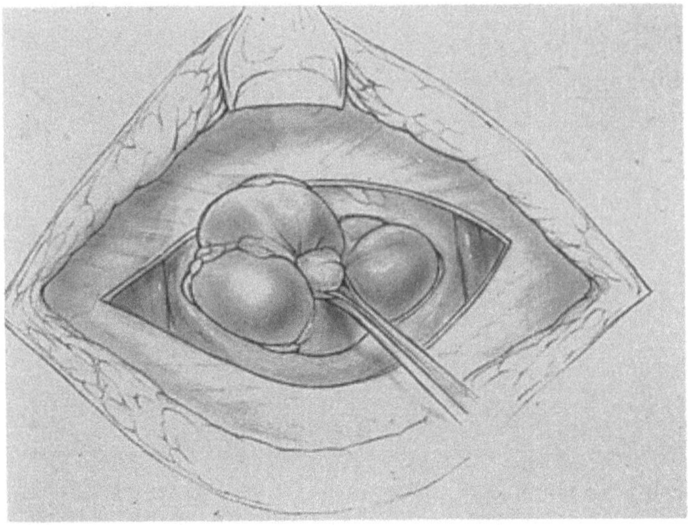

A

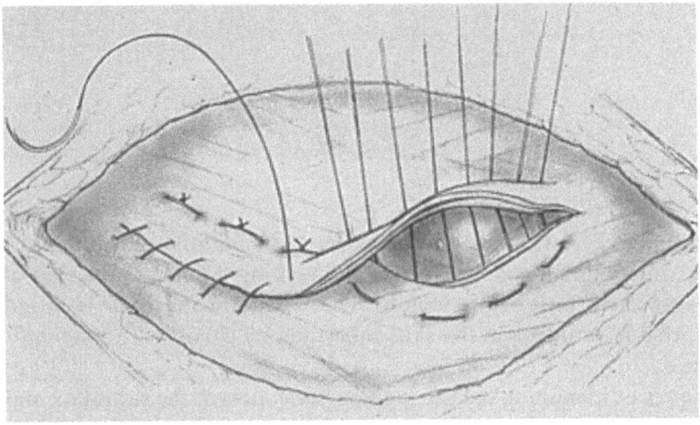

B

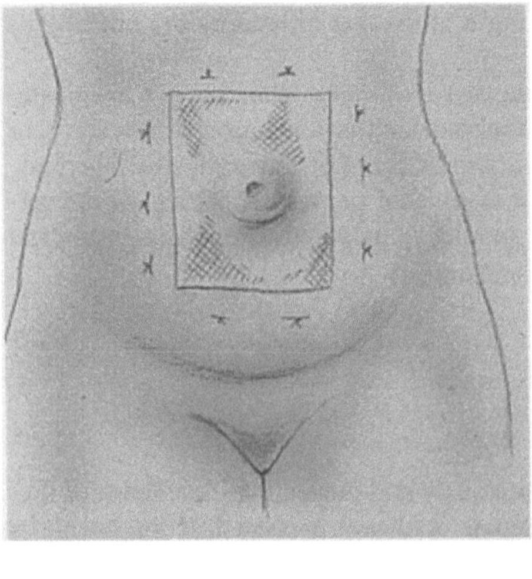

C

Fig. 5A–C. Umbilical hernioplasty.
(A): Inversion of the intact sac into the abdominal cavity; *(B)*: Classical mayo-procedure; *(C)*: Prosthetic mesh reinforcement retromuscularly

small and separated from the umbilicus, it is advisable to mark the hernia site with a skin marker with the patient erect because it can be extremely difficult to identify once the patient is anaesthetised. For solitary hernias separated from the umbilicus, a transverse incision over the hernia provides the best exposure. The incision is carried down to the protruding fat and the linea alba on all sides is dissected out. If the fat is viable, it is reduced into the abdominal cavity and the defect is closed either transversely or vertically, depending on the defect. The use of absorbable or non-absorbable sutures is debated but, as a general rule, non-absorbable sutures of appropriate strength should be used. In patients with strangulated or infected fat, it is best to excise the herniated preperitoneal fat. In patients with both a paraumbilical and umbilical hernia, the incision can be made above the umbilicus, a vertical fascial closure generally providing the best results. In patients with multiple fascial defects, the entire linea alba may have to be repaired up to the xiphoid.

23.1.4 Umbilical Hernia in Adults and Acquired Umbilical Hernias

The nonoperative technique is uniformly unsuccessful because these hernias are loculated and often only partially reducible. In elective cases, it is important to identify any associated underlying pathology and to try and improve the general condition of the patient before undertaking surgical correction. Patients with acquired umbilical hernias often have serious underlying problems and should not undergo operation unless the hernia incarcerates or becomes extremely large and the overlying skin is thinned down to such an extent that spontaneous rupture is possible. Patients with adult umbilical hernias also often have incarcerated hernias and prolonged preoperative therapy to improve their general condition may not be possible.

These high-risk adult patients are generally operated on using regional or local anaesthesia. In smaller adult umbilical hernias, a subumbilical incision can be used, but large hernias, and particularly incarcerated hernias, often require a large midline incision. Dissection is carried through the subcutaneous fat down to the aponeurotic layer above, below and on the sides of the sac. The entire mass of skin, fat and hernia is elevated while the neck of the sac is incised, because adhesions of the omentum or underlying bowel are more likely at the fundus. The incarcerated contents must be evaluated and treated as required. Richter hernias occur occasionally and must be carefully excluded. After the contents are dealt with, the peritoneal sac is repaired and an edge-to-edge closure carried out in either the transverse or vertical direction, whichever is appropriate. For small hernias (<4 cm in diameter), primary edge-to-edge apposition with nonabsorbable sutures of appropriate size is sufficient. The classical Mayo [10] approach has been to overlap the edges (vest-over-pants operation) (Fig. 5B) but Farris and coworkers [11] demonstrated that the bursting strength of the wound did not improve by imbrication and actually was impaired to a degree proportional to the amount of overlapping and tension.

The overlying umbilical skin should not be excised unless it is macerated or infected. If excision is performed, care should be taken with the creation of a new umbilicus, as recurrences may occur at the point on the linea alba where the umbilicus is created. In larger hernias (>4 cm in diameter), it is important to obtain closure without tension. To achieve this, the classical technique was to incise the anterior and posterior sheath laterally. The advent of prosthetic mesh has replaced this technique, and larger defects should be repaired with a sheet of prosthetic mesh placed retromuscularly to reinforce the fascial closure (Fig. 5C). If the fascial edges cannot be brought together, a sheet of mesh should be placed across the defect extraperitoneally, overlapping the fascial edges by at least 4 cm, and fixed in place by non-absorbable sutures. If wound sepsis is feared, the subcutaneous fat and skin should be left open and plans made for delayed primary closure.

Complications include the development of seromas, haematomas and infections. In addition to local problems, these patients often have respiratory and cardiovascular complications and may require prolonged hospitalization.

23.2 Epigastric Hernias

In children, epigastric hernias are uncommon and most of the asymptomatic hernias resolve with time. Therefore, expectant management has been recommended in young children. The decision for surgical intervention depends on the type and severity of symptoms. In adults, operative intervention is considered the only acceptable therapy.

Small, solitary defects may be approached with either a vertical or transverse incision in the midline, centred over the hernia. For larger hernias or if multiple defects are present, a vertical incision is preferred. The hernia and its contents are dissected from the surrounding subcutaneous tissues and fascia to expose the margins of the fascial defect. The superior edge of the ring is incised and the fascial edge grasped with a tissue-holding forceps to elevate the anterior abdominal wall and facilitate exposure of the hernial contents and a sac should it exist.

After the hernia is dissected free, a finger is inserted and searches superiorly and inferiorly to define any further weakness that may not be easily visible. If other defects are found, the incision in the linea alba should be extended to incorporate them so that a more complete repair can be accomplished without fear of a late recurrence. Preperitoneal fat may be excised or reduced into the abdominal cavity (Fig. 6A). If a sac exists, it is opened and any involved viscus is reduced. If evidence from the preoperative evaluation suggests an underlying abnormality, formal exploration of the abdominal cavity is carried out. This procedure is usually unnecessary and meddlesome when not warranted. The peritoneum may be closed with absorbable sutures or left open, and the formal repair is begun. For an effective closure, it is essential to adequately expose the fascia on each side of the linea alba. Closure is performed with nonabsorbable sutures, the left margin stitched to the right margin of the linea alba with simple sutures, ensuring at least 1.5-cm bites on both sides separated by about 1 cm (Fig. 6B). Careful, secure suture tying is essential. Rarely should any subcutaneous drain be placed before the skin is closed. Recurrence is unusual.

Most complications of epigastric hernia repair are not unique to this operation. They are the usual complications associated with an abdominal incision or anaesthesia, and their rate should be low. Local wound infection is especially worrisome because it greatly increases the probability of recurrence. Other factors contributing to recurrence include obesity and inadequate assessment of the linea alba, some "recur-

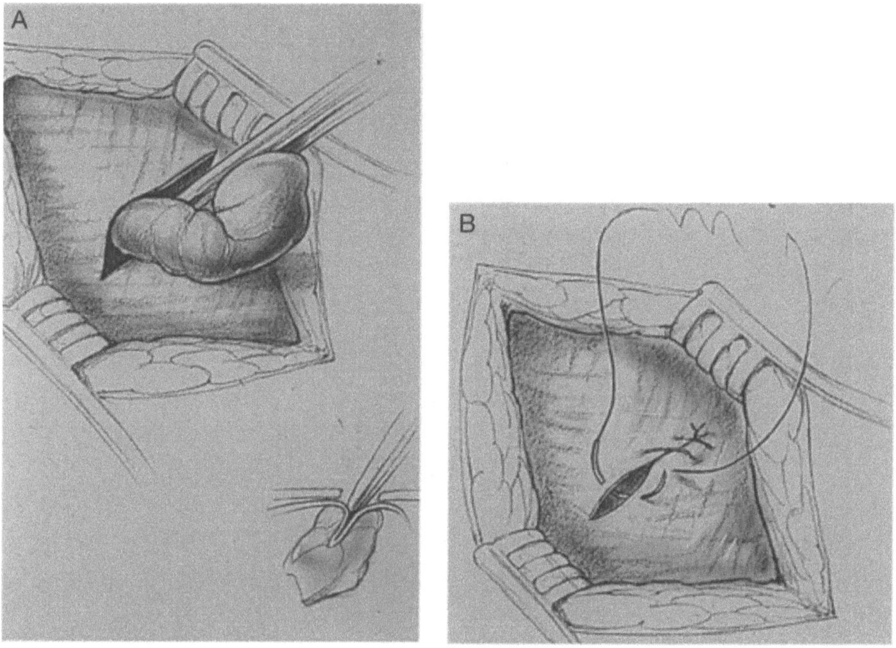

Fig. 6. Epigastric hernia repair

rences" actually representing the persistence of a second hernia or area of weakness that was overlooked at the initial procedure.

23.3 Spigelian Hernias

Spigelian hernias should be treated surgically. The use of different incisions should be considered for palpable and non-palpable hernias. In palpable hernias, a gridiron incision provides excellent exposure (Fig. 7A). After the external aponeurosis is split, the hernia is usually easy to identify (Fig. 7B). If no sac is present, the preperitoneal fat may be simply reduced. If a sac is present, it should be opened and the contents inspected (Fig. 7C) and reduced. The sac neck may then be transfixed with an absorbable suture and the sac excised (Fig. 7D). The simplest form of hernioplasty is generally sufficient; aposing the fascial edges with nonabsorbable sutures (Fig. 7E). As a rule, the hernial orifice is so small that the repair will be free of tension but, in larger defects, the repair may be reinforced with a sheet of prosthetic mesh placed in the retromuscular, extra-peritoneal plane.

If a gridiron incision is used, the incision should be extended medially to open the anterior lamella of the rectus sheath. This provides better exposure of the spigelian aponeurosis and adjacent parts of the posterior lamella of the rectus sheath, reducing the risk of an undetected intravaginal hernial offshoot. Defects in the posterior lamel-

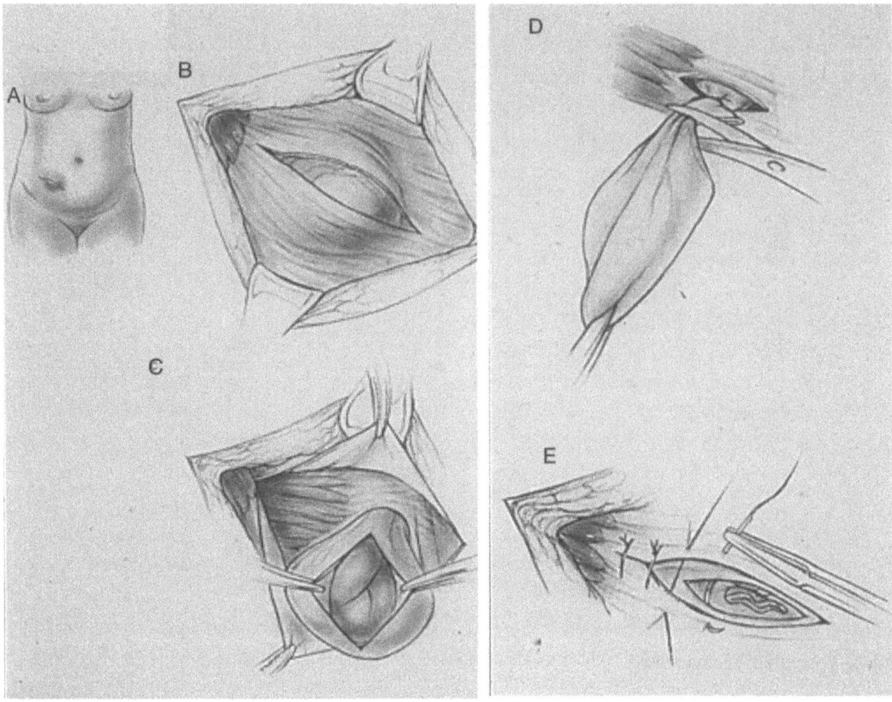

Fig. 7A–E. Spigelian hernia repair

la of the rectus sheath are common and should be closed with nonabsorbable sutures. A gridiron incision may also be used in patients without a palpable hernia or hernial orifice if computed tomography (CT) or ultrasound have shown that the sac lies between the two oblique muscles. The hernial sac is then visible when the external aponeurosis is split.

If no palpable hernia or hernial orifice is detected preoperatively but ultrasound or CT findings are consistent with a spigelian hernia, a preperitoneal dissection through a paramedian incision provides good exposure. The paramedian incision is made through the anterior lamella of the rectus sheath and the rectus muscle is retracted medially so that the posterior lamella can be split longitudinally. Preperitoneal dissection is then carried down to the spigelian aponeurosis. This enables easy inspection of the spigelian aponeurosis and the posterior lamella of the rectus sheath. The hernial orifice and additional aponeurotic defects can be exposed without difficulty and closed without cutting muscles and aponeuroses anterior to the spigelian aponeurosis.

If the internal oblique muscle is intact over the hernia, it may be difficult to locate the hernial orifice through a gridiron incision. Identifying the orifice through this incision may also be difficult in the absence of a peritoneal sac in an intubated and paralysed patient, because the orifice is usually small. An aponeurotic defect can be identified more easily by palpation from the peritoneal side. A paramedian approach facilitates hernioplasty and permits preperitoneal exploration and treatment of other abdominal wall hernias. A preperitoneal approach is also highly suitable for exploratory laparotomy which is recommended in patients with preoperative ultrasound or CT findings consistent with a spigelian hernia who have no palpable hernia or hernial orifice on physical examination. These patients, who seek medical advice because of pain, may have a quiescent spigelian hernia detected in the course of investigation. Therefore, the need to open the peritoneum to identify any other or additional causes of the patients symptoms should always be considered. A vertical incision is also a good alternative in patients with incarcerated or strangulated spigelian hernias in whom a bowel resection may be required.

Prosthetic mesh is not usually required in the repair of spigelian hernias but may be beneficial if the hernial orifice is large or the abdominal musculature/aponeurosis is thin or atrophic secondary to nerve injury. The use of prosthetic mesh should also be considered if there are several concomitant defects in the spigelian aponeurosis or if the hernia is recurrent.

An alternative technique, which is gaining support among some surgeons, is a laparoscopic, preperitoneal repair. The laparoscopic experience with inguinal hernias has demonstrated the preperitoneal approach to be safe, and the long-term results are promising. For spigelian hernias, ports are placed in the midline above and below the umbilicus, and the preperitoneal plane is dissected in the standard way. A spigelian hernia may then be identified traversing the preperitoneal space and entering a defect in the spigelian aponeurosis. The sac is reduced and the defect covered with a sheet of prosthetic mesh, which is anchored laterally with staples, care being taken to avoid any nerves associated with the ilio-pubic tract. This technique has the advantage of also being able to repair associated inguinal or femoral hernias with the addition of only one or two further ports.

Due to the low incidence of spigelian hernias, there are no significant published series of laparoscopic spigelian hernia repair, but inpatients with both inguinal and spigelian hernias, laparoscopic approach should be considered.

The results of operation for spigelian hernia are excellent, and the risk of recurrence is low.

23.4 Discussion

Devlin: Why do you say you have to repair epigastric hernias with non-absorbable material in children?

Bennett: We did not do that. It is unusual to use non-absorbable stitches in children.

Read: Can you say anything about multiple spigelian hernias, because they can appear in double or triple?

Bennett: Indeed, this is an indication for prosthetic repair. In this case, CT scan and ultrasound are important diagnostic methods preoperatively.

Read: It seems to me that spigelian hernias are lateral to the rectus sheath and therefore I do not open it. I think the hernia comes in the muscle bundles and not in the fascia.

Bennett: Yes, for a palpable hernia it is possible to go through the muscle directly on the hernia. It is the technique for nonpalpable hernias to split the rectus sheath and to look to see where the hernia is arising.

Schumpelick: From the anatomical point of view, does it make sense to use transverse incisions in huge umbilical hernias compared to incisions in the linea alba?

Bennett: I think the transverse incision is fine for small umbilical hernias, because you can dissect without opening the rectus sheath. For large primary umbilical hernias and incisional hernias, I think the midline incision is the appropriate approach.

Schumpelick: We know about the higher rate of umbilical hernias after laparoscopy. Is it better to put the trocar below or above the umbilicus, because epigastric hernias never appear below the umbilicus?

Bennett: From the literature, we have data for infra-umbilical incisions and these are the data I am referring to, but we do not have data on supra-umbilical incisions.

Schumpelick: Where is the indication for a mesh in huge umbilical hernias? If we can close the defect primarily without tension, then we should attempt to do so; if not, we should use prosthetic material.

Bendavid: I noticed that 50% of patients with umbilical hernias also have inguinal hernias. Can you comment that?

Devlin: In the literature there is no overlap.

Bendavid: How often do you find other smaller defects using a midline rather than a transverse incision?

Bennett: At the time of repair of epigastric hernias, the linea alba should be palpated proximally and distally and a midline incision should be used if multiple defects exist. I think this is one of the common causes of recurrence.

Filipi: I think it is a good approach to use a 45° laparoscope for the detection of impalpable hernias.

Stoppa: You did not mention cirrhotic patients with ascites and liver insufficiency with a high rate of bleeding and a recurrence rate of about 30%.

Devlin: In my experience, you can have extensive bleeding from big veins at the bottom of the hernias.

Hartel: Nevertheless, the combination of liver cirrhosis and umbilical hernia is not rare. Is there any specific preoperative treatment?

Bennett: There is no specific treatment. Some people use spironolactone, whereas others use preoperative peritoneal drainage of the ascites.

References

1. Nakayama DK, Harrison MR, Gross BH et al. Management of the fetus with an abdominal wall defect. J Paediatr Surg 1984; 19: 408

2. Sipes SL, Weiner CP, Sipes DR, Grant SS, Williamson RA. Gastroschisis and omphalocele: does either antenatal diagnosis or route of delivery make a difference in perinatal outcome. J Obstet Gynaecol 1990; 76: 195
3. Grob M. Conservative treatment of examphalos. Arch Dis Child 1963; 138: 148
4. Gross RE. A new method for surgical treatment of large omphaloceles. Surgery 1948; 24: 277
5. Schuster SR. A new method for the staged repair of large omphaloceles. Surg Gynecol Obstet 1967; 125: 837
6. Schwartz MZ, Tyson KR, Milliorn K, Lobe TE. Staged reduction using a silastic sac is the treatment of choice for large congenital abdominal wall defects. J Pediatr Surg 1983; 6: 713
7. Canty TG, Collins DL. Primary fascial closure in infants with gastroschisis and omphalocele: a superior approach. J Pediatr Surg 1983; 18: 707
8. Allen RG, Wrenn EI, Silon as a sac in the treatment of omphalocele and gastroschisis. J Pediatr Surg 1969; 4: 3
9. Shermeta PW, Haller JA. A new preformed transparent silo for the management of gastroschisis. J Pediatr Surg 1975; 10: 973
10. Mayo WJ. An operation for the radical cure of umbilical hernia. Ann Surg 1901; 34: 276
11. Farris JM, Smith GK, Beattie AS. Umbilical hernia: an inquiry into the principle of imbrication and a note on the preservation of the umbilical dimple. Am J Surg 1959; 98: 236
12. Canty TG. Omphalocele. In: Nyhus LM, Condon RE, eds Hernia, ed 4. Philadelphia, JB Lippincott, 1995, 340

Part VII Repair of Incisional Hernia

Mesh-Free Techniques

Mesh Techniques

CHAPTER 24

Indication and Limitations of Suture Closure – Significance of Relaxing Incisions

L. Herszage

There are two factors involved in repair to close the abdominal wall: Technical factors, which depend entirely on the surgeon and biological ones, which depend entirely on the patient as a living organism.

24.1 Technical Factors

Leaving aside the general principles of surgery, it must be noted that the closures have to be made using functional tension (not free of tension), because tension is a primary condition for repair [1]. Important points include pre- or perisurgical methods (pneumoperitoneum, relaxing incisions, prosthesis), the selection of the suture material (calibre and type) and the technical characteristic of the suture (e.g. continuous or interrupted, special stitches).

24.2 Biological Factors

The biological factors are related to immunity, in which molecular biology plays a key role. Their role in surgery begins with the first incision and the microvascular lesion, which are ultimately responsible for septic complications and dehiscence [2, 3], and does not end until many years later [4]. This role is also conditioned by pre- and perisurgical aspects.

24.2.1 Presurgical Aspects

Presurgical aspects include the skin tests used to classify the patient as normo-, hypo- or anergic, for which we use Rebuck's modified "skin window" test [5, 6]. This allows us to establish with 95% certainty the patient's ability to respond to infection and cicatrization. We use this test in all cases of recurrences and major surgery. In order for the operation to be successful, 97% of all the hypo- and anergic patients modified their skin test values by dietary and psychological measures after 21 days.

24.2.2
Perisurgical Aspects

Meticulous attention to an antiseptic state, classical care and perioperative antibiotic therapy allowed us to greatly reduce infection (0.5% of 656 operations).

24.2.3
Incisional Hernia Classification

In addition to their site, incisional hernias are also classified according to their width:
- Small (up to 3 cm)
- Moderate (up to 6 cm)
- Large (up to 10 cm)
- Extra-large (up to 20 cm)
- Enormous (those that have a tumor of more than 20 cm or a width of 20 cm or more)

24.2.4
General Remarks

The above comments show that suture closure, i.e. using a special running suture from the edges of an incisional hernia without auxiliary measures, was only able to be achieved in cases of small or moderate incisional hernia in normal patients (normoergic, without breathing difficulties or serious gastrointestinal problems). The technical indication of implanting stitches [7] of non-absorbable monofilament thread, 1–2 cm from the edges of the hernial ring, 0.5–1 cm apart, with a suture to wound ratio of 4:1, must be respected.

It is important to point out that suture closure in laparotomies is biologically different to the closure of incisional hernias. From the immunity point of view (bloody edges in laparotomy and smooth, scarred edges in incisional hernias), the union of the edges is biologically totally different.

Suture closure in incisional hernias is transformed in a running suture with excellent results. In this type of suture, each penetration by the needle leads, in microscopical terms, to the formation of a raw surface. The stitches must be placed close together (0.5–1 cm) so as to appear as one incision of interrupted cuts. This produces a surface of collagenogenesis that is able to form a strong scar. The stitches must be firm on each side, taking care that the non-absorbable thread does not come in contact with the viscera. We have seen adherence between the thread (polypropylene) and the viscera in experimental surgery and in some patients.

Under these circumstances, suture closure can have the advantage of the surgeon not wasting time separating layers in a bloody procedure, but it can only be used in moderate cases with little tension.

24.3 Auxiliary Methods

To use the same closure in large incisional hernias, auxiliary methods are usually used in surgery to diminish tension:
1. Pneumoperitoneum of Moreno
2. Relaxing incisions

Both procedures are solutions used to lessen tension, but with different mechanisms.

24.3.1 Pneumoperitoneum

Pneumoperitoneum [8] produces a progressive stretching of the muscular layers, and peritoneal irritation from the 19th day, measured by the number of macrophages, shows a rise in the cicatricial response of the immune system. Its use can be prolonged in time until the edges come close together, tension is normal, the extruded viscera can be inserted easily and breathing becomes normal. Pneumoperitoneum is essential in some patients. It can be implemented in various ways, but it is not frequently used, mainly for socio-economic reasons.

24.3.2 Relaxing Incisions

Relaxing incisions have the same objectives as pneumoperitoneum, but without previous preparation and as part of the surgery in a bloody procedure. Their function is triple:
1. To enlarge the volume of the cavity
2. To lessen the abdominal wall tension, maintaining its function
3. To allow the muscles to return to their original places

Any type of reconstruction that begins with an incision of some of the abdominal wall layers must be considered as a relaxing incision, regardless of the technique that follows. Even in moderate incisional hernias, the incision of one of the layers, usually the first, permits us to transform an ectropion into a flat edge with normal tension.

Three points should be remembered:
1. The irrigation and innervation of the compromised muscles must be preserved, regardless of pseudo-hypotrophy, because of hypofunction or partial disinsertion. Their reimplantation in functional conditions will lead to the muscles regaining their normal thickness in normoergic subjects (with an immediate neuroimmune response).
2. Repair using relaxing incisions must be planned in such a way as to ensure that two or more layers remain, forming the abdominal wall and the stretch lines that biologically form the abdominal dome. As we know, the tension lines of the three layers of the anterolateral wall of the abdomen cross, and this mechanical/physical

structure (three layers one over the other, with crossed tension lines) is used in civil engineering with maximum security and in structures subject to very high tension.
3. The transversus layer should always be spared, as its integrity guarantees closure of the abdominal cavity closure.

Relaxing incisions are indicated in the following cases:
- In chronic cases with major insufficiency of breathing
- In acute postoperative cases in which abdominal distention is the usual answer

They are usually used in the following topographical sites:
- Middle incision: in the anterior rectus sheath
- Lateral incision: on the wide muscles
- A combination of the middle and lateral incision

24.3.2.1
Middle Incision

The first well-known middle incision in surgery was Gibson's [9]. It is still used identically today. It is done by cutting the anterior rectus sheath from the edge of the rib cage to the pubis in the union of the external third with the internal two thirds.

Clutteau [10] made with an interrupted line of cuts in the anterior rectus sheath of the length required using as many lines as necessary.

24.3.2.2
Lateral Incision

Lateral incisions are used in the following cases:
- Chronic umbilical/pubican hernias. Published by Oghi, Leiro und Barbarelli [11], the cut is made in the external oblique muscle, 2 cm inside the anterior superior iliac spine, and is prolonged following the direction of its fibres from the edge of the rib cage to the inguinal region.
- Patients with acute postoperative complications. Xipho-pubic incisions are used, as published by Levy et al. [12], cutting the skin and the external oblique muscle from the edge of the rib cage to the pubis, outside the rectus sheath.
- Subcostal incisional hernias. This involves incisions disinserting the external oblique muscle 2 cm above the edge of the rib cage from the Xiphoid to the tenth rib [13].

24.3.2.3
Combined Incision

In middle incisional hernias from the xiphoid to the umbilicus and in some cases to the pubis, I use Albanese's technique, published in 1951 [14]. This technique is used for hernias up to 30 cm in width and in patients with insufficient breathing. In this technique, the middle of the abdomen is transformed into a solid shield, the abdomen is expanded laterally ("batrachian" abdomen), allowing recovery of breathing, and two muscle layers are left over the entire abdomen at the end of the operation.

The steps involved in this technique are as follows:

1. Incision of the external oblique muscle 0.2 cm over the edge of the rib cage from the xiphoid to the tenth rib, because the ninth fasciculus is the strongest.
2. From this point, downwards, we cut the external oblique muscle 2 cm inside ASIS 4 cm longer than the hernia itself.
3. Dissection of the internal flap of the external oblique muscle from the internal oblique muscle and the rectus sheath; we then cut this sheath in its external border, leaving the rectus muscle exposed from the rib cage passing the inferior limit of the hernia.
4. Introduction of the fingers of one hand under the rectus muscle, taking care to spare vessels and nerves, in order to expose the edge of the hernial ring.
5. Incision of this edge lengthwise in order to separate the posterior leaf of the sheath from the anterior one, which stays adhered to the rectus muscle.
6. Running suture of both posterior leaves, closing the abdominal cavity.
7. Running suture of both anterior leaves in the middle, joining both rectus muscles.
8. Suture of the inner part of the external oblique muscle to the outer one part of the internal oblique muscle. The abdominal wall is thus reconstructed with three layers in the middle and two laterally. These will be joined by collagenogenesis in 30 days.

24.4 Discussion

Amid: I think there is an anatomical explanation for the low incidence of incisional hernia after Pfannenstiel's incision, because as the rectus muscles go upwards into the costal margin, they diverge. So the rectus muscles are touching each other below the umbilicus, and above the umbilicus they diverge; that is the reason why diastasis recti is very rare below the umbilicus and why we have epigastric hernia above the umbilicus and very rarely below the umbilicus.

Jeekel: We are studying the incidence of incisional hernia in the lower abdominal areas; you have them there too. I think the incidence will be lower than in the upper abdominal area. You did not have any after the Pfannenstiel incision, but I agree with you that they stitch the rectus muscles together again. Their closure is different from our midline incision in the upper abdominal area, and that may be a reason; I am not sure why exactly. Is the rectus muscle strong enough to prevent a hernia occurring?

Schumpelick: I am surprised you do not have any incisional hernias after Pfannenstiel's incision. We have a lot – at least ten that I have operated on myself. It is not a typical incision of the midline; it is a low spigelian hernia, because if you tuck in too much of the rectus muscle, you have Hesselbach's triangle free of muscle coverage and then you have a hernia there. Is that true in your patients?

Jeekel: Patients come with an inguinal hernia, and you operate on them. You make an incision in the region of Pfannenstiel's incision and then you see a low spigelian or direct hernia. The direct hernia occurs spontaneously.

Schumpelick: We only see it in laparoscopic repairs.

Kingsnorth: In which layer of the abdominal wall do you place the mesh? Is it retromuscular or is it an onlay mesh?

Jeekel: Retromuscular.

Kingsnorth: Why do you think surgeons have abandoned paramedian incisions, because they used to be very popular? I think they fell into disrepute because the incisional hernias that occurred were due to poor suture material. Now we all use midline incisions and, as you have rightly pointed out, there is a huge failure rate. The results of using the lateral paramedian incision are very good. Why are surgeons still persisting in use the midline incision?

Jeekel: I like to make a midline incision and you reach the abdomen before long. It is a nice feeling. I think it may be as simple as that. I was taught the lateral paramedian incision in the United States as a student in 1966. It is amazing that it has changed so much; looking at the literature, we should not do a midline incision.

Kingsnorth: How many surgeons in the room occasionally use a paramedian incision now, or has everybody abandoned it?

Jeekel: I use transverse incisions for sigmoid.

Kingsnorth: I personally still use a lateral paramedian incision. I would say I use it in about 5%–10% of my laparotomies.

Read: There is still some confusion about what the Pfannenstiel incision is. I don't know where Pfannenstiel worked, but I think in this last paper it was mentioned correctly. As I understand it, the Pfannenstiel incision is transverse in the skin, but it is midline under the skin. Now I think some people think that it is transverse all the way through, but I think there was some confusion. Who was Pfannenstiel?

Jeekel: I am not sure; he most probably was a gynaecologist.*

Klinge: Do you have any explanation for why the size of the hernia seems to be important? Is it a problem of tensile strength of suturing, or of the surgeon? What is the reason for it?

Jeekel: My simple explanation is that you have too much tension when you close up if it is more than 4–6 cm.

Schumpelick: Why did you make 6 cm the criterion in your study, as most had shown 4 cm.

Jeekel: Good question. In the literature, 6 cm is often the size which is critical, and to get more surgeons into the study we needed a lot of centres We thought 6 cm was better, otherwise surgeons would close with a mesh.

* Both are right. Prof. Pfannenstiel was gynaecologist in Breslau (Eds.)

Schumpelick: I would like to make a proposal to all the French colleagues and to all the others. We need a classification of incisional hernia. Some say 4 cm, and some say 6 cm; some say big, and some say small. We need a classification.

Flament: Yes, I think 6 cm is not enough. You can have a very long midline incision with no retraction of lateral muscles. You can close them, but sometimes you have very small, short incisional hernias in the midline. Especially if they have been cut transversally and there is retraction of the rectus muscle, width is important, and not the length of the midline of the incisional hernia.

Jeekel: I completely agree that the width is much more important than the length, and we should have a measure for that; we should calculate that.

Kingsnorth: You mentioned that we needed a classification for incisional hernia. Could I suggest a classification of five types, type 1 being less than 3 cm, type 2, 3–6 cm, type 3, 6–10 cm, type 4, 10–20 cm, and type 5, over 20 cm. Either in the width of the defect or in the fundus itself. I think that may be a reasonable start. Does anybody have any modifications or contributions?

Jeekel: It has been said before that the width is very important. How do you measure it?

Kingsnorth: I suggest we make the measurements when the patient is standing. The size of the fundus is also very important, especially if there are trophic ulcers complicating the hernia. Do you image the abdominal wall preoperatively?

Flament: We now use a computed tomography (CT) scan in all patients, and it is very important to see the retraction of the lateral muscles for the quality of the abdominal wall and the amount of bowel outside the abdominal cavity, so CT scan is very important to classify incisional hernias. Width and length are not enough. Sometimes you have patients with what we call ladder incisional hernia; there are small bridges of connective tissue, but if you repair only one of the holes, you will get a recurrence above or below, and if you have five or six small holes less than 3 cm, we think this has to be considered as a very big incisional hernia, even if the width is only 3 cm.

Hartel: I have one question about the effect on the blood supply after a relaxing incision. You not only decrease the tension of the abdominal wall, but you also probably improve the blood supply to the ribs and the margins. Has any experimental work been done on this question? This also applies to interrupted and running sutures, because when you do a running suture and take big bites and the wound comes under tension, that might destroy the blood supply.

Herszage: We tried to calculate the intraoperative tension. We use to operate under epidural anaesthesia in critical cases, with continuous anaesthesia in the sixth dorsal space to control the breathing of the patient during the operation. We are careful not to increase the tension when we make the incision. We are careful to close with tension, but with normal tension without any kind of duress.

Schumpelick: You have a vast amount of patients. How many meshes do you use in incisional hernia using your technique of incision? Do you need any meshes?

Herszage: We use meshes in 30% of patients.

Stoppa: What is your personal experience of these complicated incisional hernias? Do you advise us to use only the relaxing incision on the rectus sheath or on the external oblique and not this complicated operation?

Herszage: We use all the techniques. In one of the cases I showed, we had a patient with an aneurysm of the aorta. He had a tumour in the bladder, and in this patient we used the left of the sac. We never resect the sac of the incisional hernia. We came to the conclusion intraoperatively about what to do. In this case, we used to cut the sac to use the two flaps - we used one flap to close the cavity, put mesh in and then used the other flap to cover the mesh. We use all the techniques we know.

References

1. Ingber D., Folkman J., Mechanochemical switching between and differentiation during fibroblast growth factor stimulated angiogenesis. Role of extracellular matrix. J Cell Biol. 1989, 109:317.
2. Badia J.M. et al. Peritoneal and systemic cytokine response to laparotomy. Brit J Surg 1996, 83:347–48.
3. Menger M.D., Vollmar B. Adhesion molecules as determinants of disease: from molecular biology to surgical research. Brit J Surg 1996, 83:588–601.
4. Mc Culloch J.M. et al. Wound Healing. Davis Co. Philadelphia 1995.
5. Rebuck J.W., Crowley J.H. A method of studying leukocytic functions in vivo. Ann NY Acad Sci. 1955, 59–757.
6. Barroetavena J., Herszage L., et al. Cirugia de las eventraciones. Ed. El Ateneo. Bs.Aires, 1988 page 6,7.
7. Chevrel J.P. Hernias and surgery of the abdominal wall. 2nd .Ed.Springer-Verlag. Berlin-Heidelberg, 1998.
8. Goni Moreno I.- Eventraciones y hernias voluminosas. Bol.y Trab. Acad Arg de Cir 1946, 30–1041.
9. Gibson Ch.L. Operation for cure of large ventral hernia. Ann Surg 1920,72:214.
10. Clutteau J.E., Premont M. Cure des eventrations latgerales por un procede plastie aponeurotique. Press Med. 1987,16:2123–24.
11. Oghi A., Leiro O., Barbarelli J.J. Eventraciones. Incisiones des descarga. Rev.Arg.de Cir. 1966, 11:197.
12. Levey E. et al. La couverture cutanée abdominale sans traction. Ann Chir 1981,32:5–99.
13. Zaidman M., Alché S. Eventracion subcostal. Prensa Med. Arg. 1965, 55:1086.
14. Albanese A.R. Eventraci6n mediana xifoumbilical gigante. Rev Asoc Med Arg 1951, 65:376.

CHAPTER 25

Significance of Fascia Doubling in the Management of Incisional Hernia

M. Decurtins

25.1 Introduction

The incidence of incisional hernia following abdominal surgery ranges from about 1% to 10% [1–3], depending on the site of the initial laparotomy. The lowest incidence (1%) has been reported after paramedian laparotomy [4], and the highest (15%) after midline incision [5, 6].

Several factors may affect wound healing and the development of wound complications, i.e., suture technique [7], need for reoperation [8], degree of operative contamination, and wound infection [9, 10]. The patients build may also be important in wound healing, and weight has been associated with the rate of both wound infection and incisional hernia [5, 11].

About 50% of incisional hernias develop within 1 year after primary operation [7]. However, 10%–18% of incisional hernias are diagnosed more than 5 years after laparotomy [12, 13] (Table 1).

The large number of surgical procedures described in the literature to repair incisional hernias documents the fact that no single technique can be considered ideal for such repair. Primary mass closure with either interrupted or continuous sutures is the oldest and still one of the most frequently employed technique in the management of incisional herniation. In 1901, W.J. Mayo inaugurated fascia doubling as a new technique for the treatment of umbilical hernia. The promising results with this method led to the adoption of fascia doubling for the cure of incisional hernia as well.

Nevertheless, recurrence rates after hernia repair with primary closure techniques remain as high as 30%–50% [14–17], with primary extrusion of sutures due to excessive closure tension being the main cause of failure [13]. Reapproximation of avascular scar tissue (which carries poor healing capacity) could be another explanation for the high recurrence rates using only primary closure [18].

Table 1. Incidence of incisional hernias [12]

Year	Patients (*n*)	(%)
1	27	44
3	22	35
5	2	3
7	6	10
9	5	8
Total	62	100

To reduce this hazard, tension-free treatment of incisional hernia either by underlaying the closure or by replacing defects with a prosthesis has been used increasingly since the introduction of polyproylene mesh (Marlex) in 1962 [19]. Although the use of meshes seemed to produce better results, the reported postoperative and long-term complications have limited its use to the repair of large or recurrent incisional hernia [20–22].

A randomized controlled trial with unselected incisional hernias would be the ideal way to demonstrate the superiority of one technique over another. However, such randomization would be unacceptable, as it would also lead to primary sutured repair of large defects under high tension with a high probability of recurrence.

The objective of this report is to analyze the significance of fascia doubling in the management of different types of incisional hernias by comparing preference and outcome of the Mayo repair with the results of others primary closure techniques (with or without mesh reinforcement).

25.2 Technique of Fascia Doubling

There are three principal methods for incisional hernia repair:

1. Primary closure (with relaxing incisions)
   a) One-layer (mass) closure
   b) Two-/three-layer closure
   c) Fascia flipover
   d) Fascia doubling
2. Reinforced primary closure
   a) With synthetic mesh
   b) With autologous tissue
3. Defect replacement
   a) With synthetic mesh
   b) With autologous tissue

Primary suture techniques are used mainly for small primary and recurrent hernias, the margins of fascia being adopted by mass sutures, by different layer sutures, by fascia padding, or by fascia doubling. Some authors have also adopted such primary closure techniques for larger defects, often in combination with relaxing incisions.

Reinforced primary sutures by different synthetic meshes or by autologous tissue (skin strip) have been employed especially for recurrent and for large hernias, and recently also for small and primary incisional hernias.

When primary suture is impossible, abdominal wall defects are bridged by synthetic prosthesis or by autogenous or homogenous tissue (fascia lata, muscle flap, cutis, or dura) [23, 24].

In 1901, Mayo developed and published a new method for the repair of umbilical hernia [25]. He advocated the overlapping of the aponeurotic structures, securing a wide area of adhesions instead of edge to edge union. His concept rapidly came into widespread use not only for treatment of umbilical hernia, but also as a standard technique for incisional hernia repair.

The operation is performed as follows:

- Excision of abundant skin over the hernia
- Clearing the surface of the abdominal wall 3–4 cm in all directions from the edge of the disrupted fascia
- Preparing the sac by dividing the fibrous coverings of the hernia
- Opening the sac, exposing its contents, and separating adhesions if intestinal viscera are present
- Peritoneal closure with running, absorbable suture
- Approximation of the margins of the fascia whichever way the overlapping is easiest
- Separating the peritoneum from the lower surface of the overlay fascia
- Doubling the fascia with nonabsorbable mattress sutures, beginning 3 cm from the margin of the overlay fascia, with the loop grasping the margin of the underlay fascia
- Fixing the free margin of the overlay fascia to the surface of the abdominal wall with nonabsorbable sutures
- Reducing excessive wound tension by relaxing incisions in aponeurosis or in rectus sheaths 5 cm lateral to the suture

25.3 Preference for Fascia Doubling in Incisional Hernia Repair

Only a few published series of incisional hernia repair were unselected, and therefore little information is available about the preference for the different methods in incisional hernia repair [1].

In 1997, Paul reported a survey in Germany of the treatment of incisional hernias following open laparotomy [26]. Analysis of the questionnaires returned by 669 different institutions revealed a predominance of the Mayo duplication technique not only for primary hernia repair, but also for the treatment of recurrent hernias of all sizes (Table 2). A total of 45% of departments exclusively use fascia doubling for primary hernia repair, whereas only 7% treat these hernias by simple mass or layered suture. For recurrent incisional hernias, the Mayo technique is preferred by 37% of surgeons. Alloplastic material is implanted for recurrent hernias by 26% of the surgeons asked.

This survey probably represents the current preference for fascia doubling in incisional hernia repair in most European countries. An explanation for this attitude could be the disappointing experience with other primary closure techniques combi-

Table 2. Method of repair used for primary and recurrent hernias

Type of hernia	Method	Use (%)
Primary hernia	Mass suture	7
	Synthetic material	8
	Mayo procedure	45
Recurrent hernia	Mass suture	5
	Synthetic material	26
	Mayo procedure	37

ned with Mayo's convincing idea of improving wound healing by ensuring a wide area of adhesions [25]. His hypothesis was supported by experimental work by Schildberg, who studied the biochemical and physical parameters of wound healing in rats after laparotomy and wound closure either by layered suture or by fascia doubling [27].

Schildberg was able to show that, after 3 weeks, the strength of doubled fascia was significantly higher than the strength of a mass-sutured wound and reached almost half of the strength of normal tissue. He explained this observation by an increase of collagen synthesis in scar tissue dependent on the tension placed on it.

25.4 Long-Term Results of Fascia Doubling for Primary and Recurrent Incisional Hernia Repair

The literature was analyzed to compare the results of fascia doubling with the outcome of primary and recurrent incisional hernia repair performed by other accepted methods.

Unfortunately, prospective and randomized studies comparing different types of incisional hernia repair are still lacking. Most of the published series retrospectively analyzed standard techniques, often used on selected patients. Only very few authors referred to selection criteria, and reliable comparisons are thus not possible.

Table 3 shows recently published recurrence rates after incisional hernia repair by primary suture techniques. Only studies with a mean follow-up of at least 5 years are listed, as primary and recurrent incisional hernias can occur 5 or more years postoperatively [5].

The overall recurrence rate after primary closure was 32.7%. Hernias treated by fascia doubling had a recurrence rate of 33.1%, and the recurrence rate in those repaired by other primary suture techniques was 28.3%.

Table 4 summarizes the almost identical recurrence rates of recurrent incisional hernia repair treated either by Mayo duplication (24.9%) or by direct mass closure of the defect (26.3%).

Table 3. Recurrence rates after incisional hernia repair by primary suture techniques

Year	Reference	Technique	Patients (n)	Recurrence (%)
1983	[27]	Mass closure	44	23
		Mayo repair	33	6
1986	[16]	Mass/layer closure	81	46
1989	[13]	Mass closure	169	24
1991	[33]	Mass closure	114	36
		Mayo repair	57	32
1992	[39]	Mass closure	55	25.4
		Mayo repair	120	25.8
1993	[29]	Various	231	41
1996	[30]	Mass closure	70	38.5
		Mayo repair	27	44.4
1997	[3]	Mayo repair	135	5.5
1997	[31]	Mass closure	33	24
		Mayo repair	58	38

Table 4. Recurrence rates after recurrent incisional hernia repair by mass closure or Mayo duplication

Year	Reference	Technique	Patients (n)	Recurrence (%)
1983	[27]	Mayo repair	15	27
1994	[1]	Mass closure	53	25
1996	[30]	Mass closure	58	27.6
		Mayo repair	35	22.8

The lower recurrence rate of primary closure techniques for recurrent incisional hernia repair compared to the outcome after primary incisional hernia treatment with the same methods probably reflects the fact that the use of meshes has become the method of choice for the repair of recurrent incisional hernia [1, 28], leaving only small, uncomplicated defects for simple mass closure or for a Mayo procedure.

25.5 Conclusion

It is generally accepted that the repair of incisional hernias and particularly of their recurrences is difficult and often unsuccessful. Standard repairs aim to approximate the edges of the hernial defect and to hold them securely until healing is complete. No matter which technique is used, this necessitates putting the tissue under tension and consequently increases the risk of tissue ischemia and suture cutout. Obviously, this hazard depends on the size of hernia defect [29] and increases by doubling the fascia from side to side.

Mayo and his imitators achieved improved outcomes after umbilical hernia repair by overlapping the aponeurotic structures instead of mass closure. This method proved to be successful mainly due to a horizontal fascia repair with little tension and also because the fascia around the hernial ring is not as avascular as it may be after laparotomy with failed wound healing. The poor overall results achieved with the fascia doubling technique for treatment of primary and recurrent incisional hernia clearly show that umbilical and incisional hernias are different entities.

Considering the documented high recurrence rates with all available primary suture techniques and in view of the promising results obtained after mesh repair of large defects [30–32, 35–38], the question remains whether or not prosthetic material is also needed for the repair of smaller hernias.

With the introduction of synthetic meshes, the concept of hernia repair has undergone revolutionary changes, and meshes are currently widely employed for primary and recurrent inguinal hernia repair, both in endoscopic and open procedures. This experience can safely be adopted for use in incisional hernia repair. Fears of increasing wound infection rates using synthetic material have not been substantiated [30].

Under these circumstances (low infection and recurrence rates with mesh implants), the time has come to reconsider the significance of the Mayo procedure in the treatment of incisional hernia. Primary mass closure reinforced by a synthetic mesh graft is also recommended for the repair of small and primary incisional hernias.

25.6 Discussion

Flament: Just one comment on the historical point of view. The Mayo paper was only for umbilical hernias, and in 1912 there was a paper by Mayo and Judd on doubling sutures, but only for lateral incisions on appendectomy incisional hernia; it was never written in the old papers before the First World War that this was for midline incisions.

Schumpelick: Either you think it is justorfied to carry out a controlled trial at least in small hernias using a prosthesis or a direct suture? I do not think that the final word has yet been spoken on small hernias. Are you saying that even for the 4-cm hernias it is justified to use a prosthesis from the beginning?

Flament: I feel that, with our results, with small hernias recurring, we should use a prosthesis in all patients, but this might just be a personal feeling, and for small incisional hernias a trial would be appropriate.

Stoppa: I agree with Flament. For medium, even small incisional hernias, we put in a mesh. In medium-sized hernias, we have up to 30%–40% recurrences in umbilical hernia, for example.

Schumpelick: Would you put a mesh in even in a small hernia on the edge of a midline incision, e.g., above the umbilicus, or a 2-cm hernia?

Stoppa: Yes, if there is an aggravating factor such as obesity, age, or something like that.

Chevrel: In one slide, we can see 46 recurrences with mesh repair. I would like to ask how you use this mesh.

Decurtins: I showed a picture where we had just put the mesh in the defect using the inlay technique.

References

1. Liakakos T, Karanikas I, Panagiotidis H and Dendrinos S: Use of Marlex Mesh in the Repair of Recurrent Incisional Hernia. British Journal of Surgery 81 (1994) 248–239
2. Stelzner F: Theorie und Praxis der fortlaufenden Laparotomienaht (Platzbauch und Narbenhernie). Chirurg 59 (1988) 654–660
3. Paul A, Korenkov M, Peters S, Fischer St, Holthausen U, Köhler L, Eypasch E: Die Mayo-Doppelung zur Behandlung des Narbenbruchs der Bauchdecken nach konventioneller Laparotomie. Zentralbl Chir 122 (1997) 862–870
4. Donaldson DR, Hegarty JH, Brennan TG, Guillou PJ, Finan PJ, Hall TJ: The Lateral Paramedian Incision – Experience with 850 Cases. Br J Surg 69 (1982) 630–632
5. Bucknall TE, Cox PJ, Ellis H: Burst Abdomen and Incisional Hernia: a Prospective Study of 1129 Major Laparotomies. Br Med J 284 (1982) 931–933
6. Wissing J, van Vroonhoven TJMV, Schattenkerk ME, Veen HF, Ponsen RJG, Jeekel J: Fascia Closure after Midline Laparotomy: Results of a Randomized Trial. Br J Surg 74 (1987) 738–741
7. Hohlbach G, Meffert R: Wundruptur – Narbenhernie. Zentralbl Chir 122 (1997) 190–192
8. Israelsson LA, Jonsson T: Overweight and Healing of Midline Incisions: The Importance of Suture Technique. Eur J Surg 163 (1997) 175–180
9. Houck JP, Rypins EB, Sarfeh IJ, Juler GL and Shimoda KJ: Repair of Incisional Hernia. Surg Gynecol Obstet 169 (1989) 397–399

10. Stelzner F: Die Bauchdeckenfunktion, die Entstehung und die Therapie von Hernien (unter anderem: Die Parakolostomiehernie). Langenbecks Arch Chir 379 (1994) 109–119
11. Pitkin RM: Abdominal Hysterectomy in Obese Women. Surg Gynecol Obstet 143 (1976) 532–536
12. Mudge M and Hughes LE: Incisional Hernia: a 10 Year Prospective Study of Incidence and Attitudes. Br J Surg 72 (1985) 70–71
13. Read RC, Yoder G: Recent Trends in the Management of Incisional Herniation. Arch Surg 124 (1989) 485–488
14. Dehne A: Narbenhernien. Chir Gastroenterol 9 (1993) 358–360
15. Ellis H, Gajraj H and George CD: Incisional hernias: when do they occur? Br J Surg 70 (1983) 290–291
16. George CT, Ellis H: The results of incisional hernia repair: a twelve year review. Ann Roy Col Surg 68 (1986) 185–187
17. Langer S and Christiansen J: long-term results after incisional hernia repair. Acta Chir Scand 151 (1985) 217–219
18. Lamont PM, Ellis H: incisional hernia in re-opened abdominal incisions: an overlooked risk factor. Br J Surg 75 (1988) 374–376
19. Usher FC, Allen JE, Crosthwait RW, et al: Polypropylene monofilament: a new biologically inert suture for closing contaminated wounds. MAMA 179 (1962) 780–782
20. Elliot MP, Juler GL: Comparison of marlex mesh and microporous teflon sheets when used for hernia repair in the experimental animal. Am J Surg 137 (1979) 342–344
21. Gilsdorf RB, Shea MM: Repair of massive septic abdominal wall defects with marlex mesh. Am J Surg 130 (1975) 634–638
22. Kaufman Z, Engelberg M, Zager M: Fecal fistula: a late complication of marlex mesh repair. Dis Colon Rectum 24 (1981) 543–544
23. Eisner L, Harder F: Narbenhernien. Chirurg 68 (1997) 304–309
24. Zimmermann G, Müller G und Haid A: Chirurgische Therapie der Narbenhernien. Chirurg 62 (1991) 656–662
25. Mayo WJ: An operation for the radical cure of umbilical hernia. Ann Surg 34 (1901) 276–280
26. Paul A, Lefering R, Köhler L, Eypasch E: Gegenwärtige Praxis der Narbenhernienrekonstruktion in der Bundesrepublik Deutschland. Zentralbl Chir 122 (1997) 859–861
27. Schildberg FW, Vatankhah und Nissen R: Chirurgische Behandlung des Narbenbruches der Bauchdecken. Langenbecks Arch Chir 361 (Kongressbericht 1983) 319–323
28. Westweber K-H, Lepique F, Haaf F, Horatz M, Rink A: Netzplastiken bei Bauchwand-Rezidivhernien – Ergebnisse. Zentralbl Chir 122 (1997) 885–888
29. Hesselink VJ, Luijendijk RW, de Wilt JHW, Heide R and Jeekel J: An evaluation of risk factors in incisional hernia recurrence. Surg Gynecol Obstet 176 (1993) 228–234
30. Schumpelick V, Conze J, Klinge U: Die präperitoneale Netzplastik in der Reparation der Narbenhernien. Chirurg 67 (1996) 1028–1035
31. Trupka AW, Schweiberer L, Hallfeldt K, Waldner H: Versorgung grosser Bauchwandbrüche durch Fremdmaterial (Gore-Tex-Patch). Zentralbl Chir 122 (1997) 879–884
32. Amid PK und Lichtenstein IL: Retromuskuläre Alloplastik grosser Narbenbrüche: eine einfache Heftklammertechnik. Chirurg 67 (1996) 648–652
33. Manninen MJ, Lavonius M and Perhoniemi VJ: Results of Incisional Hernia Repair. Eur J Surg 157 (1991) 29–31
34. Farthmann EH und Mappes H-J: Der spannungsfreie Verschluss der Narbenhernie. Chirurg 68 (1997) 310–316
35. Eypasch E, Paul A: Bauchwandhernien: Epidemiologie, Ökonomie und chirurgische Technik – Ein Überblick. Zentralbl Chir 122 (1997) 855–858
36. Rubio PA: New technique for repairing large ventral incisional hernias with marlex mesh. Surg Gynecol Obstet 162 (1986) 275–276
37. Matapurkar BG, Gupta AK and Agarwal AK: A new technique of "Marlex â-peritoneal sandwich" in the repair of large incisional hernias. World J Surg 15 (1991) 768–770
38. Stoppa RE: the treatment of complicated groin and incisional hernias. World J Surg 13 (1989) 545–554
39. Amgwerd M, Decurtins M, Largiadèr F: Die Narbenhernie – Prädisposition oder insuffiziente Nahttechnik? Helv chir Acta 59 (1992) 345–348

CHAPTER 26

Polypropylene Mesh Repair of Incisional Hernia: Marlex and Prolene Mesh

B. Devlin†

The technique of polypropylene mesh repair of incisional hernia is applicable to the large, diffuse incisional hernia when there is a tissue defect demonstrated preoperatively.

Prior to operation, the patient must be carefully appraised, the physiological status of the patient (especially cardiorespiratory function) must be optimised and the size and dimension of the defect estimated [1]. The protracted exclusion of much of the viscera from the peritoneal cavity, so-called loss of demesne, has profound physiological consequences. The dimension of the defect or defects can be measured clinically by asking patients to tense their muscles or by computed tomography (CT) scanning or ultrasound [2]. Alternatively, on-table pneumoperitoneum can be used, which assists in defining the real margins of the defect and may also reveal the presence of occult hernias [3].

It is always helpful to mark on the relaxed, anaesthetised patient, prior to making any skin incision, the anticipated outline of the mesh replacement (see below; Fig. 1).

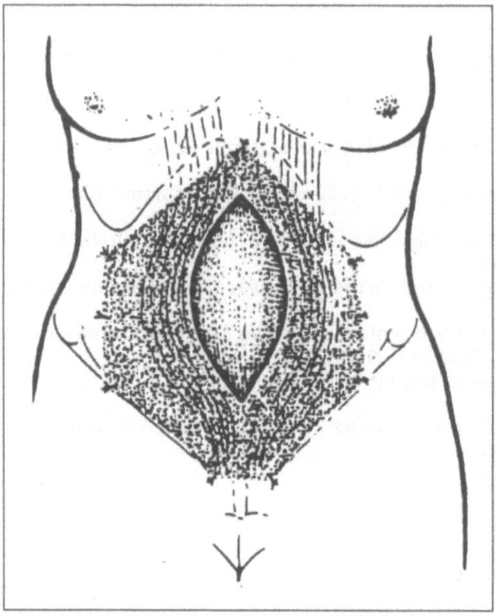

Fig. 1. The outline of the mesh replacement and the positioning of the sutures are marked on the patient prior to any skin incision. (From [1])

26.1 Incision and Dissection

An elliptical incision removing the skin cicatrix is used. It is important to remove minimal skin scar tissue at this stage; above all, at the completion of the operation, the skin must be closed without any tension that might may lead to haematoma or infection.

The dissection is carried down to the neck of the sac. If the sac needs to be opened – because it is irreducible or its contents are compromised – this is done and the peritoneal opening is then closed. If the sac does not need to be opened, and opening the sac should be avoided if possible, it is imbricated with "snaking" sutures of absorbable polymer.

If the hernia is in or near the midline, the anterior rectus sheath on either side should be mobilized by a lateral releasing incision [4]. The anterior rectus sheath is then reflected inward and sutured together with polypropylene to form the posterior layer of the repair. This reconstitutes the linea alba above the umbilicus (Fig. 2).

The lateral edges are then brought to within 3 cm of each other and sutured together with a patch of mesh to form the anterior layer. This is the "onlay technique" (Fig. 2).

If the peritoneum is deficient, e.g. in a flank hernia, and cannot be closed over the viscera, the greater omentum should be mobilised to lie over the intestines. Alternatively, a prosthetic mesh-peritoneal sandwich technique can be used so that the mesh lies between two layers of peritoneum fashioned from the overstretched hernia sac and there is no direct contact with intestine [5]. This is the preferred technique as opposed to leaving the mesh in contact with greater omentum but potentially free to adhere to intestine. The mesh should never be placed in contact with the guts (Fig. 3).

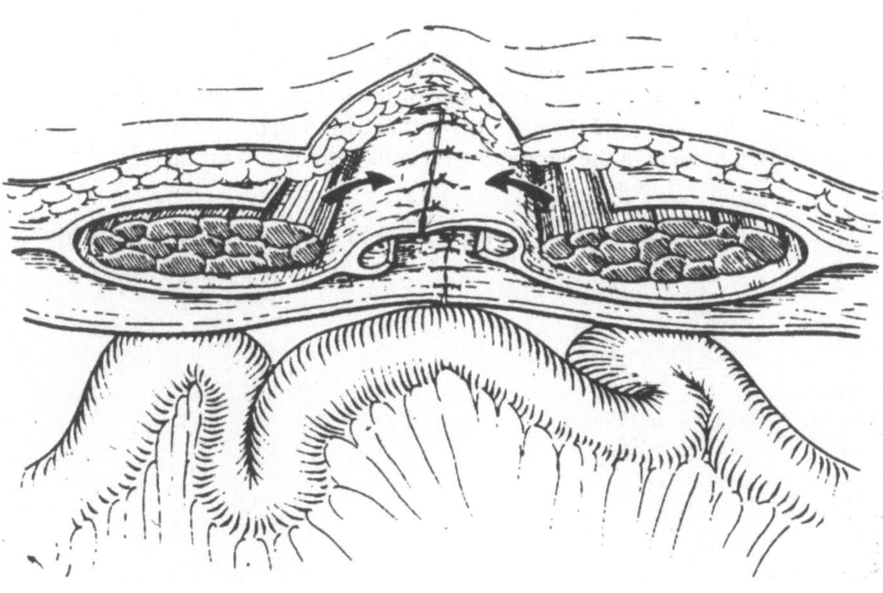

Fig. 2. Formation of an new linea alba by turning in flaps from either rectus sheath prior to onlay mesh replacement. (From [1])

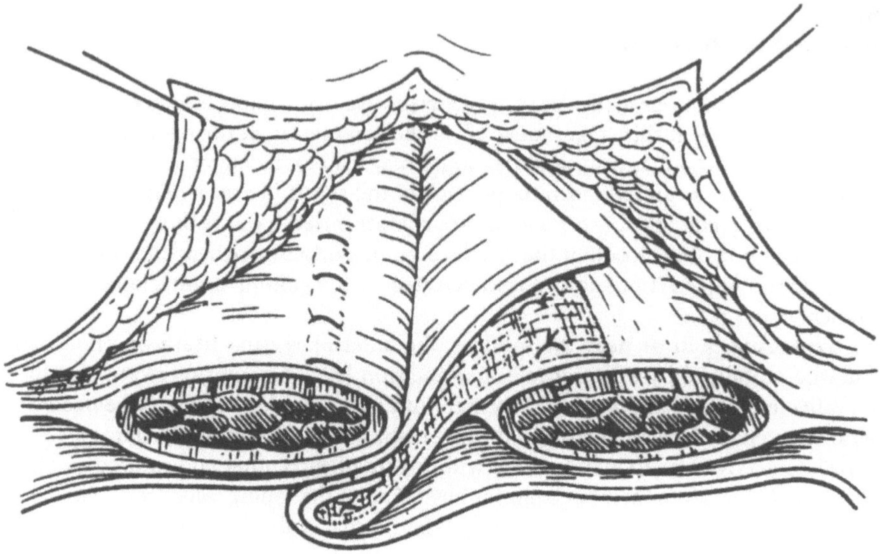

Fig. 3. A peritoneal mesh "sandwich" replacement of the deficit. (From [1])

With this technique, the sac is exposed and freed for 3–5 cm beyond the hernia ring. The sac is then incised along its midline, and the left leaf is tucked under the right leaf and the free border sutured lateral to the opposite hernia ring. The mesh is then placed superficial to this layer and sutured to overlap the margins of the hernia ring; it laid over the defect and sutured to the margin of the opposite hernia ring to complete the circumferential suture line. The right (other) leaf of the hernial sac is now stretched over the mesh and sutured to the lateral side of the left hernia ring. The aponeurotic sheath can then be closed, and the mesh lies within a sandwich of peritoneum. If this is done carefully, the extent of the hernia ring is overlapped by 2.0–3.0 cm (Fig. 4).

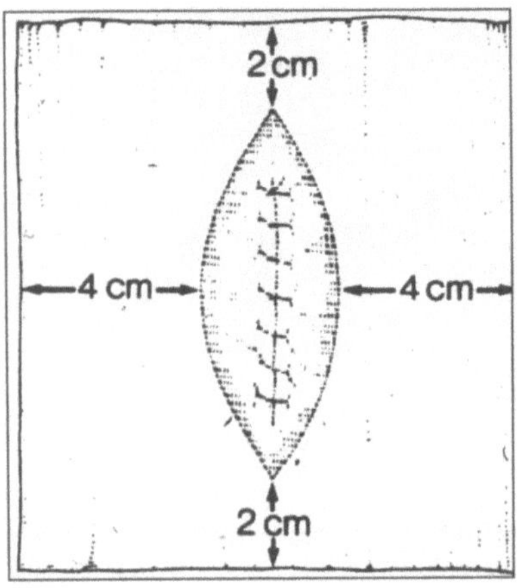

Fig. 4. Margins for overlap of the mesh. (From [1])

Mesh should never be in direct contact with the intestine, because of the risk of adhesion formation and fistulation.

The mesh should be fixed to aponeurosis around the margins of the defect. The greatest difficulty is usually to make the tension of the mesh equal all around the defect that is intended to be repaired. There are four approaches:

1. The mesh is placed over the defect and sutured in position. In this technique, the mesh is extra-aponeurotic (onlay technique).
2. The mesh is carefully cut to size and finally "railroaded" into position at the correct tension. Wagman et al. [6] recommend a "through all layers" suturing of the mesh. In this technique, first sutures are placed through all layers and the peritoneum and aponeurosis are closed. Then the sutures placed through all layers of the parietal muscle wall are pushed through the mesh, which is railroaded into position and fixed in the extraparietal plane [6] (extra-aponeurotic onlay technique; Fig. 5).
3. The mesh is divided into two halves, sutured into position and the tension adjusted by suturing the two halves together (extra-aponeurotic onlay technique; Fig. 4).
4. Each rectus sheath is incised along its medial border and opened in the midline to expose the anterior and posterior aspects of the rectus muscle. Each rectus muscle is then mobilised to its entire width along the length of the defect. The mesh is then placed posterior to the rectus muscles after first closing the posterior leaf of the sheath/peritoneum (extraperitoneal sublay technique).

The layered closure is completed by approximation of the anterior rectus sheath.

Whichever technique is employed, the mesh must overlap each margin of the aponeurotic defect by some 4 cm and must be well fixed to the aponeurosis. This can be achieved by using continuous "quilting" sutures, at least three lines, all around the defect to ensure approximation and adhesion of the mesh to the adjacent aponeurosis.

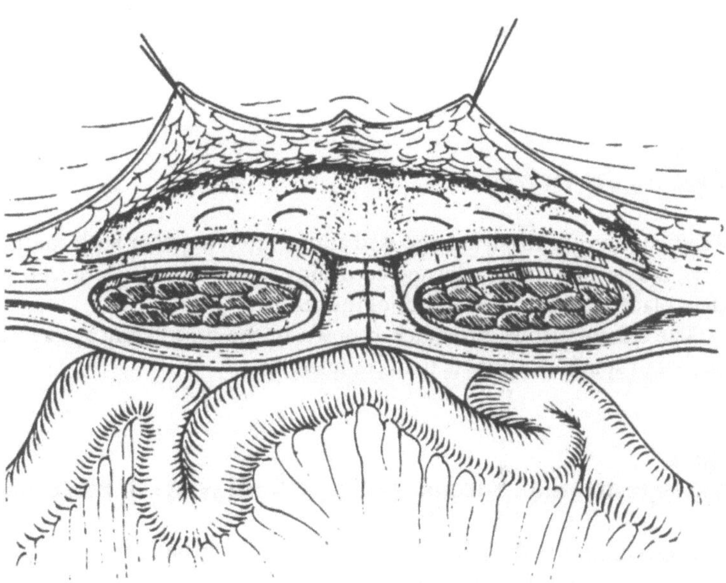

Fig. 5. Extra-aponeurotic mesh onlay technique. (From [1])

26.2 Preparation of Mesh

The mesh is cut so that it is 4 cm longer and some 8 cm wider than the defect. The rectangle of mesh may then be divided into two equal halves down its central long axis if the two-leaf technique is to be used.

26.3 Insertion of Mesh

The mesh is applied as an onlay to the external surface of the aponeurosis or the external surface of the posterior rectus sheath if the first three methods are being used and fixed with polypropylene sutures. Generally, three lines of continuous suture are placed.

In onlay mesh techniques, the farthest one is placed first, at the margin of the mesh, which should be some 3.5–4.0 cm from the edge of the aponeurotic defect. The sutures should take good bites of the aponeurosis and mesh at intervals of not more than 0.5 cm.

With the mesh spread taut by traction by an assistant, a second line of sutures 1 cm closer to the margins of the defect is placed, and finally a third line of sutures is placed at the margin of the defect.

The mesh is then put into the contralateral side using the same technique. A fine suction drain catheter is placed to lie deep to the mesh along the suture line in the peritoneum.

A technique of stapling the mesh in position has been described [7]. After placing the mesh in the preperitoneal space, the linea alba is closed; this can be facilitated by multiple buttonholes in the anterior rectus sheath. The mesh is then placed deep to the abdominal wall muscles and fixed in place with an articulating stapler at multiple points.

26.4 Closing the Defect

The two leaves of mesh are opposed and sutured together with continuous polypropylene, the tension being adjusted according to the size of the defect. A suction drain is then placed down to the surface of the mesh.

The subcutaneous fat is tacked down to the underlying aponeurosis to obliterate the "dead space". Closure is then completed.

26.5 Extraperitoneal, Subaponeurotic, Sublay Mesh Placement

Extraperitoneal (subaponeurotic) placement of mesh is the ideal to be achieved, and this can frequently be done by dissecting the extraperitoneal space only after closing

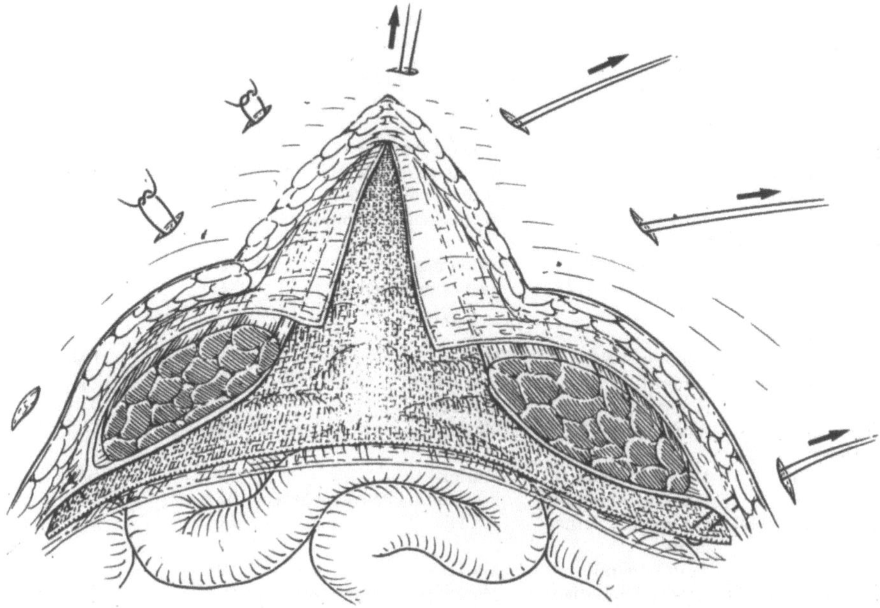

Fig. 6. Extraperitoneal, subaponeurotic placement of mesh using multiple skin wounds. (From [1])

the peritoneum. The mesh is held in position by multiple small cutaneous stab incisions around the defect and sutures of each site. It is important to tie these sutures onto the external oblique aponeurosis, and not onto the subcutaneous fat. Some experts recommend slowly absorbable sutures for this technique to avoid the long-term presence of subcutaneous knots, which patients may find tiresome [8] (Fig. 6).

This technique does not involve an extensive subcutaneous dissection or the creation of a vast dead space. It is the sole technique I have used recently and I find it works very well, particularly if care is taken with the suturing of the mesh through multiple small stab wounds.

The literature confirms the soundness of using Marlex or Prolene mesh in cases of incisional herniation with tissue deficit. A disadvantage is that some patients complain the repair is "stiff" postoperatively.

26.6 Deciding Which Technique to Use

It is impossible to compare the various techniques of repair of incisional hernias (Table 1). The outcome of these operations is often determined by the initial pathology which leads to the original surgery. However, some conclusions can be drawn by reviewing the literature: firstly, suture techniques never cure incisional hernias if there is a tissue defect; secondly, mesh techniques which use mesh to close the defect and involve suturing the mesh to the margin of the defect, so-called inlay techniques,

Table 1. Results of incisional hernia repair (adapted from [1])

Reference	Clinic	Technique	Patients (*n*)	Recurrence rate (%)
Suture of layer techniques				
Obney (1957)	Shouldice, Canada	Layered steel wire	192	12.5
Young (1961)	Warrington, UK	Rectus-relieving incision	15	6.6
Akman (1962)	Shouldice, Canada	Layered steel wire	500	1.6
Maguire and Young (1976)	Warrington, UK	Rectus-relieving incision	32	18.8
Jenkins (1980)	Guildford, UK	Nylon darn	50	8.0
George and Ellis (1986)	Westminster, UK	Keel or mass nylon	81	46.0
Graft techniques				
Usher (1962)	Houston, USA	Marlex	156	10.2
Hamilton (1968)	Louisville, USA	Fascia lata	43	7.0
Usher (1970)	Houston, USA	Marlex	48	0.0
Larson and Harrower (1978)	Providence, USA	Marlex	53	11.3
Lewis (1984)	McGill, Canada	Marlex	50	6.0
Pless (1993)	Odense, Denmark	Free fascia lata transplant	32	28
Van der Lei (1989)	Groningen, Netherlands	ePTFE	11	18
Molloy (1991)	Cork, Ireland	Marlex	50	8
Matapurkar (1991)	New Delhi, India	Marlex peritoneal sandwich	60	0
Liakakos (1994)	Athens, Greece	Marlex	102	8

ePTFE, expanded polytetrafluoroethylene.

always fail; thirdly, sepsis and haematoma formation compromise mesh repairs. The ideal is to achieve incorporation of the mesh into the fibrous tissue of the repair; polypropylene achieves this, although, like all fibrosis healing, the scar tissue will contract over time and may cause the stiffness some patients complain of [9–14].

26.7 Discussion

Chevrel: It looked very complicated what you propose. The fixing of the mesh looks very complicated to me. There is a recurrence possibility between stitches; even if you use a running suture, the bowel can still go around the side. It is very important how you fix it, and I think we should talk about that too.

Amid: Four very short points. I would like to re-emphasise the advantage of not opening the hernia sac, as Dr. Devlin mentioned. Secondly, I think, for once, Mr Flament will agree with me that the overlap should be at least 6 cm and perhaps even 8 cm. Thirdly, should the opening of the rectus sheath go inside the rectus compartment? If the opening is made on the anterior rectus sheath on each side, we lose 1–2 cm of rectus sheath and the final closure will therefore be difficult. If the opening is made in one posterior rectus sheath, the closure will be easier; that is a trick I learnt from Dr. Wantz. Finally, adapting the mesh to the size of the defect using suture closure, you have to have precise tailoring and measurements. The good thing about stapling fixation is that you do not need precise measurements; you tailor as you go.

Jeekel: Why do you say so strongly that you should not open the peritoneum, that you should try to keep it closed? Is that true?

Devlin: There are two reasons why I believe that you should not open it. If you do not open one sac at all, the incidence of adynamic ileus postoperatively is far lower.

Jeekel: Is that true?

Devlin: As far as we can see, yes.

Jeekel: Has it been proven somewhere?

Amid: Yes, if you do not get into the peritoneal cavity, the postoperative course will be much smoother.

Jeekel: You say that, but has it been demonstrated?

Devlin: It is very difficult to do a randomised trial to describe that.

Jeekel: That is why I ask whether it has been proven.

Devlin: The second reason not to open it is that, if you put the mesh in contact with the gut, you get additional fistulation, adhesions and so on.

Jeekel: We do not see fistulation, only adhesions.

Devlin: Even with polypropylene?

Flament: I would like to make a comment on this point. We have to consider incisional hernias not only as holes in the abdominal wall; they are a general disease, and we think that bowel wall adhesions are part of the disease, a part of the symptomatology, so we always open the sac. We free the bowel adhesions, and that is why I disagree with Dr. Devlin. From the anatomical point of view, you said you can put a prosthesis between the muscle and the posterior sheath, and between the muscle and the anterior sheath, but the posterior aspect is very easy to free; you just pass a finger between the layers. The anterior aspect is very difficult, because you have to cut the aponeurosis into sections. So why put the prosthesis between the muscle and the anterior sheath when it is so easy to put it between the muscle and the posterior sheath? My last comment is on one of your slides. In one slide you placed the prosthesis between the peritoneum and the posterior rectus sheath. It is also very difficult to free. Below the arcuate line it is easy to free because there is no more rectus sheath, but above the arcuate line it is very difficult to free the peritoneum from the rectus sheath. We therefore advocate prosthesis between muscle and the posterior sheath.

Simmermacher: I think what Professor Flament said was illustrated by the anatomist above who told us that the posterior sheath is easy to free. Secondly, I think we need to add an important technical point when using Marlex, and that is if you take stitches, the bite in the Marlex should always be smaller than the bite in the tissue: otherwise you get wrinkling of the Marlex by the suturing, which might be a great problem later on because of the sawing effect of the wrinkled Marlex. I think we should stress that as well.

Devlin: To some extent you are right, but the polypropylene mesh manufactured by Ethicon does not have the rigidity that Marlex does.

Amid: I think Professor Flament misunderstood my comment about opening the anterior rectus sheath. I did not mean separating the muscle from the anterior rectus sheath; I meant separating it from the posterior rectus sheath entering the rectus compartment.

References

1. Devlin HB and Kingsnorth A, Management of Abdominal Hernias, 2nd Edition Chapman &Hall, London,1998-07-09
2. Truong SN, Pfingsten F, Dreuw B, Schumpelick V, Value of ultrasound in the diagnosis of undetermined findings in the abdominal wall and inguinal region. Inguinal Hernia, Eds V Schumpelick, GE Wantz. Basel: Karger, 1995; pp.29-41
3. Winslet MC,. Obeid ML, Kumar V, On-table pneumoperitoneum in the management of complicated incisional hernias. Ann R Coll Surg Engl 1993; 75:186-188
4. Loh A, Rajkumar JS, South LM, Anatomical repair of large incisional hernias. Ann R Coll Surg Engl 1992; 74:100-105
5. Matapurkar BG, Gupta AK, Agarwal AK A new technique of "MarlexR-peritoneal sandwich" in the repair of large incisional hernias. W J Surg 1991; 15:768-770
6. Wagman ID, Barnhart GR and Sugerman HJ, Recurrent midline hernial repair. Surgery, Gynecology and Obstetrics 1985; 161:181-182
7. Wagman ID, Barnhart GR and Sugerman HJ, Recurrent midline hernial repair. Surgery, Gynecology and Obstetrics 1985; 161:181-182
8. Devlin HB, Nicholson S, Hernias of the abdominal wall and pelvis: Incisional hernias and parastomal herniation. Operative Surgery and Management, 3red ed. Eds Keen G, Farndon J. Oxford: Butterworth Heinemann, 1994.
9. Young D., Repair of epigastric incisional hernia. Br J Surg 1961;48:514-516
10. George CD and Ellis H, The results of incisional hernia repair: a twelve year review. Ann R Coll Engl. 1986; 68:185-187
11. Usher FC, Hernia repair with Marlex mesh. Arch Surg 1962; 84:73-76
12. Molloy RG, Moran KT, Waldron RP, Brady MP, Kirwan WO, Massive incisional hernia: abdominal wall replacement with MarlexR mesh. Br J Surg 1991; 78:242-244
13. Matapurkar BG, Gupta AK, Agarwal AK, A new technique of "MarlexR-peritoneal sandwich" in the repair of large incisional hernias. W J Surg 1991; 15:768-770
14. Liakakos T, Karanikas I, Panagiotidis H, Dendrinos S. Use of Marlex mesh in the repair of recurrent incisional hernia. Br J Surg 1994;81:248-249

CHAPTER 27

Prosthetic Incisional Hernioplasty: Indications and Results

G.E. Wantz, E. Fischer

Before I was aware of the retromuscular technique developed in France for the repair of major incisional hernias, I, like other American surgeons, used a hodgepodge of techniques. Although these techniques usually eliminated the hernia, they left a feeling of dissatisfaction. Visits to France in 1985 and 1986 to observe R. Stoppa in Amiens and J.B. Flament in Reims were most educational and valuable. Since then, sincere and ardent attempts have been made to teach surgeons in the United States about their methods. Herein, I, together with Eva Fischer, report with enthusiasm our experience with the technique, emphasizing indications for the procedure and results.

27.1 Materials

There were 204 patients who underwent 206 repairs for major abdominal incisional hernias (105 females, 99 males). Ages varied from 33 to 85 years, the median being 65 years for both men and women. Of the 206 incisional hernias, 125 (61%) were primary and 81 (39%) recurrent. The patients with recurrent hernias had undergone an astonishing 222 previous unsuccessful prosthetic repairs (2.8 operations per patient). In fact, one patient had 11 previous repairs, another eight, and another seven. This dismal record says something about the current state of incisional hernia repairs in my country. The locations of the primary incisional hernias were as follows: 29 supraumbilical midline, 51 subumbilical midline, 26 combined midline, four upper quadrant, eight lower quadrant, and seven flank. The locations of the recurrent incisional hernias were as follows: one epigastric, four umbilical, 19 supraumbilical midline, 25 subumbilical midline, 14 combined midline, one upper quadrant, 12 lower quadrant, four flank, and one parastomal (Table 1). Of interest was the fact that 15 patients had 23 groin hernias repaired coincidently by the prosthesis used for the repair of their incisional hernias.

27.2 Prostheses

The primary retromuscular prosthesis was Mersilene in 184 patients (89.3%) and polypropylene in 22 (10.7%). The Mersilene primary prosthesis was always sutured to the anterior abdominal wall with absorbable traction–fixation sutures, whereas when

Table 1. Location of incisional hernias

Site of recurrence	Primary hernia (n)	Recurrent hernia (n)	Total (n)	% of total	Recurrences (n)
Epigastric	-	1	1	0.50	
Umbilical	-	4	4	1.9	1
Above umbilicus	29	19	48	23.3	0
Below umbilicus	51	25	76	36.9	1
Combined midline	26	14	40	19.4	0
Upper quadrant	4	1	5	2.4	0
Lower quadrant	8	12	20	9.7	0
Lumbar	7	4	11	5.3	1 (partial)
Parastomal	-	1	1	0.5	0
Totals	125 (61%)	81 (39%)	206	-	3 (1.5%)

the primary prosthesis was polypropylene it was never anchored to the anterior abdominal wall. A secondary prosthesis was occasionally used to close the posterior and anterior rectus sheaths if they could not be approximated primarily. The posterior rectus sheath was closed with Vicryl in 49 (24%) patients, and the anterior rectus sheath was stabilized with polypropylene mesh in 26 (13%) patients. The omentum, when present, was used to intervene between the abdominal viscera and the Vicryl.

27.3 Indications for Mesh

Incisional hernias as a general rule should be repaired providing local and systemic conditions ensure a safe outcome. A prosthesis is necessary in the absence of sepsis for a successful repair in all major incisional hernias. A major incisional hernia is by definition a hernia with a diameter greater than 10 cm. Flament, Stoppa, and Verhaeghe have indicated how the prosthesis should be used in the various types of incisional hernias and we have followed their advice (Figs. 1–6).

Mersilene is the prosthesis of choice, as it is supple, flexible, and conforming. It is always fixed to the anterior abdominal wall and to Cooper's ligament, when appropriate, with absorbable sutures, while it is never sutured in place in the properitoneal and retroperitoneal spaces. However, when the mesh is attached to the ribs, very strong permanent sutures are required. Polypropylene meshes are semirigid, and large pieces of mesh are not suitable for the repair of most major incisional hernias, as they may immobilize the abdominal wall. However, they may be used in midline incisional hernias when large pieces are not required. Polypropylene mesh does not require peripheral fixation to the anterior abdominal wall if the midline is closed over the mesh or if the edges cannot be approximated and are instead sutured to the central portion of the mesh.

The primary prosthesis is positioned as follows: in upper midline hernias, the mesh is retromuscular and lays on the surface of the posterior rectus sheath; in lower midline hernias, the mesh is on the surface of the posterior rectus sheath superior to the arcuate line, and inferiorly it is in the properitoneal space and the space of Retzius; in upper quadrant hernias, the prosthesis is submuscular inferiorly, whereas superiorly it

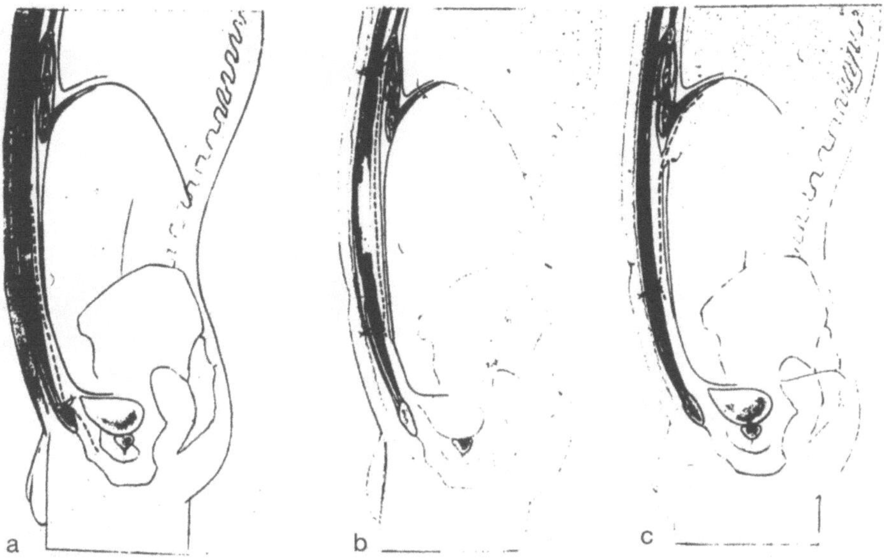

Fig. 1a–c. Parasagittal sections of the abdomen showing the position of the prosthesis in *a* subumbilical incisional hernias, *b* supraumbilical incisional hernias, and *c* subcostal incisional hernias. (Reproduced with permission from [4])

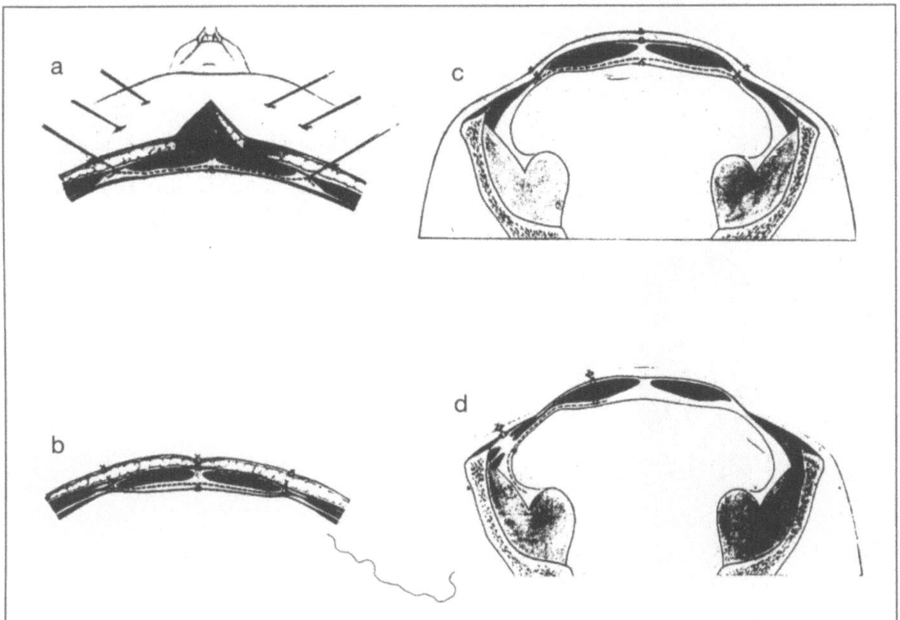

Fig. 2a–d. Transverse sections of the abdomen showing the position of the mesh *a* above the umbilicus, *b* at the umbilicus, *c* below the umbilicus, and *d* in a lower quadrant hernia. (Reproduced with permission from [4])

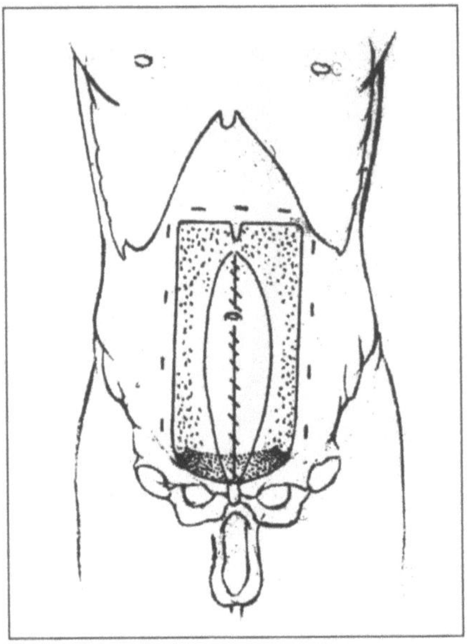

Fig. 3. Anterior view of the prosthesis in a midline incisional hernia. Above the umbilicus, the mesh needs a slit to accommodate the linea alba. (Reproduced with permission from [4])

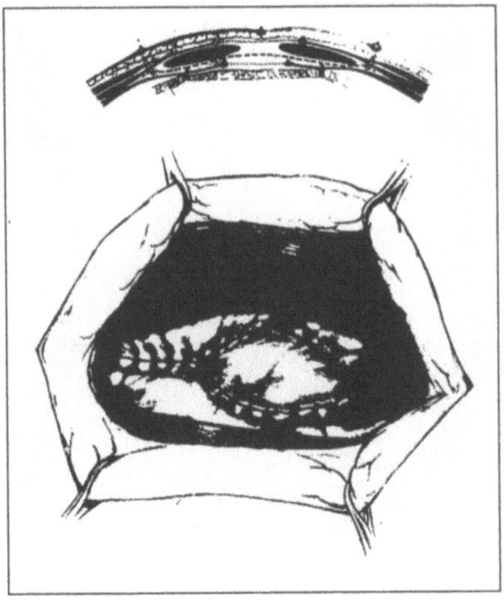

Fig. 4. It is essential that the permanent prosthesis avoids direct contact with the bowel. Omentum may be inserted between the permanent prosthesis and the bowel when available. Absorbable prosthesis such as Vicryl and Dexon may be used to close the posterior rectus sheath if its edges cannot be approximated. (Reproduced with permission from [4])

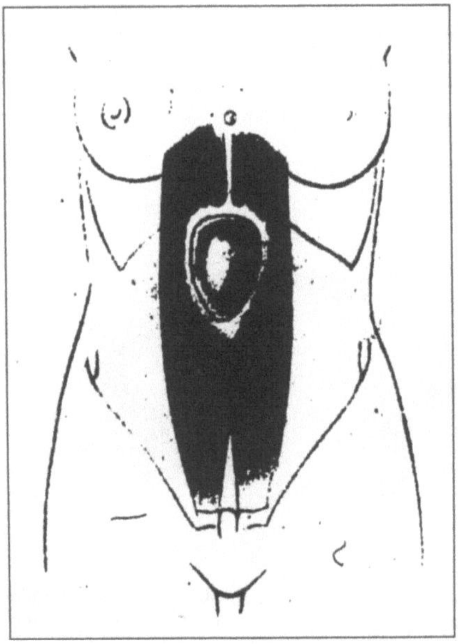

Fig. 5. If the anterior rectus sheath cannot be approximated, the anterior rectus sheath and abdominal wall can be stabilized by a permanent or absorbable prosthesis inlayed in the parietal defect. (Reproduced with permission from [4])

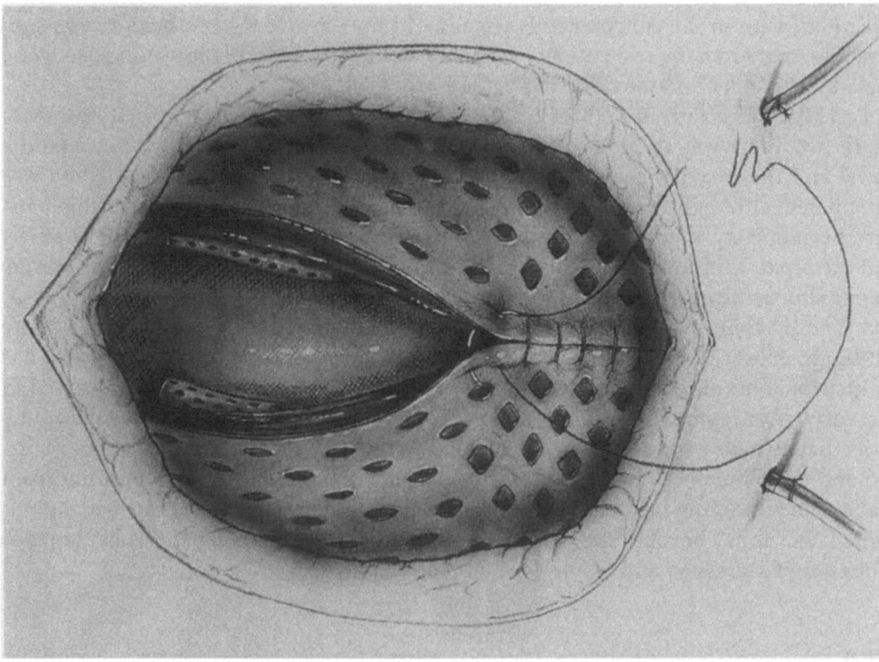

Fig. 6. Use of quincuncial relaxing incisions to facilitate closure of the midline. Closed suction drains are used to prevent seromas and should not be removed until the drainage is 10 cc or less per 24-h period. In most instances, this takes 4–5 days. (Reproduced with permission from [4])

is intraperitoneal and under the diaphragm, where it is sutured to the lower ribs with through and through permanent sutures bolstered with pledgets of polypropylene mesh to prevent tearing of the Mersilene; in lower quadrant hernias, the prosthesis is submuscular medially, and laterally it wraps around the visceral sac in the properitoneal and retroperitoneal space without fixation; in lumbar (flank) hernias, the prosthesis is both extraperitoneal and intraperitoneal superiorly and is attached to the ribs as in subcostal incisional hernias, while inferiorly and posteriorly the prosthesis is deep in the properitoneal and retroperitoneal space.

27.4 Mortality and Complications

There were two deaths from pulmonary embolism despite prophylaxis. One of the deaths occurred after discharge from the hospital. There were 13 complications, giving a complication rate of 6.3%. The complications included one delayed infection, two early infections, two skin sloughs, three fecal fistulas, one persistent pain at the traction fixation suture site that required surgical intervention, one severe hemorrhage due to hemorrhagic diathesis, two partial intermittent intestinal obstruction, and one seroma cured with 100 mg doxycycline instilled in the seroma twice. The early wound infections were in the subcutaneous tissues, did not involve the mesh, and were successfully treated. In the two patients with skin sloughs, the Mersilene was exposed; one healed completely, and the other has yet to heal.

Fecal fistulas occurred in three patients who had Mersilene as the primary prosthesis. In two, there was an intervening layer of the absorbable mesh Vicryl between the bowel and the Mersilene, and in one there was none. In one patient, the fistula was anticipated, although it occurred 18 months after the repair. At the time of this patient's hernioplasty, a granuloma was encountered. A gram stain of this was negative, and the repair with mesh was completed in the belief that the granuloma was sterile. To our shock, the culture grew staphylococci, and unfortunately long-term antimicrobial therapy could not be given because the patient was sensitive to the appropriate antibiotic drugs. The mesh was removed, the bowel repaired, and the patient still has an incisional hernia. In the other two patients with intestinal fistulas, one occurred in the early postoperative period probably at the site of an inadvertent enterotomy immediately below the access incision. Since, in this patient, the hernia has not recurred and the fistula's output is low and manageable, no attempt to correct it has been made. The remaining intestinal fistula occurred in the subcutaneous tissues of a parastomal incisional hernia repair. This was remedied by removing the subcutaneous sequestered Mersilene and moving the stoma.

27.5 Recurrences

Three patients with 206 repairs had recurrences, giving a recurrence rate of 1.5%. One was a small recurrence in a patient following an incisional flank hernioplasty in which a suture holding the mesh to the ribs failed. Another recurrence was the result of a delayed infection occurring 3 months postoperatively that required removal of sequestered mesh and later a subsequent repair. The remaining recurrence, which has not been repaired, occurred in the patient with the delayed infection and fecal fistula.

27.6 Conclusion

The favorable results speak for themselves. The deaths were disappointing and caused us to maintain subcutaneous heparin for a few more days after hospital discharge usually on the fourth to the sixth postoperative day. Fecal fistulas are well-known complications whenever the intestines become immobilized by dense adhesions to a permanent prosthesis of either polypropylene or Mersilene. Vicryl absorbable mesh does not ensure protection, especially if the bowel is denuded or contains an enterotomy. Vicryl is known to hamper healing of intestinal anastomoses. Consequently, traumatized bowel must, if possible, be positioned away from possible contact with both absorbable and permanent prostheses. Intervening omentum is always advisable, but unfortunately it is too often gone or unusable after the patient has had many laparotomies. Gram stains are unreliable and may not display bacteria that subsequently may be revealed by culture. The prudent advice is not to proceed with a prosthetic repair if a granuloma is encountered during any stage of the operation, no matter how small it is. If this advice had been followed, the serious delayed fecal fistula with infection and recurrence of the hernia would have been avoided.

In conclusion, retromuscular prosthetic incisional hernioplasty produces excellent results however measured. The preferred primary prosthesis is Mersilene, but polypropylene mesh may be used providing the piece is not too large and the hernias is in the midline.

27.7 Discussion

Schumpelick: Why do you think you have to fix the Mersilene mesh and not the polypropylene one?

Wantz: The Mersilene is elastic; when you suture the abdominal wall, it stretches out and pushes everything down. If you do that with polypropylene, it does not look the same. Polypropylene is so stiff that it does not give very much, so we just lay it in place. It will be held in place by the posterior rectus sheath. When you put polypropylene in, you cut it and trim it, but it never looks right; it never looks as good as Mersilene does.

Amid: Do you use nonabsorbable mesh as a second layer if you cannot close the defect over the deep mesh? On three occasions instead of using nonabsorbable mesh we used absorbable mesh, and all three patients had massive seroma. I wonder whether this seroma was a result of inflammatory reaction to the nonabsorbable mesh.

Wantz: Seroma is a result of not leaving your drains in long enough.

Amid: No, I left the drains in for a week to 10 days, and I sent the patient home with the drains in.

Wantz: I have no explanation for that; we just do not see the seromas that everyone is talking about. We only had one, and two on another patient not in this series of surgery, of course.

Amid: Are these two the same patients who had nonabsorbable mesh as a second layer?

Wantz: I cannot remember. I remember the small one was just with a piece of polypropylene.

Read: You put your sutures around the ribs intraperitoneally. Is that always necessary? Is it difficult to dissect the extraperitoneal plane in that area?

Wantz: Posteriorly there is plenty of space, because you are not inside the chest, but anteriorly you are in the abdomen and the stitches go through the bottom ribs.

Stoppa: Why do you put the mesh intraperitoneally in this type of hernia?

Wantz: Because there is no space next to the ribs.

Stoppa: But with hydrodissection you can separate the peritoneum from the ribs.

Wantz: I will try that next time.

Schumpelick: I would like to comment on the seroma problem. We did not have seromas until we used ultrasound, and since we have starting using ultrasound routinely, nearly all patients have seroma. Therefore I think it is a question of diagnosis; most of the seromas are not clinically apparent, but they could be the result of an infection. Therefore I think it is better to look on ultrasound to see whether there is a real seroma even in big meshes.

Wantz: We are not free to get computed tomography (CT) scans and sonograms anymore; that is a luxury that has disappeared from our practice. I agree that, if we had sonograms, we would most probably find other seromas.

Schumpelick: What is the experience of the French group? I think you use ultrasound. What about seroma formation?

Flament: I have ultrasound equipment in my own department, so we do ultrasound on every patient. We always find 1 cm of seroma around the prosthesis, and we do not know why.

Wantz: How long does that last?

Flament: I do not know. We do ultrasound before the patient leaves the hospital, but after that we do not.

Stoppa: The first step of healing is exudation, so you must have this.

Devlin: There are two points I would like to make. The first point is about splaying out the mesh superior to the umbilicus to allow the linea alba to persist. Does it matter if you get a small hernia in that area postoperatively? Because this is quite common in cardiac patients after they have undergone bypass surgery; they often get a little hernia up there and it seems to cause no trouble.

Wantz: In the cardiac patients, we just lay a piece of polypropylene mesh far enough under the defect and sew the edges of the defect to the polypropylene mesh.

Devlin: The point I am asking is whether it matters if they get a small defect.

Wantz: I do not know either, but I guess I should get a sonogram machine.

Devlin: I think you should, and a CT scanner. Another questions I would like to ask you is whether we should come out of this meeting and say that all hernias – recurrent or incisional – should be repaired in the extraparietal, retroperitoneal layer? In't that the message?

Wantz: I would not want to say that without reservation because I have not done a Chevrel procedure yet, but there is one coming up. I think these procedures are certainly indicated when you have a frozen abdomen. There are some indications to do anterior preperitoneal repair.

Klaiber: One critical point for me is the upper part of the midline incision, and I realise with bad experience that the mesh wears down in time because it shrinks and it is a stiff plate, so recurrences appear here. Do you have any experience with fixing the mesh to the bone in this part or to the xiphoid? The other new problems is incisional hernia after sternotomy for cardiac bypass. I see a lot of these patients. What do you do with them? Do you fix the mesh to the bone?

Wantz: Yes.

Bendavid: We have seen a lot of these incisional hernias lately. We always use mesh.

Bendavid: The mesh is really not that big; it is limited to the upper portion of the abdomen.

Wantz: You lay the mesh in place, bigger than the hole, sew the edges of the anterior linea to the mesh; they will not come together.

Filipi: Could you please comment on your use of doxycycline? I find that nothing works.

Wantz: Maybe we have just had good luck. We keep about ten ampoules in the office in anticipation of further incisional hernia. It works.

Filipi: Orally?

Wantz: No, you aspirate the seroma, put it in, and let it sit there; it causes an irritation and the seroma closes.

References

1. Flament JB and Rives J: Major incisional hernias. In Hernias and Surgery of the Abdominal Wall. Edited by JP Chevrel . Pp 128–158. Heidelberg Berlin New York, Springer 1998.
2. Stoppa RE: The treatment of complicated groin and incisional hernias. World J. Surg., 1989, 13:545–554.
3. Wantz GE: Incisional hernioplasty with Mersilene. Surg, Gynecol. & Obstet., 1991, 172:129–137.
4. Wantz GE: Atlas of Hernia Surgery. New York, Raven Press, 1991.

CHAPTER 28

Intermediate Follow-Up Results of Sublay Polypropylene Repair in Primary and Recurrent Incisional Hernias

V. Schumpelick, U. Klinge

The repair of incisional hernias is one of the most frequent but still problematic procedures in surgery, although the introduction of meshes has led to a marked improvement of the results. The simple repetition of the primarily failing closure technique results in disappointing recurrence rates of more than 50%. This is disastrous for both the surgeon and the patient, especially if the original operation was successful.

28.1 Indication for Meshes

The indications for meshes is determined by the recurrence rates of alternative techniques. In accordance with the literature [1], an evaluation of 245 patients with 272 incisional hernias, operated on from 1986 to 1995, revealed that both the simple closure and the doubling of the fascia (Mayo) failed in almost 50% after 5 years without any marked difference between the different techniques (Fig. 1).

In contrast to other reports, the difference in recurrence rates depending on the size of the hernia was not statistically significant (Fig. 2) (although the smaller ones have less recurrences), and similar results were seen for the number of previous hernia repairs (Fig. 3) and whether absorbable material or non-absorbable material was used (Fig. 4). Only an age of 70 years seems to affect the success rate significantly (similar interval) (Fig. 5), perhaps due to the usually more relaxed abdominal wall in elderly patients.

Thus the mesh results are barely affected by the number and the technique of previous operations, the size of the hernia, the age of the patient or the type of the used suture material [2]. Clear risk factors always leading to a failure of conventional techniques have not yet been established, although experimental studies indicate a probable defect of collagen formation [3–5].

If the primarily failing technique is repeated, both the frequently delayed development of hernias and the high rates of recurrences underline the importance of tissue response. Consequently, in the case of recurrent hernia, particularly if technical faults were not very likely, the support of the formation of a strong scar tissue is essential and is usually carried out by adding an alloplastic mesh.

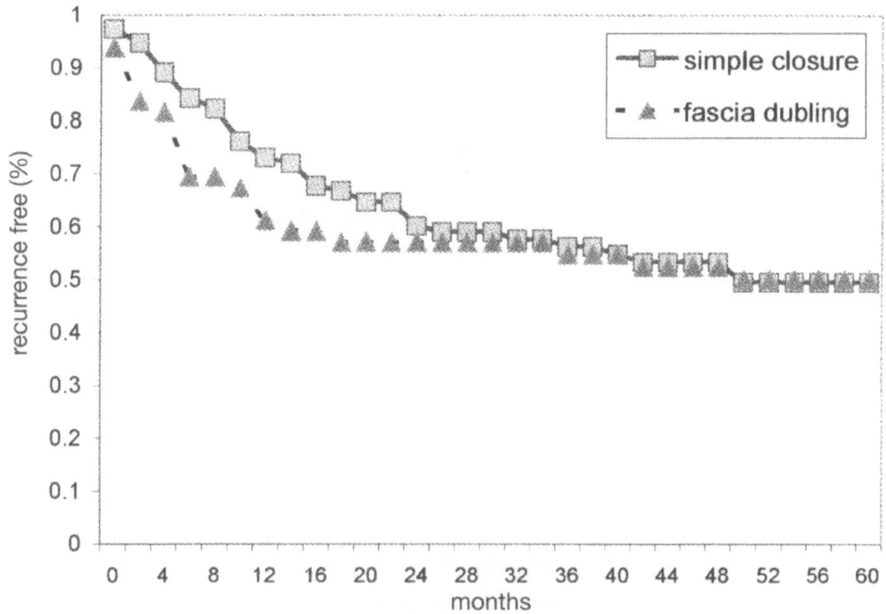

Fig. 1. Recurrence rate following mesh-free repair according to technique in 160 patients with incisional hernia from 1986 to 1995 (Kaplan-Meier). *Squares*, simple closure; *triangles*, fascia doubling

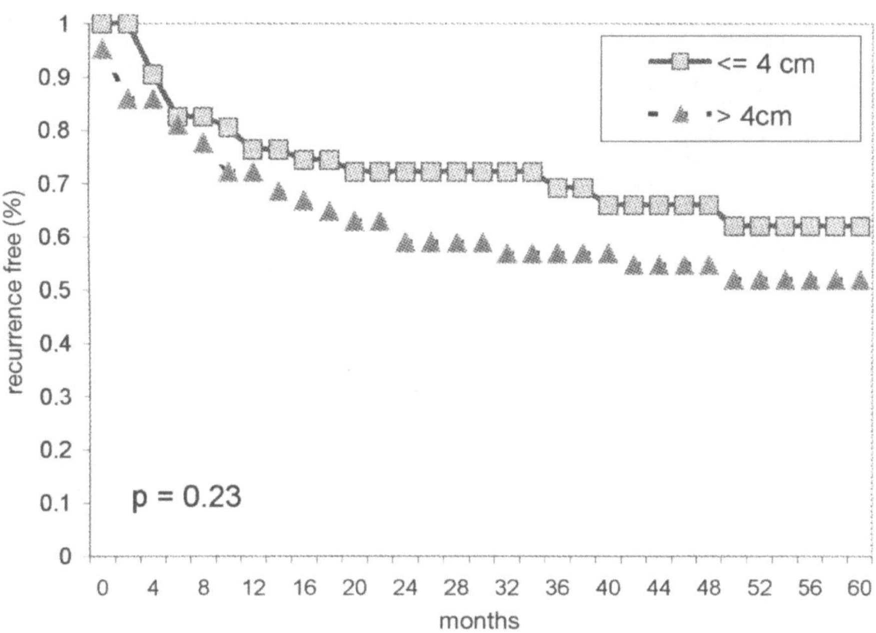

Fig. 2. Recurrence rate following mesh-free repair according to hernia size in 160 patients with incisional hernia from 1986 to 1995. *Squares*, ≤4 cm; *triangles*, >4 cm

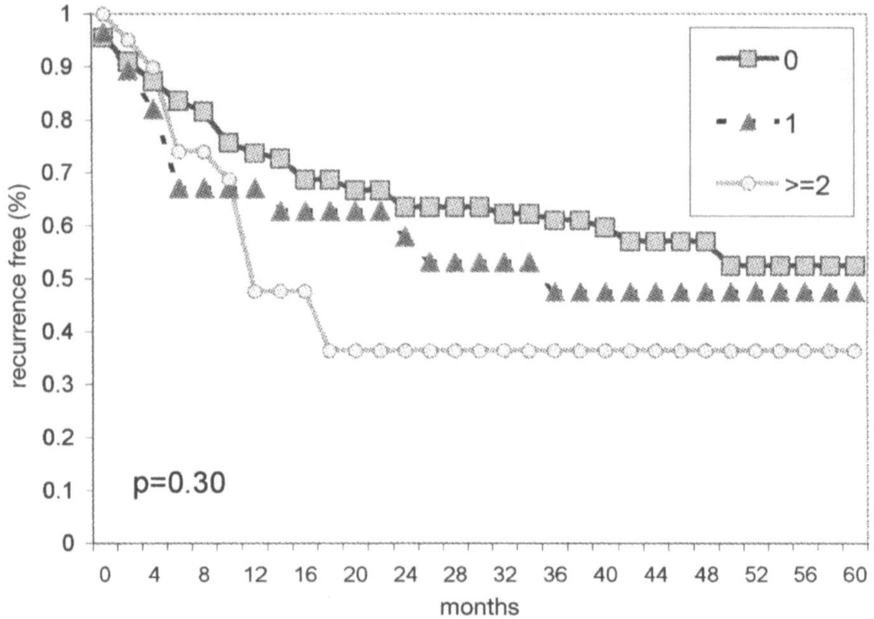

Fig. 3. Recurrence rate following mesh-free repair according to previous incisional hernia repairs in 160 patients with incisional hernia from 1986 to 1995. *Squares*, none; *triangles*, one; *circles*, two or more

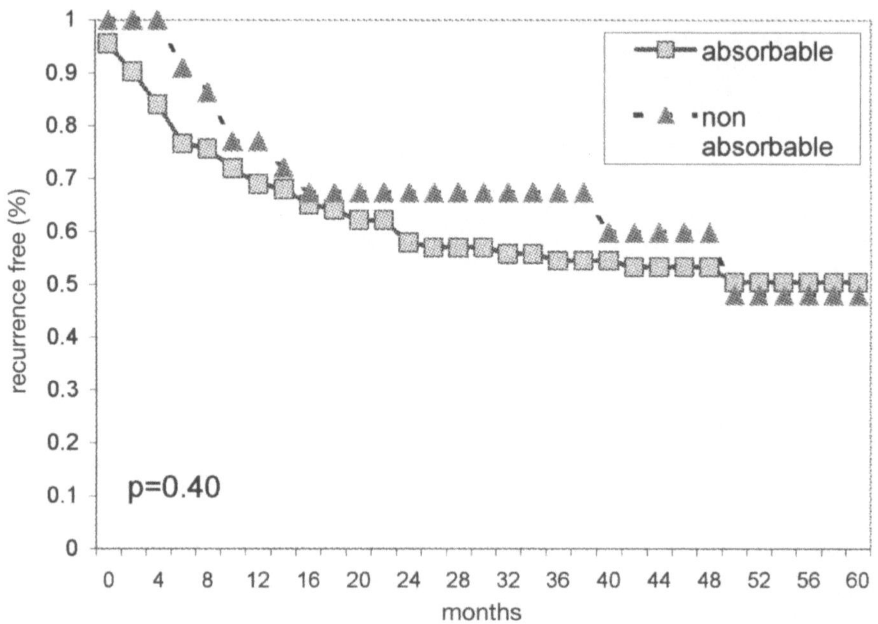

Fig. 4. Recurrence rate following mesh-free repair according to suture material in 160 patients with incisional hernia from 1986 to 1995 *Squares*, absorbable; *triangles*, non-absorbable

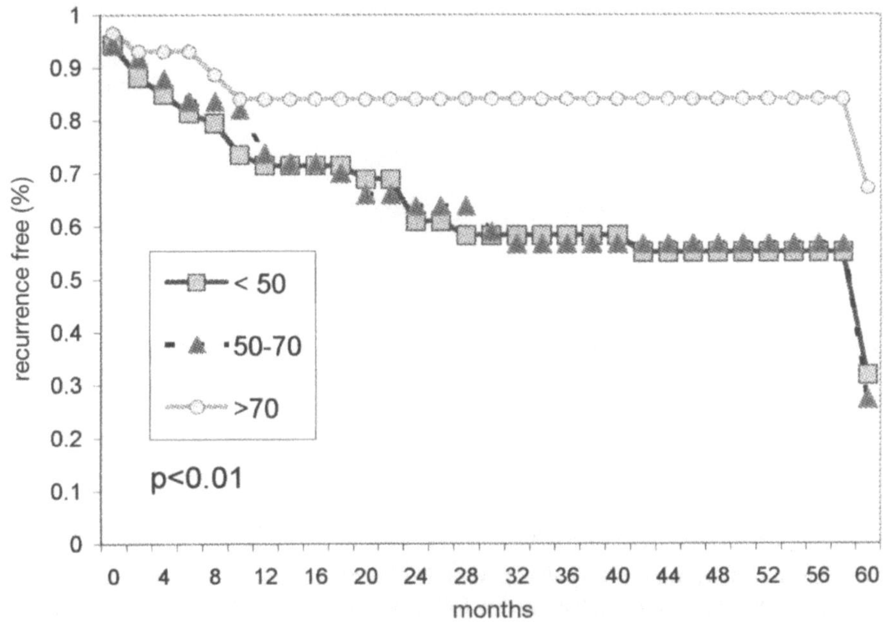

Fig. 5. Recurrence rate following mesh-free repair according to age in 160 patients with incisional hernia from 1986 to 1995. *Squares*, <50 years; *triangles*, 50–70 years; *circles*, >70 years

28.2 Implantation Technique

As a consequence of the disappointing data on mesh-free repair of incisional hernias, meshes were introduced to strengthen the abdominal wall repair. A variety of different materials and techniques were initially used: onlay, inlay and sublay with various materials (Fig. 6).

Implantation as an inlay did not achieve any strengthening of the abdominal wall in accordance with the previously described animal experiments. Recurrence rates of up to 50% have been reported [6–8].

The onlay position seem to work as long as the mesh is sufficiently fixed on the fascia. If this connection is lost, a buttonhole hernia will develop at the edge of the mesh. Two patients with an onlay mesh developed severe peritonitis caused by recurrent hernia and erosion of intestine at the mesh borders. The reported recurrence rates were comparatively low (0%–20%), but usually with a short follow-up period [7, 9–11].

In our view, the sublay position seems to be the most favourable position, because a mesh in the sublay position is fixed by the intra-abdominal pressure. Polypropylene meshes in this position is able to strengthen the abdominal wall both by mechanical sealing and by the induction of a strong scar tissue. Reported recurrence rates vary between 0% and 20%, and recurrences are mainly due to technical problems [7, 10, 12–18].

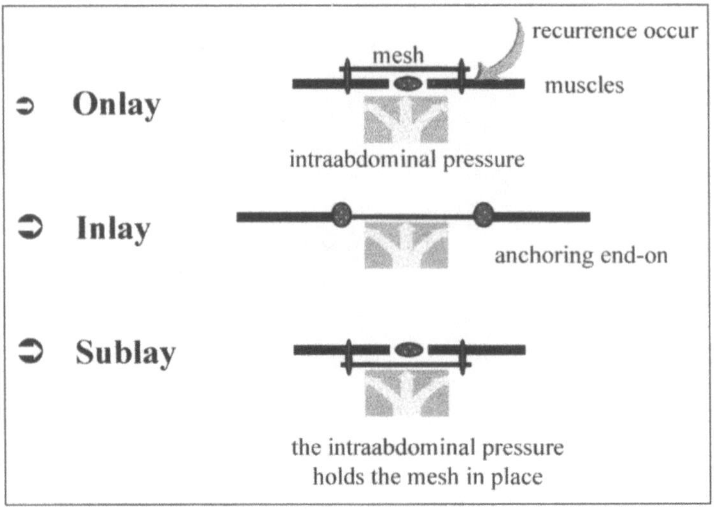

Fig. 6. Techniques of mesh implantation with regard to the mesh position

We analyzed the results in 82 patients with incisional hernias who received a mesh in the years 1986–1995 (Fig. 7). The mean follow-up was 19 months. All patients underwent a physical examination.

The main problem of hernia surgery, the resulting recurrence rate, partly confirms the published reports. The implantation of meshes in a sublay position failed only in

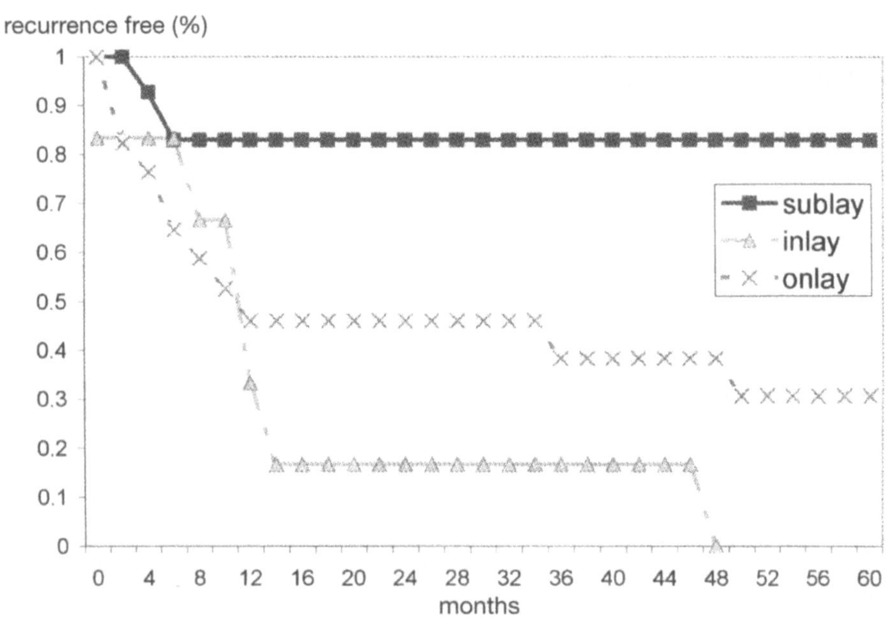

Fig. 7. Recurrence rate following mesh repair in 82 patients with incisional hernia from 1986 to 1995. *Squares*, sublay; *triangles*, inlay; *crosses*, onlay

10%, whereas five of 11 patients with a mesh in the onlay position developed a recurrence (45%). Recurrences always appeared at the edge of the formerly implanted mesh, which usually appeared shrunk and folded.

Compared to conventional repair, the rate of early complications following mesh implantation showed a significant increase in slight seromas and haematomas. These were not usually clinically apparent, but could be detected by postoperative ultrasound. A seroma was confirmed if the volume of liquid exceeded 10 ml. Patients with seromas are significant heavier ($p<0.01$). Seroma frequently appear after re-incisions as a consequence of the extended destruction of the lymph vessels but also indicate the inflammatory power of the implanted alloplastic materials.

The infection rate was similar even in the presence of alloplastic material. Only one haematoma following mesh implantation required a revision. In the literature, the rate of early complications is not usually specified, but varies between 0% and 40%, mainly due to seroma and haematoma [9, 14, 15, 19–22) (Table 1).

With regard to the causal importance of scar formation, a repair of the whole scar is advisable, particularly if multiple hernias are present. Furthermore, the obligate shrinkage of the wound and the mesh area of about 40% [23] requires sufficient subduction of the mesh material of at least 5–8 cm. The mesh is placed in the preperitoneal space underneath the posterior sheet of the rectus (Figs. 8–12). As the dissection of

Table 1. Early complications in 242 patients operated on for incisional hernia 1986–1995

Complication	Without mesh	With mesh
Recurrence	44	8*
Seroma	14	27**
Haematoma	5	12***
Infection	4	5****

*$p<0.01$; **$p<0.05$; ***$p=0.08$; ****not significant.

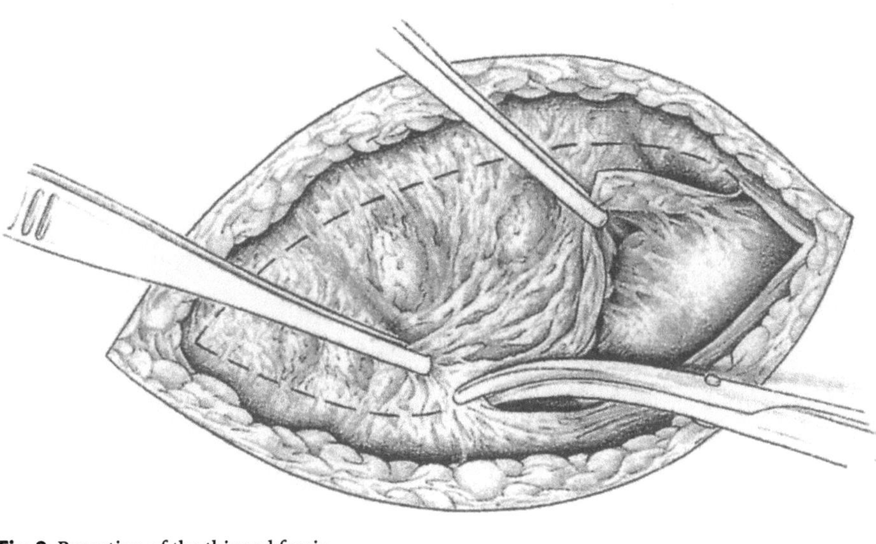

Fig. 8. Resection of the thinned fascia

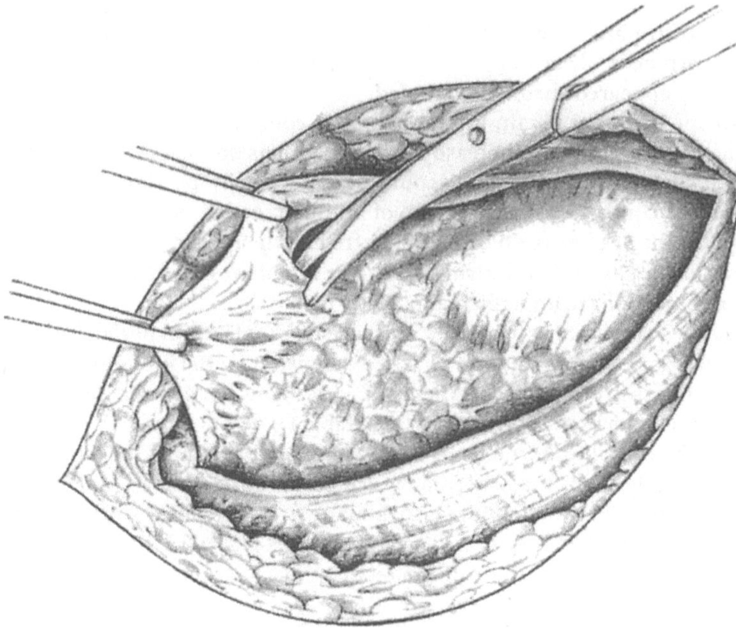

Fig. 9. Preparation of the fascial borders of the hernia gap with separating of the peritoneum

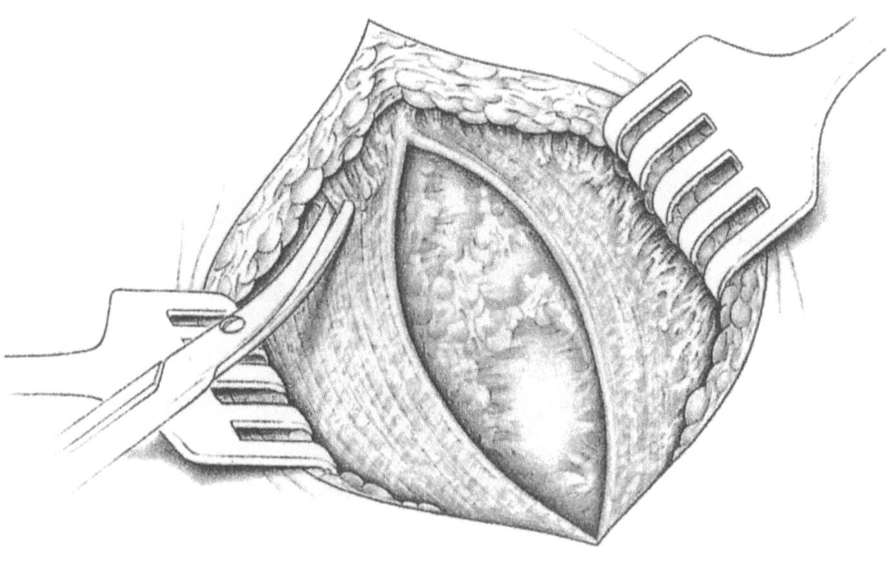

Fig. 10. Prepared hernia gap before repair

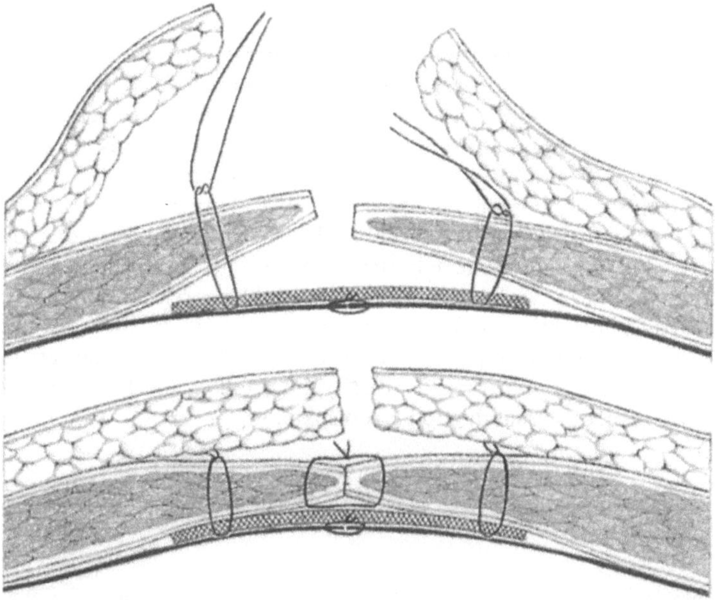

Fig. 11. Careful closure of the peritoneum, sublay position of the mesh, which is fixed either to the muscle or (better) only to the posterior sheath of the rectus muscle with absorbable single stitches (3/0), closure of the fascia continuously, absorbable, end-to-end

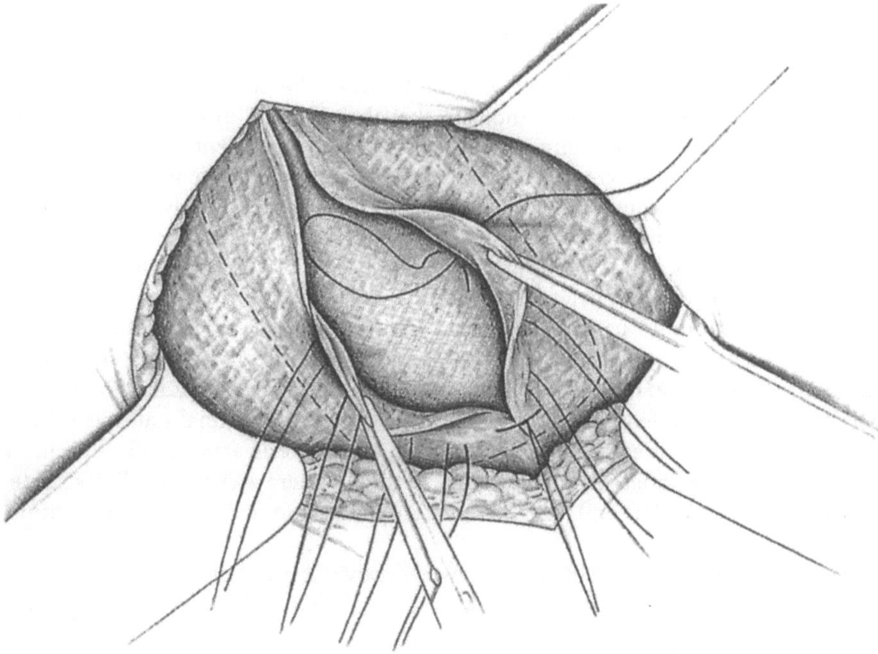

Fig. 12. Closure of the fascia after placement of the mesh in a sublay position with an underlap of at least 5–8 cm on each side. The here shown transmuscular V-sutures are abandoned for I/O CGS single sutures to the posterior rectus muscle sheath

this area usually is difficult, it is advisable to place the mesh underneath the rectus muscle onto the posterior sheet. As protection against early dislocation, the edges of the mesh are fixed with single sutures (3/0 absorbable). Technical problems can appear proximal to the bones (rips, pelvis) or if the incision crosses the semilunar line. The mesh should always be completely covered by peritoneum to prevent direct contact between mesh and intestine. If this is not possible, it is advisable to insert omentum or, if this is not possible, an absorbable mesh (small pore size).

Two drains were usually placed adjacent to the mesh, with an additional one under the cutis. They were usually removed after 48 h. Seroma formation is controlled by regular ultrasound scan, and larger volumes should be released by aspiration to prevent a capsule formation and to ease the penetration of the scar tissue. The strength of meshes makes it impossible for a recurrent hernia to penetrate the mesh. Thus the appearance of a recurrence is usually the result of a technical failure (either the mesh has shrunk or the subduction is too sparse).

28.3 Mesh Material

The implantation technique determines the recurrence rates, whereas the type of selected mesh material markedly influences the rate of local wound complications and the discomfort that patients experience [24].

Expanded polytetrafluoroethylene (ePTFE) does not lead to a stronger connective tissue reaction and cannot be fully integrated into scar tissue. The material can usually still be removed from the wound after years without any problem, and permanent reinforcement of the abdominal wall with this material therefore cannot be expected. The long-term histological results indicate that these "films" probably cause severe problems. After some disappointing results (five out of six patients who received an ePTFE mesh showed a recurrence), we completely abandoned this material.

Most of the meshes commonly available consist of polyester or polypropylene. Due to the known long-term degradation of polyester [25–30] and the lack of preserved strength over decades as well as the extensive production of fibrous seroma within the first week, we prefer polypropylene as mesh material.

With the exception of patients with recurrent hernias, 97% of the patients with a polypropylene mesh in the sublay position were fully satisfied with the results of the operation, although nearly half of them have discomfort or complaints (Table 2). A total of 29% of our patients felt that the mobility of their abdominal wall was restricted during daily activities, and 5% even in rest. Paraesthesia was significantly more frequent in younger patients under 50 years ($p<0.05$). There was no significant correlation between complaints and mesh size or complaints and duration of implantation, respectively.

Vestweber [21] and McLanahan [20] have recently published similar results. Corresponding figures following giant prosthetic reinforcement of the visceral sac (GPRVS) vary between 14% and 25% [14, 31–34].

Measuring the abdominal wall mobility using a three-dimensional stereography technique [35] in comparison to 23 healthy controls, we were able to show an increase in stiffness following the implantation of a Marlex mesh (Table 3). This decrease of

Table 2. Complaints in 53 patients with a Marlex mesh as sublay (follow-up, 17 months)

Complaint	(%)
No complaints	46
At rest	7
During daily activities	29
During heavy work	17
Paraesthesia	54

mobility correlates significantly to the complaints, but both seemed to be independent of the mesh size or the follow-up interval. It is interesting that eight out of nine patients with incomplete fascia closure were completely free of complaints.

The implantation of a large amount of plastic material in an extended area causes an intense reaction of the recipient tissue, as was demonstrated some days ago. The extent of inflammation is mainly determined by the type, the structure and the amount of material used. Large pores seem to be favourable to prevent the formation of an all-embedding scar plate, as was previously described.

Regarding the overestimated strength of meshes compared to the physiological strength, the obviously material-dependent inflammatory reaction with seromas and shrinkage as well as the restriction in abdominal wall mobility that sometimes occurs make it reasonable to reduce the alloplastic material. We therefore started to implant the newly developed Soft Hernia Mesh (SHM) [36] within a prospective clinical study. The mesh has a decreased polypropylene part (PP) of less than 30% compared to the well-known Marlex mesh. The reduced amount of material permits a construction with very large pores, ensuring a preserved elasticity even with penetrating scar tissue. The mesh is very flexible with a high transparency. To improve handling and to decrease the inflammatory response of the tissue, filaments of absorbable polyglactin are added.

The preliminary results of the implantation of SHM seem to confirm that a decrease in material is followed by a decrease in the rate of seromas of more than 10 ml (not significant, $p=0.35$) from 40% with Marlex mesh, 35% with Atrium mesh (70% of the PP of Marlex) and 28% with SHM. Although only a small number of patients were studied, the volume of the liquid in the patients with a seroma was significantly decreased ($p<0.05$) with SHM (16±13 ml) compared to Marlex mesh (34±33 ml) and Atrium mesh (31±16 ml). Three-dimensional stereography showed a decreased stiffness compared with Marlex mesh, although the measurements after SHM were made soon (6 weeks) after operation (Table 4, Fig. 13).

Table 3. Three-dimensional stereography of patients with a Marlex sublay (follow-up, 17 months) in comparison to healthy controls

Group	Patients (n)	Height difference (cm)[a]	Maximum curvature[b]	Radius at maximum excursion[c]
Control	21	5.5	6.2	41
Marlex sublay	41	3.1*	3.7*	69*

[a] Difference in height at maximum abdominal wall excursion (maximum minus minimum).
[b] Decrease in curvature (1/100 cm) at maximum indicates an increase in stiffness.
[c] Calculated best-fitting radius in the area over the mesh; a large radius indicates increase in stiffness.
* $p<0.01$.

Table 4. Abdominal wall compliance following mesh implantation, measured with three-dimensional stereography

Group	Patients (*n*)	Curvature at maximum excursion (1/100 cm)	Radius at maximum excursion (cm)	Height difference (cm)
Control	21	6.2	41	5.5
Marlex mesh	41	3.7	69	3.1
SHM	8	4.5	52	4.0

SHM, Soft Hernia Mesh.

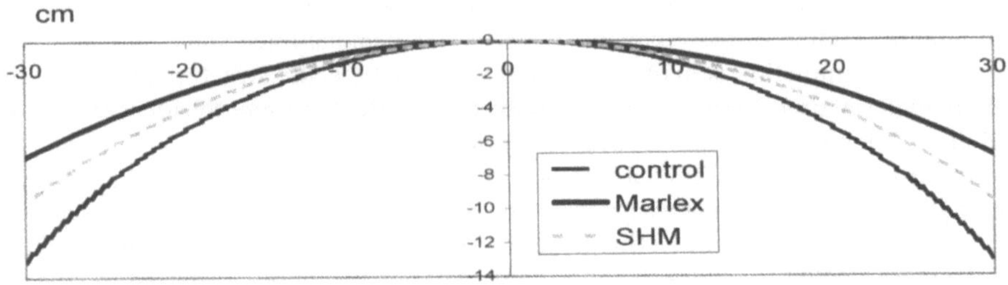

Fig. 13. Calculated radius of the abdominal wall following mesh implantations. *Thick black line*, 41 patients with Marlex mesh after 17 months; *faint dashed line*, eight patients with Soft Hernia Mesh (SHM) after 6 weeks; *dark gray line*, 21 controls

Our results indicate that the type of mesh used influences the clinical results and the patients' comfort. In general, it seems to be advantageous to use as much material as necessary but as little material as possible. Our early experiments underline the effect of the mesh material selected on the rate of local wound complications and the discomfort experienced by patients. The use of a mesh with a reduced amount of polypropylene and a large pore size of more than 5 mm seems to improve the clinical results.

28.4 Conclusion

Meshes are essential and indispensable for the repair of incisional hernias. However, with regard to their consequences concerning abdominal wall mobility, the unknown long-term histologic tissue response and the problem of durable mesh fixation to prevent dislocation and fistula formation, mesh implantation should be restricted to patients in which satisfactory mesh-free techniques are not available, particularly in young patients. Thus, in principle, we cannot recommend laparoscopic repair or even a Lichtenstein repair. If mesh implantation is necessary, the mesh should be made of polypropylene with large pores and with the smallest amount of material as possible.

28.5 Discussion

Wantz: One of the things I would like to see is a very compliant soft polypropylene mesh; there is a company in Lille in France that makes a lot of mesh. An entrepreneurial American got hold of these meshes and sent them to me, and we have already tried one – a very compliant polypropylene mesh that looks thinner than Mersilene. We have only used it once, as we have only had this mesh for 2–3 weeks, but I would certainly welcome some lighter-weight polypropylene.

Schumpelick: I do not think it is important which material is used – it can be Mersilene or it can be polypropylene – but I think the architecture of the mesh is important. I think we only need augmentation of the wall, and not total replacement.

Hartel: I found it surprising that you had such good results in patients over 70. Perhaps this group contains quite a number of private patients, who are usually very disciplined and active?

Schumpelick: Firstly, I do not think that private patients are less active than non-private ones. The first question my private patients ask me is, when am I allowed to play golf again? I think golf is a sport you need your abdominal wall for, and there is no distinct distribution of private and non-private patient in this group. I think it is not only a question of activity, but also a question of compliance, because some of these patients will not come back if they are not called, but all these patients have a follow-up.

Klaiber: May I ask you why you chose multifilament mesh, because there is no real advantage in my opinion?

Schumpelick: I think there is no real difference between multifilament and monofilament mesh if you have a large pore size; we looked at infection studies and there was no difference. I think multifilament mesh is more flexible in this situation; it is a question of producing the mesh, which is very difficult. I did not know how to make a mesh before, but I now know that it is easier to make a multifilament flexibel one.

Klaiber: What we need is a mesh which is very elastic at the side, because the main problem of meshes is at the border. You have a stiff material touching a flexible material, and this border should be smooth. We would like the industry to produce a mesh in which the border thins out so that the border is not so stiff.

Schumpelick: You are absolutely right, but this mesh has the same elasticity as the abdominal wall. That means that there is no difference between the elasticity of the wall and that of the mesh.

Klaiber: Not initially, but after 1 year it is stiffer.

Flament: I want to ask a question about mortality. In all the statistics we have seen up to now, mortality is zero. No one has ever died. We had a 0.7% mortality rate in 500 huge hernia treatments; three patients died. Why has nobody spoken about mortality with this huge operation?

Schumpelick: I think it is because most of this mortality is not concerned with hernia, but is related to different co-morbidity, e.g. lung disease, heart disease. If you do intestinal resection, that would increase mortality, but most hernias do not involve intestinal resections.

Wantz: We had two deaths from pulmonary emboli, which was very disappointing. We now send our patients home with subcutaneous heparin. They go home after 4–5 days, and they are not out of the dangerous period then. We teach them how to use it, and they keep it up for another week.

Schumpelick: The normal stay in hospital is in the range of 8–10 days, and they are fit then.

Jeekel: When you talk about compliance, it is important how you place your mesh. I used to keep it rather round, not flat and straight, but to have it a little bulging.

Schumpelick: We place it during operation, i.e. relaxation, and we do not put any tension on the mesh.

Jeekel: Why is there so much concern about seroma if it does not cause the patient any problems?

Schumpelick: Because we are always concerned about the possibility of infection. We do not have any infection here, but I think seroma could predispose a patient to infection.

Skandalakis: Do you give antibiotics in the operating room and for perhaps 48 h afterwards?

Schumpelick: Not routinely.

Simmermacher: I would like to ask Dr. Scott about seroma formation. In laparoscopic extraperitoneal hernia repair, you place a mesh in the extraperitoneal gauze. People come back complaining that they have a recurrence and then what you feel is that there is a seroma in the original space where the bulge was, which will go away after about 6 weeks. That is the experience I have had in several patients, and I want to ask if you have had the same experience? Then you have to tell the patient that this is not a recurrence, but either a haematoma or seroma, which will be drained.

Scott: Yes, we do see some seromas; we see them more commonly in large direct hernias, and we do a step to try to decrease that. We tell all patients that they are going to get a bulge down there, although 95% do not. We have not drained any of them, and they have all gone away satisfied. In our experience at least, they have not caused the patients any significant amount of pain, and we have not put the patients on antibiotics postoperatively because of seroma formation or presence.

Kingsnorth: When you do your prospective double-blind randomized trial, which mesh or meshes are you going to compare with SHM?

Schumpelick: We have started a randomized trial comparing Atrium with SMH. Atrium is polypropylene in a milder version than Marlex.

Kingsnorth: Why not include Mersilene in the trial, because Dr. Wantz is achieving such spectacular results, with no seroma and very good compliance? We would like to have the information from your computer about compliance with Mersilene.

Bendavid: What evidence do you have that seromas are in fact a pre-infectious stage? As you know, Coutts from Austria has established that 100% of mesh operations have a seroma, be it deep or superficial to the mesh itself; they all have it, and you can follow them. They are definitely there, but we do not see an incidence of infection that is in keeping with the incidence of seroma. We never drain ours.

Schumpelick: I think that seroma is a response of the body to a foreign body, and if the foreign body causes little seroma it might be better. Thus, seroma are an indicator for foreign body reaction. We used to drain seromas, but now we know that we do not have to. I think it was important in the development of meshes for us to see that one particular foreign body is not accepted as well as another one.

Skandalakis: If you keep drains there for 24–48 h or sometimes 4–5 days, you do not give any antibiotics?

Schumpelick: No.

Skandalakis: You are a brave man.

Schumpelick: No, we do not do it because it is not necessary

Stoppa: Have you investigated the principle of making a sort of aponeurotic tendon for reinsertion of the lateral belt, as proposed by Flament yesterday?

Schumpelick: All we want to do is correct the stability of the abdominal wall, whatever happens.

References

1. Luijendijk R, MHM Lemmen, WCJ Hop, ICJ Wereldsam. Incisional hernia recurrence following "veest-over-pants" or vertical Mayo repair of primary hernias of the midline. World J Surg 1997;21:62–66.
2. Klinge U, Prescher A, Klosterhalfen B, Schumpelick V. [Development and pathophysiology of abdominal wall defects]. Chirurg 1997;68(4):293–303.
3. Friedman D, CD Boyd, P Norton, RS Greco, AH Boyarsky, JW Mackenzie, SB Deak. Increases in type III collagen gene expression and protein synthesis in patients with inguinal hernias (see comments). Ann Surg 1993;218,6:754–60.
4. Ajabnoor MA, Mokhtar AM, Rafee AA, Taha AM. Defective collagen metabolism in Saudi patients with hernia. Ann Clin Biochem 1992;29(Pt 4):430–6.
5. Berliner SD. An approach to groin hernia. Surg-Clin-North-Am 1984;64(2):197–213 issn: 0039–6109.
6. Amgwerd M, M Decurtins, F Largadèr. Die Narbenhernie – Prädisposition oder insuffiziente Nahttechnik? Helv Chir Acta 1992;59:345–8.
7. Loh A, JS Rajkuma, LM South. Anatomical repair of large incisional hernias. Ann Royal Coll Surg Engl 1992;74:100–5.
8. Read RC, Yoder G. Recent trends in the management of incisional herniation. Arch-Surg 1989;124(4):485–8 issn: 0004–0010.
9. Molloy RG, Moran KT, Waldron RP, Brady MP, Kirwan WO. Massive incisional hernia: abdominal wall replacement with Marlex mesh. Br-J-Surg 1991;78(2):242–4 issn: 0007–1323.
10. Liakakos T, Karanikas I, Panagiotidis H, Dendrinos S. Use of Marlex mesh in the repair of recurrent incisional hernia [see comments]. Br-J-Surg 1994;81(2):248–9 issn: 0007–1323.
11. Bellon JM, Contreras LA, Sabater C, Bujan J. Pathologic and clinical aspects of repair of large incisional hernias after implant of a polytetrafluoroethylene prosthesis. World J Surg 1997;21(4):402–6.
12. Read RC. Preperitoneal herniorrhaphy: a historical review. World-J-Surg 1989;13(5):532–9; discussion 539–40 ISSN: 0364–2313.

13. Sugerman HJ, Kellum JM, Jr., Reines HD, DeMaria EJ, Newsome HH, Lowry JW. Greater risk of incisional hernia with morbidly obese than steroid-dependent patients and low recurrence with prefascial polypropylene mesh. Am J Surg 1996;171(1):80–4.
14. Temudom T, Siadati M, Sarr MG. Repair of complex giant or recurrent ventral hernias by using tension-free intraparietal prosthetic mesh (Stoppa technique): lessons learned from our initial experience (fifty patients). Surgery 1996;120(4):738–43.
15. Sitzmann J, DW McFadden. The internal retention repair of massive ventral hernia. Am Surgeon 1989;55:719–23.
16. Eisner L, F Harder. Narbenhernien. Chirurg 1997;68:304–9.
17. Schumpelick V, Conze J, Klinge U. [Preperitoneal mesh-plasty in incisional hernia repair. A comparative retrospective study of 272 operated incisional hernias]. Chirurg 1996;67(10):1028–35.
18. Kung C, U Herzog, JP Schuppisser, C Ackermann, P Tondelli. Abdominal cicatricial hernia – results of various surgical techniques. Swiss Surg 1995;6:274–8.
19. Stoppa R. The treatment of complicated groin and incisional hernias. World J Surg 1989;13:545–554.
20. McLanahan D, King LT, Weems C, Novotney M, Gibson K. Retrorectus prosthetic mesh repair of midline abdominal hernia. Am-J-Surg 1997;173(5):445–9 issn: 0002–9610.
21. Vestweber K, Lepique F, Haaf F, Horatz M, Rink A. [Results of recurrent abdominal wall hernia repair using polypropylene-Mesh]. Zentralblatt für Chirurgie 1997;122:885–888.
22. Rohr S, Vogt F, Thiry CL, Dai B, Meyer C. [Parietal prosthetic mesh in the treatment of large incisional hernias]. J-Chir-Paris 1993;130(1):37–40 issn: 0021–7697.
23. Klinge U, Klosterhalfen B, Müller M, Öttinger A, Schumpelick V. Shrinking of polypropylene-meshes in-vivo (an animal study). EJS 1998:in press.
24. Amid P. Classification of biomaterials and their related complications in abdominal wall hernia surgery. Hernia 1997;1:5–8.
25. Riepe G, Loos J, Imig H, et al. Long-term in vivo alterations of polyester vascular grafts in humans. Eur J Vasc Endovasc Surg 1997;13(6):540–8.
26. Pourheydimi B, Wagner D. On the correlation between the failure of vascular grafts and their structural and material properties: a critical analysis. J Biomed Mat Res 1986;20:375–409.
27. Berger K, Suavage L. Late fiber deterioration in Dacron arterial grafts. Ann Surg 1980;193(4): 477–491.
28. Koopmann M, Brands L. Degenerative changes in Dacron external velour vascular prostheses. J Cardiovasc Surg 1980;21:159–162.
29. Maarek J, Guidon R, Aubin M, Prud'homme R. Molecular weight characterization of virgin and explanted polyester arterial prosthesis. J Biomed Mat Res 1984;18:881–894.
30. Sladen J, Gerein A, Miyagishima R. Late rupture of prosthetic aortic grafts. Am J Surg 1987;153:453–458.
31. Langer I, Herzog U, Schuppisser JP, Ackermann C, Tondelli P. [Preperitoneal prosthesis implantation in surgical management of recurrent inguinal hernia. Retrospective evaluation of our results 1989–1994]. Chirurg 1996;67(4):394–402.
32. Beets GL, van Geldere D, Baeten CG, Go PM. Long-term results of giant prosthetic reinforcement of the visceral sac for complex recurrent inguinal hernia. Br-J-Surg 1996;83(2):203–6 issn: 0007–1323.
33. Read RC, Barone GW, Hauer Jensen M, Yoder G. Properitoneal prosthetic placement through the groin. The anterior (Mahorner-Goss, Rives-Stoppa) approach. Surg-Clin-North-Am 1993;73(3): 545–55 issn: 0039–6109.
34. Bittner R, Leibl B, Kraft K, Daubler P, Schwarz J. [Laparoscopic hernioplasty (TAPP)–complications and recurrences in 900 operations]. Zentralbl Chir 1996;121(4):313–9.
35. Klinge U, Müller M, Brücker C, Schumpelick V. Application of three dimensional stereography to assess abdominal wall mobility. Hernia 1998;in press.
36. Klinge U, Klosterhalfen B, Conze J, et al. A modified mesh for hernia repair adapted to abdominal wall physiology. Eur J Surg 1998;in press.

CHAPTER 29

Polyester Mesh for Incisional Hernia Repair

J.P. Chevrel, A.M. Rath

29.1 History

The development of prostheses of a polymer of polyester composed of ethylene glycol and terephthalic acid dates back to 1939. It was in 1946 that the first publication appeared in the United States proposing the use of these prostheses in the treatment of major hernias [10]. Polyester prostheses are also known by the name of dacron prostheses and marketed by Ethicon under the name Mersilene. In 1956, Wolstenholme [16] reported in the *Archives of Surgery* the use of these prostheses in 15 cases of inguinal hernia and four cases with loss of abdominal wall substance.

In 1962, Adler [1], again in the *Archives of Surgery*, reported the use of the dacron prosthesis in reinforcing the suture of 31 ventral incisional hernias; in one case, the prosthesis had been used to fill out a loss of substance which had led to a recurrence. In the following years, the dacron prosthesis was increasingly used in hernia repair, as shown by a report on 3000 cases by Bellini in 1969, for example. Shortly afterwards, this prosthesis appeared in France, and articles were written by Jean Rives and his assistants in 1971 relating to 17 cases of major incisional hernias and again in 1973, and there have subsequently been many other reports. Since this date, numerous reports have been made, both by American authors [4, 5, 8, 10] and by French authors [2, 6, 11, 55], to list only the major ones.

29.2 Material and Methods

To illustrate the use of these polyester prostheses, we reviewed a series of 418 major abdominal incisional hernias operated on between 1979 and 1997 and studied retrospectively the indications and results obtained with Mersilene prostheses.

Out of 418 operations, 161 repairs were made by herniorrhaphy or hernioplasty (38.51%), while in 257 reinforcement of the parietal repair was done by using a prosthesis (61.48%). Of these 257 prostheses (including both absorbable and non-absorbable prostheses, some polyester and some polypropylene), 126 were fixed by vaporisation of fibrin glue (49%). The retrospective study of our case records revealed a preferential use of polyester prostheses between 1980 and 1990, with a preference for polypropylene prostheses since 1991 (see Fig. 1). The reasons for abandoning Mersilene in favour of a Prolene prosthesis are associated with the fact that we had to treat

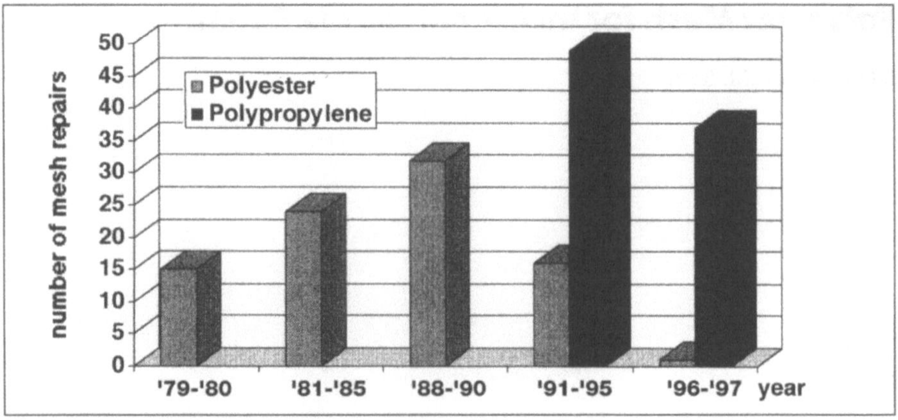

Fig. 1. Non-absorbable mesh repairs (personal series)

three cases of postoperative recurrence of an abdominal incisional hernia in which a Mersilene prosthesis had been used, which we found to be torn in its middle portion, explaining the recurrence. In one of these three cases, each half of the Mersilene prosthesis had perforated an intestinal loop at either margin of the incisional hernia. This led us to perform a double resection of the small intestine and to repair the wall by a herniorrhaphy reinforced by an absorbable polyglycolic acid (Dexon) prosthesis. We also found in the literature an identical case of tearing of a Mersilene prosthesis reported by Gautier Benoït in 1993. The possible finding during operation of a tear in the Mersilene prosthesis led us to conduct an experimental study in 1996 in 130 rabbits divided into five groups: one control group of ten rabbits, a group of 30 rabbits which had a laparotomy where closure was reinforced by an onlay polyester mesh, another group of 30 rabbits in which the laparotomy was reinforced by the insertion of an onlay polypropylene mesh, a further group of 30 rabbits in which the prosthesis used was made of polyglactin 910, and finally a group of 30 rabbits in which we used a composite prosthesis of dacron and polyglactin. This study was monitored by tests of tensile strength and bursting strength and by histologic studies to assess strength by studying fibrosis and to assess tolerance by measuring the inflammatory and foreign body reactions.

The results of this experimental study, which were published in *Chirurgie* [12], are shown in Figs. 2–4 and Table 1. This study led us to conclude that, after repair of the linea alba by suture or plasty, the reinforcement of this repair by an onlay polyester or polypropylene prosthesis led to relatively early maximal solidity (4–6 weeks). The polypropylene prostheses appeared to have a better resistance than those of polyester, which subsequently led us to adapt the choice of prosthesis to the morphotypes of the

Table 1. Histological findings: tolerance

Reaction	Polyester	Polypropylene
Foreign body reaction	Intense and constant	Mild
Inflammatory reaction	None	Intense at 30 days, mild and 60 days and absent thereafter

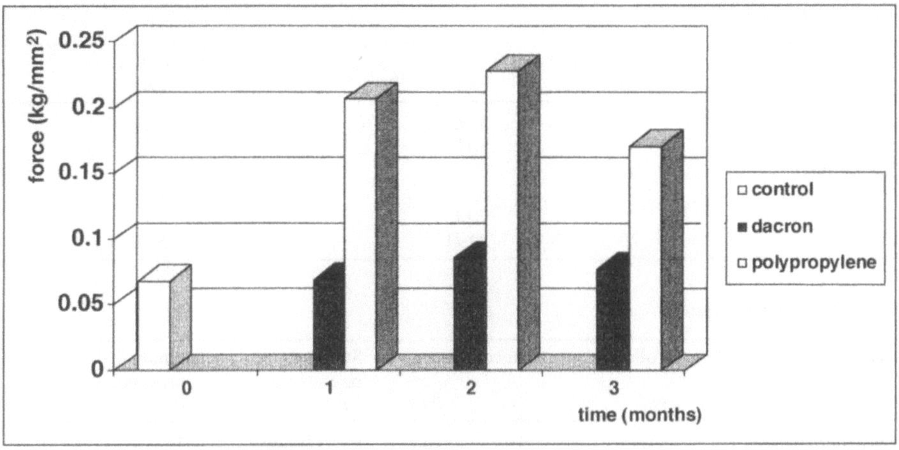

Fig. 2. Results of tensile strength tests

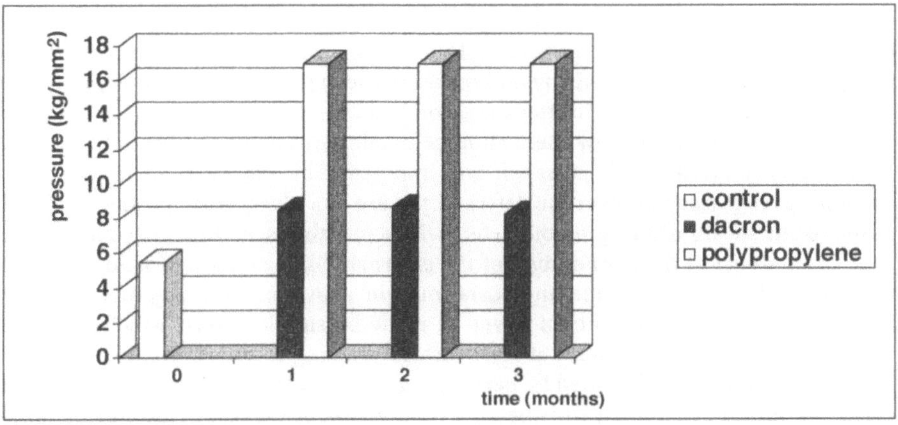

Fig. 3. Results of bursting strength tests. The bursting strength of polypropylene was superior to the device's maximum capactiy (17 kg/cm²)

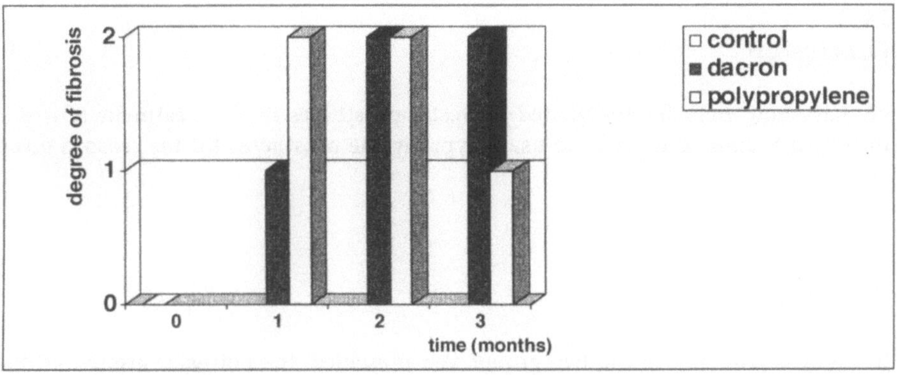

Fig. 4. Histological findings: degree of fibrosis. 0, none; 1, mild; 2, intense

Table 2. Morbidity

Morbidity	Polyester (n=98)		Polypropylene (n=85)	
	(n)	(%)	(n)	(%)
Sepsis	8	8.16	1	1.17
Seromas	5	5.10	2	2.35
Hematomas	0	0	1	1.17
Skin necrosis	0	0	1	1.17
Chronic sepsis	7	7.14	0	0
Total	20	20.41	5	5.88

Table 3. Long-term results

Material	Follow-up	Recurrences		Successful operations	Final recurrences	
	(%)	(n)	(%)	(n)	(n)	(%)
Polyester (n=98)	94.9	10	10.2	6 (with polypropylene mesh)	4	4
Polypropylene (n=85)	97.6	3	3.5	3	0	0

patients, in particular by the preferential use of polypropylene prostheses for obese patients. We have not observed any differences between the dacron and polypropylene prostheses as regards tolerance after the second month.

We will now briefly review the technique employed. The linea alba is practically always reconstructed, and such repair was impossible in only four out of 418 cases, when it was necessary to cover the defect by the use of a plasty with the anterior layer of the rectus sheath or bridging the defect with a prosthesis. A wide dissection of the superficial aspect of the aponeurosis of the external oblique muscle is made as far as the axillary line at either side, the costal margin above and the inguinal ligament below. The parietal repair should never be made by simple suture, which gives the worst results, but should always at least include relaxing incisions if suture is done, and the best results are obtained by performing suture of the linea alba by means of a plasty reinforced by an onlay prosthesis. A comparison of the results after using polyester and polypropylene prostheses is given in Tables 2 and 3.

29.3 Conclusion

We have now virtually abandoned polyester prostheses in the treatment of major incisional hernias and prefer to use polypropylene prostheses for the reasons given above.

29.4 Discussion

Jeekel: It is true that in the two groups you presented, the polyester group and the polypropylene group, you used an onlay prosthesis in all cases, and why did you use an onlay? Was it perhaps because you used a rectal flap to provide sufficient extra protection, so you did not need the onlay prosthesis?

Chevrel: No, I said I only use a prosthesis in 50% of cases. I think we can obtain the same results if we use one layer of suture after returning the anterior rectus sheath, but I prefer to make an overlapping flap where the Mersilene sandwich goes, and the choice of reinforcement is Mersilene. Prosthesis or no prosthesis, that depends on the value of the rectus muscle, because when you have made a large, wide relaxing incision, I think its important to reinforce this area of the abdominal wall because it is possible to have recurrence in the place where you have made the relaxing incision.

Wantz: Where were these recurrences when they occurred? And in these burst abdomens, was the mesh the only thing maintaining the integrity of the bowel, or was the mesh a part of an intact abdominal wall? It is hard for me to believe that Mersilene will break in two with an intact abdominal wall, a repaired abdominal wall.

Chevrel: You can see one example of the mesh in two parts. I had to remove two loops of small bowel, and in each loop we had one part of the prosthesis. I had two other cases with lateral incisional hernia in the same circumstances, and the Mersilene mesh was in two parts. In the literature, Gautier Benoit, a French surgeon, published the same case. It is exceptional, but I think when we have to repair an obese woman it is preferable to use Prolene mesh.

Kingsnorth: Regarding compliance of mesh, in the two groups of patients – one with Mersilene and one with Prolene – do you have any idea whether there is any difference, whether the patients felt that one type of mesh was stiffer than the other?

Chevrel: There is no difference.

Kingsnorth: Did both groups feel it was comfortable?

Chevrel: Sometimes with the Prolene for 2–3 months after the operation, patients had some discomfort. I found no clinical difference between the two meshes. I have presented these two groups only to try and answer the question about the use of Mersilene, because I used Mersilene at the beginning, but for 8 years I have preferred to use Prolene.

Jeekel: May I ask you about the girdle around the abdomen, which your patients wear for 1–2 months?

Chevrel: Often when I see the patient after the operation, at 2–3 months, he or she can remove the girdle. I prefer patients to keep it on in the day because I think support for the abdominal wall incision is important, but after 3–4 months they remove it first at night and then during the day as well.

Jeekel: Perhaps they do not need it?

Chevrel: I do not know of another girdle that is able to maintain all the abdominal wall from the xiphisternum to the pubis; all the other girdles are too small.

Wantz: Have you noticed any buckling with the polypropylene mesh? Have you seen any buckling or pleating? We have seen buckling of Prolene mesh in tension-free repair in the groin.

Chevrel: No. I think it is a feature of this technique, because when we fix the mesh, it is very easy to adjust the tension so that the repair is tension free. This buckling of the mesh was confirmed by CT at 12 months.

Schumpelick: Dr. Chevrel, we all learned the mesh repair of the abdominal wall for incisional hernias from the French surgeons, and we are all grateful for that, but we now have to learn from your mistakes. I would like to hear whether recurrences happen. You have a lot of recurrences, so where do they happen? The mesh was broken, but the other recurrences must be beyond the mesh.

Chevrel: I think the recurrences are always on the edge of the mesh, because at the beginning we used smaller mesh. It is good to use a mesh like a bridge; it is necessary to use a mesh overlapping the lateral abdominal wall widely. The three recurrences I had happened at the edge of the mesh because it was too small, I think.

Filipi: What type of an overlap do you use then to prevent lateral recurrence? How many centimetres do you go beyond your rectus muscle?

Chevrel: Five centimetres laterally and 5 cm superiorly over the inferior ribs and over the pubis.

Wantz: May I ask another question about the fibrin glue? We do not have this in the United States. I see there is quite a difference in recurrence rates between when you use it and when you do not. How long does it last? How effective is it? How do you spray it on? What is the gadget you use?

Chevrel: I am sure we have the best results if we use the prosthesis to reinforce the reconstruction of the linea alba and when this mesh is fixed with a running absorbable suture plus fibrin glue. A total of 1418 patients have 4.6% recurrence. Using a prosthesis without fibrin glue, I have had four or five recurrences, and using a prosthesis fixed by fibrin glue in the last series of 110 patients, there was only one recurrence.

Wantz: So it is absolutely essential to use it.

Chevrel: Yes.

Bendavid: Your operation looked so good that I wondered whether you needed the mesh at all on top of this repair. If you are going to have a recurrence through such a repair, it would be much like the tension-free repair, and it would most probably occur behind the mesh anyway. You have had some cases that you have done exactly that way, but without mesh. Is there any difference between the two sets of results?

Chevrel: Sometimes when you have made the flaps, the overlapping flap tears. You have rectus muscles that are as thin as paper, and I am not sure that the thickness of one transverse muscle is sufficient, so I prefer to reinforce this part of the anterior rectus muscle where we have no sheath because we used one sheath to reconstruct the linea alba. Athletic men have good rectus muscles, but I often operate on small women who come from North Africa. These women do not have a good rectus muscle, and there is a risk of recurrence in this area.

References

1. Adler RH. An evaluation of surgical mesh in the repair of hernias and tissue defects. Arch Surg 1962 85:156
2. Adloff M, Arnaud JP. Surgical management of large incisional hernias by an intraperitoneal Mersilene mesh and an aponeurotic graft. Surg Gynecol Obstet 1987; 165:204.
3. Bellis CJ. Immediate unrestricted activity after inguinal herniorrhaphy. Intl Surg 1969; 52:107.
4. Bendavid R. Prostheses and Abdominal Wall Hernias. 1994 R.G. Landes Company, Austin.
5. Casebolt BT. Use of fabric mesh in abdominal wall defects. J Missouri St Med Assoc 1975; 72:71.
6. Chevrel JP. Traitement des grandes éventrations médianes par plastie en paletot et prothèse. Nouv Presse Méd 1979; 8:695.
7. Chevrel JP, Flament JB. Rapport présenté au 92ème Congrès Français de Chirurgie. Paris, Masson 1990; pp 149–168.
8. Durden JG, Pemberton LB. Dacron mesh in ventral and inguinal hernias. Am Surgeon 1974; 40:662.
9. Flament JB, Olivier F, Palot JP, Delattre JS. Histoire du traitement des éventrations. Monographie GREPA 1968,8:1–6. Lab. Bruneau Ed.
10. Haskey RS, Bigler FC. Difficult hernias. J Kansas Med Soc 1975; 76:239
11. Lardennois B, Benoist M, Hibon J, Flament JB. Résultats de l'utilisation d'une étoffe en dacron dans le traitement des grandes éventrations. Acta Chir Belg 1971; 70:287.
12. Rath AM, Zhang J, Amouroux J, Chevrel JP Les prothèses pariétales abdominales. Etude biomécanique et histologique. Chirurgie 1996; 121:253.
13. Rives J, Lardennois B, Pire JC, Hibon J. Les grandes éventrations, importance du volet abdominal et des troubles respiratoires qui en sont secondaires. Chirurgie 1973; 99:547.
14. Rives J, Pire JC, Flament JB, Convers G. Le traitement des grandes éventrations (à propos de 133 cas). Bordeaux Med 1976; 26:2115.
15. Stoppa RE. The treatment of complicated groin and incisional hernias. World J Surg 1989; 13:545.
16. Wolstenholme JT. Use of commercial Dacron fabric in the repair of inguinal hernias and abdominal wall defects Arch Surg 1956; 73:1004.

CHAPTER 30

Polytetrafluoroethylene Repair of Incisional Hernia: Development and Results

R.K.J. Simmermacher

30.1 Introduction

Tetrafluoroethylene is a gas becomes liquid at a temperature of –35°C. By polymerization, a paste-like substance can be obtained called polytetrafluoroethylene (PTFE). After further manufacturing processes, PTFE threads can be made. These threads can be used either singly or doubly as sutures to make a woven (cloth) or braided (mesh) prosthesis for different surgical applications [1]. Due to its chemical structure, any product made of PTFE is chemically inert and heat resistant up to 27°C. Besides these qualities, it is also resistant to all acids, lyes (except trifluoridchloride), and enzymes, is hydrophobic, and is electronegatively charged. All the products made of PTFE are available under the brand name Teflon [2]. In 1972, W.L. Gore and Associates (Flagstaff, Arizona) developed a special manufacturing process which made it possible to stretch the PTFE, resulting in expanded polytetrafluoroethylene (ePTFE), which is better known under the name Gore-Tex. ePTFE is made of tiny knots of PTFE which are interconnected by thin flexible fibrils of the same material. The length of the interconnecting fibrils determines the pore size, which is usually between 1 and 200 μm. ePTFE was originally used for the production of vascular prostheses, which have been applied successfully [3]. The vascular prosthesis appeared to be biologically inert, not modified by tissue fluids, noncarcinogenic, and with a high patency rate [49.

Abdominal wall defects secondary to trauma, infection, or tumor resection which lack sufficient (healthy) fascia to achieve primary closure require the insertion of nonabsorbable prosthetic material [5]. Many different materials have been used for this purpose more or less successfully [6–8]. Since its introduction in 1958 by Usher, polypropylene mesh (PPM; Marlex) has been the most widely used material in abdominal wall repair [9, 10]. However, the formation of extensive visceral adhesions and occasional fistulization are well-known drawbacks [11, 12]. After the successful introduction as a material for vascular prosthesis, the ePTFE patch (Gore-Tex Soft Tissue Patch) was introduced in 1984 for the repair of abdominal wall defects [13]. Up to 1989, only two reports were published in English on the use of this material, involving 29 patients [14, 15], with promising results. However, Van der Lei et al. [16] then reported on 11 abdominal wall defects which were reconstructed with ePTFE. His study underlined the clinical usefulness of ePTFE for the reconstruction of large, uncontaminated abdominal wall defects, but he also advised using a double row of sutures because he had noticed so-called buttonhole hernias in two of three patients where single running sutures had been used without overlapping the fascial margin. Histologic analysis of the removed patch in one patient showed absence of ingrowth of fibrocollagenous tissue into the patch. Because of this clinical experience, an experimental study was undertaken to compare ePTFE and polypropylene mesh (PPM) in the repair of abdominal wall defects in rats. The study confirmed the existence of buttonhole hernias, which were found in 60% of the ePTFE group, while there were none in the PPM group [17]. Again, histologic examination showed that there was no ingrowth of fibrocollagenous tissue into the pores of ePTFE patch, indicating that there was no anchorage of the ePTFE patch to the adjacent tissue by incorporation. Such anchorage is completely dependent on the way that the patch is sutured to the adjacent tissues, something which has been found before [14, 18] and later [5, 19–25]. The study also confirmed the low number of visceral adhesions described in the other studies [26].

In order to increase the clinical usefulness of the ePTFE patch, it was modified in different ways and tested. Modifications of the ePTFE are either physical or chemical or concern the macrostructure, microstructure, or the surface structure of the material.

30.2 Physical Modification

ePTFE can be physically modified by pretreating the material with 96% ethanol, which has been successfully applied in vascular prostheses [27]. In an experimental study, ePTFE patches were pretreated with ethanol prior to subcutaneous implantation in the back of male rats. Histologic examination 8 weeks after implantation, however, also showed no ingrowth of fibrous tissue into the material, indicating no improvement in the anchorage of these patches [28].

30.3 Macroscopic Structural Modification

Perforated ePTFE vascular prosthesis showed better long-term patency [29], and perforated ePTFE patches implanted subcutaneously in rats showed ingrowth of fibrous tissue through the patches at the perforation sites which was continuous to the surrounding connective tissue [28]. An experimental study was therefore undertaken in which abdominal wall defects in rats were closed with ePTFE patches that were perforated at the rim with a 22-gauge needle and then implanted in an inlay fashion with a 5-mm overlap. Macroscopic and microscopic evaluation after 12 weeks showed buttonhole hernias in 60% of the cases, whereas the number of visceral adhesions at the abdominal side of the patch had increased. Furthermore, the adhesions themselves had become stronger, especially at the site of the perforations of the patches. At the sites where there were no buttonhole hernias, however, there was ingrowth of fibrous tissue into the perforation site. It was suggested that perforation of the ePTFE patch improves anchorage of the patch once ingrowth of tissue into the perforation has taken place. However, the subsequent increase in the number of visceral adhesions is an important drawback, which would rule out this ePTFE modification for the repair of large abdominal wall defects [30]. Nevertheless, in cases where there is no contact between viscera and patch, as in the totally extraperitoneal repair of groin hernia, this modification might improve the anchorage of the ePTFE patch to the adjacent tissues. Such a ePTFE patch now is commercially available (Mycromesh).

30.4 Microscopic Structural Modification

The production process of ePTFE enables the manufacturer to produce a microporous material of any desired pore size by influencing the length of the interconnecting fibrils. ePTFE is commercially available with a pore size of about 1–20 μm for use in cardiac surgery [31], with a pore size of 30–60 μm, which is the standard size of the ePTFE Soft Tissue Patch intended to bridge large abdominal wall defects, and with a pore size of 60–90 μm, which is used in vascular prostheses [32, 33]. As the pore size of the ePTFE Soft Tissue Patch clinically and experimentally does not initiate ingrowth of fibrous tissue into the material, whereas several reports in vascular surgery showed sufficient ingrowth of tissue into their material, experiments were undertaken to study anchorage of vascular prostheses used for the repair of abdominal wall defects in rats. ePTFE vascular prostheses with a pore size of 90 μm were cut open and implanted in abdominal wall defects in rats in an inlay fashion sutured to the surrounding tissue with interrupted nonabsorbable sutures in a single row. After 8 weeks, herniations were seen in only 13% of the cases, which appeared to be significantly less than in the group treated with a standard ePTFE patch. However, although the number of adhesions was the same in the standard Soft Tissue Patch group and the vascular prosthesis group, the grade of adhesions was clearly higher in the latter [30]. It was therefore concluded that the use of the ePTFE vascular prosthesis as a bridging material in abdominal wall defects results in better anchorage of the patch and also in a more pronounced adhesion formation.

This was histologically due to ingrowth of fibrous tissue into the patch from both the visceral and the abdominal side of the patch.

30.5 Chemical Modification

ePTFE is electronegatively charged and hydrophobic, with water contact angles of about 109° [34]. ePTFE patches which are positioned in a plasmode discharged unit for oxygen glow charge under argon pressure become hydrophilic with a water contact angle of about 20°–40° [35]. ePFTE patches in which one side was made hydrophilic were used to repair abdominal wall defects in rats with the hydrophilic side facing the abdominal wall. Histology showed a moderate foreign body response, with definite tissue ingrowth resulting in no herniations at the fascia patch interface [30].

Ion beam etching for 45 min followed by oxygen glow discharge results in an ePTFE patch which is more hydrophobic than the standard one, with a water contact angle greater then 140° [34]. Patches treated like this with the superhydrophobic layer facing the viscera were also used to bridge abdominal wall defects with astonishing results. There was a persistent inflammatory reaction around the patch, with layers of macrophages and foreign body giant cells visible after 1 week and a maximum reaction after 8 weeks. In about 30% of cases, infection persisted. Afterwards, the foreign body reaction diminished, but from the fourth week ingrowth of tissue could be observed. Electromicroscopic investigation showed an unexpected concomitant structure modification of the patch, resulting in a "hairy" surface of the ePTFE patch, thus significantly enlarging the surface of the ePFTE patch and resulting in more adhesions [34] (Figs. 1, 2).

30.6 Double-Layer Principle

Abdominal wall defects lacking sufficient healthy fascia to be closed primarily should be bridged using a nonabsorbable prosthesis. In most cases, PPM or polyester mesh are adequate. However, in cases in which there is no peritoneum or greater omentum left to protect the viscera from the prosthetic material, the two above-mentioned materials are unsuitable due to the fact that they both initiate firm visceral adhesions, which might result in serious clinical problems such as ileus or possible fistula formation. In these rare cases, a prosthesis should be used that avoids formation of visceral adhesions. In contrast, in all cases in which prosthetic material is used to repair abdo-

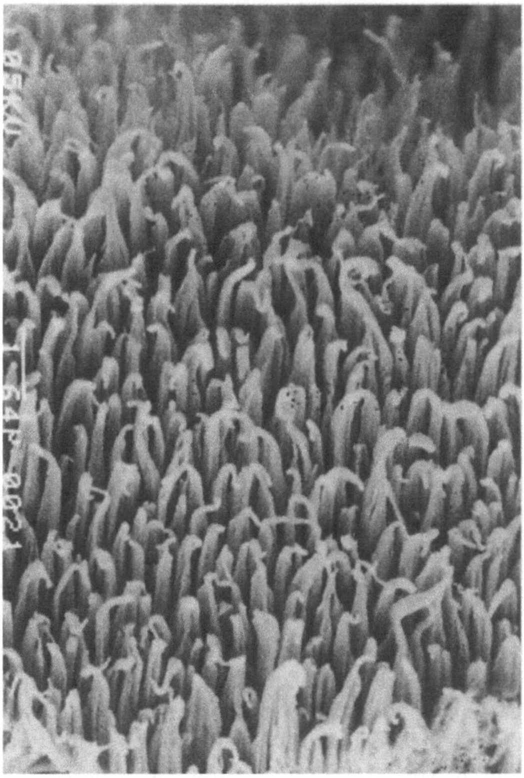

Fig. 1. Scanning electromicrograph of a superhydrophobically modified expanded polytetrafluoroethylene (ePTFE) patch, demonstrating the hairy appearance of the top of an ePTFE node

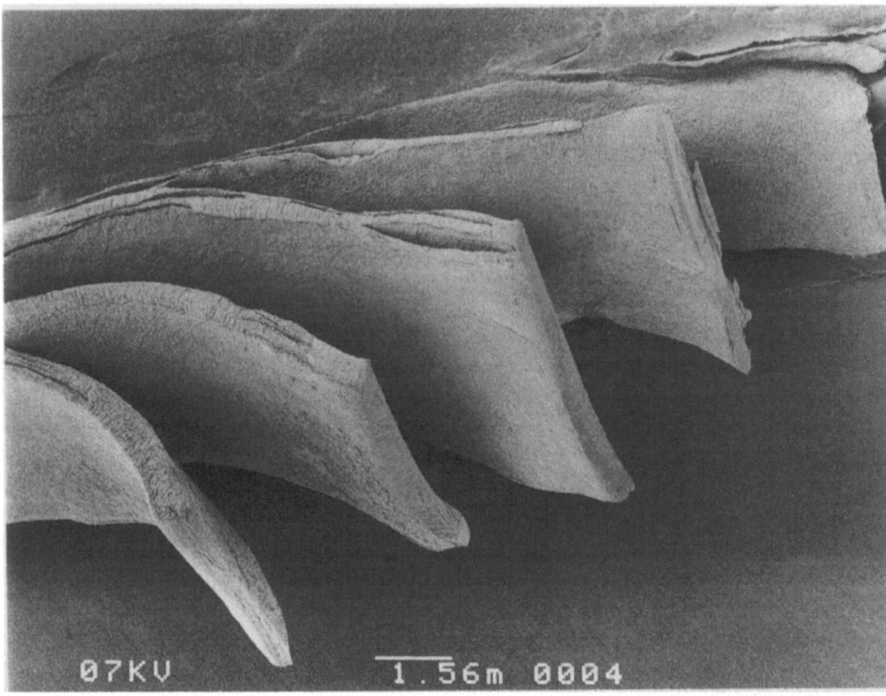

Fig. 2. Scanning electromicrograph of an infected expanded polytetrafluoroethylene (ePTFE) patch demonstrating its separation into different layers

minal wall defects, incorporation of the material into the adjacent fibrous tissue is required to obtain anchorage of the prosthesis, regardless of the type of sutures used. Both anchorage of the prosthesis to the surrounding tissue and the formation of visceral adhesions depend on ingrowth of any kind of tissue into the material. Ingrowth into any material depends on several factors, one of which is the pore size of the material used.

So far, all prostheses used for the repair of abdominal wall defects are homogenic, exerting the same qualities on both sides of the implant. However, theoretically, the ideal prosthesis for bridging abdominal wall defects should show ingrowth of fibrous tissue on the abdominal or outer side of the prosthesis, while there should be no possibility of ingrowth of any kind of tissue on the visceral or inner side of the prosthesis. This means that the ideal prosthesis should have different qualities on either side. This can only be achieved by either using composite meshes [36] or by using a functional double-layer patch. In order to validate this idea, experimental studies have been undertaken in which a composite mesh and a functionally double-layer prosthesis were used to bridge abdominal wall defects in rats. The composite mesh was made of an inner ePTFE layer upon which a macroporous polyurethane mesh was glued (Epigard) [37]. The functional double-layer patch was created by using an ePTFE standard Soft Tissue Patch, the abdominal side of which was made hydrophilic by glow discharging it. The results of the study [30] confirmed the idea by showing no herniations with the modified ePTFE patch and 26% herniations in the Epigard group. The latter herniation rate was caused by breakage of the material, not at the suture side. This is due to the fact that this prosthesis was never intended to bridge abdominal wall defects, but is used as a temporary protection of skin wounds [37]. The number of visceral adhesions and the extent of these adhesions in both groups were identical to the numbers and extent observed when using a standard ePTFE patch. It was therefore concluded from these studies that, in abdominal wall defects lacking peritoneum or greater omentum to protect the viscera from the patch, a prosthesis should be used which functionally or actually consists of two layers. In 1995, Amid supported this idea when reporting about composite meshes in the repair of abdominal wall defect in rabbits [38]. In the literature, there are reports that the composite meshes might be different from what is presupposed, probably due to unexpected chemical interactions between the two different materials [20, 36, 39]. Gore has now introduced a functional double-layer patch, the so-called Dual Mesh, which has to be studied in clinical trials; theoretically, the material is homogenous, but the surfaces are different.

30.7 Future Developments

It therefore seems that we will be able to find the ideal prosthesis for the repair of abdominal wall defects in the near future. However, this is not really true yet, due to the fact that there are other drawbacks, albeit apparently minor ones, to the use of ePTFE in abdominal wall repair. There have been a few reports on the use of ePTFE in a contaminated area, all of which show that this is very unsuccessful, necessitating removal of the ePTFE patch due to the inability to defeat the persisting infection [20, 25, 40, 41]. Another problem that has not yet been clarified is alleged hypersensitivity to ePTFE, which in some cases appears to be very difficult to treat [16, 42]. Last but not least, there are also different reports questioning long-term implantation of ePTFE due to the apparent breakdown of the microstructure of the material, showing rupture of the fibrils only 1 year after implantation [43].

30.8 Conclusion

ePTFE, currently available as the ePTFE Soft Tissue Patch (Goretex), is a suitable prosthesis for the repair of large, noncontaminated abdominal wall defects lacking peritoneum or greater omentum to protect the viscera, but it is not yet the ideal prosthesis for that purpose. According to Amid's classification of biomaterials in abdominal wall hernia surgery, ePTFE is a type II prosthesis, being suitable to house bacteria and showing inadequate pore size [44]. Experimental and clinical studies showed that its main drawbacks are the lack of ingrowth of fibrocollagenous tissue into the material resulting in anchorage of the patch, which is solely dependent on the type of suture material used. In order to improve the ePTFE patch, experimental studies showed that the standard ePTFE patch can be turned into a functionally double-layer patch by modifying its outer or abdominal side by ion beaming and glow discharge to form a hydrophilic layer, which permits ingrowth of tissue into the pores. This modification is not yet commercially available, and studies should be carried out to achieve this goal via other means.

30.9 Discussion

Wantz: It is surprising how much Gore-Tex is used in the United States. The company woos residents and takes them out to dinner, and for one reason or another, the residents decide to use Gore-Tex to fix groin hernias and fix incisional hernias. It is beyond me why anyone uses it at all.

Devlin: I have done three cases with Gore-Tex and all of them ended in a catastrophe. The first patient got sepsis, so I had to take the mesh out; the second patient got a localized allergy over it, just over the site of the Gore-Tex, so that had to come out too; and the last one got all screwed up.

Simmermacher: Yes, I agree.

Jeekel: My congratulations on your research; it is very interesting and teaches us a lot. Why did you go this way? Because you were worried about adhesions and you were looking for another material? Did you chose very expensive material in preference to polypropylene (Marlex) to try to avoid getting adhesions? Why not cover it with something? We learned last year that there is a significant difference in the occurrence of adhesions, especially in the postoperative period, if you use Sepra film in the abdominal wall. Why don't you put a Sepra film on top of the Marlex, for example?

Simmermacher: The first thing to say is that this was a choice which was made because we presented our results to the manufacturers and they asked us whether we would be able to modify it and do some research on that; it was purely practical. We were thinking about modifying Marlex, which appeared to be more difficult, because one of the problems was what is going to happen when it wrinkles due to wound contraction. We also followed another path; we were able to get one firm to agree to make a patch for us that was microporous on the visceral side and porous when open to the abdominal side. We had quite good results with that, but due to financial problems the firm stopped making it.

Schumpelick: Dr. Jeekel, why do you think that Sepra film will prevent adhesions in the long term? I do not know of any convincing studies on that, only at the beginning, and not over a period of many years.

Jeekel: It prevents adhesions in a certain percentage of cases, and that in the long term and the short term. If you prevent adhesions in the first year, you prevent them completely, but there is a significant difference in the number of adhesions and in the grade of adhesions; however, you still get quite a number of adhesions, so yes, we would like to prevent adhesions in 100%.

Schumpelick: I was asked by this company whether we could combine a Marlex mesh with Sepra film to solve all problems, but there is no proven result to show that there is any convincing way to do it. We do not know at the moment; we only know that some of the acute adhesions are prevented.

Jeekel: No, I do not agree with you; they are the acute and long-term adhesions. Still, it is not enough, I agree with that.

Schumpelick: Was it not available 10 years ago?

Jeekel: Of course.

Flament: On the subject of adhesions, do you know the rate of adhesions to the posterior aspect of the primary closure? Because when we operate on patients who have had a laporotomy many years ago, we always find adhesions, so what is the rate of adhesions in any primary closure? Secondly, about your experiment, why did you not use running sutures and why not Gore-Tex sutures to prevent adhesions, because we have seen stitches that are not made of Gore-Tex on your slides?

Simmermacher: The answer to the first question is that we did sham operations and we did not have any adhesions. I realize that in human beings it is quite different, and I think we can talk about adhesions for about a week. There is no need for adhesions to be a problem. From the start we were afraid of visceral adhesions, and I clearly stated that in the beginning we were looking at those abdominal wall defects where there is no peritoneum and no greater omentum available, because we are afraid of the adhesions of viscera to the patch. The second thing is that we deliberately did not use a running suture because we were afraid that, if the running suture broke, then due to the fact that you do not get any anchorage, you get a big gap, so we chose the interrupted suture. I do not think they were nonabsorbable sutures, Prolene, and we think it makes no difference whether you use a nonabsorbable suture anyhow. We might discuss why there is a big space between the stitches, but we were really looking for this model because we wanted to see anchorage and whether or not it was quick anchorage, so it was done deliberately.

Kingsnorth: We have been discussing a problem of an undefined size. No one so far has presented any data at this meeting showing how frequent intestinal obstruction is following the use of different types of mesh. Dr. Wantz has a very big series with zero incidence of intestinal obstruction or problems with adhesions; Dr. Flament has published a series, again a very big series with not a single case of adhesive obstruction. Why are we worried about it?

Simmermacher: With respect to Marlex in an unprotected abdominal wall defect, I think there are several reports in the literature indicating that you get fistula formation. Sometimes you get ileus, which is difficult to define, but there is evidence that there might be fistula formation due to wrinkling of the Marlex mesh, and this is a very nasty complication to have. The other thing is that the patients returned after the repair, which was formally wrong because it was an inlay, and they complained about nausea.

Schumpelick: I would like to report that we have reopened patients with Gore-Tex meshes after 8 years, and we have reoperated on three of these patients because of intestional obstruction with adhesions on the margins. They are not absolutely safe.

Amid: I just wanted to mention that Gore-Tex sutures really have no advantage over braided suture, because Gore-Tex sutures are porous. I did a small study on Gore-Tex sutures, and they are exactly like the Gore-Tex patch; they are not monofilament. The answer to your question why Dr. Wantz does not have that problem is because he does not put it inside the peritoneal cavity. He puts his mesh outside the peritoneal cavity and that is why he does not have intestinal obstruction problems, but if you have to put it inside the peritoneal cavity for any reason, or if you do not have enough peritoneum, then the bowel comes into contact with whatever biomaterial you use, and that is when you get that kind of problem.

Wantz: We always get the peritoneum closed in the pelvis. The position of Vicryl is always up in the epigastrium, where we cannot close the posterior rectus sheath; that may explain a lot why we do not have intestinal obstruction, because the adhesions are high in the abdomen. However, we did have two patients with transient small bowel obstruction that had to be treated and the patients had to be admitted to hospital.

Simmermacher: But these are very rare occasions where you have no peritoneum left, about 1%.

Filipi: I have a question that may not be totally related, but I understand the Gore pericardial membrane has been quite successful and that they have not had problems with pericardial adhesions. I have not heard of any allergy problems or infection. Are you aware of their experience with that?

Simmermacher: Personally, I have not any experience with it. You have told us that they have good results and no problems. I think that is because they normally did not operate in a contaminated area. If you have a slight small bowel opening, you might get some contamination, and that is disastrous if you use a PTFE patch. Normally, thoracic surgeons are afraid of any kind of contamination of wounds, so they do not have to deal with that aspect, and as far as I know, there are no adhesions of the heart, because the heart is still moving and the diameter of the pores is very small – it is about 1 μm.

Filipi: Has there been any work with impregnating antibiotics into PTFE?

Simmermacher: Not as far as I know. The problem is the formula. Application of any kind of thing on the PTFE patch is very difficult. That was the problem with the patch. I showed you where a polyurethane layer was glued on the PTFE. We did not trust this because we were afraid that there might be separation of one or two layers, because the firm itself says you cannot put anything on the PFTE patch.

Jeekel: There was a question about the incidence of adhesions after primary closure of the abdominal wall. We did a prospective study in 435 patients looking at adhesions, and the incidence after primary closure of the midline abdominal wall was 97%, so in nearly all cases you get adhesions after just closing the abdominal wall as well as with a mesh, but very rarely obstructive problems after a mesh operation. It might be that one adhesion is not the adhesion that caused it and it may not be the adhesion to the mesh, but it is very difficult to say that the mesh in the abdominal cavity is a great danger.

Read: It seems to me that with all your experiments you have covered nearly all the options available with this mesh. What makes you think that the new product they are bringing out is going to be better than the products that you have already investigated?

Simmermacher: We are just thinking about it because they offered us this dual patch. We are going to talk about whether we are going to use it and whether we are going to do the study, because these are very rare cases and it will be very difficult to get enough numbers to do a study in humans. We will probably start with animal studies so that we can get results from them.

References

1. Stoltz M, Verwendung von expandiertem Polytetrafluoroethylen (ePTFE) als medizinisches Implantat – Structurvarianten zur Lösung chirurgischer Probleme. Chemie 1988;10
2. Rosenthal D and Walters MJ, Preperitoneal synthetic mesh placement for recurrent hernias of the groin. Surg Gyn & Obstet 1986;163:285–6
3. Soyer T, Lempinen M, Cooper P, Norton L, Eiseman B, A new venous prosthesis. Surgery 1972; 72:864–72
4. Cuadros CL, One hundred percent patency of one-millimeter polytetrafluoroethylene (Gore-tex) grafts in the carotid arteries of rats. Microsurgery 1984;5:1–11
5. Amid PK, Shulman AG and Lichtenstein IL, Selecting synthetic mesh for the repair of groin hernia. Post Gen Surg 1992;4:150–5
6. Pans A and Pierard GE, A comparison of intraperitoneal prostheses for the repair of abdominal wall defects in rats. Eur Surg Res 1992;24:54–60
7. Savioz D, Ludwig C, Leissing C, Bolle JF, Bühler L, Morel, Repeated macroscopic haematuria caused by intravesical migration of a preperitoneal prosthesis. Eur J Surg 1997;163:631–2
8. Rath AM, Zhang J, Amouroux J and Chevrel JP, Les protheses parietales abdominales. Chirurgie 1996;121:253–65
9. Usher FC, A new plastic prosthesis for repairing tissue defects of the chest and the abdominal wall. Am J Surg 1959;97:629–33
10. Bellon JM, Bujan J, Contreras L, Hernando A and Jurado F, Macrophage response to experimental implantation of polypropylene prostheses. Eur Surg Res 1994;26:46–53
11. Kaufman Z, Engelberg M, Zager M, Fecal fistula: a late complication of Marlex mesh repair. Dis Colon Rectum 1981;24:543–4
12. Voyles CR, Richardson JD, Bland KI, Tobin GR, Flint LM, Polk HC, Emergency abdominal wall reconstruction with polypropylene mesh: short-term benefits versus long-term complications. Ann Surg 1981;194:219–23
13. Berliner SD, Clinical experience with an inlay expanded polytetrafluoroethylene soft tissue patch as an adjunct in inguinal hernia repair. Surg Gyn & Obstet 1993;176:323–6
14. Bauer JJ, Salky BA, Gelernt IM, Kreel I, Repair of large abdominal wall defects with expanded polytetrafluoroethylene (PTFE). Ann Surg 1987;206:765–9
15. Hamer-Hodges DW, Scott NB, Replacement of an abdominal wall defect using expanded PTFE-sheet (Gore-tex). J R Coll Surg Edinb 1985;30:65–7
16. Van der Lei B, Bleichrodt RP, Simmermacher RKJ, van Schilfgaarde R, Expanded polytetrafluoroethylene patch for the repair of large abdominal wall defects. Br J Surg 1989;76:803–5
17. Simmermacher RKJ, Schakenraad JM, Bleichrodt RP, Reherniation after repair of the abdominal wall with expanded polytetrafluoroethylene. J Am Coll Surg 1994;178:613–6
18. Wantz GE, Giant prosthetic reinforcement of the visceral sac. Surg Gyn & Obstet 1989;169:408–17
19. Bebawi MA, Moqtaderi F and Vijaj V, Giant incisional hernia: staged repair using pneumoperitoneum and expanded polytetrafluoroethylene. Am Surg 1997;63:375–81
20. Pans A, Desaive C. and Jacquet N, Use of a preperitoneal prosthesis for strangulated groin hernia. Br J Surg 1997;84:310–12
21. Bellon JM, Bujan LA, Contreras LA, Hernando A, Jurado F, Similarity in behaviour of polytetrafluoroethylene (ePTFE) prostheses implanted into different interfaces. J Biom Mat Res 1996;31:1–9
22. Bellon JM, Bujan J, Contreras LA, Hernanado A, Integration of biomaterials implanted into abdominal wall: process of scar formation and macrophage response. Biomaterials 1995;16:381–7
23. Bellon JM, Contreras LA, Sabater C, Bujan J, Pathologic and clinical aspects of repair of large incisional hernias after implant of a polytetrafluoroethylene prosthesis. World J Surg 1997;21:402–7

24. Gillion JF, Begin GF, Marecos C, Fourtanier G, Expanded polytetrafluoroethylene patches used in the intraperitoneal or extraperitoneal position for repair of incisional hernias of the anterolateral abdominal wall. Am J Surg 1997;174:16–9
25. DeBord JR, Wyffels PL, Marshall JS, Miller G, Marshall WH, Repair of large ventral incisional hernias with expanded polytetrafluoroethylene prosthetic patches. Post Gen Surg 1992;4:156–60
26. Haney AF, Hesla J, Hurst BS et al, Expanded polytetrafluoroethylene (Gore-tex surgical membrane) is superior to oxidized regenerated cellulose (Interceed TC7) in preventing adhesions. Fertil & Steril 1995;63:1021–6
27. Trudell LA, Boudreau L, Van de Water JM, Jaurequi H, Richardson PD, Galetti PM, Alcohol-treated PTFE vascular grafts. Trans Am Soc Artif Intern Organs 1978;24:320–3
28. Simmermacher RKJ, Van der Lei B, Bleichrodt RP, Schakenraad JM. Improved tissue ingrowth and anchorage of expanded polytetrafluoroethylene by perforation. Biomat 1991;12:22–4
29. Kusaba A, Fischer CR, Matulewski TJ, Matsumoto T, Experimental study of the influence of porosity on development of neointima in Gore-tex (R) grafts. Am Surg 1981;47:347–54
30. Simmermacher RKJ, Biomaterials in the repair of abdominal wall defects (thesis). Groningen (NL), 1994
31. Amato JJ, Cotroneo JV, Galdieri R, Alboliras E, Antillon J, Vogel RL, Experience with the polytetrafluoroethylene surgical membrane for pericardial closure in operations for congenital cardiac defects. J Thor Cardiovasc Surg 1989;97:929–34
32. Jorgensen LN, Kallehave F, Karlsmark T, Gottrup F, Reduced collagen accumulation after major surgery. Br J Surg 1996;83:1591–4
33. Zacharias RK, Kirkman TR, Clowes AW, Mechanism of healing in synthetic grafts. J Vasc Surg 1987;6:429–36
34. Schakenraad JM, Stokroos I, Bartels H, Busscher HJ, Patency of small caliber superhydrophobic ePTFE vascular grafts. Cells and Materials 1992;2:193–9
35. Busscher HJ, Stokroos I, Golverdingen JG, Schakenraad JM, Adhesion and spreading of human fibroblasts on superhydrophobic FEP-Teflon. Cells and Materials 1991;1:243–9
36. Soler M, Verhaeghe P, Essomba A, Sevestre H, Stoppa R, Le traitment des eventrations post-operatoires par prothese composee. Ann Chir 1993;47:598–608
37. Vaubel E, Gorkisch K, Linke K, Polyurethan-Hautersatzmaterial zur temporaren Wunddeckung. Fortschritte der Medizin 1980;98:1351–6
38. Amid P, Shulman G, Lichtenstein I, Sostrin S, Young J, Hakakhan M, Evaluation preliminaire de materiels composites pour la reparation des eventrations. Ann Chir 1995;49:539–43
39. Cristaldi M, Pisacreta M, Elli M, Vago GL, Danelli PG, Sampietro GM, Taschicin AM, Femoropopliteal bypass occlusion following mesh plug for prevascular hernia repair. Hernia 1997;1:197–9
40. Bleichrodt RP, Simmermacher RKJ, Van der Lei B, Schakenraad JM, Expanded polytetrafluoroethylene patch versus polypropylene mesh for the repair of contaminated defects of the abdominal wall. Surg Gyn & Obstet 1993;176:18–24
41. Walter C, Gugenheim S, Bartlett A, The selection of implant material for facial augmentation with special reference to Gore-tex. Face 1993;3:151–7
42. Bhat DJ, Tellis VA, Kohlberg WI, Driscoll B, Veith FJ, Management of sepsis involving expanded polytetrafluoroethylene grafts for dialysis access. Surgery 1980;87:445–50
43. Geiger G, Krempien B, Structuranalyse von Expanded Polytetrafluoroethylene Prothesen nach Langzeitmplantation beim Menschen. Angio 1988;10:169–78
44. Amid PK, Classification of biomaterials and their related complications in abdominal wall hernia surgery. Hernia 1997;1:15–21

CHAPTER 31

Plastic Reconstruction of Abdominal Wall Defects

A. Berger, J. Liebtau

31.1 Introduction

If all conventional surgical options are limited to ensuring closure of recurrent abdominal wall hernia or abdominal defects, a microsurgical technique might be used to reestablish abdominal wall stability. We use the m. latissimus dorsi as a muscle or a myocutaneous free flap with a microsurgical neurovascular transfer. A microanastomosis from the thoracodorsal nerve to a motoric branch of the femoral nerve in the recipient area is performed. A total of 12 patients have been treated successfully up to now.

Abdominal wall weakness and abdominal wall hernias usually constitute a surgical problem which can be solved in the majority of cases by conventional methods of abdominal wall surgery or by local flaps. Large abdominal wall hernias mainly result from impaired wound healing processes. They are often accompanied by defects of muscle and fascia. Many patients have postoperative local infections, resulting in scar tissue with impaired blood supply. Abdominal wall defects can occur after tumor resection, chronic ulceration after radiotherapy, or after trauma. Many operative methods have been used [4, 11]. These include simple closure, fascia doubling, and replacement of the defect with autologous or foreign material [6]. In the literature, a recurrence rate of 27%–57% is mentioned [7]. Even with omentum plasty and corium plasty, there is a 8% recurrence rate.

There is a small group of patients with multiple courses of recurrent hernia after surgery or defects due to tumor, radiotherapy, or trauma. The innervated abdominal wall muscles and the fascial structures are destroyed, and a reconstruction with local methods, implants, or omentum transplant is not possible [9]. Based on the experience of microsurgical tissue transfers and on our experience with free muscle transfer and reinnervation, we have used this technique for reconstruction of the abdominal wall [1, 10].

We therefore employed neurovascular muscle transfer in special cases [2, 3]. We take the m. latissimus dorsi, which we are used to transferring in other fields such as injuries of the extremities.

31.2 Material and Methods

The harvesting of the m. latissimus dorsi with vessel and nerves, forming a pedicle as long as possible up to 14 cm, is performed together with preparation of the hernia, the abdominal wall defect, the inguinal vessels, and a motoric branch of the n. femoralis. The abdominal defect is closed with corium plasty. The m. latissimus dorsi is placed upon the defect and fixed to the fascia and the pelvic bone. The artery and vein of the m. latissimus dorsi are microsurgically anastomosed end to end or end to side to a side branch in the inguinal region [1].

The thoracodorsal nerve is coaptated with 10/0 filament end to end with a motoric branch of the femoral nerve. Before doing this procedure, we check that the innervation of the femoral nerve is sufficient without this branch. If there is enough skin, it is closed above the muscle. Alternatively, a skin island of the latissimus may be used, and a myocutaneous latissimus flap is used to cover the remaining defect.

Precise postoperative flap monitoring is important. A bodice must be used to stabilize the abdominal wall. Reinnervation cannot be expected before 6–8 months. After this time, the abdominal wall may be trained like any other muscle.

31.3 Results

In the last 9 years, we have operated on 15 patients suffering from recurrent abdominal wall hernia. There were recurrent incisional hernias in nine patients, which were always second or third recurrences, e.g., a 25-year-old patient after multiple laparotomies who showed an abdominal wall hernia peri- and infraumbilically, who was treated with a latissimus dorsi flap (Fig. 1). Another 26-year-old patient presented with an extended hernia in the right lower abdomen and paramedian. He had a myocuta-

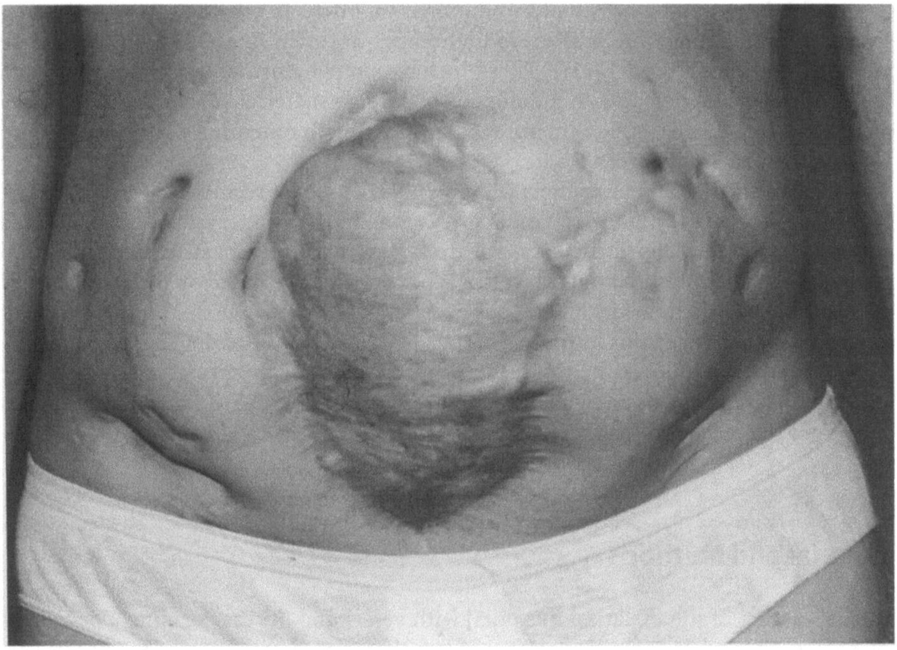

Fig. 1a.

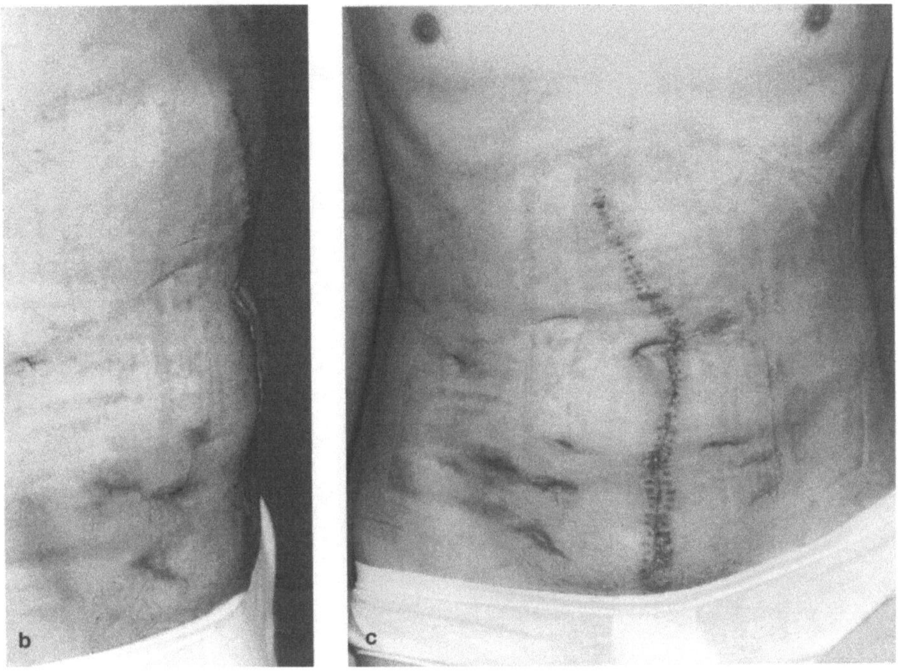

Fig. 1a–c. A 25-year-old patient after multiple laparotomies with an abdominal wall hernia peri- and infraumbilically; the patient was treated with a latissimus dorsi flap

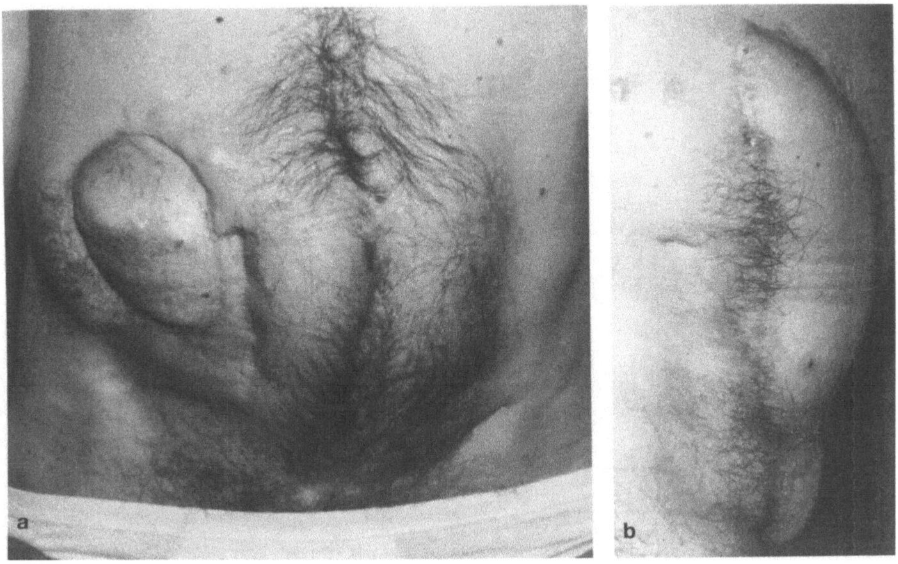

Fig. 2a, b. A 26-year-old patient with an extended hernia in the right lower abdomen and paramedian; the patient was treated with a myocutaneous latissimus dorsi flap

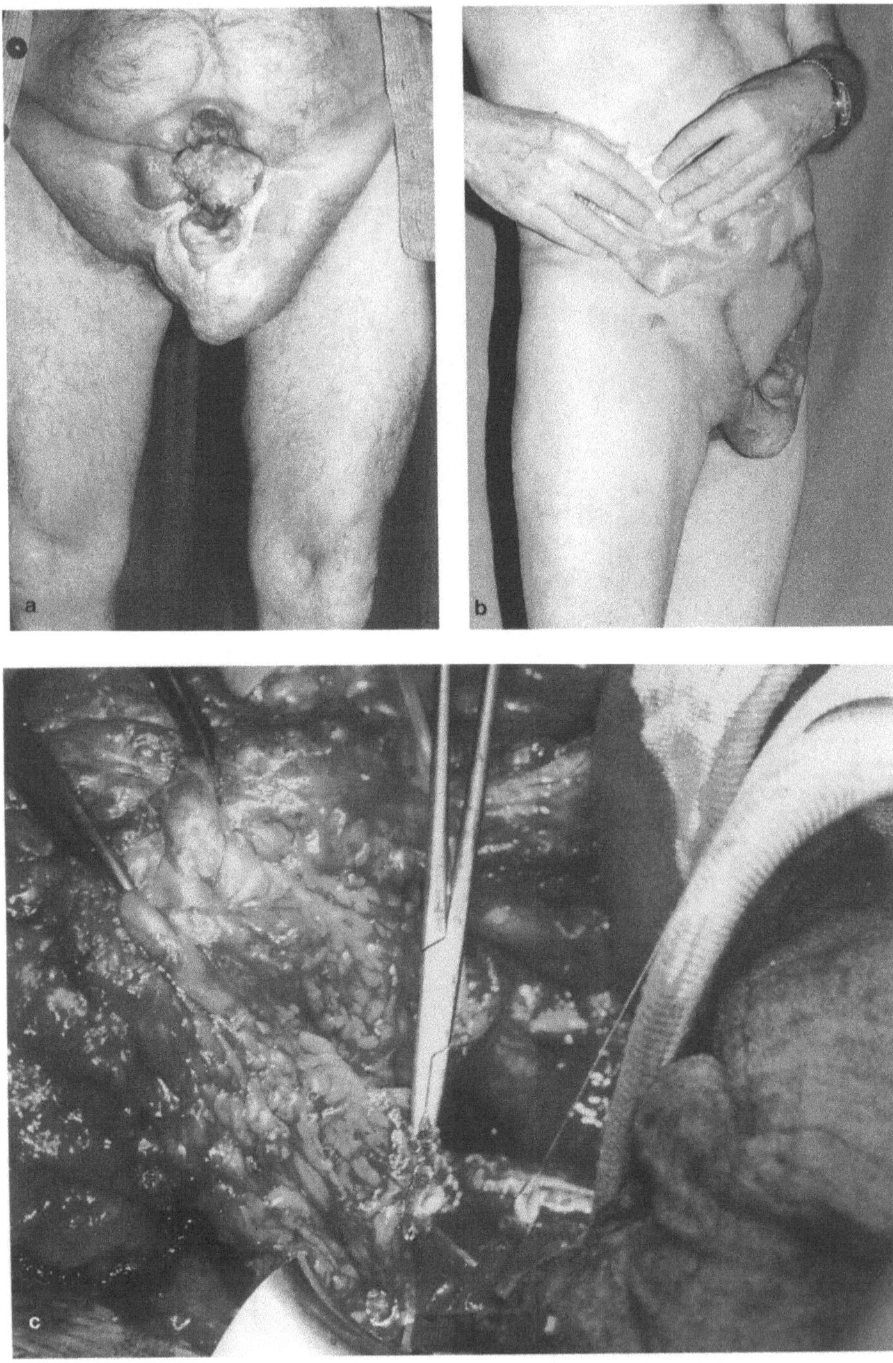

Fig. 3a–c. A 53-year-old patient with extended carcinoma of the bladder who received a latissimus dorsi free flap after radical tumor resection

neous latissimus dorsi flap with a good functional result (Fig. 2). One patient had the fifth recurrence of a hernia. In four patients, abdominal wall reconstruction was necessary after tumor resection, and two of these were urological tumors, e.g., a 53-year-old patient with extended carcinoma of the bladder. This patient received a latissimus dorsi free flap after radical tumor resection and had stable postoperative results (Fig. 3). One patient suffered from chronic ulceration and severe scar formation and fistula after radiation therapy following a gynecological operation. Another patient had a reconstruction following a severe car accident with good reinnervation.

Of the 15 patients, 12 (80%) obtained a sufficient reinnervation 2 years after the abdominal wall reconstruction. No active abdominal wall contraction was seen in two patients. One patient suffered a complete flap failure and had a corium plasty covered by a skin graft.

31.4 Conclusion

Primary abdominal wall defects include umbilical, epigastric, and spigelian hernia, and secondary ones include incisional hernias following laparotomy, tumor resection, radiation therapy, or trauma. If all conventional methods fail, such as duplication of the fascia and the use of synthetic material, e.g., mesh implants [5], or autologous material, e.g., corium plasty, with or without mesh [8], free tissue transfer is a possible method of reconstruction.

Reconstruction of the fascial structure with muscle transfer is possible with a neurovascular muscle or a myocutaneous transfer. Only a few carefully selected patients are considered for this special method. The technique described enables us to reconstruct the abdominal wall in a physiological way. The problem of muscle activity during rest remains to be solved. Innervation of the branch of the femoral nerve can be trained. However, there might be unintended innervation of the abdominal wall when leg muscles are used. Our patients were able to learn a separate intended movement of the leg and the abdominal wall.

In conclusion, reconstruction of a severe abdominal wall defect can be performed using a microneurovascular technique, transferring a large muscle such as the latissimus dorsi muscle. The abdominal wall can be reconstructed in its muscular fascial content and function using this technique. The indication and operative technique of this method might be able to be extended.

31.5 Discussion

Bendavid: There are cases after nephrectomy where you lose innervation of the flank muscles. You do not have a hernia, but you do have a bulge that resembles a hernia. I have also seen it in three primary cases associated with diabetes. I am wary of doing anything. Is there anything that you could offer in the way of a flap?

Berger: What we have seen for a long time now in microsurgery and in diabetic patients is that there is not much difference between a normal and a diabetic patient. You have to be very careful in selecting the vessels that you need for microvascular tissue transfer; this depends on the chronically infected area. You must also be aware that you should never go from small vessels onto big vessels. In this way you can use the microvascular method, even in very difficult cases. We have just operated on a 52-year-old woman who has had a severe radiation ulcer for 32 years in the lower part of the abdominal wall that was becoming malignant and severe diabetes for 40 years. The only solution was to remove the whole thing using the latissimus dorsi in the groin on the femoral artery and it worked.

Skandalakis: When the femoral nerve leaves the iliopsoas with all its branches, most of them will be destroyed. What do you do about innervation?

Berger: Yes, absolutely right, these are the main problems, not only in abdominal wall reconstruction (or in other neurovascular muscles). You find easier vessels, but it is very often problematic to find the nerve. In one case, although not a very powerful reinnervation, we took a graft to the intercostals. In the intercostal after the 12th and 11th, you can go up, and we used them for the innervation of the upper arm. You need a graft, and this is not so good for the abdominal wall; it is too long and takes too long to reinnervate. So if I cannot find any nerve on this side, I would do a graft beforehand.

Schumpelick: You said that in these cases with a monolayer or with a material layer intestinally, it is difficult to remove the skin from the intestine. We have a lot of these cases. After leaving the abdomen open in peritonitis, we put a Vicryl mesh in and later a mesh graft and after 0.5–1 year we remove the skin and close the abdominal wall defect. There is no problem to remove the skin from instestine. Might Vicryl be the reason?

Berger: It takes at least 6 months until this muscle starts to be reinnervated, so in 6 months the stricture can easily be stretched in the wrong way. If the external support is not safe enough, we thought it was better to have a reinforcement of the abdominal wall itself. The muscle then has time to become reinnervated.

Schumpelick: You wait 6 months?

Berger: Yes.

Willis: It is absolutely fascinating what you showed us, but if we have an incisional hernia and make a primary closure, we also cover the gap with a perfectly innervated muscle, with the rectus. It is not enough and we always have to use a prosthesis, so my question is whether it is probably necessary to take a prosthesis for your free muscle flaps?

Berger: These are very special cases. These patients usually already have a weakness of the abdominal wall, and the rectus muscle is already not working well; that is the reason why we see them. The prosthesis might not have worked well enough against herniation here. In these cases, if you use the muscle pedicle, you have the muscle immediately innervated, and then you would need no prosthesis, no dermis. However, if you use it as a free muscle, you need a protection for 1 month until the muscle is innervated.

References

1. Berger A, Flory PJ, Schaller A (1990) Muscle transfer in brachial plexus lesions. J Microsurgery 6 (2): 113–116
2. Berger A, Hierner R, Pallua N (1993) New ways with reinnervated muscle transfer for abdominal wall reconstruction. Reconstructive microsurgery Current trends 67–68
3. Berger A, Schneider We (1993) Neue Wege mit mikrochirurgisch transferierten innervierten Muskellappen zur Rekonstruktion der Bauchwandbrüche. Langenbecks Arch Chir Suppl (Kongreßbericht 1993) 276–281
4. Klein P (1993) Die Inlay/Onlay-Technik als funktionelle Rekonstruktion der Bauchwand nach Narbenhernien und Narbenhernienrezidiven. Kurzreferate DGCHH 110. Kongreß, Demeter Verlag Nr. 181
5. Klinge U, Conze J, Klosterhalfen B, Limberg W, Obolenski B, Öttinger A P, Schumpelick V (1996) Veränderungen der Bauchwandmechanik nach Mesh-Implantation. Langenbecks Arch Chir 381: 323–332
6. Piza-Katzer H, Meissel G, Stachen G (1979) Rekonstruktion von Bauchwanddefekten mit Corium. Chirurg 50:775
7. Schildberg F-W, Vatankhah M, Nissen R (1983) Chirurgische Behandlung des Narbenbruches der Bauchdecken. Langenbecks Arch Chir 316:319–323
8. Schütter F-W, Kiroff P (1995) Die netzverstärkte Kutisplastik. Langenbecks Arch Chir 380: 249–252
9. Stelzner F (1993) Das Fascienskelett der Bauchhöhle-Hernien und andere Störungen. Kurzreferate DGCH, 110. Kongreß, Demeter Verlag Nr. 178
10. Tizian C, Berger A (1987) Reconstruction of muscle function in extremities after traumatic loss-using free myocutaneous flaps. Proc 2nd Vienna Muscle Symposion 6/1985
11. Wilker D (1988) Narbenbruchoperationen. Breitner Chir OP-Lehre Brand III, Chirurgie des Abdomens 86–96

Part VIII Recurrent Inguinal Hernia

Suture Repair

Mesh Repair

Laparoscopic and Endoscopic Techniques

CHAPTER 32

Experience of the Shouldice Clinic in Recurrent Inguinal Hernia Repair

R. Bendavid

32.1 Introduction

The unrelenting march of events in hernia surgery has led to the introduction of prosthetic materials for every possible type of herniorrhaphy. Prostheses, however, are not a panacea. Their use should be judicious and justified. The reliance on prefabricated prosthetic devices will not supplant a good knowledge of anatomy or the understanding of the causative pathology.

32.2 Background (Past)

The Shouldice Hospital has set an enviable record since 1945 in the treatment of hernias, and particularly groin hernias. Statistics reveal that to date more than 250,000 operations have been performed. Every year, 7000 or more operations are carried out. Although the overall recurrence rate of the Shouldice repair may range from 0.5% to 2.2% [1], these data do not reflect the true nature of the problem of re-recurrences.

A study carried out by Obney and Chan [5] looked at 964 patients undergoing 1057 operations for recurrences. Details reveal that 37% of patients had an indirect inguinal hernia, 8% had a femoral hernia, 10% had two or more hernias present, and 45% had a direct inguinal hernia.

These patients underwent a standard Shouldice repair between 1970 and 1972 and were re-evaluated in 1983, at a time when prosthetic materials were not yet in use at the Shouldice Hospital.

The survey established a recurrence rate ranging from 2.3% to 20%, depending on the number of previous attempts at repair (Table 1). Results since the introduction of prostheses, however, have considerably improved, as is shown in the tables.

Femoral hernias represent an even more difficult problem that has long been underestimated. A study carried out at the Shouldice Hospital in 1989, covering 508 operations on 493 patients, confirmed that recurrence rates varied between 11.8% and 75%, depending on the number of previous attempts (Table 2) [2]. Here, again, the introduction of prostheses in the form of an umbrella has largely corrected the problem [3].

Table 1. Re-recurrence rate following the Shouldice repair [5]

Recurrence	Total (n)	Re-recurrence (n)	(%)
1st	775	18	2.3
2nd	212	15	7
3rd	49	6	12
4th	14	1	7
5th	5	1	20

Table 2. Recurrence and re-recurrence of femoral hernias [2]

Recurrences (n)	Operations (n)	Recurrences (n)	(%)
Primary femoral hernia	251	15	6.1
1st	144	17	11.8
2nd	72	25	34.7
3rd	26	9	34.6
4th	10	3	30
5th	4	3	75
6th	1	0	–

32.3 Background (Present)

As of November 1983, it became evident that prosthetic materials would be incorporated in our treatment of groin hernias. For inguinal hernias, a fascia transversalis replacement would be used [4], for femoral hernias, an umbrella [3].

To appreciate the improvement in results since the introduction of mesh, the year 1995 was chosen for its statistics. Table 3 shows a distribution of primary and recurrent inguinal hernias. Table 4 reveals that all hernias having a femoral component predict a poor outcome unless treated aggressively. Table 5 shows that 54 primary repairs and 118 recurrent hernias required prostheses. Tables 6 and 7 show the need of these prostheses as a percentage and hence a better indication of that need for the specific type of hernia. Table 8 shows the rate of re-recurrence, revealing that in some instances where indigenous tissue is of good consistency, a Shouldice repair can still be of value. However, for femoral hernias, a re-recurrence rate of 15.4% would indicate that mesh is still not used frequently enough. Table 9 shows a recurrence rate of 1.7%

Table 3. Types of hernias: primary and recurrence treated surgically during 1995

Type	Primary	Recurrence	Total
Indirect inguinal hernia	3594	259	3853
Direct inguinal hernia	1942	350	2292
Femoral hernia	55	47	102
Indirect-direct femoral hernia	30	23	53
Inguinofemoral hernia	0	5	5
Prevascular hernia	3	6	9
Total	5624	690	6314

Table 4. Percentage of hernias presenting as a recurrence (1995)

Type	Total	Recurrence	
	(*n*)	(*n*)	(%)
Indirect inguinal hernia	3853	259	6.7
Direct inguinal hernia	2292	350	15.2
Femoral hernia	102	47	46
Indirect-direct femoral hernia	30	23	76.6
Inguinofemoral hernia	5	5	100
Prevascular hernia	9	6	66.6

Table 5. Use of prostheses in various hernias

Type	Primaries	Recurrences (1st to 5th)
Inguinal hernia (direct/indirect)	7	50
Femoral hernia	14	34
Indirect-direct femoral hernia	30	23
Inguinofemoral hernia	0	5
Prevascular hernia	3	6
Total	54	118

Table 6. Use of mesh in primary repairs

Type	Total	Mesh used	
	(*n*)	(*n*)	(%)
Inguinal hernia (direct/indirect)	5536	7	0.12
Femoral hernia	55	14	25.0
Indirect-direct femoral hernia	30	30	100
Inguinofemoral hernia	0	0	-
Prevascular hernia	3	3	100

Table 7. Use of prostheses in recurrences

Type	Total	Prostheses used	
	(*n*)	(*n*)	(%)
Inguinal hernia (direct/indirect)	609	50	8.2
Femoral hernia	47	34	72.3
Indirect-direct femoral hernia	23	23	100
Inguinofemoral hernia	5	5	100
Prevascular hernia	6	6	100

Table 8. Re-recurrences for operations performed without mesh

Type	Total	Re-recurrence	
	(*n*)	(*n*)	(%)
Direct inguinal re-recurrence	559	7	1.6
Indirect inguinal re-recurrence	559	2	
Femoral re-recurrence	13	2	15.4

Three direct recurrent hernia repairs recurred as femoral hernias.

Table 9. Re-recurrence following mesh use

Total (n)	Re-recurrence
(%)	(n)
172	3[a]
1.7	

[a] Two direct inguinal hernias and one prevascular hernia.

in a class of hernias that is particularly difficult and where the extent of coverage could perhaps be wider yet.

In summary, it can be stated that the use of prosthetic material was of the order of 0.96% (54 out of 5624) in primary hernias and 17.1% (118 out of 690) in recurrent hernias.

32.4 Conclusion

Whereas the Shouldice Hospital used to emphasize surgery without prosthetic material, a review of our statistics has compelled us to view prostheses with a more liberal attitude. The results undeniably support this new attitude.

32.5 Discussion

For a discussion, please see Chap. 33.

References

1. Bendavid, R.: Expectations of hernia surgery (inguinal & femoral) in: Principles and practice of surgical laparoscopy. Paterson-Brown, S.; Garden, J. (Eds) W.B. Saunders, 1994, pp 387–414.
2. Bendavid, R.: Femoral hernias: primary vs recurrence. Int Surg 1989; 74: 99–100.
3. Bendavid, R.: A femoral "Umbrella" for femoral hernia repair. Surg Gynec & Obst, Aug 1987, Vol 165, pp 153–156.
4. Bendavid, R.: New techniques in hernia repair. World J. Surg 1989; 13:522–531.
5. Obney, N., Chan, C.K.: Repair of multiple time recurrent inguinal hernias with reference to common causes of recurrence. Contemporary Surg. Vol 25, Dec 1984, pp 25–32.

CHAPTER 33

Shouldice Repair for Recurrent Inguinal Hernia – A Ten-Year Follow-Up

K.H. Treutner, G. Arlt, V. Schumpelick

33.1 Introduction

For nearly a century, the Bassini repair was the treatment of choice for inguinal hernias in Germany [2]. The Shouldice technique, first published in 1945, was introduced to Germany at the beginning of the last decade [7, 8]. Within 10 years, it became the standard procedure for primary and recurrent inguinal hernias in more than 50% of the hospitals in Germany [10].

The low recurrence rates after the Shouldice hernioplasty are well known and have been reported in a number of publications [1, 3, 9, 12]. The recurrence rates after repair of recurrent hernias are higher than those after surgery of primary hernias. In addition, recurrence rates are closely related to the location and size of the fascial defect [5]. This prompted follow-up studies on the Shouldice repair for recurrent inguinal hernia focusing on the recurrence rates and complications and on determining the limitations of this procedure with respect to the different types and sizes of the hernial orifice.

33.2 Patients and Methods

From January 1986 to December 1987, we operated on 130 recurrent inguinal hernias in 126 patients. The 112 men and 14 women (male to female ratio, 8:1) who presented with a hernia recurring for the first to fifth time were between 21 and 80 years of age (mean, 54.2 years). All of them underwent Shouldice hernioplasty using polypropylene sutures predominantly under local anesthesia [4]. In case of bilateral hernias, surgery started with the location of the highest number of recurrences or the most complaints. Repair of the contralateral side was performed after an interval of 48 h. All of the above-mentioned patients received a letter inviting them to a follow-up examination at our department 10 years after they had undergone recurrent inguinal hernia repair. Upon presentation, a history was taken, focusing on complaints and re-recurrences following repair. Furthermore, the patients were subjected to a thorough clinical and sonographic examination of the groin region [11].

Another group of patients were operated on for recurrent inguinal hernia during an extended period of time between 1986 and 1992. They underwent Shouldice repair using the same thread and anesthesia. Follow-up examinations, however, were carried out after intervals ranging from 5 to 10 years after hernioplasty. In this latter group, the location and size of the fascial defect was determined and measured intraoperatively according to our own classification (the Aachen classification of groin hernias).

In this classification system, the site of the hernial orifice is described by the letters L for lateral (indirect) or M for medial (direct). Femoral hernias are given the letter F. The diameter of the fascial defect is given in Roman numerals, with I being less than 1.5 cm, II 1.5–3.0 cm, and III greater than 3.0 cm. The diameter of the tip of the index finger serves as the standard in open surgery. Combined hernias are classified as M, as this is part is of major importance for the development of recurrences. They receive the index c and the sizes of the two orifices are summed up [5, 6].

33.3 Results

Of 126 patients, 97 (77%) accounting for 101 of 130 (78%) repairs came to the follow-up examination 10 years after recurrent inguinal hernia repair. Testicular atrophy (0.9%), chronic inguinal pain (3.0%), and persistent hypesthesia were recorded as late postoperative complications. Although 86% of the patients had no complaints and felt physically strong, 25% reported that they avoided hard physical labor for fear of another recurrence.

The overall recurrence rate after 10 years in the 101 recurrent inguinal hernia repairs that were followed up was 6.9% (seven out of 101). The recurrences occurred at different intervals after surgery at our department. In four cases, re-recurrence was diagnosed within 1–5 years, two appeared 6–7 years after the operation, and another one developed after 8–10 years.

In the second group, 370 Shouldice repairs of intraoperatively classified recurrent hernias were followed up for 5–10 years. The results show that there were no re-recurrences following repair of small and medium-sized lateral hernias (LI–II) or medial hernias less than 1.5 cm (MI). Recurrence rates for large indirect (LIII) and medium direct (MII) hernias were 1.9% and 1.6%, respectively. Shouldice repair of recurrent inguinal hernias classified MIII (2.4%) and McII (2.6%) resulted in slightly higher figures. Follow-up of hernioplasty for large combined hernias with a total fascial defect greater than 3 cm (McIII) revealed a re-recurrence rate of 7.7% (Table 1).

Table 1. Results of Shouldice repair for recurrent inguinal hernia according to the Aachen Classification of groin hernias [5, 6]

	Recurrences (%)		
	I	II	III
L	0	0	1.9
M	0	1.6	2.4
Mc		2.6	7.7

Table 2. Results of Shouldice repair for primary and recurrent inguinal hernia

Reference	Year	Follow-up (years)	Recurrences (%)	
			Primary hernia repair	Recurrent hernia repair
[3]	1984	>10	1.1	3.1
[12]	1989	1–18	1.3	7.2
[9]	1993	5	1.4	3.7
[1]	1995	2–20	1.3	2.6
Schumpelick (underlying study)	1997	10	2.3	6.9

33.4 Conclusion

The Shouldice procedure is the gold standard for inguinal hernia repair. It can be performed as outpatient surgery using local anesthesia [4, 5]. Overall recurrence rates for primary and recurrent inguinal hernia are 1.1%–2.3% and 2.6%–7.2%, respectively [1, 3, 9, 12]. These results depend on the duration of the follow-up period. Even between the sixth and the tenth year after surgery, a considerable number of recurrences are diagnosed [5] (Table 2).

The observation of elevated recurrence rates after Shouldice repair for recurrent inguinal hernia raises the question whether this procedure is indicated in all these patients. The analysis of our second group of patients clearly demonstrates a relation between the type and size of the hernia and the long-term outcome. Those patients with large direct and combined hernias are considerably more prone to recurrence than those with lateral and small to medium-sized medial fascial defects (Table 1). As a consequence, we introduced a new regimen for surgical treatment of recurrent inguinal hernia. Whereas hernias classified as LI–III and MI–II are still being repaired by the Shouldice procedure, direct hernias with an orifice greater than 3.0 cm and all combined hernias are now operated on using mesh material. The results of this modified regimen are presented in Chap. 37.

33.5 Discussion

Bendavid: Dr. Treutner, can you tell us whether these recurrences were femoral or indirect?

Treutner: I cannot divide them up into direct or indirect now, but they were true recurrences, and not femoral hernia after repair of an inguinal hernia.

Flament: Dr. Bendavid, we have seen patients concerned about hard physical work, 25% in your experience. How long do you ask your patients to rest after a Shouldice procedure and how much physical work do you let them do in the first week?

Bendavid: We do not impose any limitations whatsoever. We tell them to go and do anything they wish to do as soon as they want. The only limitation is comfort. If you are comfortable in whatever you want to do, please go ahead and do it.

Read: Which of those approaches, the inferior or the Bassini transinguinal approach, do you prefer or which one do you use more frequently?

Bendavid: I think I have usually used the approach from above, in other words going through the floor of the canal using an inguinal approach. But there is no doubt in my mind – it has been my experience and I think it is also reported in the literature – that if the defect is large enough, and especially in females, that unless you have clinical evidence of an inguinal hernia, surgically you may not usually find it. If you are sure in females, it is simple. Otherwise, which means 95% of cases, depending on the size of the defect and invariably if you can identify Cooper's ligament from below, it will take one or two sutures; in fact, I insert the sutures first and then put in the mesh. You can simply thread the end of the sutures through the interstices of the mesh and anchor it. That would save more extensive dissection through the floor of the canal. Otherwise, it can be done by spreading the floor of the canal, inserting a pair of callies from below, grasping the stem of the umbrella, pulling it down (it positions itself), and then anchoring it.

Devlin: Should we be talking about just recurrences or should we be following the pattern that Schumpelick and Treutner have followed of looking at all the outcomes after surgery in the groin? For instance, should we know 100% of those patients who have recurrences, persistent pain, testicular atrophy, and so on? Surely this is a more realistic way of looking at a population-based study?

Bendavid: It is a good attitude, although it may be overdone, I think, because a lot are simple primary cases.

Devlin: How many of those simple primary cases have complications?

Bendavid: In my experience, the minority of them.

Devlin: Have you examined them all?

Bendavid: No, that would be impossible. But certainly of those I have examined, only a minority have had complications.

Devlin: You need to examine them all because the ones you might not examine might be the ones with the complications.

Bendavid: That is a point that would be well taken up in most series. No, I have not examined them all, but certainly we have one of the most assiduous systems of following up patients. I send out about 100,000 letters on a yearly basis on top of the ones that we actually see in our offices and on top of the ones we see at an annual check-up, which accounts for about 1500 cases. It is always a very difficult issue to discuss, and the one of the figures that I showed was interesting in the sense that those who do not respond or those who do not come for an examination are the group that you wonder about. But certainly, within the small group of 500 cases, 20% could not be bothered to answer and certainly did not add a single recurrence to the entire series. You still have another 15% that did not answer, so I am not sure whether your question can be answered.

Hartel: Dr. Bendavid, you said that after the operation you let patients do what they want whenever they feel comfortable. But is there no special exercise you could recommend to prevent recurrences? This question may be important for other abdominal wall hernias, too. Is there any special physiotherapy for the abdominal wall?

Bendavid: I certainly have no experience and have not followed up whether any particular exercise is recommended. Within our hospital, we do implement a regiment of exercise. But this is simply to promote the circulation and prevent any stiffness while patients are in the hospital. I am certainly not aware of any exercise that is going to reinforce the abdominal wall or that is going to improve the situation.

Schumpelick: We have very good connections with the Shouldice Hospital, but my feeling is, and Treutner showed this, that in some cases the Shouldice repair of large direct hernias is undertreatment. That means that in these cases we would do better to put a mesh in. Is this your experience, too, since you have a huge amount of direct hernias and recurrences?

Bendavid: In fact, when I went to the Shouldice Hospital, mesh was unheard of. I looked at the statistics and what I saw, and my impression was that the Shouldice repair was not enough in certain cases. This is one thing that has always been important to me. This is probably what made Belraft one of the greatest surgeons. He was probably the first one to say "I killed that patient because I did this," and this is very important in hernia as well.

Scott: Our findings in our series as far as types of hernias go are remarkably similar to yours. And we see many other series where you find a rate of femoral hernias of under 1% or very low; I am thinking of Rutkow's series and others, in particular. How do you explain that?

Bendavid: I think I said at the beginning that I do not know the answer. I am certain the follow-up is not there. Most people see one or two a year; you have to rely on emergencies, which may not be the same. It is difficult to account for and to explain, as you can see in our experience, and I am talking of hundreds of thousands. Each year an average of 50% of all our cases are recurrences. And over the last 20 years it has also been 50%. It is not because we are a particular referring center, and in fact most of the femoral hernias are actually seen in emergencies. If you are only doing elective surgery, you are going to have only 2%.

Kingsnorth: There is one important difference between these two series. In the Shouldice Clinic, it has been known for many years that after inguinal hernia repair a significant number of recurrences in the groin are femoral hernias. Some people have accused you of causing femoral hernias after a Shouldice repair. But I noticed in the Aachen series that all the recurrences are inguinal hernias. Can we explain the difference between the two series?

Bendavid: This is true. In fact, if you look at our own recurrences on a yearly basis, two thirds of our own recurrences (and we have about 70 cases a year) are femoral hernias. This was originally pointed out by Glassow. He tried to figure it out; probably 1 in 500 cases may in fact be a complication of the Shouldice repair. And the reason for it may well be because you have an overzealous surgeon who wants to do a good, tight repair along the inguinal ligament and thus invariably applies a little more tension than you would like to the femoral triangle and perhaps promotes a femoral hernia.

Whether we have missed them is another interesting issue. Because a lot of people do not examine adequately for a femoral hernia, and I missed them myself. What is a femoral hernia at the time of surgery? Once you have split the floor of the canal, you can insert your finger, and there is invariably the impression medial to the femoral vein where often you will feel the so-called Cloque lymph node. And very often you will also see some fat below the inguinal ligament. Should you disturb it? We have seen this with two surgeons in particular, Dr. Hoffny and Dr. Georgewski, who always made a point of removing anything and putting in a suture or two, and they had the highest recurrences of femoral hernias. So the tip is to leave things alone or, if you have femoral fat from below, simply leave it alone, do not disturb it, as it serves the purpose of plugging.

Treutner: I would certainly agree that the fat is very important for plugging, and you should by no means try to disturb the natural anatomic architecture beside the femoral vein. But a careful look is important so that you do not get so-called false recurrences, i.e., overlooked femoral hernias after inguinal hernia repair. In our group, we did not see any femoral recurrences, either true or false, after inguinal hernia repair.

Skandalakis: We always tell residents to read the OR report prior to a recurrence to be sure that a repair was done in the femoral area. We also ask them to always see whether they can find any stitches there or any repair which was done at the femoral ring.

Schumpelick: If we had the possibility to differentiate the huge direct hernia from the other groups before the operation, would you agree that this might be a group for stratification in the laparoscopic approach primarily? Or would you say that your Rives procedure or our transinguinal preperitoneal prosthesis (TIPP) procedure is better even in these cases because of local anesthesia and costs?

Bendavid: It will certainly be difficult to sit down with a laparoscopic surgeon and argue that. I feel that the size of the hernia itself is not factor, because we are always limited at the base of the defect essentially by the floor of the canal and it is very rarely the peritoneal defect, no matter how big it is. I have seen them coming down to the knees; when you can reduce it, essentially the defect is not that big. You certainly would have a far more secure repair in my experience using an open anterior approach, and I am getting to see far too many laparoscopic recurrences; we should have a series. We very often find that the meshes are too small, too highly placed, and often detached from the ligament of Cooper. If I am going to put a mesh in using the open method, as we do, I know that it is going to be there and it is going to stay there and is not going to move. I can do it very securely. I am sure some laparoscopic surgeons can do as good a job, but I find it very difficult to do something as secure as what I insert.

Schumpelick: Do you think that the tension of the Shouldice repair is responsible for recurrences?

Bendavid: There is no doubt that a lot of people have stated that there is a lot of tension. I therefore do not hesitate to use a relaxing incision. It was never part of the original Shouldice repair, but I have certainly done it in over 2000 cases, and it is already a series to report. I have never seen one recurrence caused by a relaxing incision. I know that some surgeons do a relaxing incision and cover it with mesh. I have never had to do this. There is some tension, but it is really not that much because with time there is some relaxation of the tissue as well.

Devlin: In Europe, we work in general hospitals and see large numbers of acute femoral hernias; at least 50% of them are acute, and these are obviously not the same sort of cases that you are treating, they are very different. We are treating very different patient populations compared to Toronto. We must appreciate that the first principle of surgery is to do no harm. I therefore think that the Aachen classification and just operating on the type of hernia that presents is better than this massive opening of what you call the floor of the inguinal canal (we call it the posterior wall). To open it is probably adding to the problem and probably gives you some of these femoral hernias at follow-up in your cases.

Bendavid: Opening the posterior wall of the canal does not represent that much of an invasion, especially in a femoral hernia, and I must be very specific here: more than any other hernia, this is the one type of hernia where I will be most aggressive. There is no doubt in my mind, and I do not consider it an invasion. In fact timewise (I am considering the nature of the anesthetic), we are only talking about 10 min, and if you look at the emergencies, I think we should have an adequate examination.

Chevrel: Dr. Treutner, I saw on your slide 3% of chronic pain. I would like to know what the best treatment is for this chronic pain. What treatment do you use?

Treutner: The term "chronic pain" is often very hard to define because sometimes patients report chronic pain while in hospital or in the examination room, but when you look at them when they do not feel supervised they might carry out their work disregarding the pain. However, there is certainly a small number of patients with severe chronic pain. The first thing we do is to try to locate it and to treat it with repeated injections of local anesthetics. If this does not help, after a series of injections you have to consider a surgical reintervention with dissection of the ilioinguinal nerve.

Bendavid: I saw that in your series you reported 4.6% of hyperesthesia or anesthesia following surgery. We do not pay attention to the nerves. If they need to be divided, we do not hesitate to divide all the nerves, including the ilioinguinal/hypogastric block if they happen to be in the way or do not facilitate surgery. We have been cutting them very liberally. Following up a lot of these cases, we find that at the very most there is only an area which is no bigger than a 25-cent coin that is actually anesthetized. You can confirm this with a needle.

Treutner: The problem of hypesthesia is pointed out on the slides of our series just to mention all aspects of this topic. When you look at a number of studies, this problem is often disregarded completely. This is really a minor problem. Patients in their everyday life do not complain about it. Only if you especially ask about it and thus draw the patient's attention to this problem you might hear that there is a certain difference between the sensations between the right and left side. But this does not impair sports or hard labor.

Schumpelick: How many patients have been reoperated on because of chronic pain?

Treutner: None of the patients reported in this series.

References

1. Barwell, N.J.: The technique of Shouldice repair in Great Britain. in: Schumpelick V, Wantz GE (eds): "Inguinal hernia repair", Karger, Basel, 135 (1995)
2. Bassini, E.: Sulla cura radicale dell'ernia inguinale. Arch Soc Ital Chir 4: 380 (1887)
3. Glassow, F.: Inguinal hernia repair using local anaesthesia. Ann R Coll Surg Engl 66: 382 (1984)
4. Peiper, C., Töns, C., Schippers, E., Busch, F., Schumpelick, V.: Local versus general anesthesia for Shouldice repair of inguinal hernia. World J Surg 18: 912 (1994)
5. Schumpelick, V., Treutner, K.H., Arlt, G.: Inguinal hernia repair in adults. Lancet 344: 375 (1994)
6. Schumpelick, V., Treutner, K.H., Arlt, G.: Klassifikation von Inguinalhernien. Chirurg 65: 877 (1994)
7. Schumpelick, V.: Leistenbruchreparation nach Shouldice. Chirurg 55: 25 (1984)
8. Shouldice, E.E.: Surgical treatment of hernia. Ontario Med Rev 12: 43 (1945)
9. Töns, C., Kupczyk-Joeris, D., Pfingsten, F.P., Schumpelick, V.: Die Shouldice-Reparation als Qualitätsmaßstab für Neues in der Hernienchirurgie: Fünf-Jahres-Ergebnisse der prospektiven Shouldice-Studie für Primär- und Rezidivhernien. Langenbecks Arch Chir Suppl (Kongressbericht) 293 (1993)
10. Töns, C., Muck-Töns, A., Schumpelick, V.: Leistenhernienchirurgie in Deutschland 1992: Eine Umfrage an 1656 deutschen Kliniken. Chirurg 64: 635 (1993)
11. Truong, S.: Sonographie und Doppler-Sonographie. in: Schumpelick, V. "Hernien", Enke Verlag, Stuttgart, 1996, pp. 41–44
12. Wantz, G.E.: The Canadian repair: Personal observations. World J Surg 13: 516 (1989)

CHAPTER 34

Suture Repair of Recurrent Inguinal Hernia – A Review of the Literature

C. Töns

34.1 Introduction

In the past, many investigations have been published concerning surgical repair of recurrent inguinal hernia. However, many of these publications do not meet scientific standards and therefore cannot be used to define criteria of surgical approach to recurrent groin hernia.

To meet scientific standards, a study should include the following criteria:

- An exact and sufficiently high (more than 100) number of performed operations
- A defined and standardized repair technique
- A defined and standardized follow-up concept
- A sufficient follow-up period (at least 1 year) with repeated follow-up examinations (preferably by physical examination)
- A discrimination between short-term and long-term complications
- An exact re-recurrence rate

To give a current survey in the field of open approach in recurrent inguinal hernia surgery, a Medline research was performed. Between 1990 and 1998, 162 studies dealing with open surgery for recurrent inguinal hernias were published (Tables 1–3).

Altogether, only 47.5% of these papers display precise distinction regarding the outcome of the surgical procedure as mentioned above.

In about 14% of the investigations, more than 100 were treated and controlled during a follow-up period. In contrast, in about 61% of the studies, the exact number of treated patients is not mentioned.

Table 1. Literature quality: assessment of follow-up in 77 preselected publications from 1990 to 1998

Criterion	(%)
Time of follow-up	
No information	62.3
Not specific ("up to" etc.)	9.1
<1 year	1.3
1–4 years	19.5
>4 years	7.8%
Kind of follow-up	
No information	89.6
Questionnaire	1.3
Physical examination	9.1

Table 2. Sutured procedures without alloplastic augmentation

Procedure	Author	Year	Follow-up (n)	Time (years)	(%)	Kind	Re-recurences (%)
Bassini	Kux	1994	-	2	-	-	13.5
	Herzog	1990	295	-13	70	Q	30.0
	Guthy	1983	70	-11	97	PE	35.3
	Witte	1983	160	-10	-	PE	27.5
McVay	Alexandre	1996	142	?	?	?	0
	Barbier	1989	95	-17	71	PE/Q	9.5
	Rutledge	1988	127	-25	97	PE/Q	2.4
	Horn	1984	35	-8	?	PE	14.0
	Halverson	1970	580	-22	?	?	5.5
Transversalis repair	Kuttel	1991	124	>1	91.7	PE	5.9
	Chevalley	1989	394	0.5	76.0	Q	7.5
	Berliner	1984	171	2	100	?	4.3
Shouldice	Schippers	1996	197	5	83	PE	3.1
	e-Silva	1995	102	-10	66	?	4.9
	Kux	1994	-	2	-	-	7.6
	Jan	1992	22	-5	94	PE	4.5
	Wantz	1989	639	-18	-	?	7.2
	Berliner	1984	272	-11	-	PE/Q	5.9
	Obney	1984	1057	11	?	?	3.9
	Glassow	1984	2524	>10	?	PE/Q	2.5

PE, follow-up with physical examination; Q, follow-up using questionnaire.

Table 3. Open approach using alloplastic augmentation

Procedure	Author	Year	(n)	Time (years)	(%)	Kind	Re-recur rences (%)
Lichtenstein	Fuchsjäger	1995	55	2.5	?	?	3.6
	Gilbert	1997	412	2–5	88	?	0.24
	Rutkow	1998	1313	4	?	?	0
	Law	1990	52	-4	96	PE	10.0
Mesh plug	Lichtenstein	1993	1500	-5	87	?	1.6
	Amid	1992	1400	?	?	?	1.0
	Shulmann	1991	1402	?	90	?	2.0
TIPP/Rives	Schumpelick	1996	54	-2	95	PE	0
	Munegato	1992	121	?	?	?	5.7
	Bendavid	1992	280	5	?	?	3.2
	Flament	1993	586	10	90	?	1.7
Wantz	Hoffmann	1993	52	3.5	?	?	0.5
	Fong	1992	827	-10	?	PE	0.5
	Schaap	1992	98	-13	87	PE/Q	25.0
	Mozingo	1992	100	-5	92	PE/Q	3.0
Stoppa	Beets	1996	126	5.7	100	PE	1.0
	Langer	1996	58	2.9	100	?	12.0
	Wantz	1993	108	?	?	?	8.3
	Beaten	1990	150	-5.5	100	?	0.75
	Stoppa	1989	270	-10	75	?	1.1

TIPP, transinguinal preperitoneal prosthesis; PE, follow-up with physical examination; Q, follow-up using questionnaire.

A defined and standardized repair technique is used in 69% of the performed studies, while 12% use various techniques with only small study groups or without a classification. Finally, almost 20% specify the used repair method only superficially or not at all.

Even more shortcomings may be found when the follow-up data is presented. The length of the follow up-period is not presented in 62% of the articles. In about 8%, the follow up-period is of undefined length or its termination is described by "up to." Only about 30% of the investigations present a sufficient follow-up period of 1–4 years (21%) or more than 5 years (9%).

Besides the history-taking or a questionnaire, a physical examination should be included in every follow-up assessment. However, only 9% of the studies report the performance of a physical examination, while more than 90% of the authors do not specify the follow-up protocol.

The exact number of followed cases is reported in only 16% of the evaluated articles. Furthermore, some investigators present a follow-up rate of 100% over several years, which may indicate that suspicion is warranted.

In summary, the number of comparable and usable articles is small.

34.2 Results of the Open Approach

34.2.1 Bassini Technique

The recently published investigations by surgeons using the classical technique for repair of a recurrent groin hernia included a follow-up period of 10 years and a careful follow-up examination. A re-recurrence rate is reported in between 27.5% and 35% of the cases [9, 11, 29]. A lower recurrence rate of only 13.5% was reported by Kux [14]. However, the follow-up period in this study was only 2 years.

In conclusion, the re-recurrence rate using the Bassini repair is unacceptably high.

34.2.2 McVay Procedure

The other classical method of recurrent hernia repair is not used very frequently at present. A review of the literature does not lead to comparable results: Rutledge [20] and Halverson [10] found a low re-recurrence rate of 2.4%–5.5% after a follow-up period of 20 years, while Barbier [2] and Horn [13] reported a substantially increased number of relapses (9.5% and 14%, respectively).

34.2.3 Transversalis Repair

The recurrence rate of the transversalis repair method using a double-layer technique by continuously sutured fascia transversalis ranges between 4.3% and 7,5% [3, 5]. These are acceptable results; nevertheless, a follow-up period of 2 years does not permit a final conclusion.

34.2.4 Shouldice Technique

The use of the Shouldice technique to treat recurrent groin hernias has been carefully evaluated in numerous studies with high numbers of patients. A few well-known investigations with up to 2500 participating patients and an observation period of 10–18 years report a re-recurrence rate ranging between 2.5% and 7%. Relevant studies performed in nonspecialized hospitals reported a recurrence rate no higher than 4.5% and 7.6% when the Shouldice method was applied to recurrent groin hernias.

A completely different approach is the use of alloplastic material in the repair of recurrent hernia.

34.2.5 Lichtenstein Technique

If the mesh is used with the onlay technique using the inguinal approach, the currently reported recurrence rates vary. The rate ranges between almost 0% [19] and 10% [15], which may be explained by the very different case numbers and follow-up concepts.

34.2.6 Mesh Plug

Excellent results are reported when the mesh-plug method is used in specialized centers. These centers report recurrence rates of less than 2%; however, in some cases, the follow-up protocol has not been specified sufficiently.

34.2.7 Preperitoneal Mesh Layer Using the Inguinal Approach (Transinguinal Preperitoneal Prosthesis/Rives Procedure)

In selected cases, some surgeons advocate a preperitoneal alloplastic augmentation of the fascia transversalis. Although this has been performed in highly selected and problematic patients, the re-recurrence rate after a 10-year observation period was no higher than 0%–5.7%.

34.2.8
Preperitoneal Mesh Layer Using the Extrainguinal Approach (Wantz Technique)

When a preperitoneal approach cranial to the inguinal canal is used with preperitoneal mesh implantation, the re-recurrence rate ranges between 0.5% and 5.3% after an observation period of up to 10 years [6, 12, 17]. In contrast to these favorable results, Schaap et al. [21] demonstrated an unacceptably high recurrence rate of 25% after a follow-up of 13 years. All study groups used a follow-up protocol including physical examination and a questionnaire.

34.2.9
Stoppa Procedure

Divergent results are also reported for the Stoppa technique. Some authors report excellent recurrence rates of 1% after up to 10 years of follow up [26], whereas others found recurrence rates of 8.3%–12.0%.

34.3
Conclusion

With respect to the surgical approach to recurrence groin hernia, a review of the literature does not lead to definite answers. This is mainly due to the fact that many articles cannot be use, since fundamental scientific standards are not met. However, even if standards are met, as mentioned above, the results still remain divergent.

The Shouldice repair of recurrent groin hernias is certainly the best evaluated method, as numerous studies with high numbers of patients have been performed. The recurrence rates ranged between 2.5% and 7%. Relevant studies performed in nonspecialized hospitals reported a recurrence rate no higher than 4.5%–7.6%.

These results were only surpassed when alloplastic material was used. The method of alloplastic augmentation bears obvious advantages in selected cases. The divergent results of the performed investigations, however, point to persisting substantial technical problems.

Several questions remain to be answered, including the kind of recurrent groin hernia that really needs alloplastic augmentation and which material should be used and which technique.

After standardized techniques have been established, even nonspecialized centers should be given the opportunity to use alloplastic material safely in appropriate cases and using a proper technique with proven material.

34.4
Discussion

Amid: One of your slides showed a recurrence rate of 1.6% reported by Lichtenstein. I just want to mention that the recurrence rate is for the time that Dr. Lichtenstein was doing tissue repair. It does not reflect the recurrence rate of the tension-free repair. Also, for the method of follow-up for Lichtenstein and myself, you have a question mark, which means you could not establish which method of follow-up was used. I find this surprising, because our method of follow-up was published in the *American Journal of Surgery*. It is a computerized system but involves physician examination, and it was published in 1987. I am surprised that you have not come across that.

Töns: I think it was in older studies, and I did not find those papers. I do not remember the exact year, but it was not described in these papers.

Amid: I will give you a copy of the most recent article in *Der Chirurg*, where the method of follow-up is also described.

Jeekel: You have seen the whole literature. I would like to have an opinion from you on what the best treatment is for recurrent hernia, also taking into consideration the ease of the technique (mesh might be much easier) and what it means to the patient postoperatively.

Töns: It is not a good thing for research to ask for an opinion, but we have no better alternative. There are no studies that have been really well done. Third recurrence and MIII should be tested with the Shouldice against the TIPP procedure. So I can give you only my personal opinion. In a first recurrence with a smaller gap, I would prefer Shouldice repair with local anesthesia. If it is a recurrence that has already occurred more often, I would place a preperitoneal mesh using the inguinal procedure. And if recurrence has already occurred more often on both sides, I would do a Stoppa procedure.

Nilsson: You have gone through the literature and you have commented on the ways of following up hernia patients. What advice would you give to the general surgeon in a large or middle-sized hospital on how patients should be followed up? We know that is almost impossible year after year to ask patients in a rigorous manner to come back. How do we get the information? Have you any suggestions?

Töns: I think the best way is physical examination if the people are living close to the hospital. We would try to do it after 1 and 5 years at least. If you are unable to do a physical examination, you can call them and ask them on the phone, not by a questionnaire, and ask people who have doubts about their answers to come in for a physical examination.

Nilsson: So as a second alternative, you would choose questionnaires with selective follow-up depending on the questionnaire?

Töns: A phone call is better than a questionnaire.

Filipi: Some of the patients are going to be a distance away from the surgeon, but I think the best way, especially for reluctant patients, is a house call, i.e., to go out to the house and examine the patient. I know that it is not en vogue these days, but a house call is still appropriate under some circumstances.

References

1. Amid, P.K., Shulman, A.G., & Lichtenstein, I.L. (1993). Critical scrutiny of the open "tension-free" hernioplasty. Am J Surg, 165, 369–371.
2. Barbier, J., Carretier, M., & Richer Jp. (1989). Cooper Ligament Repair: An Update. 01 XV 413 World J Surg, 13, 499–505.
3. Berliner, S.D. (1984). An Approach Of Groin Hernia. 01 XV 062 Surg Clin North Am, 64, 197–213.
4. Berliner, S.D. (1993). Clinical experience with an inlay expanded polytetrafluoroethylene soft tissue patch as an adjunct in inguinal hernia repair. Surg Gynecol Ostet, 176, 323–326.
5. Chevalley, J.P., Rothenbühler, J.M., & Harder, F. (1989). Erste Erfahrungen mit der Transversalisplastik in der Behandlung der Leistenhernie. Helv Chir Acta, 56, 221–224.
6. Fong, Y., & Wantz, G.E. (1992). Prevention of ischemic orchitis during inguinal hernioplasty. Surg Gynecol Ostet, 174, 399–402.
7. Gilbert, A.I. (1992). Sutureless repair of inguinal hernia. Am J Surg, 163, 331–335.
8. Glassow, F. (1984). Inguinal Hernia Repair Using Local Anaesthesia. 01 XV 020 Ann Roy Coll Surg Engl, 66, 382–387.
9. Guthy, E., & V.D.Boom, H. (1983). Das Mehrfachrezidiv beim Leistbruch. 01 XV 362 Langenbecks Arch Chir, 361, 315–318.
10. Halverson, K., & Mc Vay, C.B. (1970). Inguinal And Femoral Hernioplasty. 01 XV 088 Arch Surg, 101, 127–135.
11. Herzog, U. (1990). Das Leistenhernienrezidiv. Schw Rundschau Med (Praxis), 79, 1166–1169.
12. Hoffman, H.C., & Traverso, A.L.V. (1993). Preperitoneal prosthetic herniorrhaphy. Arch Surg, 128, 964–969.
13. Horn, J., & Paetz, B. (1984). Rezidiveingriffe nach Leisten- und Schenkelbrucheingriffen. 01 XV 130 Chirurg, 55, 558–563.
14. Kux, M., Fuchsjäger, N., & Hirbawi, A. (1993). Verstärkung des Peritonealsacks mittels großer Prothese (Operation nach Stoppa). Chirurg, 64, 329–333.
15. Law, N.W., & Ellis, H. (1990). Preliminary results for the repair of difficult recurrent inguinal hernias using expanded PTFE patch. Acta Chir Scand, 156, 609–612.
16. Lichtenstein, I.L., Shulman, A.G., & Amid, P.K. (1993). The cause, prevention and treatment of recurrent groin hernia. Surg Cl of North Am, 73, 529–544.
17. Mozingo, D., Walters, J., Otchy, D., & Rosenthal, D. (1992). Properitoneal synthetic mesh repair of recurrent inguinal hernias. Surg Gynecol Ostet, 174, 33–35.
18. Obney, N. (1984). Application Of Shouldice Technique In Large Scrotal Hernias And Sliding Hernias. 01 XV 406 Contemporary Surg, 25, 11–16.
19. Rutkow, I.M., & Robbins, A.W. (1993). "Tension-free" inguinal herniorrhaphy: a preliminary report on the "mesh plug" technique. Surgery, 114, 3–8.
20. Rutledge, R.H. (1993). The cooper ligament repair. Surg Cl of North Am, 73, 471–484.
21. Schaap, H.M., van de Pavoordt, H., & Bast, T.J. (1992). The preperitoneal approach in the repair of recurrent inguinal hernias. Surg Gynecol Ostet, 174, 460–464.
22. Schumpelick, V., Kupczyk-Joeris, D., Töns, C., & Pfingsten, F.P. (1990). Reparation der Rezidivleistenhernie. Taktik, Technik und Ergebnisse. Chirurg, 61, 526–529.
23. Schumpelick, V., Treutner, K.H., & Arlt, G. (1994). Inguinal hernia repair in adults. Lancet, 344, 375–379.
24. Shulman, A.G., Amid, P.K., & Lichtenstein, I.L. (1990). The 'Plug' Repair Of 1402 Recurrent Inguinal Hernias. 20-Year Experience. Arch Surg, 125, 265–267.
25. Shulman, A.G., Amid, P.K., & Lichtenstein, I.L. (1992). Prosthetic mesh plug repair of femoral and recurrent inguinal hernias: the American experience. Ann R Coll Surg Engl, 74, 97–99.
26. Stoppa, R.E., & Verhaeghe, P. (1995). Results after Stoppa Procedure. In V. Schumpelick & G.E. Wantz (Eds.), Inguinal hernia repair. (pp. 399–402). Basel: Karger Verl.
27 Wantz, G.E. (1989). The Canadian Repair: Personal Observations. 01 XV 414 World J Surg, 13, 516–521.
28. Wantz, G.E. (1995). The technique of giant prosthetic reinforcement of the visceral sac performed through an anterior groin incision. Surg Gynecol Ostet, 176, 497–500.
29. Witte, J. (1983). Die Rezidivleistenhernie im Erwachsenenalter; Operationsindikation, Verfahrenswahl, Ergebnisse. 01 XV 361 Langenbecks Arch Chir, 361, 309–313.

CHAPTER 35

Causes and Treatment of Recurrent Inguinal Hernias

P.K. Amid

Recurrent inguinal hernias can be grouped into two broad categories: recurrence after tissue approximation repair and recurrence after mesh repair.

Recurrence after tissue approximation repair is caused by (a) tissue failure due to degenerative nature of inguinal hernias and (b) technical failure such as tension at the suture line. Recurrence after mesh repair is caused by: (a) mesh failure such as shrinkage of prosthetic materials [1] and (b) technical failures such as inadequate mesh size, inadequate mesh fixation, inadequate overlap (mesh tissue interface beyond the inguinal floor), inadequate laxity of the mesh (to account for the increase in intra-abdominal pressure and future shrinkage of the mesh), and inadequate dissection and exploration.

35.1 Treatment

For more than 20 years, our preferred method of repairing recurrent inguinal hernias was the mesh plug technique. The idea of the mesh plug technique was based on the assumption that the recurrent inguinal hernias occur through a single defect in an otherwise intact inguinal floor, requiring minimal dissection limited to the area of the defect for the repair. This assumption was proved wrong by Greenburg's study, which showed that 10% of the recurrent inguinal hernias consisted of more than one defect [2]. Furthermore, insertion of a plug behind the fascia transversalis and into the small space of Bogros places the plug in close proximity to the iliac vessels. Figure 1 shows a collapsed preformed mesh plug (Perfix plug) herniated from the internal ring into the inguinal canal with its base firmly attached to the iliac vein, requiring operative room consultation with a vascular surgeon for its removal. In addition, erosion of the plug into the iliac artery has been reported [3]. Therefore, because of the failure of the mesh plug repair due to (a) missing a second defect as a result of inadequate dissection, (b) failure of the repair due to shrinkage of the plug (see Chap. 13, Fig. 3), and more importantly (c) due to serious complications such as migration of the rock-hard and abrasive shrunken plug into the inguinal canal (Fig. 1) and scrotum(Fig. 2) and erosion of the plug into the bladder [1], intestines [4], and iliac vessels[3], the mesh plug repair was completely abandoned in 1996 and all recurrent inguinal hernias were repaired by the tension-free patch technique, similar to the repair of primary inguinal hernias.

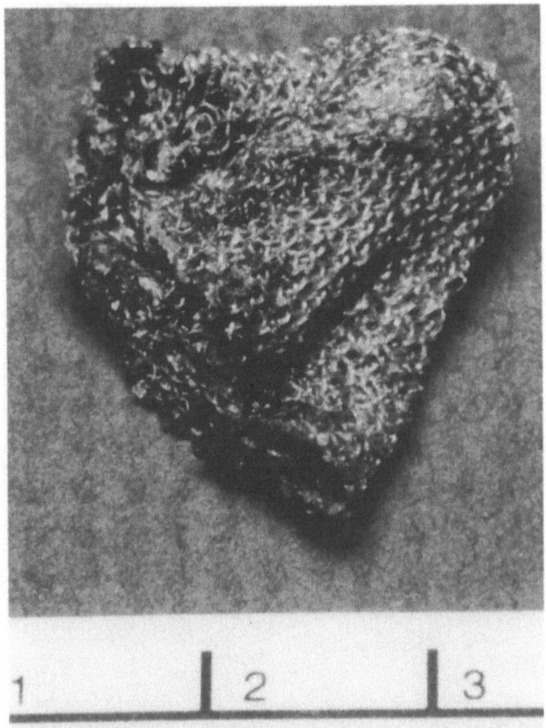

Fig. 1. Shrunken Perfix mesh plug herniated through the internal ring into the inguinal canal removed after its separation from the iliac vein

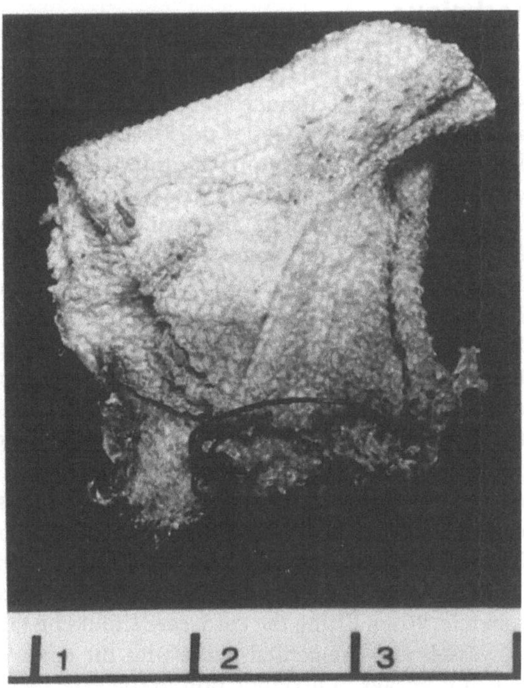

Fig. 2. A shrunken Perfix mesh plug removed from the patient's scrotum

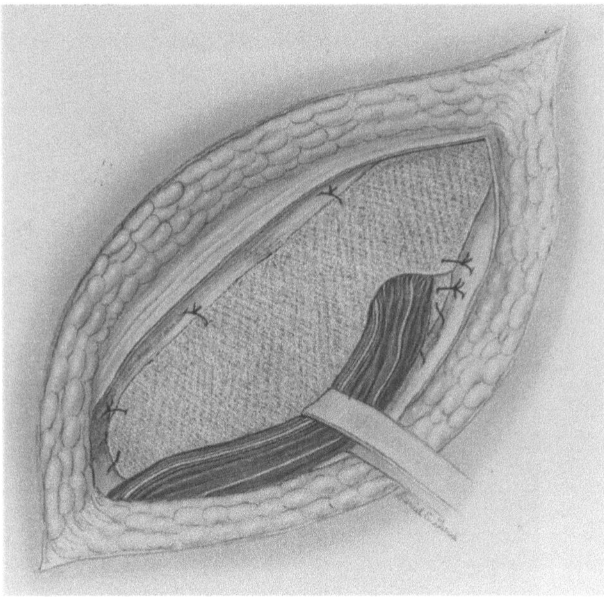

Fig. 3. Complete reinforcement of the inguinal canal with an adequate mesh–tissue interface and construction of a new internal ring

35.2 Technique

The tension-free procedure is performed under local anesthesia administered in a simple four-step technique [5] and consists of reinforcement of the inguinal floor by an adequately large sheet of prosthesis in order to provide a sufficient tissue–mesh interface beyond the inguinal floor [6] (Fig. 3). As a result, the entire inguinal floor is completely and permanently protected from all future mechanical or degenerative adverse affects. Therefore, the operation has a dual effect, therapeutic and prophylactic. A 5-cm skin incision, which starts from the pubic tubercle and extends laterally within the Langer's line, gives an excellent exposure of the pubic tubercle and the internal ring. After skin incision, the external oblique aponeurosis is opened and its lower leaf freed from the spermatic cord. The upper leaf of the external oblique is then freed from the underlying internal oblique muscle and aponeurosis for a distance of 3 cm above the inguinal floor. The anatomical cleavage between these two layers is avascular, and the dissection can be done rapidly and nontraumatically. High separation of these layers has a dual benefit, as it visualizes the iliohypogastric nerve and creates ample space for insertion of a sufficiently wide sheet of mesh that can overlap the internal oblique by at least 3 cm above the upper margin of the inguinal floor. The cord with its cremaster covering is separated from the floor of the inguinal canal and the pubic bone for a distance of about 2 cm beyond the pubic tubercle. When lifting the cord, care should be taken to include the external spermatic vessels and the genital nerve with the cord. This ensures that the genital nerve, which is always in juxtaposition to the external spermatic vessels, is preserved. The ilioinguinal and iliohypogastric nerves should also be preserved. To explore the internal ring, for indirect hernia sacs, the cremasteric sheath is incised transversely (if thick) or longitudinally at the level of the deep ring. Indirect hernial sacs are freed from the cord to a point beyond the neck of the sac and inverted into the abdomen without ligation. In the event of direct hernias, if large, the direct sacs are inverted with an absorbable suture. A sheet of mesh 8x16 cm is used. The preferred choice of mesh is one of the monofilament polypropylene meshes (such as Atrium, Marlex, Prolene, Surgipro "monofilament," and Trilex), because their surface texture promotes fibroplasia and their monofilamented structure does not promote or harbor infection [1]. The medial end of the mesh is rounded to the shape of the medial corner of the inguinal canal. With the cord retracted upwards, the rounded corner is sutured with a nonabsorbable monofilamented suture material to the aponeurotic tissue over the pubic bone, overlapping the bone by 1–1.5 cm. The periosteum of the bone is avoided. This suture is continued (as a continuous suture with up to five passages) to attach the lower edge of the patch to the inguinal ligament up to a point just lateral to the internal ring. If there is a concurrent femoral hernia, the mesh is also sutured to Cooper's ligament 1–2 cm below its suture line, with the inguinal ligament to close the femoral ring. A slit is made at the lateral end of the mesh creating two tails, a wide one (two thirds) above and a narrower (one third) below. The upper wide tail is grasped with a hemostat and passed toward the head of the patient from underneath the spermatic cord; this positions the cord between the two tails of the mesh. The wider upper tail is crossed and placed over the narrower one and held with a hemostat. With the cord retracted downward and the upper leaf of the external oblique aponeurosis retracted upward, the upper edge of the patch is sutured in place with two interrupted absorbable sutures, one to the rectus sheath and the other to the internal oblique aponeurosis, just lateral to the internal ring. Using a single nonabsorbable monofilamented suture, the lower edges of each of the two tails are fixed to the inguinal ligament just lateral to the completion knot of the lower running suture.

This creates a new internal ring made of mesh. The excess patch on the lateral side is trimmed, leaving at least 5 cm of mesh beyond the internal ring. This is tucked underneath the external oblique aponeurosis, which is then closed over the cord with an absorbable suture.

Since 1992, 360 recurrent inguinal hernias have been repaired utilizing Lichtenstein's tension-free patch technique; except for large, nonreducible hernias, all operations were performed under local anesthesia. The patients were discharged from the hospital between 1–3 h after the operation. The postoperative analgesic requirement was 0–20 tablets (mean, eight) of hydrocodone or Ibuprofen. Return to routine daily activities or unrestricted work activities was possible 2–14 days depending on the patient's occupation. Complications included less than 1% wound infection and seroma formation, and one case of orchitis, which did not lead to testicular atrophy. There was one recurrence in the parapubic region in a patient who had a previous open prostatectomy. Similar results have been reported by Horeyseck in a series of 115 Lichtenstein patch operations for the repair of recurrent inguinal hernias [7].

35.3 Discussion

For a discussion, please see Chap. 36.

References

1. Amid PK. Classification of biomaterials and their related complications in abdominal wall hernia surgery. Hernia 1:12–19,1997.
2. Greenburg AG. Revisiting the recurrent groin hernia. Am J Surg 154:35–40,1987.
3. Cristaldi M, Pisacreta M, Elli M, et al. Femoro-poplieteal by-pass occlusion following mesh-plug for prevascular femoral hernia repair. Hernia 1(4):195–199,1997.
4. Danielli PG, Kurihara H, Montecamozzo G, et al. Le complicanze dei plugs: Infezioni e recidive. Hernia 1(1):55,1997.
5. Amid PK, Shulman AG, Lichtenstein IL. Local anesthesia for inguinal hernia repair step-by-step procedure. Ann Surg 220(6):735–737,1994.
6. Amid PK, Lichtenstein IL. Aktuelle Einschätzung der spannungsfreien hernienreparation nach Lichtenstein. Chirurg 68:959–964,1997.
7. Horeyseck G, Pohl C. Lichtenstein-patch repair of recurrent inguinal hernia. Hernia 2(1):S6,1998.

CHAPTER 36

European Experience with the Lichtenstein Repair for Recurrent Inguinal Hernia

A.N. Kingsnorth

36.1 Introduction

Except for one abstract presented at the American Hernia Society in 1998, there are no published results from European centres concerning the experience with the classical Lichtenstein patch repair for recurrent inguinal hernia. A postal survey of expert herniologists undertaken in Europe revealed results from only three countries, i.e. Sweden, Germany and England.

It is several years since Chevrel observed that, although the present tendency is increasingly towards the use of pre-peritoneal prostheses in France, there is still room for re-operative surgery by the inguinal route incorporating a prosthesis in some cases [1]. However, before any further discussion on this topic, it is worth considering a proposed classification and surgical strategy for treating recurrent inguinal hernia proposed by Campanelli and colleagues in 1996[2]. An R1 recurrence is a first relapse of an indirect type less than 2 cm in size in a non-obese patient, and the plug operation was recommended for this type. An R2 recurrence is a first relapse of a direct type less than 2 cm in size in a non-obese patient, and the pre-peritoneal unilateral Wantz/Trabucco repair was recommended in this type. The R3 recurrence covers all other types, for which the Stoppa technique or laparoscopic repair was recommended.

36.2 Lichtenstein Plug Operation

The Lichtenstein plug operation is not the classic Lichtenstein patch repair, but will be considered briefly to discard it as a major strategy for utilisation in the repair of recurrent inguinal hernias. The plug is a cylindrical polypropylene prosthesis consisting of a rolled-up length of prosthesis measuring approximately 5x20 cm. Fuchsjager and colleagues repaired 55 recurrent inguinal hernias out of a total of 245 recurrences during the period 1990–1994[3]. At a median follow-up of 30 months, two hernias had re-recurred (3.6%). The authors recommended that the plug repair was suitable for stage 1 and 2 recurrences (St. Moritz I classification) with a maximal defect of 2–3 cm.

36.3 Lichtenstein Patch Repair

Not satisfied with the plug operation, Horeyseck and colleagues concluded that it was unsuitable for the majority of recurrent inguinal hernias because the defect is a hole in a flat surface rather than a tunnel [4]. During the period 1993–1997, 115 patients had recurrent inguinal hernias repaired by the Lichtenstein operation. Of these 60 were indirect, 43 direct, ten pantaloon and four femoral; 94 were first-time recurrences, of which nine had been initially laparoscopic repairs. A total of 25 operations were performed under local anaesthesia. At a median follow-up of 23 months, there were no recurrences; there were four complications, of which one was an ischaemic orchitis and one a neuralgia.

The present author's personal experience from 1992 to 1997 is as follows: of 156 patients treated for recurrent inguinal hernia, 48 underwent Lichtenstein patch repair (31%). These patients were selected on the basis that the recurrence was a first-time recurrence, the first operation had been uncomplicated, mesh had not been used and the hernia was clinically small and reducible. Only 62% of patients were followed up, at a median of 37 months. One recurrence was found, which was a lateral recurrence in an obese patient. The complications included three patients with ischaemic orchitis (6%) and four with a significant neuralgia (8%).

Nilsson reported the results from the 1992–1996 Swedish register by personal communication. During that period, 2050 operations were performed for recurrent inguinal hernia, and the method utilised was classified as being Lichtenstein or mesh operation in 359 patients. Of these, the Lichtenstein operation was specifically identified as the method in 136 patients, and mesh alone was identified as the method in 223

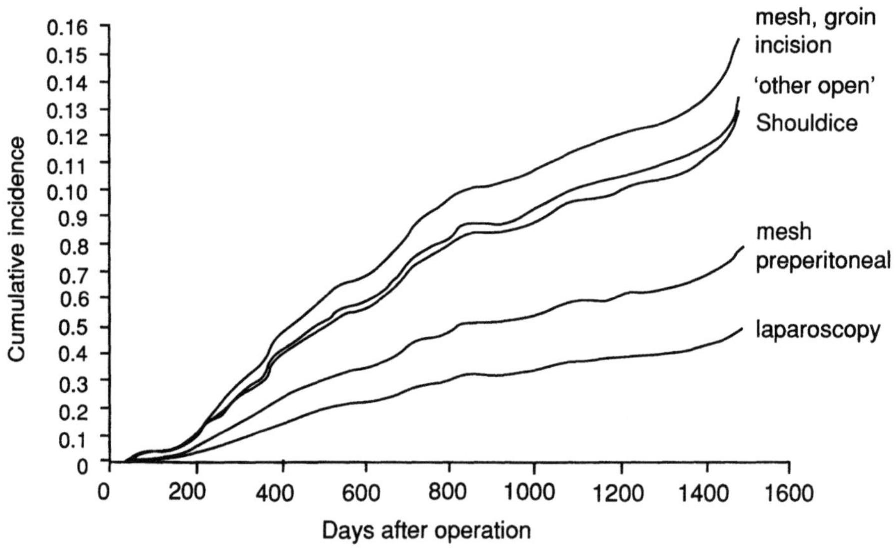

Fig. 1. Risk of recurrence following operation for recurrent hernia

patients. At 3 years, the cumulative instance of re-operation was 13%. By comparison, the re-recurrence for other methods was 7.5% in 316 patients where pre-peritoneal mesh had been applied and 4.5% in 444 patients in whom the laparoscopic method was used (Fig. 1).

36.4 Conclusion

In conclusion, the European experience with the Lichtenstein repair for recurrent inguinal hernia provides insufficient data to make specific recommendations. However, the preliminary data suggests that, in the excessively scarred groin or where mesh has been utilised in a previous repair, such situations may be contraindications. There is a need for classification of recurrences so that the repair utilised may match the type of recurrence.

36.5 Discussion

Read: I was interested in your historic reference, Dr. Amid. I think that the paper Dr. Wantz sent you was written by Sheetle in 1921. There was another surgeon who was plugging before Sheetle, and that was Dr. Kelly at Johns Hopkins, who put a marble into the femoral canal in 1896; he was very proud of this. His approach was the intra-abdominal approach, because as a gynaecologist he was operating on the ovaries, and if he found an incidental femoral hernia he put a marble into the femoral canal. I think that is an earlier plug than Sheetle's saphenous vein.

Jeekel: Dr. Amid, you presented some data which where sort of casuistic, and you had a problem with the bladder where the hard plug was introduced. That is so incidental, I think, that I am not sure that it has ever been presented in the literature. But were there no other reasons for changing your method? What was the incidence of recurrence after the plug, and did that change your ideas?

Amid: First let me tell you that there are actually more cases reported. There is a report from the University of Milan by Dan Jely about two or three erosions of the plug into the intestine in the last issue of Prof. Chevrel's book. There is one report of intestinal erosion by Arthur Gilbert. I showed you the one where the plug was eroded into the femoral artery. Now, why did we change our method? Let me give you an example. For many years, for the repair of incisional hernias we put Marlex mesh in, until we started seeing scattered isolated reports of intestinal fistula. Even at this time, if you do a thorough search you will not find more than, say, 20 or 30 isolated reports of intestinal fistula from putting mesh inside the abdominal cavity. We stopped doing that based on these isolated cases, because in the USA, if I put mesh inside the abdominal cavity and someone gets a fistula, I have no excuse. There are now reported cases of plug erosion into the different organs, and if I get one of those complications, legally I have no excuse. The recurrence rate in the original paper we published on plug repair was about 2.4%, but that was before we started seeing more and more recurrences. I think the overall recurrence rate is about 4%–5% of the old plug repairs that we did.

Jeekel: Dr. Kingsnorth, why are you so keen to have a staging procedure? Perhaps there is a method that covers any recurrent hernia? Why do you want to have a perfect staging? I can see that it is easier to read the literature if you know that it is comparable with a hernia that you are treating, but there might be a treatment that covers any stage.

Kingsnorth: I think it is essential for outcome studies to stratify patients, because we cannot compare a tiny little medial recurrence with some huge inguinal-scrotal recurrence. I think we have to stratify the groups and look at the outcomes in terms of the treatments, and I think most of us probably would agree that are a variety of options open to treating recurrent inguinal hernias.

Jeekel: I do agree, I asked the question because I wanted to hear your arguments. Is there not a possibility that it is more complicated than staging, that it is a kind of progress in weakness of the wall and more like a disease than one stage at a certain time?

Kingsnorth: Yes, I think I agree with that. Again, a personal opinion, I do not believe the plug is suitable for direct inguinal hernias or particular recurrences because the posterior wall collapses with age. Once it has given way in one area, I feel that there is a great potential for giving way in another area. So hernias get bigger and press.

Muschawek: You told us there are often two small defects in the posterior wall. Do you then put two plugs into these two separate defects? Surely the main point is where you put the umbrella in and where you do the suture, in which layer? The original technique is to put the umbrella in the hole and make four single sutures in the muscle. I think this is one of the points where the umbrella can go. I have never had to remove an umbrella.

Amid: Well, let me answer your first question. When we were doing plug repair, we never used more than one plug. If we encountered two defects, we did a formal patch repair. With regard to insertion of the sutures, those are all related to movement of the plug and recurrence of the hernia. And that is not really my main concern, because we can live with recurrence. The plug that went to the bladder was exactly in the same place that my partner put it. It did not leave its original place to go to the bladder. These are not migrations, they are erosions. The plug is next to the femoral artery, and it does not leave its place and migrate, it just erodes into it.

Muschawek: So you have to know where to put a plug in and where to make a suture?

Amid: In the space of Bogros, because of the size of that space is, if you put a plug there, you are close to all these structures, the bladder and the vessels. If you put a plug into the internal ring, especially in a sliding hernia, the plug is right over the bowel. I do not really know a way to put a plug into the small space of Bogros and make sure that it is not close to the bladder or a major vessel.

Schumpelick: Do we have really proven, controlled 10-year follow-up data concerning Lichtenstein recurrence rates? I missed your data; you did not show your long-term results.

Amid: You mean Lichtenstein repair of recurrent hernia? We really do not have a good track of those isolated Lichtenstein patches that we did while we were doing plug operations. But from 1992, which is when we started doing much more patch operations, we do have an accurate follow-up. In 360 operations, we had only one recurrence.

Schumpelick: I asked this question because I have seen your figures and those of Horasek, in the last 2 years I reoperated in at least 25 cases after a so-called Lichtenstein repair in Europe. There is a switch to Lichtenstein because it is easy, not harmful and less invasive. I even operated on two of Horasek's cases that I did not see on the slides. Is it justified at the moment to switch completely to the Lichtenstein repair in Europe on the basis of the data currently available?

Kingsnorth: For recurrent inguinal hernia, I do not think it is. There is a very small amount of data in terms of outcomes. I am certainly backing off it because of my problems with ischemic orchitis.

Schumpelick: I was impressed by the last slide showing the difference pre-peritoneal and Lichtenstein approach. There was a big difference between those. In Miami, there was a paper from your clinic, Dr. Read, showing that there is no difference. Can you explain this, because it was the first prospective trial?

Read: That was not in recurrent hernia, it was in primary hernia.

Amid: Approximately 20%–25% of the operations we do are for recurrence. And I make every effort to study the original surgeon's report. It is unbelievable to see what surgeons do and then call it a Lichtentein operation. As you know, before 1984 Lichtenstein was doing a Bassini procedure with a relaxing incision for indirect hernia and mesh for direct hernia. That is called a Lichtenstein operation. A plug operation is called a Lichtenstein operation. Every time a surgeon uses a piece of mesh, it automatically becomes the Lichtenstein operation. In those cases the surgeon classifies as a Lichtenstein operation, the surgeon usually uses a 1x4-inch mesh. I am talking about the real Lichtenstein operation based on the publications after 1992. Because anything before 1992 was a preliminary report, and at that time we used only a 5-cm mesh. So people who are well trained and know exactly how to do the operation do get good results. It is important to know what is meant by the Lichtenstein operation.

Klinge: Do you have any age restrictions for the patients receiving meshes?

Kingsnorth: No, I do not. If you look at the age incidence of hernias, you see that there is a big peak in infancy which then drops off to a trough after the age of 2 years. And the peak age for the incidence of a hernia is between the ages of 55 and 85. I usually get asked the question what I would do about an 18-year-old. The incidence in 18-year-olds is minute. You might operate on one 18-year-old with an inguinal hernia in a year. I probably do not even operate on one a year. So we are talking about very small numbers of patients here, inguinal hernias at a young age. And I would agree that some of them just have a very small internal ring and a small indirect sack, and I think it is appropriate for them just to close the ring and do nothing more. But certainly in any hospital where I have worked, many people neglected hernias. So you sometimes get a young man in his twenties who presents with a large inguinal-scrotal hernia. I would definitely put mesh in. So I think it is not the age I look at, it is the type of hernia.

Amid: We do not use mesh in patients younger than 18–20 years old. You want to see the patient fully grown. And if you ask me why – I really do not know.

Jeekel: If you look for a technique of surgery, you should look at a technique that is easy for the patients and easy for the surgeon and has good results. We are moving toward laparosocopic surgery because it is easier for the patient and I am sure we are moving toward the Lichtenstein technique, because it is easy for both the patient and the surgeon. When we look at results, we should look at results where the general surgical population is doing well and not a group of surgeons which are very experienced and can do difficult operations and have nice results. Shouldn't we really look at the Lichtenstein operation? And I am convinced that in the future it will have to be either the laparoscopic or the Lichtenstein procedure. I think that is where we have to compare the results. We did a prospective randomized study and finished it 2 years ago; we will look at the data 1 year from now comparing the Lichtenstein to the Bassini/McVay technique for primary and recurrent hernia. So in 1 year we will know in a prospective manner whether the Lichtenstein procedure is better than the Bassini/McVay technique. But shouldn't we really look at the laparoscopic versus the Lichtenstein technique, and isn't the older Shouldice technique too difficult for most surgeons in general practice?

Kingsnorth: I have to disagree with just about everything you just said. The laparoscopic operation is a very difficult operation for the surgeon. It has a long learning curve, and we do not let our trainees undertake the operation unsupervised. While I am here at this conference for a week, I am perfectly happy for my residents to be doing Lichtenstein operations unsupervised on their own, and I know they will have a good outcome because they are well trained. It is a difficult operation for the patient as well. I do not think it is an easier operation, particularly because there are many of us here who can do the Lichtenstein operation very simply under local anaesthesia and have patients out of the hospital in 2–4 h. And certainly our data indicate that 80% of our patients are not taking analgesics after 24 h. We have to have a prospective double-blind randomized trial. It can be done, because it has been done for cholecystectomy. I do not believe that laparoscopy is the future for hernia repair.

Skandalakis: I do not think that we can say dogmatically that we have to do one or the other. The virginity in this area is gone totally and completely, so I think it wrong to say that this is always the right procedure. We have to choose the procedure that the local catastrophe permits us to do. I agree with you about the laparoscopic procedure, although I have no experience there. But just to say that the Lichtenstein operation is the only procedure that we can do on recurrence is wrong, although I have a profound respect for my friend Amid.

Amid: I do not think that is the only procedure to be done. The fear of testicular injury with anterior repair for recurrent hernia belongs to tissue repair, because when we do tissue repair, we are dealing with two different tissues, spermatic cord (we cannot compromise that) and the fibroconnective tissue (and we cannot compromise that either). So we have to be in between just when we do lysis of adhesions. But if we do mesh repair, we do not care about fibroconnective tissue of the groin. We can stay away from the cord and compromise tissue for the sake of the cord; this is the same thing as you do in bowel lysis, where you compromise peritoneum for the sake of the bowel. So you stay away from the cord and compromise the tissue. Of course, you do not have any tissue to close, but you do not need that tissue because you are using mesh. That is why I think you do not have testicular problems with the recurrent operation because we make a wide berth around the cord. And we had only one case of orchitis which did not lead to testicular atrophy in these 360 patients.

Skandalakis: Imagine you have an debilitated old man like me and I have a second or third recurrence. Are you going to remove my testicle?

Amid: No, there is no reason to.

Kingsnorth: My previous comments applied to primary hernias. For recurrent inguinal hernia, I think there is a lot of debate we need to progress through in terms of the different techniques and the different types of recurrence. And I am not advocating the Lichtenstein patch operation for all recurrences. It can be done in selected cases. Laparoscopy I do believe has a role to play because I believe recurrences should be in the hands of experts. And therefore I think there is a place for the laparoscopic expert in repairing recurrent inguinal hernias. Likewise, I think that the pre-peritoneal operations are not as simple as a lot of people make out. Again, I think recurrences by the pre-peritoneal route should be done by experts. So I think there are different types of recurrences, and people with a special interest should be repairing them. There is a variety of techniques out there, and we have got to find out which technique suits which type of recurrence.

Bendavid: There has been such an emphasis on what you are doing when you do a Lichtenstein repair. And yet it is the simplest procedure; it takes 15 min and there is absolutely nothing to it as long as you cover the floor of the canal.

Amid: There is a difference between knowing how to do something and being able to do it after you know how to do it. Let's take laparoscopic repair as an example. After you know how to do a laparoscopic repair by reading several articles and watching experts doing it, when you start doing it you still have a learning curve. But with a Lichtenstein repair, as long as you know how to do it, and all it takes is reading five articles or watching one video, then you can do it. In those cases that I tell you people call a Lichtenstein operation and when you read the operative report you find it was not a Lichtenstein operation and you read that the surgeon used a little tiny mesh or did not fix the mesh where it is supposed to be fixed, that is not a learning curve, that is not knowing how to do it. That is the difference between the two.

Kingsnorth: I am very disappointed in human nature. You can get surgeons out there who mess up the simplest operation. Whether the Lichtenstein operation is messed up less often than any other remains to be seen. I agree with you, people put scrubby little bits of mesh in and then put them improperly or stitch them in there and call it a Lichtenstein patch operation, which it clearly is not. I think that the results of a genuine Lichtenstein operation, which is relatively simple compared with other techniques, are excellent. But a long-term follow-up outside the Lichtenstein Clinic is not yet available.

Simmermacher: I fully agree with Skandalakis, who said that you should not be dogmatic. You should consider whether to place a mesh using the anterior or the posterior approach. I also agree with Professor Kingsnorth that the laparoscopic approach (although I prefer it myself) is quite a nice one to do but it is difficult and ultimately it is probably costly. Some of you will know that we have already started an alternative approach in Holland to the pre-peritoneal space to place a mesh as in a laparoscopic approach by a grid iron incision. I will hopefully be able to present results on that compared to a laparoscopic approach within 1 year. So there are other ways to get there, and laparoscopy is nice to do but I think sometimes it is very difficult to do, as you said. So I do not think that there is such a future for laparoscopic hernia repair.

Filipi: I just want to mention that we need to think of the ease of the operation from the perspective of a first-year resident. We all have done many open hernia repairs and are familiar with the anatomy of the groin, but for a first-year resident, especially if there is a large sliding hernia or something more complicated than a small indirect hernia, the anatomy and the orientation is not easy. And so I do not agree totally that the Lichtenstein repair is easier. I am talking from the perspective of a first-year resident, and I think it takes time; you need to be in the groin 40 or 50 times before you really understand where the cord is in relationship to the sack and how to dissect the sack and those types of things. Maybe there is a way for us to teach our residents and new surgeons a better way before they start operating laparoscopically or even in the groin so that we know that they know some of the basic things that we assume they know.

Skandalakis: I wonder what Bassini would say if he was in this room. The statement that you made was that it is difficult after my operation to say that there will be other procedures. Bendavid reported 160 techniques for the repair of inguinal and femoral herniation. So I do honestly feel that we cannot say that we must use the same procedure for every patient. It depends what we find there anatomically, and then we have to choose the right procedure.

Muschaweck: Prof. Kingsnorth, I would not agree that we should only do the easiest operation that could be done, because if you get mesh (Lichtenstein), you have the mesh for your whole life, and if you see the results of the Shouldice Hospital with a recurrence rate of 0.3%, why shouldn't you do this operation? And perhaps you can do the Lichtenstein operation when the patient is older? But if you do the Lichtenstein operation, you cannot remove the mesh at all, and why should you do this in the beginning, for the primary hernia?

Kingsnorth: There are three ways in which we have to look at any type of hernia operation. The first is the efficacy, in other words, how well it can be done by the expert. And we have more than enough data that any of these specialized techniques are efficacious and can be done well by the experts. The second is to look at effectiveness; that means how well the operation is done by everybody else. And we now have information that the Shouldice operation fails at least five times more often with all of us out here than it does with Bendavid, and it may even be more than that. So it is not effective in the hands of surgeons in general. And the third thing is looking at cost-effectiveness, and that probably is the biggest issue for the health care industry, because the costs have gone out of control. And if we are looking at such a common operation, 700,000 a year in the USA, 105,000 a year in the UK, if you just add $100 to each operation, it will cost the health care system an enormous amount of money. So I think we have to look very carefully at whether to use a plug that costs £80 or a patch that costs £15. No one would deny anybody an operation if it were five times better than any other operation, we would pay for it. But when the benefits are marginal, you have to look very carefully at the costs. So we have to look at efficacy, effectiveness and cost-effectiveness.

Amid: I am a firm believer in the Shouldice operation. Shouldice repair is not really a herniorrhaphy, it is a hernioplasty, a muscle transfer hernioplasty; you bring the triple layer of Bassini and you make a new floor out of muscle or you convert a male groin to a female groin, or an adult groin to a baby groin; it is covered by muscle.

Flament: You are speaking of recurrent hernias, but I agree with Filippi that the difficult time in a recurrent hernia is the beginning of the procedure, recovering a normal anatomy. So you cannot ever say that recurrent hernia using the anterior approach can be easy. Sometimes you have to dissect a big peritoneal sac with bowel inside, and recurrent hernia is not always an easy procedure. When you have recovered a normal anatomy with the sac reduced into the abdominal cavity or resected and the spermatic cord freed, after that any procedure can be easy, but the previous time may be long.

Amid: I agree with you completely. There are times when I spend 2 h doing a Lichtenstein repair for a recurrent inguinal hernia. But it could be done safely.

Schumpelick: We reported a series of 101 patients with a proven recurrence rate of 6.9% after 10 years. We are not a specialized clinic, and 45 surgeons have performed these operations. That means the Shouldice procedure cannot be so difficult that is only appropriate in specialized centres. I have a more philosophical question. Is it justified to say we should make an operation so simple that in can be done in any clinic, or should we have some centres of excellence? I do not mean hernia centres, but centres with proven good long-term results achieved by a good method.

Kingsnorth: I tend to agree with you. I think that recurrent herniation in the groin is a difficult problem. The way I would put it, the patients should be referred to people with a special interest, not necessarily regarded as experts because people feel a bit wary about experts in groin hernia surgery. But they should be treated by surgeons who have a variety of skills at their disposal, so they can do a Lichtenstein, a pre-peritoneal repair, can deal with giant hernias, and they have the backup to deal with it.

Skandalakis: Can you explain to me the difference between hernioplasty and hernia repair?

Amid: Herniorrhaphy is a rhaphing procedure, and hernioplasty is reconstruction. This is really semantic. If you want to change it to something else, that is fine with me. But herniorrhaphy refers to the tissue approximation repair, because you are suturing the things together. Mesh repair is reconstruction, so it is a plasty rather than a rhaphy.

Nilsson: May I just take the opportunity of adding some information with reference to the Swedish register. We have to make the distinction that there is a difference between what is done in general practice with one technique and what is done in centres of excellence. This is the difference again between effectiveness and efficacy. I just want to underline this with reference to the Swedish data. They are effectiveness data; they are what was performed by Swedish surgeons thinking that they were doing the Lichtenstein procedure; they noted it and we took the records but it might have been an inadequate Lichtenstein procedure, and in many cases it certainly was.

References

1. Chevrel JP, Perez M, Lumbroso M, Morice P. Recidives herniares. La Presse Medicale 1991; 20: 1543–7
2. Campanelli G, Cavagholi R, Bottero L, DeSimone M, Pietri P. Hernies recidivees de l'aine. Propositions de classification et de tactique chirurgicale, J Chir Paris 1996; 133: 270–3
3. Fuchsjager N, Feichter A, Kux M. Die Lichtenstein-plug-Methode zur Reparation von Rezidivleiste in Hernien: Indikation Technik und Ergebnisse. Der Chirurg 1995; 66: 409–12
4. Horeyseck G, Pohl C. Lichtenstein-patch repair of recurrent inguinal hernia. American Hernia Society, 1998 (abstract)

CHAPTER 37

Transinguinal Preperitoneal Prosthesis Placement Under Local Anesthesia – Management and Follow-Up of 100 Patients

G. Arlt, V. Schumpelick

In recurrent hernia surgery today, there are numerous procedures used in routine clinical practice. The procedures can be classified as suture repairs, (Shouldice, Bassini, or McVay), open mesh repairs (Lichtenstein, Wantz, and Stoppa repair, Rives/transinguinal preperitoneal prosthesis technique, TIPP), and endoscopic techniques (transperitoneal or extraperitoneal mesh repair, TAPP/TEP). Most of these techniques are used according to the principal of "one method fits all types of hernia" for both primary and multiply recurrent hernias, thus losing several of the individual advantages of each procedure. For example, all suture repairs are suitable for an operation under local anesthesia, but not all recurrent hernias can be definitively cured by these procedures. On the other hand, a giant mesh prosthesis might reduce the re-recurrence rate in general, but such a procedure seems to be an overtreatment in small lateral recurrences.

37.1 Development and Technique

Evaluation of the results of the Shouldice repair using the Aachen classification of groin hernias (Schumpelick 1994) shows a quite detailed distribution of the recurrence rates. In recurrent hernia, the re-recurrence rate exceeded the 2% margin in MIII and combined hernias (McII–III). The recurrence rate was unacceptable high, especially in huge combined hernias (McIII) with a defect of the entire posterior wall (7.7%). Consequently, in large or combined recurrent hernias, the additional placement of a preperitoneal polypropylene prosthesis (Fig. 1) has been under evaluation since January 1994.

The TIPP technique represents a slight modification of the mesh repair described by Rives [9]. The hernia is prepared using an open transinguinal approach under local anesthesia. The decision whether to carry out a conventional (Shouldice) repair or a TIPP procedure depends on the intraoperative classification of the hernial defect. In general, the TIPP technique is indicated in all recurrent hernias with a medial defect of more than 3 cm in diameter (MIII) and in cases of a combined recurrence with a medium (1.5–3 cm = McII) or large (>3 cm = McIII) hernial orifice.

After classification of the defect, the posterior wall is completely opened and the preperitoneal fat is widely dissected away from the fascia transversalis. A polypropylene mesh of 15x10 cm with a lateral slit, two thirds above and one third below, is placed in the preperitoneal space. A new internal ring is created by closing the slit laterally to

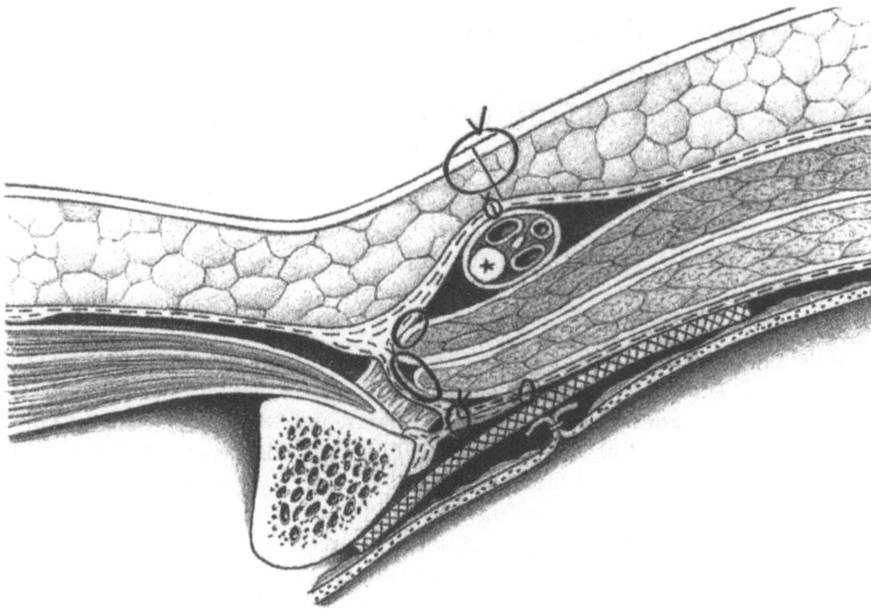

Fig. 1. Transinguinal preperitoneal prosthesis (TIPP) repair: mesh position in a cross-section

the spermatic cord with interrupted polypropylene sutures (Fig. 2). The medial lower edge is sutured to Cooper's ligament. The upper edges are fixed transfascially and transmuscularly to the ventral abdominal wall (Fig. 3). The procedure is then completed by reconstruction of the posterior wall mostly using the two-row Shouldice technique [5].

37.2 Local Anesthesia

Local anesthesia is the routine anasthesia method at the Surgical University Clinic in Aachen. The current percentage of repairs done under local anesthesia is about 92% in primary hernia and 55% in recurrent repairs. With increasing experience in management, the conversion rate is very low (0.26%). Comparing the intra- and postoperative course under general and local anesthesia, the advantages of the latter in our hands are as follows:

- Reduction of patients' total time in the operating room from 115±38 min to 92±25 min
- Decrease in the rate of nonspecific postoperative complaints (*n*ausea and vomiting, urinary retention, headache) about three- to fourfold under routine use of local anesthesia
- Reduction of postoperative inguinal pain and immediate postoperative mobilization

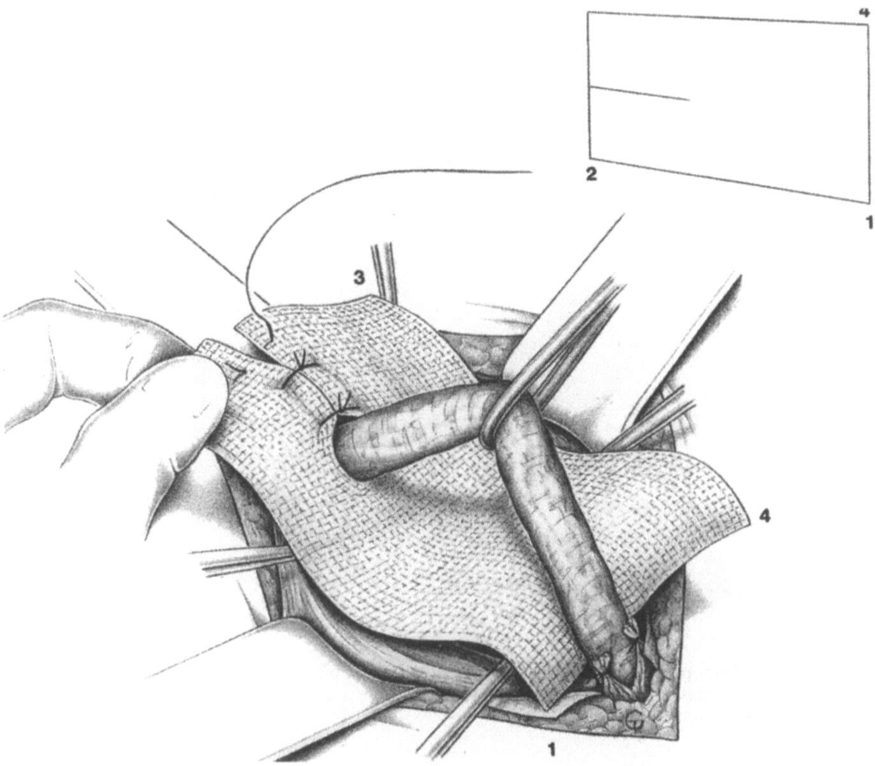

Fig. 2. Transinguinal preperitoneal prosthesis (TIPP) repair: creation of a new internal ring by closure of the lateral slit with interrupted sutures

Apart from these advantages, the rate of early and late postoperative complications is not affected by the type of anesthesia. Patients' acceptance of local anesthesia is positive, and about 96% of patients would choose local anesthesia again for a second hernia repair.

37.3 Patients

From January 1994 to December 1996, 380 recurrent hernias (first to eighth recurrence) were operated on in 364 patients at the Surgical University Clinic in Aachen. A Stoppa or Wantz repair was done in those cases with a preoperative diagnosis of bilateral or very large recurrences (n=52). In 228 hernias, the decision whether or not a mesh repair was necessary could not determined preoperatively. These cases were prepared to undergo an open transinguinal repair, using local anesthesia in the majority of them (n=203, 62%). After intraoperative classification, 94 recurrences were candidates for a TIPP repair (Table 1). The recent repair was a Bassini procedure in most of

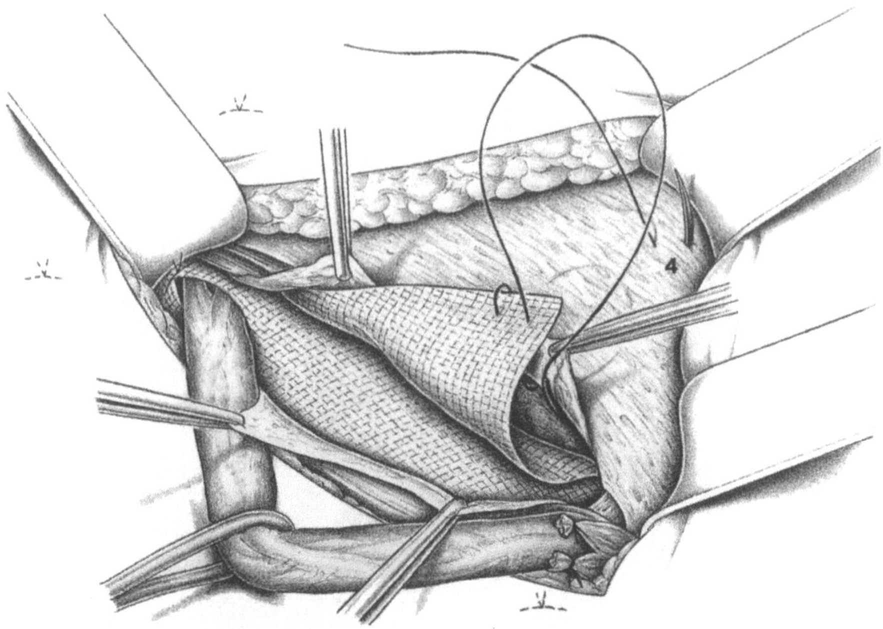

Fig. 3. Transinguinal preperitoneal prosthesis (TIPP) repair: placement of the mesh in the preperitoneal space and transfascial–transmuscular fixation

Table 1. Recurrent inguinal hernia surgery (380 first to eight recurrences in 364 patients) at the Surgical University Clinic of Aachen 1994–1996

Procedure	Operations (*n*)	Local anesthesia	
		(*n*)	(%)
Stoppa/Wantz	52	–	–
Shouldice	234	151	65
TIPP/Rives	94	52	55

TIPP, transinguinal preperitoneal prosthesis.

these cases (*n*=31), followed by a Bassini-Kirschner (*n*=18) and a Shouldice repair (*n*=15) (Table 2).

All patients had a follow-up examination at 12 and 24 months postoperatively. A total of 322 cases were evaluated by a questionnaire, and 42 patients with complaints were examined clinically and by ultrasound.

37.4 Results

In the 94 TIPP/Rives repairs, the placement of the prosthesis required an additional operation time of about 15 min for the first ten operations. After this learning curve,

Table 2. Recent procedure and classification in 94 transinguinal preperitoneal prosthesis (TIPP)/Rives repairs

Procedure	Operations (*n*)	Class of recurrence
Bassini	31	MIII
Bassini-Kirschner	18	LIII
Shouldice	15	MIII/FIII
McVay	8	MIII/McIII
Vicryl mesh	13	McIII/FIII
ePTFE patch	3	MIII
Lichtenstein	6	FIII/McIII
Total	94	–

ePTFE, expanded polytetrafluoroethylene.

the additional operation time decreased to 5–8 min during routine use. Conversion of the type of anesthesia – from local to general anesthesia – was not necessary in any case. There were no procedure-related intraoperative complications.

Early postoperative complications were hematoma in three (3.2%), subcutaneous infection in one (1.1%), and an ischemic orchitis in another one case (1.1%). Seroma around the prosthesis was a frequent finding by ultrasound, requiring repeated punctures in 12.8% of cases.

Two recurrences were found 12 and 24 months after the TIPP/Rives repair (2.1%). The patient with an ischemic orchitis developed a testicular atrophy (1.1%).

37.5 Comments

Our detailed analysis of the recurrence rate after recurrent repair showed that there might be unsatisfactory and unacceptable results in certain types of hernia. Most of the lateral and the small medial recurrences can be repaired using the Shouldice technique [1, ,12], but large medial or combined recurrences require an additional reinforcement of the posterior wall for permanent closure of the defect. A preperitoneal mesh prosthesis placed by an open approach or endoscopically are the alternative procedures under current evaluation [3, 4, 6, 7, 11]. In order to reach a classification-related intraoperative decision whether or not an additional mesh is necessary, we recommend open preperitoneal mesh placement (TIPP/Rives) under local anesthesia [2]. By following such a policy, the mesh repair can be restricted to those cases that really need a mesh and save the others from any type of overtreatment.

The routine use of local anesthesia offers additional advantages: intraoperative demonstration of the hernia and testing of the repair, safe anesthesia for the elderly and those with cardiac or pulmonary disease, decrease in the rate of urinary retention even in the prostate age-group, reduction of time in the operating room, immediate postoperative mobilization, and reduction of direct costs (Peiper 1994).

37.6 Discussion

Flament: Preperitoneal preparation was first described by Rives in 1965, but I was not able to find a publication by Rives from that year. Now we have 32 years of experience with this technique and we actually do about 25% of our hernia repair using the Rives technique. Indications are huge primary and huge recurrent inguinal hernia. We have not found that entering the preperitoneal space is difficult by the anterior approach. It is just the same as in laparoscopic repair. In recurrent repair, our re-recurrence rate is 1.7%. About 65% of the repairs are done under spinal anesthesia.

Arlt: The type of anesthesia may be determined by the personal experience of the surgeon and policy of the clinic. I think you use just the same indications as we do. We also did the TIPP repair in some huge primary hernias; I did not mention that because it is not the topic today. Concerning the preparation, it is a question of whether you have to repair a primary hernia or operate on a multiple recurrence. In the latter, the transinguinal approach is really difficult. Preparation of nerves and vessels from scars carries a substantial risk of damage and troublesome postoperative complications, such as chronic inguinal pain and testicular atrophy.

Bendavid: We now have nearly 400 cases operated on by the Rives technique. The risk of mesh migration is very low when you place the mesh by the open technique using a proper fixation to Cooper's ligament. I have never seen a mesh migration in our series.

Schumpelick: The TIPP technique is a kind of reinvention of the Rives procedure. We first developed the technique in our clinic and later found it already described in the literature. Our modification of the Rives procedure is the lateral slit in the mesh, which works like an additional fixation at the internal ring. Using meshes, we had the impression that a proper fixation is mandatory. We saw two recurrences in the TIPP series, both at the medial side and both due to insufficient fixation and insufficient size of the mesh.

Read: We also like this type of operation, and I would like to mention that we always try to preserve the epigastric vessels, because they might be important in cases of heart surgery using the mamaria interna. We do not use a lateral slit and we fixate the mesh only at Cooper's ligament, but mesh migration has never been a problem in our patients.

Filipi: Dr. Arlt, have you ever seen problems with the caudal and lateral mesh fixation at the iliopubic tract?

Arlt: We fixate the mesh laterally at the inguinal ligament. We do not go below this structure, and we have never seen complications at this step of the operation.

Skandalakis: Since there are wide variations in the anatomy and tissue condition in our patients, there cannot be only one operation for all hernias. Surgeons have to be familiar with several procedures and choose the right one for the individual patient.

Arlt: I totally agree with you. As I pointed out, we use four different procedures (Shouldice, TIPP, Wantz, Stoppa) in recurrent hernia repair. And we will add endoscopic repair (TEP) in the very near future.

References

1. Arlt G, Peiper Ch, Schumpelick V: Ausführung und Ergebnisse der Standardtechnik nach Shouldice. Akt Chir 33 (1998):7–10
2. Arlt G, Schumpelick V: Transinguinale präperitoneale Netzplastik (TIPP) in der Versorgung der Rezidivleistenhernie. Chirurg 68 (1997):1235–1238
3. Arregui ME, Davis CJ, Yucel O, et al.: Laparoscopic mesh repir of inguinal hernia using a preperitoneal approach: A preliminary report. Surg Laparosc Endosc 2 (1992):53
4. Barkun JS, Wexler MJ, Hinchey EJ, et al.: Laparoscopic versus open inguinal herniorrhaphy: Preliminary results of a randomized controlled trial. Surgery 118 (1995):703
5. Berliner SD: An approach to groin hernia. Surg Clin North Am 64 (1984):197–213.
6. Felix EL, Michas CA, Gonzalez MH: Laparoscopic hernioplasty – TAPP vs TEP. Surg Endosc 9 (1995):984
7. Nyhus LM, Pollak R, Bombeck Th, Donahue Ph: The preperitoneal approach and prosthetic buttress. Repair for recurrent hernia. Ann Surg 208 (1988):733
8. Peiper C, Töns C, Schippers E, Busch F, Schumpelick V: Local versus general anesthesia for Shouldice repair of the inguinal hernia. World J Surg 18 (1994):912 -916.
9. Rives J: Surgical treatment of the inguinal hernia with Dacron patch. Principles, indications, technique and results. Int Surg 47 (1967):360
10. Schumpelick V, Treutner K-H, Arlt G: Klassifikation von Inguinal-Hernien. Chirurg 56 (1994):877–879.
11. Stoppa RE, Rives JL, Warlaumont CR, et al.: The use of dacron in the repair of hernias of the groin. Surg Clin North Am 64 (1984):269
12. Wantz GE: The Canadian repair: Personal observations. World J Surg 13 (1989):516–521.

CHAPTER 38

Experience with the Mesh Umbrella Repair of Recurrent Inguinal Hernia

U. Muschaweck

38.1 Introduction

In cases of inguinal hernia relapses, it is of eminent importance to minimize the surgical preparation. The tension-free closure of the defect by application of so-called plugs of a knit monofilament polypropylene netting material is the essential aspect of this technique.

38.2 Personal Experience

38.2.1 Case Rate

Throughout the period from August 1989 to November 1993, we have operated on 695 hernia patients in the Rechts der Isar clinic (Munich), and in the period from December 1993 to December 1997 on 4055 hernia patients in the Arabella Clinic (Munich), using the original Shouldice technique with local anesthesia in all cases.

Among the patients who were operated on in the latter clinic, roughly 690 (16.1%) suffered from an inguinal hernia relapse, of which 82% experienced a first relapse, 13% a second relapse, and 5% a third or even higher-grade relapse.

38.2.2 Perioperative Patient Management

The family physician or a medical adviser is responsible for preoperative treatment, which includes the determination of laboratory parameters, electrocardiogram (ECG), and – in patients aged 50 years upward – a chest radiograph.

A clinical examination is performed when the patients come to see us for a first consultation. The sonographic examination of the testes, with a documentation of their size, is a mandatory element of this initial examination.

The patients are then comprehensively informed about details of the surgical technique and about potential complications, and they are advised about how to behave before and after the operation.

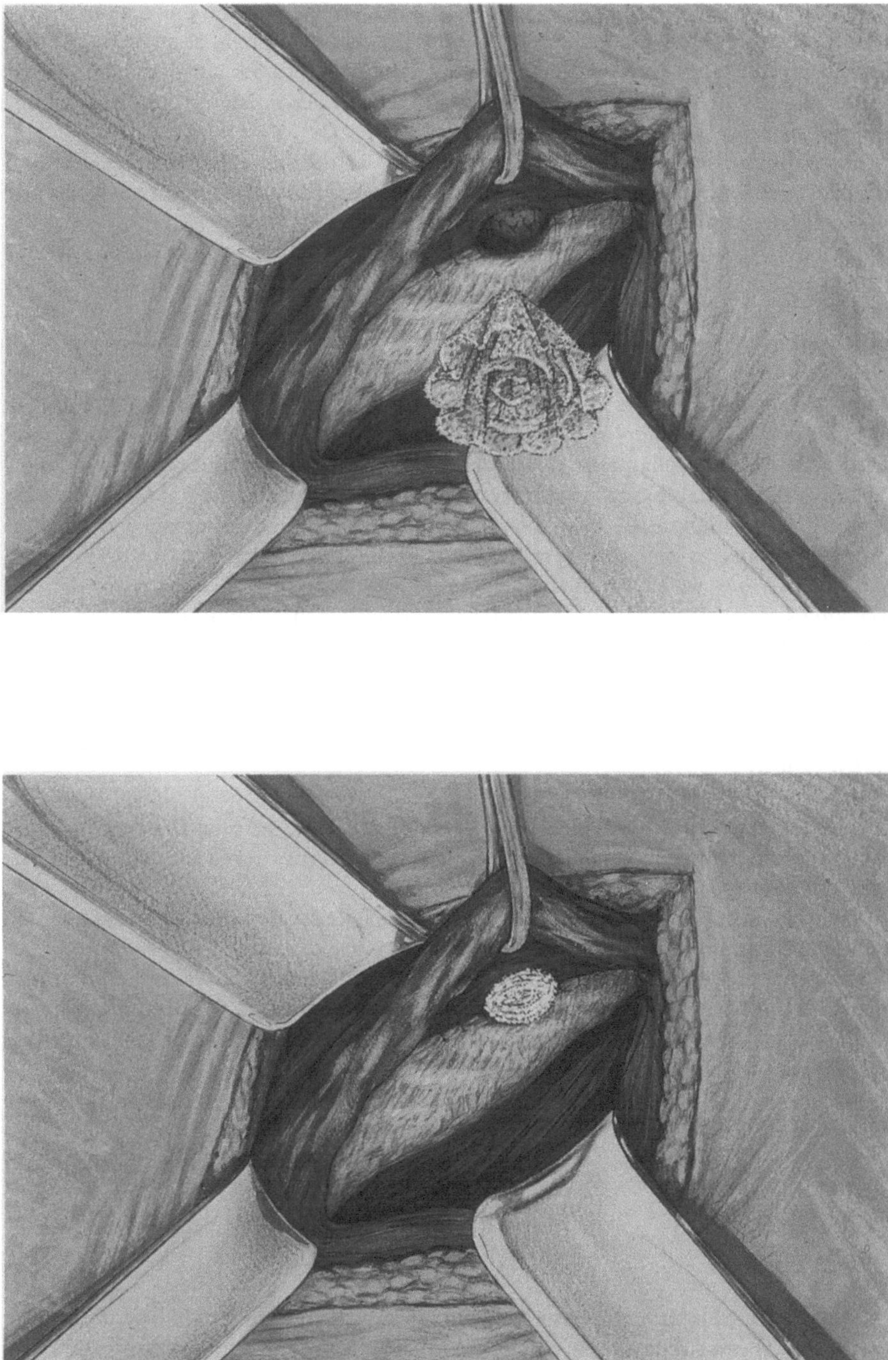

Fig. 1. Mesh Umbrella

In the morning, between 6.45 and 9.45 a.m., on the day of the operation, the patients then come to the clinic without any breakfast. A single-shot cephalosporin dose is administered to all patients roughly 15 min before the surgical intervention begins in order to prevent infection. We do not usually administer prophylaxis against thrombosis except in high-risk patients.

The patients are discharged around 5.00 p.m. on the same day, if necessary after postoperative orchiosonography and comprehensive information about analgesia and recommendations on how to behave after the operation.

38.2.3 Indication

If only a localized defect is involved, with a sufficiently stable bottom that is intact in all other respects, we employ a so-called mesh umbrella for "tension-free" closure of the defect; this umbrella permits reinforcement of the bottom and obviates the need for a resection of stable cicatricial sections. We have substituted the flat Marlex netting by this form of implant, because this netting always required major parts of the bottom to be opened as well, which resulted in an unintended increase in the defect.

Since July 1995, we have implanted a total of 230 mesh umbrellas in the 307 patients receiving surgical treatment of inguinal hernia relapses throughout this period, which corresponds to a rate of almost 75%.

38.2.4 Methodology

The surgeon provides for topical anesthesia in the form of medial nerve blocking above the anterior iliac spine. Injections are then administered individually under each nerve in steps.

A physician specialized in anesthesia is responsible for due care at the "head end," including comprehensive monitoring (with ECG, pulse oximetry, RR checking).

Following a circular preparation of the base of the hernial sac, the resection is performed. In the area of the hernial orifice, the transverse fascia is seized by means of small clamps along a circular line and is then mobilized. Subsequently, the umbrella is introduced and fixed by a circular suture.

We use a mesh umbrella in approximately 80% of all patients suffering from a relapse of inguinal hernia.

38.2.5 Results

After the surgical intervention, the patients are almost free from pain, and in terms of sports they do not require any convalescent treatment. The application of the mesh umbrella in cases of relapse of inguinal hernia successfully reduces the period for which patients are written off sick even further.

In the vast majority of patients, a strict convalescence period of 0–4 days is prescribed, and only in isolated cases (if patients have to carry out heavy work) do we allow a convalescence period of up to 2 weeks.

With a relapse risk in cases of inguinal hernia of less than 1.5%, we have so far observed only a single case of relapse after the implantation of a mesh umbrella throughout the past 11 months. We have not observed a single wound infection after mesh umbrella implantation. Occasionally, a seroma occurs, which we tap under sterile conditions.

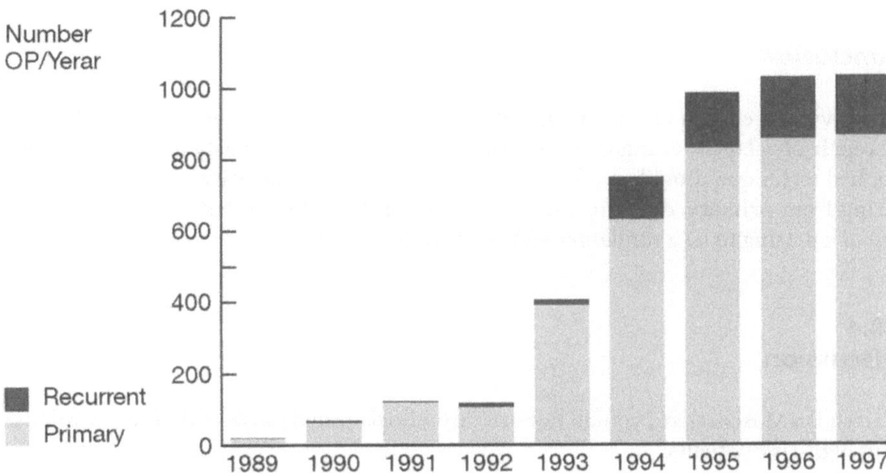

Fig. 2. Inguinal Hernia 1989–1997

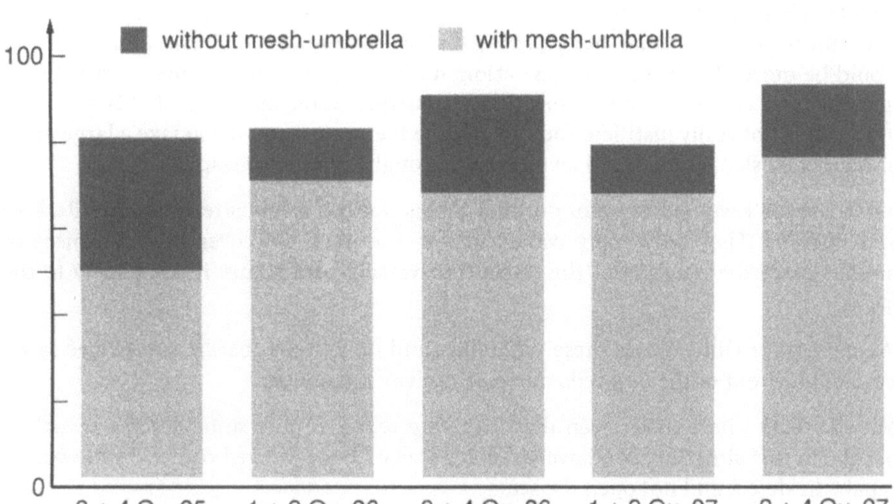

Fig. 3. Application of Mesh Umbrella for recurrent Groin Hernia

38.2.6 Comparison of Conventional Shouldice Versus the Flat Netting and Mesh Umbrella Techniques

In the classical Shouldice technique, stable parts of the bottom must be opened again, and even when flat nettings are implanted it is necessary to incise marginal areas, which involves an undesirable enlargement of the defect. The application of mesh umbrellas, by contrast, allows for a tension-free repair.

38.3 Conclusion

In our view, the mesh umbrella implant ensures a substantial improvement in the field of repair of relapses of inguinal hernia. The displacing fascioplasty as the exclusively applied technique provides sufficient stability in the large majority of all patients suffering from primary, direct or indirect hernia, and we therefore do not consider the use of a netting to be a fundamentally justified technique.

38.4 Discussion

Hartel: Dr. Muschaweck, you do not use thrombosis prophylaxis routinely. Do you use it in high-risk patients?

Muschaweck: Yes, we only use prophylaxis in patients with a positive history of thrombosis and in selected patients with obesity and varication.

Bendavid: You use the term "umbrella." I think in your operation it is not an umbrella but rather a plug, the same that is propagated by Rutkow and Robbins. A real umbrella would be more effective in that operation. It opens up the preperitoneal space, becomes flat and creates a preperitoneal layer. Furthermore, the price of this so-called umbrella is not really justified. You can achieve the same result if you take a large piece of Marlex mesh and cut it into 20 pieces. This might be much cheaper.

Muschaweck: I wanted to point out that this is not the original technique of Rutkow and Robbins. They only apply two sutures to the plug and cover it with a piece of mesh. I place the plug under the fascia transversalis and suture it completely to the fascia.

Wantz: Arthur Gilbert uses these umbrellas, and he told me that he sometimes saw a kind of blow-out of the umbrella during Valsalva's maneuver.

Muschaweck: I have never seen that. The plug repair is only suitable for a recurrent hernia. In this situation, you have an intact scar with an isolated defect. I just want to repair the defect and not open the scar.

Bendavid: I do not accept the concept of putting a plug into a hole in hernia surgery. When repairing a recurrent hernia, we have to deal with the whole floor of the inguinal canal. It is not sufficient to repair a punched-out whole and ignore the rest of the posterior wall.

Flament: We have little experience with plug repair, but we saw two cases of plug migration into the canal. Now we use a new mesh device (Ethicon Prolene Hernia System), which is associated with minimal patient discomfort and so far excellent clinical results in 53 patients.

Muschaweck: The most important detail is the fixation of the plug. If you suture it to the muscles, it will migrate, but if you suture it under the fascia transversalis using the whole circumference of the defect, you will achieve a stable repair.

CHAPTER 39

Prosthetic Repair of Recurrent Groin Hernias

R. Stoppa, F. Ralmiaramanana, X. Henry, P. Verhaeghe

39.1 Introduction

Recurrent groin hernias expose a patient to the complications of all groin hernias. At the same time, they are more difficult and hazardous to repair.

The frequency of recurrent groin hernias observed in global series of groin hernia varied, with rates of 10% [4, 7], 12% [14], 18% [30], 20% [22], and 30% [13, 31] being reported. During long postoperative follow-up studies (of well-known differences in complexity of procedures), the recurrence rates were less than 1% in a Shouldice series [7] and after Stoppa's giant prosthetic repair [27], 3.5% in McVay's series [17], 6.8% after 3 years of follow-up in Marsden's series [16], and 8.6% after 10 years in the series of Palumbo and Shape [20]. It is known that the skill and the specialization of surgeons lower recurrence rates, and the Shouldice series [11] demonstrates this concept. The recurrence rates at that hospital were 18.8% in 1945, 12% in 1946, 6% in 1947, 3% in 1948, and less than 1% since 1951. In our series, the recurrence rates for giant prosthetic repairs by the abdominal approach were 3.3% in 1974, 1.2% in 1983, and 0.56% in 1986.

The time to recurrence varies, and it has been as long as 25 years [11]. In our review of multiple techniques of repair, 5.6% of recurrences appeared during the first postoperative month, 39.1% during the first year, and 23.5% after the tenth year. After prosthetic repair, recurrences take place during the first postoperative year and are associated with incorrect technique; after herniorrhaphy, they are dispersed over a long postoperative period, with an incorrect technique associated with worsening results. Halverson and Mc Vay [8] proposed a formula for determining the predictable recurrence rate at the 25th year by multiplying the first-year recurrence rate by 5, the 2-year rate by 2.5, the 5-year rate by 1.5, and the 10-year rate by 1.2.

Among 459 recurrent groin hernias reported by the Shouldice Hospital [7], 60% were inguinal hernias and 40% were femoral hernias. Femoral hernias recurred most often (2.2% in men, 1.3% in women) and sliding hernias were second (1%). In the AFC inquiry [9], femoral hernias recurred most often (8.2%), followed by inguinal eventerations (7.9%). Some authors have shown a higher recurrence rate after operations for recurrences. One initial recurrence rate was 7%, and these hernias recurred in 19% of the patients after the recurrence was treated [16]. Clear [6] reported a failure rate of 39% for repairs of recurrent hernias. Thus recurrences must be considered as new lesions, partially produced by previous operations. The preferable treatment is with a prosthesis. This recommendation has been upheld by surgeons at the Shouldice Hospital [3] faced with recurrent femoral hernias.

The mechanisms of recurrence after a repair are difficult to identify when the recurrence is late and when the previous operation has been performed at another hospital. Even during the reoperation, the previously used procedure is often not identifiable. Houdard and Stoppa [10] classified recurrence factors as one of three types: incorrect technique, a large hernial defect, and miscellaneous factors.

Incorrect technique is responsible for most recurrences during the first postoperative year. Examples include not dissecting or not finding a sac [7], leaving too long a peritoneal stump [22], incorrect closure of the hernial orifice, as demonstrated by the frequency of indirect recurrences, and suture under tension, which is most involved in direct recurrences. [10]. Some techniques are more likely than others to lead to a recurrence. These include totally pre- or retrofunicular repairs and procedures using Cooper's ligament without a McVay transition suture on the vessel sheath.

Large hernias recur twice as often as small ones, and careless management results in a recurrence. Extended dissection or traumatic sutures may change a contractible inguinal wall into a fibrous wall exposed to progressive rupture [10].

Other risk factors, independent of the quality of the operation, are the patient's general condition and age, abdominal wall weakness, and obesity [5]. The most dangerous factors are postoperative sepsis and chronic cough. Early activity or return to work is no longer blamed for recurrences. Eighty percent of recurrent hernias are independent of heavy work [22]. Individuals with sedentary occupations suffer more recurrences (17.6%) than those performing heavy labor (9.1%) [10]. Marsden [16], Rives and Hibon [23], and Houdard and associates [9] support that finding. In Warlaumont's series [30], 56% of recurrences appeared in the absence of any effort, and only 15% after extreme exertion.

Recurrences after prosthetic repair result exclusively from technical mistakes and thus appear during the first postoperative year. In our series, no recurrences appeared after the end of the first year. During the postoperative course, serohematomas must be distinguished from recurrent hernias. The classical clinical signs can be confirmed by echography. Recurrences that take place after placement of a giant prosthesis through a midline subumbilical approach are usually caused by insufficient size or displacement of the prosthesis. Slitting a prosthesis to let the cord pass through predisposes it to breakage, so we prefer to avoid the risk by walling off the cord components [26, 27].

39.2 Treatment

To repair a recurrent inguinal hernia, the surgeon has to choose between an inguinal incision or a preperitoneal approach. The inguinal route requires a larger incision [18]. Local anesthesia can be used, and Poupart's and Cooper's ligaments are often intact, but the surgeon has to be prepared for a more or less difficult dissection, a certain risk of injury to the cord (a factor in sequelar testicular atrophy), and a possible regional nerve lesion. When damaged inguinal structures are exposed, a prosthesis can be used, but there are more difficulties than with the preperitoneal approach.

The preperitoneal approach for the placement of a giant polyester mesh prosthesis is a simple operation in which the surgeon progresses through normal, unmodified anatomy and cannot miss any other hernia. It is an almost absolutely fail-safe weapon against recurrence, but sepsis must be relieved, and preparation must be made for a mandatory aseptic operation. For recurrent groin hernias, we routinely use a bilateral giant prosthesis of polyester mesh, widely interposed between the peritoneum and the abdominal wall. Through Pascal's hydrostatic principle, intra-abdominal pressure (the force that provoked the hernia) is used to eliminate recurrence. Because of its large dimensions, the giant prosthesis is instantly and definitively set in place and does not require any direct fixation. Walling off the cord components makes it unnecessary to slit the prosthesis for their passage through it, allowing the operation to be simple and safe. This original personal technique has been discussed in numerous publications [25, 29]. Thorough understanding of the procedure is recommended before it is undertaken, but no exceptional experience is necessary for regular results.

Recurrences after placement of a prosthesis by an inguinal approach may be indirectly or directly caused by partial breakage of the prosthesis fixation stitches. A preperitoneal approach is preferable for easy retroparietal dissection and for the placement of a preperitoneal prosthesis. Recurrences after placement of a giant prosthesis by the preperitoneal route are related to insufficient size, slitting the mesh, or not spreading it far enough. When the recurrent hernia is lateral, a suprainguinal incision, as described by Nyhus [19], can be used to place another piece of mesh laterally to complement the previously placed prosthesis. For a central or inferior recurrence, an inguinal incision allows the surgeon to find the inferior border of the prosthesis and fix it to Cooper's ligament.

39.3 Results

In a personal series of 349 recurrent groin hernias (15.7% of patients treated for groin hernias), the bilaterality rate was 42.2%. Four techniques were used: the Bassini operation in two patients (0.6%), Cooper's ligament repair in 30 patients (8.6%), prosthesis insertion by the inguinal route in 39 patients (11.2%), and placement of a giant prostheses through a midline incision in 270 patients (77.4%). An excellent postoperative course was observed after both Bassini operations, after 28 Cooper's ligament repairs, after 31 inguinal prosthesis placements (79.5%), and after 261 placements of giant prostheses by the midline approach (96.7%). Hematomas occurred after two Cooper's ligament repairs and nine placements of giant prostheses (3.3%). Sepsis occurred after 6.6% of the Cooper's ligament repairs, after 7.7% of the inguinal prostheses were placed, and after 3% of the giant prostheses were placed (no prosthesis was removed, and all patients healed). One re-recurrence took place after a Bassini operation, five after a Cooper's ligament repair, four after inguinal placement of prostheses (10.3%), and three after placement of giant prostheses by the midline approach (1.1%). Thus, in our experience, the placement of giant prostheses by the midline approach to treat recurrent or re-recurrent hernias has less morbidity and better results than other techniques.

39.4 Discussion

For a discussion, please see Chap. 40.

References

1. Abrahamson J: Factors and mechanisms leading to recurrence: in Bendavid R, Prostheses and abdominal wall hernias. Landes Company, Austin, 1994: 139–170
2. Beets GL: On the repair of inguinal hernia. Scientific thesis, Universitaire Pers, Maastricht, 1997
3. Bendavid R : A femoral umbrella for femoral hernia repair. Surg Gynecol Obstet 1987,165: 153
4. Borgeskow S, Skeie E: Preperitoneal herniorraphy. Acta Chir Scand, 1973, 139: 45
5. Borgstrom S: Recurrence rates of lateral inguinal hernia in adults. Acta Chir Scand., 1951, 139:429
6. Clear J: Ten year statistical study of inguinal hernia. Arch Surg, 1976, 46:70
7. Glassow F: Recurrent inguinal and femoral hernia: Br Med J, 1970, 1:215
8. Halverson K, McVay CB: Inguinal and femoral hernioplasty: A 22 year study of the author's method. Arch Surg, 1970, 101:127
9. Houdard C, Berthelot G, Carles JF: Réflecions à propos de 46 récidives de hernie inguinale. Ann Chir, 1971,25:1235
10. Houdard C, Stoppa R: Le traitement des hernies de l'aine. Monographie de l'Association Française de Chirurgie, Paris, Massson Ed., 1984
11. Iles J: The management of elective hernia repair. Am J Plast Surg, 1979, 6: 538
12. Kald A: Audit of groin hernia repair. Scientific thesis. Tryckeriet, Lincköping, 1997
13. Koontz AR, Kimberley RC: Tantalum and Marlex mesh. An experimental and clinical comparison. Am Surg, 1960, 151: 7936
14. Ljungdahl I: Inguinal and femoral hernia: an investigation on 502 own operated cases. Acta Chir Scand., 1973, Suppl. 439:81
15. Lowham AS, Filipi CJ, Fitzgibbons RH, Stoppa R, Wantz CE, Felix EL, Crafton WB: Mechanisms of hernia recurrence after preperitoneal mesh repair. Traditional and laparoscopic. Ann Surg, 1997, 225/4: 422–431
16. Marsden AJ: Inguinal hernia. A three years review of 2000 cases. Br J Surg, 1962, 49:384
17. McVay CB: Groin Hernia. Cooper ligament repair. In Hernia, 3rd edition, L.M. Nyhus, R.E. Condon editors, Philadelphia, J.B., Lippincott, 1989: 119–131
18. Myers RN, Shearburn EW: The problem of the recurrent inguinal hernia. Surg Clin North Am, 1973, 53:55
19. Nyhus LM, Klein MS, Rogers FB: Inguinal hernia. Current Problems in Surgery, 1991, XXVIII/6: 403–450
20. Palumbo LT, Shape WS: Primary inguinal hernioplasty in the adult. Surg Clin North Am, 1971, 57:1293
21. Read RC: Bilaterality and the prosthetic repair of large recurrent inguinal hernias. Am J Surg 1979, 138:788
22. Ryan EA: Recurrent hernias. An analysis of 369 consecutive cases of recurrent inguinal and femoral hernias. Surg Gynecol Obstet, 1953, 96: 343
23. Rives J, Hibon J: Hernies d l'aine. Ecycl. Med.Chir.Paris, 1974, 9:90095–10
24. Schumpelick V, Wantz GE: Inguinal hernia repair. Karger, Basel, Freiburg, Paris, 1995
25. Stoppa R, Petit J, Abourachid H: Procédé original de plastie des hernies de l'aine. L'interposition sans fixation d'une prothèse en turlle de dacron par voie mèdiane sous-pèritonèale. Chirurgie, 1973, 99:119
26. Stoppa R, Warlaumont C, Verhaege P:, Henry X: Dacron mesh in the repair of groin hernias. Surg Rounds, 1983, 6:38
27. Stoppa R, Warlaumont C, Verhaege P: Prosthetic repair in the treatment of groin hernias . Int. Surg, 198671:154
28. Stoppa R, The treatment of complicated groin and incisional hernias. World J Surg, 1989, 13:545–554
29. Stoppa R, Hernia of the abdominal wall. In: Chevrel JP (ed) Hernias and surgery of the abdominal wall. Springer, Berlin Heidelberg New York, 1998, pp 255–264
30. Warlaumont C: Les hernies de l'aine: Place des prothèses en tulle de Dacron dans leur traitement. Thèse Méd., Amiens, 1982
31. Zimmermann LM, Zimmermann JE: The history of hernia treatment. In Hernia, 2nd ed, LM Nyhus, RE Condon (eds) Philadelphia, J.B. Lippincott, 1979: 3–10

CHAPTER 40

Indications and Results of Open Preperitoneal Mesh Repair for Recurrent Groin Hernia

A.G. Greenburg

40.1 Introduction

Despite recent technical and technologic advances in the surgical repair of groin hernias, there continues to be a problem with recurrence. Many of the newer techniques have not been tested over a sufficient number of years to assess a true rate of recurrence. The issue of recurrence as a measure of outcome for repair of any hernia is considered appropriate, as it reflects the quality of the initial repair as well as its durability. Just how well these newer approaches will perform has yet to be established.

Estimates regarding the failure rate of primary groin hernia repairs range from 0.5% to as high as 15%. Failure rates for the repair of recurrent groin hernias range from 1% to as high as 25%, depending on the series and the technique reported. Few could dispute that there is a need to define an approach to the repair of recurrent groin hernias that is safe, effective, and durable. That such a repair should be based on anatomic principles and the physiology of wound healing is a given. In addition, the issue of using mesh or other synthetic or natural tissue as a means of further strengthening the repair should be addressed.

It is also apparent that the basis for the occurrence of a groin hernia is not well established. There is the obvious potential for the presence of a metabolic defect in the healing process or a genetically determined, possibly programmed, failure of the tissue. Although there can be no good teleological rationale to support the latter, it remains a possibility. Whatever the underlying tissue defect, if there is one, the repair of a recurrent groin hernia presents the surgeon with a challenge. To properly deal with the challenge, the surgeon needs an armamentarium of knowledge, skills, tools, and options to resolve the problem in the most effective manner with the lowest risk and highest quality of outcome. The latter obviously corresponds to low rates of recurrence.

40.2 Patients and Methods

In 1987, I reported on a series of 413 recurrent groin hernias repaired using the preperitoneal approach [1]. Since then, I have used the approach in an additional 238 recurrent hernias and over 300 primary repairs. Thus the experience with the repair of recurrent groin hernia is 651 cases between 1973 and December of 1997. This represents a fraction of about 10% of the more than 6500 inguinal hernia repairs in that time frame. The surgical approach used is essentially that described by Nyhus in 1960 [2]. In this prospective and sequential single-surgeon series of 413 recurrent groin hernias repaired, mesh was required in only 6% of the cases. On inspection of the defect associated with the recurrence, mesh was judged to be indicated when primary tissue approximation without tension could not be effected, the tissues were felt to be too weak, or the patient's occupation put him or her at risk for recurrence on the basis of movement. When the data from the last 10 years were added to the original series for a total of 651 repairs, there were no significant changes in the data values or results obtained in all areas of inquiry.

40.3 Results

The use of the preperitoneal approach afforded the opportunity to catalogue the defects as seen in this series of 651 hernias repaired. The most striking feature of this exercise was, of course, the variety of defects seen. The traditionally accepted adage that half are "direct" and half "indirect" really does not apply. There is great variation in the appearance, size, shape, and location of the defects seen. Moreover, there are combinations of recurrences that are only obvious if a view of the entire groin area is obtained. It is these combinations that may lead to the high incidence of recurrence following repair of a recurrent hernia if not noted at the time of the operation, and it would reflect poorly on the technique if indeed a repairable defect were to be "missed."

Twenty-six percent of the recurrent defects were "indirect." In other words, the only peritoneal sac noted was into the internal ring; the direct floor and femoral areas were solid and without evidence of fascial defect.

Fifty-eight percent of the defects were considered "direct hernia" by virtue of being found in the posterior inguinal floor between the tubercle and the internal ring, but not involving the latter. Of these, only 11.4% involved the entire floor. The remaining defects were distributed as follows: 41.9% at the pubic tubercle, 28.6% in the midfloor, and 15.2% lateral, near the internal ring but medial to the inferior epigastric vessels. Multiple defects of the direct floor were noted in 2.8% of the cases.

In this series, there was an incidence of 6% femoral hernia as the only defect noted. In the complex or multiple defect group, there were combinations of indirect or direct hernia with a femoral component noted. Indeed, about one third of the complex defects had a femoral component identified. Thus the incidence of a femoral hernia could be as high as 9% as identified in this series.

The complex defects comprise about 10% of all defects seen in this series. If a different approach had been used, it is possible that some defects would have been missed, later appearing as a re-recurrence. It is in the ability to assess the entire floor at the time of the repair for recurrence that this approach is most rational.

In the 1987 report [1], a recurrence rate of 1.7% for repairs of first-recurrence groin hernia repair was reported. There has been no essential change in incidence since that report. The operation, without mesh, using tissue approximation is safe and effective and apparently durable across the population served. That has been the experience in the more recent decade as well. Given an effective repair with tissue to tissue approximation, the issue becomes defining when to use mesh as part of the repair and how to insert it for maximum effect.

40.4 Techniques

Tissue approximation of the edges of the defect to the iliopubic band, Cooper's ligament, the periosteum of the iliac bone, or the fascia of the femoral vessels is generally preferred. The superior tissue is the transversus arch or fascia, easily recognized from the preperitoneal vantage. Suture material is nonabsorbable synthetic monofilament inserted in either a running or interrupted fashion, depending on the findings. As many of the defects are small, this is sufficient to effect the repair [3].

In those instances where mesh is required, about 6% of the time, a nonabsorbable monofilament synthetic is preferred. This is secured inferiorly to a number of structures in either running or interrupted fashion, tailored to the anatomic findings at the time of the operation. The "buttress support" is elected for a variety of reasons. First, the tissue approximation is considered the primary repair and is expected to be a major part of the prevention of a recurrence. As the tissue approximation has by itself a very good record of treating and preventing recurrence, this is a necessary first element of any repair. It is the closure of the defect, with living tissue, that forms the basis of the repair. Mesh is used to reinforce the primary repair and not to serve as the repair per se. Given the defect is approximated, the mesh becomes a posterior reinforcement of the floor of the inguinal canal, adding strength and support not only to the repaired defect but also to a larger area. It is in this reinforcement of the larger aspect of the posterior floor that there may be additional benefit to the use of mesh. Placed between the fascia transversalis and the peritoneum, the mesh is positioned to be incorporated well and safely in the healing process. From this position, the mesh also reinforces the area of the defect as well as a broader surface area, depending on the perceived need. It is the concept of reinforcing the primary tissue repair that is important in this approach.

The placement of mesh into the preperitoneal space, unsecured to the iliopubic tract or Cooper's ligament, has been previously reported first by Stoppa and then in variations by others [4–6]. Nyhus used a variant of this technique and reported it in 1988 [7], where the mesh was sutured into place.

It is a combination of these concepts that has been used, when indicated, to aid and assist the repair of recurrent groin hernia in the series presented here. The mesh is secured to the iliopubic band or Cooper's ligament, sewn to the fascia transversalis at least 3 cm above the closure of the defect, and then secured to the fascial closure of the incision of the internal and external abdominal oblique aponeurosis, well above the defect and its repair. By placing the mesh in the preperitoneal space, securing it inferiorly to a fixed and solid structure, and then attaching it to the anterior abdominal wall some 10–14 cm away, with some laxity to conform to the shape of the abdominal wall in this area, the goals of reinforcement and tension-free mesh placement are achieved.

Of note is the fact that many of these techniques are described for use in the very large or giant recurrent hernias of the groin. As was noted in the series reported in

1987, many of the recurrent defects are small, the majority less than 4 cm. Thus the use of large mesh patches to cover small defects beyond a certain level of reasonableness does not make much sense given the potential for complications with mesh placement.

40.5 Comments

Clearly there are different patterns of defects associated with the recurrent groin hernia. It is my contention that the repair should be tailored to the findings. It is further my view that the use of mesh should be considered an option rather than a requirement in the repair of a recurrent groin hernia. Moreover, mesh should be used to buttress a primary tissue repair and not be used to "span the defect" or "plug the hole," as these latter approaches do not withstand a critique based on solid and sound surgical principles. We are living in a technologic era when new developments appear promising but are often untested by time. A problem with evaluating much of hernia surgery is a lack of randomized trials used to establish better ways to accomplish our goals. What we do have are large, well-supported and documented serial sequential studies with excellent results for many of the current approaches.

Of note is the fact that these results are not apparently easily transportable, because they have not been consistently duplicated or validated when tried by other experienced surgeons. The fact is that surgeons are most comfortable with familiar techniques and are not willing to alter or change their behavior for fear of a complication or a less desirable result. In an atmosphere of intensified risk if there is a failure, it is doubtful whether a meaningful trial comparing hernia repairs to establish any method as preferable can be done.

The argument for a tailored approach to the management of groin hernia has been made [8]. A similar argument is being made for the management of the recurrent groin hernia. Although the recurrent hernia may share characteristics with others, the potential for uniqueness and differences always remains. It is for that possibility that the open preperitoneal approach with primary closure of the defect and mesh reinforcement, if necessary, is preferred. This is an anatomic repair with all of the options to add the benefits of technology if they are needed.

40.6 Discussion

Amid: The incidence of femoral hernias always used to be very low, but the incidence seems to have increased with the use of preperitoneal and laparoscopic repairs. Might this phenomenon be the negative consequence of removing the fat from the femoral orifice?

Greenburg: A femoral hernia is present when you find a peritoneal sac in the femoral orifice, and only in these conditions should a femoral hernia repair be undertaken.

Kingsnorth: Which type and what size of hernia requires a large preperitoneal mesh repair? What do you mean by peritonealization of the cord, and is there any harm for the testicular blood supply?

Stoppa: Indications for the giant mesh are not only large recurrences, but also smaller bilateral hernias. Concerning the blood supply of the testis, there is really no increased risk. You can even divide the vessels in the retroperitoneal space without a subsequent ischemic orchitis.

Greenburg: What I do is exactly the same preparation of the preperitoneal space as Dr. Stoppa. In cases of indirect hernias, the sac always lies superior and lateral to the structures of the cord, and at that level it is never a problem to dissect these structures from the sac.

Schumpelick: Dr. Greenburg, we have had bad results when we closed incidental hernias using only some internal stitches during colonic surgery, for example. Now you tell us to do hernia repair using exactly these sutures from inside. And you have good results. What is the reason for this difference?

Greenburg: I think it is the surgeon. If you prepare and identify the landmarks, inguinal ligament, Cooper's ligament etc. and suture the hernial orifice as I showed, you will achieve good results. But if you just close a peritoneal sac with some sutures from the inside, you will have further recurrences.

Schumpelick: What do you think about doing your operation laparoscopically? Preparation of the defect, suturing, not putting a mesh. Do you think this would achieve good results?

Greenburg: I do not do laparoscopic hernia repair by myself. If somebody is going to develop such a suture repair, he or she should contact me.

Skandalakis: There has been a discussion concerning the femoral ring. What do you think about putting one or two sutures to the femoral ring in every preperitoneal repair routinely?

Greenburg: A femoral hernia should be repaired only if it is present. Sutures to the femoral ring are not harmless at all. They might promote thrombosis or lesions of the vein. Suturing the femoral ring must be restricted to the presence of a femoral hernia.

Bendavid: Dr. Stoppa, you mentioned that the vessels can be dissected at the preperitoneal level without any harm to the testis. We always preserve the vessels very precisely and yet still have cases of testicular atrophy. Can you comment on this?

Stoppa: I do not divide the vessels in my operations, but I know that some urologists do this for varicoceles without atrophy resulting.

Skandalakis: Some years ago in a paper by Jordan from Tennessee, it was pointed out that division of the cord without bringing up the testis results in an atrophy rate of 2%. However, by bringing up the testis from the scrotum, the five collateral vascular routes are destroyed and a cord division leads to testicular necrosis.

Flament: Dr. Stoppa, what are the indications for your giant mesh repair? Do you put the mesh in every inguinal hernia?

Stoppa: No, I do the giant mesh repair only in about 20% of all inguinal hernia repairs.

Schumpelick: Dr. Stoppa, is there any age limitation for your mesh?

Stoppa: Yes, I never put a mesh in patients under 40 years of age.

Bendavid: Dr. Greenburg, your technique, the preperitoneal suture repair, was published by Nyhus with a recurrence rate of at least 12%, which is rather high. In your series, you put a mesh only in about 6% of cases and your recurrence rates are much better. Do you not believe that the preperitoneal repair is only successful when a mesh is used?

Greenburg: I showed that the preperitoneal suture repair works in my hands. I have a recurrence rate of 1.2%. I think the additional mesh placement can be restricted to cases with a high recurrence risk. An increased risk is likely in defects of more than 4 cm in diameter and in patients with bad connective tissue.

References

1. Greenburg, A.G. Revisiting the recurrent groin hernia, Am J Surg 154:35–40, 1987.
2. Nyhus, L.M., Condon, R.E., Harkins, H.N. Clinical experience with preperitoneal hernia repair for all types of hernia of the groin. Am J Surg 100:2234–40, 1960.
3. Greenburg, A.G. Pre-peritoneal repair of recurrent groin hernia. Perspectives in General Surgery 2:43–57, 1991.
4. Stoppa, R., Petit, J., Henry, X. Unsutured Dacron prosthesis in groin hernias. Int J Surg 60:411–412, 1975.
5. Wantz, G.E. Giant prosthetic reinforcement of the visceral sac. Surg Gynecol Obstet 169:408–471, 1989.
6. Read, R.C. Bilaterality and the prosthetic repair of large recurrent inguinal hernias. Am J Surg 138:788, 1979.
7. Nyhus, L.M., et al. The preperitoneal approach and prosthetic buttress repair for recurrent hernia. Ann Surg 208:733–737, 1988.
8. Shahinian, T.K., and Greenburg, A.G. Hernias. Current Practice in Surgery, Levine, B.A., Copeland, E.M., Howard, R.J., Sugerman, H.J., Warshaw, A.L. (Eds), Section XIII, Chapter 26, Churchill Livingstone, New York, 1993.

CHAPTER 41

Laparoscopic Treatment of Recurrent Hernias

Z.T. Awad, C.J. Filipi

41.1 Introduction

Repair of recurrent hernias has always been a challenge for surgeons. The search for the optimum method for repairing inguinal hernias has been ongoing since Bassini introduced the anterior repair over 100 years ago [1]. Bassini's repair gained universal acceptance and widespread application in a very short period. Many variations, however, have been introduced in an attempt to reduce morbidity, recurrence rates, and duration of hospitalization. Since his original description, more than 80 approaches for anterior repair of inguinal hernia and femoral hernias have been reported [2]. Bassini's repair and its many modifications share the reinforcement of the floor of the groin by overlapping or approximating adjacent viable tissue. The success of the technique is based on the strength of the suture material and the resulting scar. It is noteworthy that Bassini's incidence of recurrence was only 3% [3]. Today, the incidence of recurrence with this approach by other surgeons is between 1.9% and 32% [4, 5].

Although heuristic techniques are available for selection by surgeons, two methods of anterior herniorrhaphy, the Shouldice repair and the Lichtenstein repair, appear to produce the best results. The Shouldice technique, which involves multilayered suturing of the floor of the inguinal canal, was introduced in 1946. It achieved outstanding results [6]. However, strict analyses of the Shouldice Clinic data shows that, at the beginning of their experience (1945), they observed a recurrence rate of 17%. Their technique has been modified to include division of the cremasteric muscle, resulting in a more accurate identification of often overlooked small indirect hernia. In addition, care to identify a concomitant femoral hernia and selective use of the repair has assisted in reducing the recurrence rate. After modifications, their recurrence rate dropped to 1% [7], which is still achieved today. Certainly, this exceptional result reflects a precise understanding of groin anatomy and the pathophysiology of hernia formation.

The Lichtenstein "tension-free" hernia repair uses an onlay prosthesis to reconstruct the inguinal floor. This eliminates suture line tension, the main disadvantage found in the Bassini repair and its many modifications. Lichtenstein reported a recurrence rate of 0.4%. The main causes of recurrence were attributed to undersized mesh or its improper fixation to the tuberculum suprapubicum [8]. It is thought that early recurrence after anterior repair results from either technical errors (failure to dissect or identify the sac) or tension on the suture line (approximation of normally unapproximated structures). The latter results in a new hernia formation. Late recurrence often results from inherent weakness in the groin secondary to a collagen deficit [8, 9]. The Lichtenstein repair addresses all of these mechanisms of recurrence.

Nevertheless, it is estimated that the overall recurrence of primary hernia repair is 10% and that of recurrent hernias is 25% [10]. Repair of recurrent hernias is difficult due to obscured anatomy, making tissue dissection difficult, which in turn increases the incidence of complications. Additional concerns include the presence of already attenuated tissues and the cost to individual patients and society as a whole. Surgeons and their patients therefore need a simpler solution to the problem of recurrent hernias.

41.2 Evolution of the Preperitoneal Approach

Another important contribution to the armamentarium of herniorrhaphists is the posterior repair with mesh buttressing [11–13]. This has reduced the incidence of failed herniorrhaphy because it eliminates the effect of many of the underlying causes of recurrence. Inspecting the posterior aspect of the inguinal floor allows evaluation of the entire inguinal region and all potential hernia sites, therefore avoiding missed hernias. In addition, it allows the surgeon to perform a tension-free repair of the entire posterior floor, thus avoiding the problem of possible late recurrence due to intrinsic collagen deficit, since the entire myopectineal orifice is covered with mesh.

Stoppa has accomplished great success by using the giant prosthetic reinforcement of the visceral sac (GPRVS), which covers all potential groin hernia sites and Fruchaud's myopectineal orifice [11]. The prosthesis is placed between the peritoneum and the inner side of the abdominal wall and is held in place by the intra-abdominal pressure and subsequent ingrowth of connective tissue. Hernias are eliminated as the peritoneum can neither stretch nor extend through the myopectineal orifice and adjacent areas of weakened tissues. Stoppa's recurrence rate for primary hernia repair is reported as 0.56% for complex hernias and 1.1% for recurrent hernias. This method provided the operative principles for the present-day laparoscopic preperitoneal herniorrhaphy.

With nearly 500,000 operations performed annually in the United States for primary and recurrent hernias [14] and the enthusiasm following laparoscopic cholecystectomy, it seems logical that attempts to repair groin hernias laparoscopically would be developed. Early reports of laparoscopic hernia repair utilizing intraperitoneal closure of the hernial sac or a mesh plug and patch technique revealed an unacceptably high recurrence rate [15]. Thereafter, the lessons learned from the open preperitoneal herniorrhaphy of Stoppa were applied laparoscopically. The two most commonly performed techniques of laparoscopic herniorrhaphy are the transabdominal preperitoneal (TAPP) and the totally extraperitoneal (TEP) repair. Comparative studies showed that the overall incidence of complications, recurrence rate, and return to normal daily activities were not significantly different between the two types of repair.

The TEP repair has several advantages over the TAPP, which include the following:

1. The peritoneum is kept intact, thus avoiding possible complications of bowel injury and the risk of postoperative intraperitoneal adhesions
2. Reduced operative time as the peritoneum does not require opening or closing

3. Avoidance of peritoneal adhesions in patients with previous abdominal surgery
4. Elimination of the risk of herniation through the peritoneal closure

The advantages of TAPP include the following:
1. Less technically demand
2. Facilitates identification of the inguinal hernia type
3. Ease of dissection of complex and recurrent hernias, as exposure is easily achieved
4. Allows easy confirmation of proper mesh positioning and flattening

Some surgeons advocate what is termed the laparoscopic "sandwich" method for the repair of hernias [16]. This combines the advantages of both the TAPP and the TEP repair. Laparoscopy is performed to identify the type of hernia followed by extraperitoneal dissection. The hernial sac is then removed intraperitoneally by a pre-tied ligature or it is simply inverted. The mesh is placed in the preperitoneal space, covering the three possible hernia sites, and secured with a stapler. The laparoscope is reinserted into peritoneal cavity to ensure an adequate and flat mesh position in the preperitoneal space.

Prospective trials comparing laparoscopic herniorrhaphy with the open anterior technique revealed that patients who underwent laparoscopic herniorrhaphy experienced less postoperative pain than patients with anterior open repair, required less postoperative analgesia, and were quicker to return to their daily activities and work [17, 18]. Filipi, in a randomized prospective study on transabdominal preperitoneal laparoscopic herniorrhaphy versus the tension-free Lichtenstein repair, demonstrated a modest decrease in pain during the early postoperative period for patients undergoing laparoscopic hernia repair [19]. This, however, did not influence postoperative convalescence, as there was no significant difference in postoperative disability between groups.

41.3 Causes of Recurrence After Anterior Herniorrhaphy

Recurrences are classified as early or late and as indirect, direct, femoral, or combined. The type of recurrence is helpful in understanding the different mechanisms of recurrence for each specific type of hernia.

41.3.1 Indirect Recurrence

Indirect recurrence is usually a complication of a primary indirect hernia repair [20]. Postlethwait, in a series of 300 indirect recurrences, found 234 cases in which the sac was within the cord with no evidence of purse-sting suture, indicating a missed hernia [21]. Remnants of a purse-string suture were seen in others at one side of the sac at the level of the internal ring. Incorrect purse-string suture placement (i.e., leaving wide gaps between each suture application) favors indirect recurrence through the tissue gaps created [21]. Mehnert reported 122 indirect recurrences; 30% were funicular, i.e., the hernia sac arose at the internal ring within the confines of the spermatic cord coverings and descended within the inguinal canal, while 70% were juxtafunicular [20]. These hernias originate in the indirect area (lateral to the inferior epigastric vessels) and may carry attenuated fascia transversalis ahead of them as they advance. The line of sac progression is adjacent to and alongside the cord. Mehnert believes that funicular recurrences represent missed hernias, while juxtafunicular recurrences are probably the result of failure to accurately identify the boundaries and snugly reconstruct the internal ring [20]. Precise identification of the edges of the internal ring is difficult in the presence of a thick cremasteric muscle mass. Postlethwait recommends excision of the cremasteric muscle for better anatomical delineation and closure of the internal ring [21].

Schumpelick, in a prospective controlled study in two centers, found that there were no indirect recurrences in 237 Shouldice repairs with resection of the cremasteric muscle, while there were four indirect recurrences (2.6%) in 153 Shouldice repairs without cremasteric resection [22].

Some techniques are more likely than others to lead to recurrence. Halsted's repair involves subcutaneous transplantation of the cord and imposes the external ring upon the weakened internal ring, thus placing them directly in the line of intra-abdominal forces [20]. In Bassini's repair, there is conversion of the normal obliquity at the internal ring to one of right angles to the abdominal wall, as the lower border of the internal oblique is sutured to Poupart's ligament beneath the cord [20]. This creates a potential weakness in the abdominal wall identical to that of Halsted's repair, except for the outer buttress of the external oblique aponeurosis, which is sutured over the cord rather than beneath it.

41.3.2 Direct Recurrence

A direct recurrence is the result of either a missed hernia, tension at the suture line, or inherent weakness of the posterior wall. A missed hernia indicates an incomplete anatomical dissection. To avoid missing unexpected direct hernias or weakness of the posterior wall, Glassow tests the strength of the posterior wall by inserting a finger at the internal ring and passing it extraperitoneally, medially, and deep to the transversalis plane [23]. Postlethwait's technique involves incision of the indirect sac and intraperitoneal finger evaluation of Hesselbach's triangle and the femoral ring [21].

Suture line tension is the result of attempting reapproximation of normally unapproximated structures [33]. If in excess, this is a clear violation of surgical principles, but intraoperative tissue tension measurement is currently not available. Postlethwait, in a series of 241 direct recurrent hernias, noted recurrences as a localized defect in the fascia transversalis just lateral to the symphysis pubis in 144 cases [21]. He thought they were probably related to sutures placed too far apart, a single suture breaking or untying. Glassow noted that the typical site for direct hernia recurrence is medially near the pubic bone [23]. These were often small, consisting mainly of extraperitoneal fat, and were considered to be a technical error.

41.3.3 Femoral Recurrence

As examination of the femoral area has become a routine in modern groin hernia surgery [23], few cases of femoral hernia are missed. The majority are either new hernia formation or hernias created by the original repair. The latter is a potential sequela in methods applying tension, resulting in a weakened femoral region.

41.4 Causes of Recurrence After Open or Laparoscopic Preperitoneal Herniorrhaphy

Factors leading to recurrence after preperitoneal hernia repair, whether conventional or laparoscopic, are unique to the posterior approach. The following technical pitfalls must be avoided.

41.4.1 Incomplete Dissection

Incomplete dissection is the most common cause of recurrence after laparoscopic herniorrhaphy [10]. It results in poor overall assessment of the groin, missed hernias, and insufficient delineation of the fascial structures. Incomplete dissection leads to recurrence by a number of mechanisms, including inadequate space for mesh placement leading to mesh folding, inadequate mesh overlap, and small prosthesis size. Lipomatous hernia recurrence results from protrusion of preperitoneal fat through a direct defect. It appears in the immediate postoperative period. Lipomatous hernia recurrence can be avoided if the fascia transversalis underlying Hesselbach's triangle is completely cleaned of preperitoneal fat.

41.4.2 Inadequate Mesh Size

Initially, laparoscopic surgeons compromised mesh size. Recurrence rates have dropped as mesh size increased, which was also due to the experience of surgeons performing open preperitoneal repair. A large piece of mesh must cover not only the hernia, but also other potential sites, thereby preventing late recurrences. A small prosthesis placed over an isolated defect leads to recurrence as a result of shrinkage of the prosthesis and/or subsequent enlargement of the defect. A 10%–20% decrease in mesh surface area is seen after fibroblast ingrowth. Surgeons have yet to agree on the optimum size of the mesh. We think that 15x12 cm mesh is required for patients with unilateral groin hernia.

41.4.3
Inadequate Overlap

Complete dissection must fully define the fascial edges of the hernial defect to allow accurate mesh placement. It is thought that all defects should be overlapped in every direction by at least 2 cm if stapled and 3 cm if not stapled. Mesh placed only to the margin of a defect will invariably result in a recurrence.

41.4.4
Mesh Slitting

Slitting should be avoided, as it has been documented as a mechanism of recurrence. Originally, the slit was designed to accommodate cord structures that serve as an anchor for the mesh prosthesis and to allow better apposition of the mesh to the inguinal floor. Stapled reapproximation of the slit edges can be less than ideal, or the whole size for cord structures is overestimated and a recurrence can result. Parietalization of the vas deferens and gonadal vessels will allow flat and secure mesh placement without use of a slit. Felix believes mesh slitting is necessary to accommodate the cord structures as they tend to elevate the mesh off the inguinal floor. To prevent possible recurrence at the slit site, he uses a double-buttress technique, which is probably the most secure method if slitting is felt necessary.

41.4.5
Missed Hernias

A missed hernia indicates a poor technique as a result of incomplete dissection of the preperitoneal space. If no peritoneal sac is evident, a small direct hernia that contains only preperitoneal fat (lipomatous hernia) should be looked for. A lipomatous hernia results from protrusion of extraperitoneal fat through a direct defect. It is apparent in the early postoperative period.

41.4.6
Mesh Displacement

Displacement of the prosthesis with uncovering of a hernial defect leads to recurrence and usually results from improper fixation. Stapled fixation of an adequately sized prosthesis to Cooper's ligament is required to prevent medial and lateral mesh displacement before collagen ingrowth. Fixation above the iliopubic tract is helpful in obtaining a flat prosthesis. It is important to note that the genitofemoral nerve or lateral femoral cutaneous nerve occasionally passes through the iliopubic tract. Fixation to Cooper's ligament is necessary to prevent lifting of the inferomedial angle and subsequent medial recurrence.

Recurrence after preperitoneal herniorrhaphy is usually at the inferolateral angle. This is due to mesh lifting secondary to folding, curling, or hematoma formation.

Adequate size prosthesis is important; however, the most common reason for poor mesh apposition to the inguinal floor is incomplete dissection. During TAPP repair, the flat application of mesh can be confirmed by viewing the prosthesis with the peritoneum lifted and under tension. In the TEP repair, a final intraperitoneal view after CO_2 gas has escaped from the preperitoneal space will ensure flat mesh placement.

41.5 Transabdominal Preperitoneal Repair (TAPP)

In the TAPP procedure, the patient is placed in the supine position and a catheter is placed in the urinary bladder. A 2-cm subumbilical incision is carried down to the linea alba. The peritoneum is then opened and a sealing Hasson-type trocar is introduced into the peritoneal cavity. A pneumoperitoneum is created with CO2 insufflation through the trocar. The pressure ranges between 12 and 15 mmHg. Diagnostic laparoscopy is followed by insertion of a 10-mm port at the level of the umbilicus in the anterior axillary line. A mirror-image 5- to 10-mm port is inserted in the contralateral side. The patient is put in a Trendelenburg position, allowing the bowel to fall away from the pelvis. The dissection starts by making a peritoneal incision 4–5 cm superior to the internal ring and through the medial umbilical ligament. The incision extends 4–5 cm lateral to the internal ring. Reflection of the posterior peritoneal flap from the inguinal floor is accomplished by blunt and sharp dissection. Using important anatomical landmarks such as Cooper's ligament, the inferior epigastric vessels are then dissected, revealing the transversus abdominis aponeurosis and iliopubic tract. The floor is cleared of fat and preperitoneal tissue to expose any hidden defects. Scar tissue from previous surgery is dissected with great care to avoid peritoneal tears and injury to the vas deferens and spermatic vessels. If present, an indirect hernia is completely dissected from the cord and inverted into the abdominal cavity. If large, the sac is transected and the distal part left in situ. Direct hernia sacs, however, are not ligated or excised because of risk of injury to the bladder. The round ligament in females may be divided. Normally, we parietalize the cord structures as described by Stoppa. Scar formation often requires sharp dissection, and thus a precise understanding of the relationship of the vas deferens to the surrounding landmarks along with proximal and distal confirmation of its position prior to dissection of the vas from scar tissue is necessary. A single piece (15x12 cm) of polypropylene mesh is introduced through one of the ports to cover the entire inguinal floor. It must cover each defect by at least 2 cm and extend medially beyond the symphysis pubis, superiorly above the internal ring, and inferiorly below Cooper's ligament (Fig. 1). Mesh slitting is avoided. Staples are applied to Cooper's ligament and to the transversus abdominis anterior to the iliopubic tract. No staples are applied posterior to the iliopubic tract to avoid injury to the genitofemoral nerve and lateral femoral cutaneous nerve of the thigh. The peritoneum is closed with staples. If peritoneal openings remain, the intraperitoneal pressure is decreased and staple or suture closure is completed. A meticulous closure of each defect is necessary to prevent retroperitoneal hernia formation. The skin is closed with 4/0 absorbable suture after administration of local anesthetics.

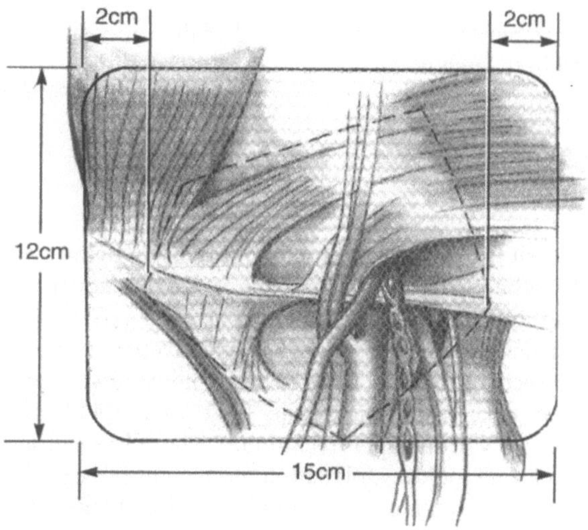

Fig. 1. Superimposed mesh over the myopectineal orifice. Note the 2-cm overlap in all directions

41.6 Totally Extraperitoneal Repair (TEP)

A 2-cm incision just below the umbilicus and off the midline is made down to the anterior rectus sheath. Two small retractors are inserted and the anterior rectus sheath is incised, exposing the rectus muscle. The medial attachments of the rectus muscle to the linea alba are divided by sharp dissection, thus entering the retrorectus space. The balloon dissector is inserted between the posterior aspect of the rectus muscle and the posterior rectus sheath and advanced beyond the line of Douglas until the pubis is felt. Under direct vision, the extraperitoneal space is exposed by the expanding balloon. It takes 30–40 compressions of the bulb to inflate the balloon completely. The balloon is left in place for several minutes, which helps tamponade any bleeding vessels. The balloon is deflated and replaced by a sealing Hasson-type cannula. The retroperitoneum is inflated using CO2 with a pressure limit of 12–15 mmHg. A 30°- to 45°-angled laparoscope is used. In the midline, a 10-mm trocar is inserted just above the symphysis pubis and a 5-mm trocar is inserted midway between the umbilicus and the pubis. The surgeon stands on the side opposite the hernia. The next step is to identify Cooper's ligament by bluntly dissecting the proportional fat off the ligament from the symphysis pubis to the iliac vessels, care being taken to avoid any underlying vessels. The space lateral to the epigastric vessels is then dissected, revealing the transversus abdominis muscle, the iliopubic tract, and the cord structures. A space is created between the cord and the iliac vessels that lie behind. Blunt dissection with one jaw of an open atraumatic 5-mm grasping forceps works well. If the peritoneum is inadvertently opened during dissection, it is ligated with an endoloop or a suture. Alternatively, a plastic cannula can be introduced into the peritoneal cavity to vent CO_2 gas. If too many openings or a large rent occur, venting is futile and conversion to a TAPP repair is necessary. To avoid this, the vas deferens and spermatic vessels must be carefully identified, as they are often encased in scar tissue secondary to the previous repair. One must dissect with scissors when freeing the peritoneum, which requires experience and an understanding of the anatomy. After complete dissection, the mesh is unfolded and fixed to the preperitoneal structures, as in the TAPP repair.

An intraperitoneal look at the end of the procedure will ensure flat apposition of the mesh in the pelvis.

41.7 Comments

Although the role of laparoscopic surgery in primary groin hernia is controversial, we believe the laparoscopic approach is the procedure of choice for patients with recurrent groin hernias in the same way as open extraperitoneal repair has been advocated for patients with recurrence. The effectiveness of hernia repair is usually determined by its recurrence rate. Table 1 shows the results of laparoscopic surgery for recurrent hernias when using either the TAPP or the TEP method, and Table 2 showed the results for various open techniques. The increased length of follow-up for the latter group is one logical explanation for a slight increase in recurrence rates. Interestingly, in only 94 of 796 recurrent hernias repaired laparoscopically was the TEP repair utilized. This is presumably because the TEP repair was developed after the TAPP. It also may reflect the increased difficulty in preserving peritoneal integrity when dissecting scar from the peritoneal surface. Recurrence was observed only in four cases (0.5%) after secondary repair, with two being the result of technical failure. In one case the mesh was undersized. The other was the result of an inability to redissect the floor, as the mesh from the previous operation was adherent to the bladder. These are convin-

Table 1. Laparoscopic repair of recurrent hernias

Reference	Recurrent hernias (*n*)	Type of repair	Recurrence rate (%)	Follow-up (months)
[28]	124	TAPP	0.8	24
	49	TEP	0	24
[24]	210	TAPP	0.95	6–36
[25]	200	TAPP	0.5	9–31
[26]	117	TAPP	0	3–36
[27]	51	TAPP	0	1–31
[34]	45	TEP	0	–[a]

TAPP, transabdominal peritoneal repair; TEP, totally extraperitoneal repair.
[a]No specific data.

Table 2. Open repair of recurrent hernias

Reference	Recurrent hernias (n)	Type of repair	Recurrence rate (%)	Follow-up (months)
[11]	270	GPRVS	1.1	24–144
[30]	201	Preperitoneal mesh	1.7	6–120
[8]	1500	Plug repair	1.6	26–240
[29]	100	Preperitoneal mesh	3	6–60
[31]	127	Cooper's ligament repair	2.4	108
[32]	1874	Shouldice	1.0	>120
[39]	189	GPRVS	3.7%	-[a]

GPRVS, giant prosthetic reinforcement of the visceral sac.
[a]No specific data.

cing results considering that laparoscopic hernia surgery is only 6–7 years old. All of these recurrences appeared within the first year.

Felix, in a repair of 173 recurrent hernias, reported 80% incidence of bilateral disease [28]. Complex hernias (hernias with more than one defect in the wall) occurred in 28% of cases. Stoppa, however, reported a 42.2% bilateral rate in 349 recurrent groin hernias [11]. The incidence of complex hernia during open repair for recurrent hernias ranges from 2%–15% [9, 31]. This wide difference between the results obtained by Felix and other series may indicate better visualization of the preperitoneal space when viewed laparoscopically.

In 1990, Schultz reported a recurrence rate of 25% as a result of limited dissection and failure to identify all the components of complex hernias [379. In his second report in 1994, in which the entire floor was dissected, recurrences were eliminated [38]. The exceptional results of Glassow with the Shouldice repair are unlikely to represent what occurs in everyday practice [35, 36], but do represent the complete and precise method by which the Shouldice Clinic surgeons dissect the inguinal floor [32]. In a repair of 1874 recurrent groin hernias, Glassow reported recurrence in 18 patients. In 12 of those who underwent further operation, there were seven direct, one indirect, and four femoral recurrences. The total number of recurrences was 91 (0.62%) in 14,586 repairs (primary and recurrent), with 51 of 91 recurrences being femoral. This figure is significant, as these femoral recurrences are either missed hernias, are due to technical error in dealing with the lower transversalis flap, or are the result of tension.

Recurrence after open preperitoneal mesh repair results exclusively from technical errors and usually manifests itself within the first year. Stoppa repaired 270 recurrent hernias by GPRVS, and the recurrence rate was 1.1% (n=3) [11]. Recurrences after placement of a giant prosthesis are usually caused by mesh that is undersized, displaced, or has split to let the cord pass through, leading to breakage. Nyhus' recurrence rate in a series of 201 recurrent hernias was 1.7% (n=2); one was indirect and the other was lateral to the mesh [30]. No further recurrence has developed since he started to use mesh to bolster the anatomical repair. Mozingo had three recurrences following repair of 100 recurrent hernias, all due to technical factors as the hernia defect was not completely covered with the mesh [29]. In Wantz' report on the repair of 189 recurrent hernias by GPRVS, there were seven recurrences in 108 cases undergoing a bilateral repair and none in 81 cases undergoing a unilateral repair [39]. There were no recurrences when Marlex mesh was used, while recurrence with Prolene (four out of 18) was the result of lateral border mesh folding or curling. A Gore-Tex recurrence (one out of 19) was due to poor adherence, as the mesh was found lying unattached within the peritoneal cavity. The intra-abdominal pressure forced it to slip through the unrepaired defect in the abdominal wall. Wantz believes that Mersilene is the best synthetic material to be used for GPRVS. The recurrences (four out of 68) when using the latter were the result of technical problems, as the mesh was incorrectly unfolded or it was imprecisely placed.

The basic principle of a Cooper's ligament repair is the closure of the deficiency in the posterior inguinal wall effected by suturing the upper margin of the defect, represented by the aponeurosis of the transversalis plus its investing fascia, downward to its insertion to Cooper's ligament along the superior ramus of the pubis lateral to the pubic tubercle. A relaying incision in the anterior rectus sheath is necessary due to tension on the suture line.

Rutledge had three recurrences (2.4%) in the repair of 127 recurrent hernias, all occurring in those operated on in the period before 1972 [31].

Lichtenstein, in a series of 1500 recurrent hernias, noted that recurrences are mainly found at either end of the sutured repair (at the pubic tubercle or at the internal ring) and where approximated tissues under tension are not supported by adjacent buttressing sutures on both sides [8, 40]. Using the plug repair, he reported a recurrence rate of 1.6% [8]. The cause of recurrence was either that the plug was too loose or too small, too few sutures were applied, or there were unrecognized defects. Lichtenstein's view is that attempting extensive dissection destroys the intact portion of the previous procedure, thereby converting a small defect into a large one [40]. The plug is easy to handle and completely occludes the defect, and its light protrusion into the peritoneal cavity prevents herniation of bowel or omentum into the cul-de-sac that an onlay mesh might create [40].

Lichtenstein uses a defect diameter of 4 cm as the cutoff point for the plug repair and utilizes the onlay patch for larger defects [8]. He advocates the preperitoneal approach for complete disruption of the inguinal floor.

41.8 Conclusion

Laparoscopic herniorrhaphy is eminently qualified for the repair of recurrent groin hernias. It eliminates one of the common causes of recurrence, the missed hernia, and allows the surgeon to identify those patients with a so-called complex hernia. It should work over the long term as it reduces tension, covers the entire myopectineal orifice, and buttresses the intrinsic collagen deficit, the cause of late recurrence. The key to maintaining these good results is the avoidance of technical errors.

41.9 Discussion

For a discussion, please see Chap. 42.

References

1. Bassini E. Nuovo Metodo Sulla Cura Radicale dell'Ernia Inguinale. Arch Soc Ital Cir. 1887; 4:380.
2. Corbitt J.D Jr. Laproscopic herniorrhaphy. Surg Laparosc Endosc. 1991; 1:23–25
3. Bassini E. Uno nouvo metodo per la cura radicale dell' ernia inguinale. Padua, 1889
4. Stoppa RE; Warlaumont CR. The Preperitoneal approach and prosthetic repair of groin hernia. Nyhus LM; Conden RE (eds) Hernia. JP Lippincott, Philadelphia, PA.1989: 199–225
5. Welsh DRJ. Inguinal hernia repair: a contemporary approach to a common procedure. Modern medicine 1974; 2: 49–54
6. Bendavid R. New techniques in hernia repair. World J Surg 1989; 13(5): 522–531
7. Felix EL; Michas CA; Mcknight RL. Laparoscopic repair of recurrent hernias. Surg Endosc. 1995;9(2):135_139
8. Lichtenstein IL; Shulman AG; Amid PK. The cause, prevention and treatment of recurrent groin hernias. Surg Cling North Am. 1993;73(3): 529–543
9. Postlethwait RW. Causes of recurrence after inguinal herniorrhaphy. Surgery 1971; 69(5):772–775

10. Lowman AS; Filipi CJ; Fitzgibbons, RJ.Jr; Stoppa R; Wantz GE; Felix EL; Crafton WB: Mechanisms of Hernia Recurrence after Preperitoneal Mesh Repair. Ann Surg. 1997, 225(4):422–431
11. Stoppa RE. The treatment of complicated groin and incisional hernias. World J Surg. 1989; 13:545–554
12. Wantz GE. Preperitoneal hernioplasty with unilateral giant prosthetic reinforcement of the visceral sac. Contemp Surg. 1994; 44(2):83–89
13. Nyhus LM; et al. The preperitoneal approach and prosthetic buttress repair of recurrent hernia. Ann Surg. 1988; 208 : 722–727
14. Rutkow IM. Laparoscopic hernia repair: The socieoeconomic tyranny of surgical technology. Arch Surg. 1992; 11.1271
15. Schultz LS; et al. Transabdominal preperitoneal laparoscopic herniorrhaphy: Lessons learned and modifications. In: Arregui ME, Nagan RF, eds. Inguinal Hernia : Advances or controversies? Oxford, England: Radcliff Medical Press. 1994: 301–306
16. Urushihara T. Laparosc Surg Update 1997; July: 82
17. Kozol R; et al. A prospecive randomized study of open vs. laparoscopic inguinal hernia repair. Arch Surg: 1997; 132(3):292–5
18. Leim MS; et al. A randomized comparision of physical performance following laparoscopic and open inguinal hernia repair. Br J Surg. 1997; 84(1):64–7
19. Filipi CJ.; et al. An assessment of pain and return to normal activity. Laparoscopic herniorrhaphy vs open tension free Lichtenstein repair. Surg Endosc. 1996; 10:983–986
20. Mehnert JH; et al. Indirect recurrence of inguinal hernias: Am J Surg. 1963; 106:958–965
21. Postlethwait R.W. Recurrent inguinal hernia. Ann Surg. 1985; 202:777.
22. Töns C; et al. Controlled study of cremateric resection in Shouldice repair of primary inguinal hernia. Zentralbl. Chir 1991;116(12):737–43
23. Glassow F. Recurrent inguinal and femoral hernia. Br Med J 1970; 1(690): 215–216
24. Leibel B; et al. Endoscopic hernia surgery (TAPP)-gold standard in the management of recurrent hernias? Chirurg. 1996 Dec;67(12): 1226–30
25. Sandbichler; et al. Laparoscopic repair of recurrent inguinal hernias. Am J Surg. 1996; 171(3):366–8.
26. Birth M; et al. Laparoscopic transabdominal preperitoneal hernioplasty: results of 1000 consecutive cases. J Lap Surg. 1996; 6(5): 293_300
27. Stancanelli V; et al. Laparoscopic repair of bilateral and /or recurrent hernia. G Chir. 1994 Nor-Dec; 15(11–12):519–23
28. Felix EL; et al. Laparoscopic repair of recurrent hernia. Am J Surg 1996; 172:580–584
29. Mozingo DW; et al. Properitoneal synthetic mesh repair of recurrent inguinal hernias. Surg Gynecol Obstet. 1992; 174(1): 33–5
30. Nyhus LM; et al. The preperitoneal approach and prosthetic buttress repair for recurrent hernia. Ann Surg. 1988; 208:733–737
31. Rutledge RH. Cooper's ligament repair: A 25 years experience with a single technique for all groin hernias in adults. Surgery 1988; 103:1–10
32. Glassow F. Inguinal hernia repair: A comparison of the Shouldice and Cooper's ligament repair of the posterior abdominal wall. Am J Surg. 1976; 131:306
33. Lichtenstein IL; Shulman AG; Amid PK. The cause, prevention and treatment of recurrent groin hernias. Surg Cling North Am. 1993;73(3): 529–543
34. Gadacz T; et al. Totally Preperitoneal laparoscopic inguinal herniorrhaphy using balloon dissection. Surg Rounds 1995; March : 107–112
35. Schumpelick V. Shouldice repair in inguinal hernia. Chirurg . 1984; 55(1): 25–8
36. Wantz GE. The Canadian repair: Personal observation. World J Surg. 1989; 13(5): 516
37. Shultz L; et al: Laser laparoscopic herniorrhaphy : a clinical trial – preliminary study. J Lap Surg. 1990; 1(1):41_45
38. Shultz L; et al. Transabdominal preperitoneal procedure. Semin Laparos Surg. 1994; 1(2): 98–105
39. Wantz GE. Giant prosthetic reinforcement of the visceral sac. Surg Gynecol Obstet. 1989; 169(5): 408–17
40. Shulman AG; et al. The Plug repair of 1402 recurrent inguinal hernias. Arch Surg 1990; 125:265–267

CHAPTER 42

Endoscopic Repair: Totally Endoscopic Preperitoneal Prosthesis in Recurrent Inguinal Hernia

C. Klaiber, M. Banz, A. Metzger

In a sense, laparoscopy has revolutionized the field of hernia surgery. Established methods of hernia repair have been questioned and the interest among general surgeons has greatly increased.

Among the endoscopic techniques available, two methods have evolved to become standard techniques, the laparoscopic transabdominal preperitoneal prosthesis (TAPP) and the totally endoscopic preperitoneal prosthesis (TEP). Both use a large prosthesis (mesh) to cover all possible defects and reinforce the abdominal wall. The origin of these procedures is the open mesh repair, as conceived by Stoppa, whereas the preperitoneal endoscopic approach more closely resembles the original method. The technique is also in accordance with the principle of tension-free repair. The usual way of learning is to start with the transabdominal approach, which is technically more accessible. Although more demanding, we now favor the preperitoneal approach, because the peritoneum and the abdominal cavity remain intact.

The overall recurrence rate of open hernia repair varies from 0.4% to 25%; the re-recurrence rate is many times higher, because the new repair is performed in an weakened area. For this reason, endoscopic techniques seem particularly suited for the repair of recurrent hernias, since the former operative field with its scar tissue of poor quality is avoided. Furthermore, the mesh constitutes the repair and does not depend on a healing process in the initial phase.

42.1 Aarberg's Strategy for Inguinal Hernia Repair

Our concept depends on the following factors: age of the patient, tissue quality, size of the hernia, suitability for anesthesia, and primary or recurrent hernia. The following are guidelines which are individualized to meet the requirements of each patient (bilateral hernias, heavy labor, sports, and patients' preferences):

1. Shouldice repair: primary hernias in men younger than 35 years and in women of childbearing age
2. TEP repair: primary hernias in men over 35 years; all recurrent hernias in patients in which growth is completed (approx. 18 years)
3. Lichtenstein repair: patients over 35 years not fit for general anesthesia

Young patients with primary hernias have good tissue quality and therefore do not need a reinforcing mesh. Since very long follow-up after mesh implantation (more than 30 years) is not yet available, we like to err on the safe side in young and very young patients.

The older the patients gets, the greater the need becomes for some kind of reinforcement. In our opinion, the good results after mesh repair outweigh any possible, not yet known late complications.

Recurrent hernias represent a failure of both tissue and possibly technique. Both can be corrected by the use of mesh through another approach, e.g., TEP. In exceptional cases we use TAPP for very large hernias (primary or recurrent), since we feel that reduction of the hernia contents can be performed more safely under direct vision.

42.2 Operative Technique

We usually obtain patients' consent to explore and, if necessary, repair the contralateral side. Before patients are taken into the operation room, they are asked to empty their bladder. We only use a Foley catheter if, for some reason, patients are not able to empty their bladder spontaneously. General anesthesia is established and the patient placed supine with their arms tucked in.

An transverse incision is made distal to the umbilicus over the rectus muscle on the side of the hernia. The anterior fascia is opened, the muscle fibers are displaced laterally, and a 10-mm trocar sleeve with a blunt trocar is introduced into the preperitoneal space. Insufflation of CO_2 follows (10 mmHg). Gentle sideways and forward and backward movements of the endoscope (25°-angle view) further open the space until the symphysis is seen (Fig. 1). A 5-mm port is introduced in the midline about 5 cm distal to the lens port. The posterior rectus sheet is incised laterally with scissors, while the underlying peritoneum is pushed dorsally. The lateral abdominal wall is thus exposed. At the level of the umbilicus in the anterior axial line, a 12-mm port is introduced (Fig. 2).

The hernial sac is now exposed and reduced using two graspers. The peritoneum is pushed cranially and the spermatic cord parietalized. Cooper's ligament, an important landmark, is fully exposed. In the case of larger direct hernias, the protruding fascia transversalis is grasped, reduced, and fixed with staples to Cooper's ligament. Regardless of the hernia type (direct or indirect, primary or recurrent), a standard polypropylene mesh of 15x13 cm is trimmed, inserted in the preperitoneal space, and positio-

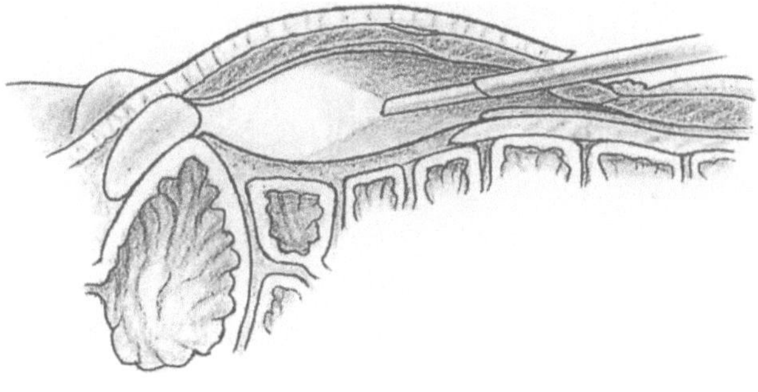

Fig. 1. Operative technique: the endoscope is moved gently forwards and backwards and from side to side to reveal the symphysis

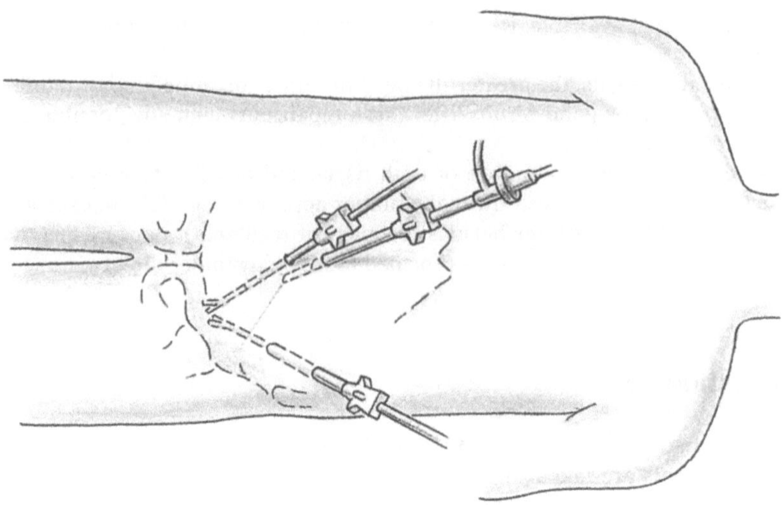

Fig. 2. Operative technique: a 12-mm port is introduced at the level of the umbilicus in the anterior axial line

ned. It covers the whole inguinal region, including the parietalized spermatic cord. The mesh is fixed to Cooper's ligament and to the abdominal wall by staples (Fig. 3).

We close holes of the peritoneum larger than 1 cm, either with staples or with a running suture, and we routinely drain the space with a small suction drain in order to avoid hematomas and seromas, which could easily displace the mesh. The drain remains in place for 24 h.

While CO_2 escapes at the end of the procedure, a grasper holds down the mesh while the visceral sac expands, thus preventing the mesh from folding up. We then close the rectus sheet and the skin.

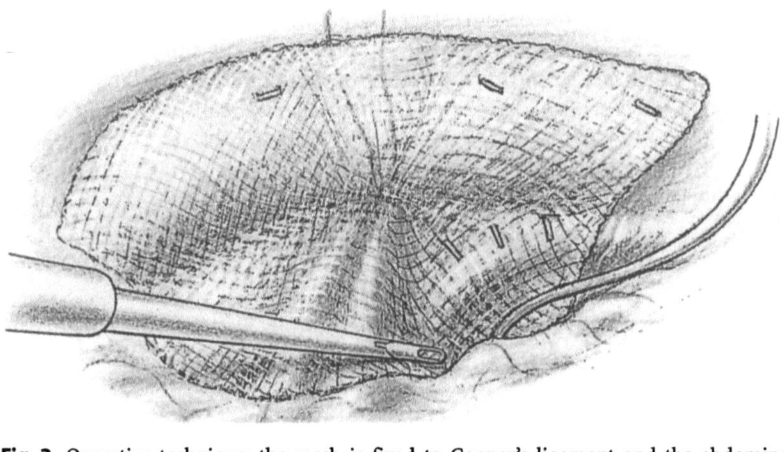

Fig. 3. Operative technique: the mesh is fixed to Cooper's ligament and the abdominal wall using staplers

The drain is withdrawn the next morning and the patient discharged. Physical activity is not restricted at all after the operation.

42.3 Aarberg's Results

We present the results of a prospective study with a follow-up of 1 year. Patients were examined by an independent physician, and the follow-up rate was 94%. From April 1994 to December 1996, 421 hernias were repaired in 285 patients (270 male, 15 female). The mean age was 55.4 years (range, 21–87 years). There were 363 primary and 58 (14%) recurrent hernias, of which 46 were first recurrences and 12 second, third, or fourth recurrences. The mean operative time was 65 min for primary hernias and 75 min for recurrent hernias. There were no conversions of TEP to an open procedure, but in three cases we switched from TEP to TAPP. Intraoperative complications are shown in Table 1. The mean hospital stay was 3.7 days. Complications during the first 30 days are shown in Table 2. Late complications occurred in nine patients (2%). There were no significant differences between patients operated upon with primary or

Table 1. Intraoperative problems and complications in363 primary and 58 recurrent hernias

Complication	Total (*n*)	Primary hernia (*n*)	Recurrent hernia (*n*)
Hemorrhage	3	2	1
CO_2 emphysema	1	1	–
Lost needle	1	1	–
Bladder injury	1	1	–
Intestinal injury	1	–	1
Total complications(*n*)	7 (1.7%)	5 (1.4%)	2 (3.4%)

Table 2. Early postoperative complications (30 days) in 363 primary and 58 recurrent hernias

Complication	Total (*n*)	Primary hernia (*n*)	Recurrent hernia (*n*)
Seroma/hematoma	7	6	1
Orchitis	–	–	-
Pneumonia	2	2	-
Pulmonary embolism	1	1	-
Diarrhea	1	1	-
Dysuria	1	–	1
Total complications	12 (2.9%)	10 (2.8%)	2 (3.4%)

Table 3. Results after 1 year in 242 primary and 43 recurrent hernias

Criterion	Total (*n*)	Primary hernia (*n*)	Recurrent hernia (*n*)
Reoperations (*n*)	3[a]	3[a]	0
Return to work (days)	23.3	23.7	20.8
Sporadic discomfort (%)	–	20.2	23.2
Pain (visual analogue scale)		27/100	1.3/100

[a] Umbilicus (*n*=1), neurolysis (*n*=2).

Table 4. Late complications (1 year) 363 primary and 58 recurrent hernias

Complication	Total (*n*)	Primary hernia (*n*)	Recurrent hernia (*n*)
Recurrences	1 (0.25%)	1	–
Umbilical hernia	2	2	–
Deep sinus umbilicus	1	1	–
Neuralgia	2	1	1
Hydrocele	2	1	1
Testicular atrophy	1	1	–
Total complications	9 (2%)	7 (1.9%)	2 (3.4%)

recurrent hernias (Tables 3, 4). There have been three reoperations for minor problems (neurolysis, deep sinus).

42.4 Conclusion

In contrast to open techniques, where the re-recurrence rate increases with additional repairs, our results for TEP repair of recurrent hernias are as good as those for primary hernias and also compare favorably with respect to short- and long-term complications to most series of open techniques. Therefore we conclude that TEP is an excellent technique for the repair of both primary and recurrent hernias. In our view, TEP should become the standard procedure for the repair of recurrent hernias in the hands of experienced endoscopic surgeons.

42.5 Discussion

Skandalakis: Dr. Klaiber, why did you fix the age limitation for your procedure at 35 years of age?

Klaiber: Twenty years ago, a mesh repair was restricted to patients of more than 50 years of age. Now we put the limit at 35 years. Dr. Stoppa indicated 40 years today. I think it is still arbitrary.

Schumpelick: Dr. Stoppa, all the laparoscopic operations are related to your procedure. Are you really convinced by the laparoscopic methods? Do they mimic your procedure by a minimally invasive approach?

Stoppa: My procedure is a complete wrapping of the entire visceral sac, so laparoscopic repair is different. The mesh is smaller, and some surgeons do incisions to the mesh. The anatomy is the same, but the procedure is not the same.

Kingsnorth: Dr. Klaiber and Dr. Filipi, who apart from you is doing the operation in your department?

Klaiber: Only three surgeons do this procedure in my department. There are about 1000 surgeons in Switzerland, and I think about 50 do the totally extraperitoneal mesh repair.

Filipi: We restrict the procedure to the experienced residents. In general, they have to perform 25 procedures under supervision. Then they are allowed to do the laparoscopic repair on their own.

Kingsnorth: I am quite concerned about the great number of new contralateral hernias with the laparoscopic approach. Dr. Filipi reported 46% of new contralateral hernias detected intraoperatively. I think a hernia has to be repaired if the patient is aware of it because of pain or something or if the surgeon finds a contralateral hernia during the preoperative examination.

Filipi: I do not know what the laparoscopic definition of an asymptomatic hernia is, but if we see a direct hernia, we feel that it should be repaired, and in indirect hernias a defect of more than 2 cm can be classified as a hernia.

Klaiber: Before we started using the TEP repair, we did about 200 TAPP repairs, and in that series we found about 20% unexpected contralateral hernias. For me, a hernia is now a hole where there is normally no hole.

Kingsnorth: Concerning the size of the mesh, I speculate that you only put such large pieces of mesh in because you are afraid of the mesh moving, folding, and curling. Perhaps it is overdoing it to put a 15x12 cm mesh in for a 2-cm defect?

Filipi: First of all, the laparoscopic repair is based on what other hernia surgeons used to do, i.e., it mimics something like the Stoppa procedure. Furthermore, we have learned that we can do a wide overlapping at the pubic bone etc. without causing any harm to the patient.

Flament: What you showed us is surgery for experts. In our department, only three surgeons can do that. How can the surgical society accept this?

Filipi: It is not necessary to be an outstanding surgeon to do this. You have to learn the method like any other surgical procedure; it is mostly experience.

Simmermacher: Do you believe that the hernia is a preperitoneal problem? Dr. Filipi, why do you make three holes in the peritoneum to close one? And Dr. Klaiber, why do you switch from the TAPP to the TEP?

Filipi: A hernia is an extraperitoneal problem. It is not difficult for a laparoscopic surgeon to put a laparoscope into the peritoneal cavity. The TAPP procedure is somewhat easier to do than the TEP, so I prefer to teach the TAPP. But in principal I believe that the TEP is the more elegant way to do the repair.

Klaiber: It is more logical to use the TEP than the TAPP. You do not have to suture the peritoneum. Using the TEP, our operation time decreased by 10 min.

Amid: Dr. Felix, an experienced laparoscopist, mentioned that the learning curve for the TEP is 200 cases. Dr. Klaiber reported a learning curve of 100 cases. Calculating the learning curves for all Swiss surgeons (1000), you get the number of all Swiss people at risk of developing a hernia. Do you believe that this is justified?

Klaiber: There are several types of hernia repair, and the patient can choose between them. It is not necessary for every surgeon to be able to perform the TEP, but it is necessary for the patient to have a choice.

Schumpelick: In Germany, the average number of recurrent hernia repairs per year is less than 30 in each hospital. This is far from the learning curve of 100 or even 200 recurrent repairs. Several surgeons therefore do their learning curve not on recurrent, but on primary hernias. Is it the same in Switzerland?

Klaiber: I think surgeons become more and more specialized. Thus the number of learning operations is limited, because not every surgeon has to do the endoscopic hernia repair.

Filipi: The number of learning operations in open surgery is not zero. Residents have to do at least 20 open repairs using a single method to become familiar with the procedure. For an experienced surgeon, it is not so difficult to switch to another method for the same disease. The same is true in laparoscopic surgery. Starting with the method, you need a lot of training operations. Once you are experienced, the learning curve may be much smaller.

Jeekel: I agree with Dr. Filipi. If we were to ask our residents how many operations they require to become familiar with the laparoscopic repair, I am sure the number would be far less than 100.

Filipi: My residents told me that they need about 25 procedures.

Bendavid: In 1992, the expected number of hernias to be repaired laparoscopically in 1997 in the USA was about 50%. The true percentage at the beginning of 1998 is about 8%. The future will show us the real significance of laparoscopic hernia repair.

References

1. C. Klaiber, A. Metzger: Manual der laparoskopischen Chirurgie. Verlag H. Huber, 1995
2. V. Schumpelick, G.E. Wantz, ed: Inguinal hernia repairs. Karger Verlag, 1995
3. M.W. Büchler, E. Frei, C. Klaiber, A. Metzger, ed: Laparoscopic Hernia Repair: A New Standard? . Progress of Surgery, Vol 21; Karger Verlag 1995

Part IX Pitfalls, Complications and Quality Control

CHAPTER 43

Complications of the Suture Repair of Incisional Hernia

R.C. Read

43.1 Introduction

Historically, suture repair of incisional herniation has been beset by complications. These have included hematoma, seroma, sepsis, evisceration, dehiscence, and recurrence. Whereas evisceration and dehiscence have been all but eliminated by the introduction of figure-of-eight permanent sutures [1] and their facilitation by continuous, single-layer mass suturing, the incidence of recurrence remains too high.

Interestingly, concern regarding the high recurrence rate after incisional herniorrhaphy was not raised until the 1970s, 40 years after Andrews [2] recommended non-operative treatment for direct inguinal herniation since failure of the corrupted Bassini repair was almost shamefully common. Since there is no evidence that in response to wound tension, modern sutures are breaking or their knots are slipping, the only remaining possibility is that they are tearing out. The suture-holding capacity of tissues has classically [3] been considered to depend upon three variables: the direction of the fibers (sutures inserted at right angles hold better), the distance from the cut edges at which they are inserted (the deeper the bite, the stronger the hold), and finally, the bulk of the tissue embraced (the larger the purchase, the more secure). Whereas these considerations have been increasingly adopted as implicit assumptions, the normality of the tissue proximate to the herniated ring has only rarely been questioned. The evidence available regarding this latter risk factor will be reviewed.

43.2 Scar

All repairs of incisional hernias are by definition performed through scar tissue. Thus primary repair of incisional herniation is equivalent to herniorrhaphy for recurrent inguinal hernias with its increased risk of failure. Even though the skin portion of the previous wound is routinely removed, the musculoaponeurotic scar is not for fear of increasing suture tension in the subsequent repair. Because the original wound failed to heal properly and its edges separated, the amount of scarring is increased over normal.

Since infection with necrosis is a strong risk factor for recurrence, this adds to the degree of scarring, as does the persistence of the original sutures (foreign body reaction). The role of this overlooked problem was examined in 1988 by Lamont and Ellis

[4], the latter being widely recognized as the doyen of investigators who have examined the problem of incisional herniation. They found an increased and significant hazard of herniation after relaparotomy (12%) and repair of incisional herniation (44%) compared to the fresh incision group (6%). They suggested that "there is an inherent defect in the reincised wound itself that encourages subsequent incisional herniation, which is unrelated to the type of surgery or the incidence of complications occurring in the patient who undergoes surgery through previous scar tissue." However, the incidence of wound infection in incisional hernias which recurred in this study was over twice that of sound repairs, indicating microbes may lurk in the scar, interfering with wound healing.

43.3 Buttonhole Herniation

In 1987, Krukowski and Matheson [5] reported on two patients with multiple small paramedian hernias presenting several years after midline laparotomy closure with continuous nonabsorbable suture. Their observations were soon confirmed [6]. The development of herniation long after a wound has matured was difficult to explain. Concepts that collagen could stretch later or that localized deep infection could lead to such defects had previously, in other circumstances, been considered unacceptable by Ellis et al. [7]. Krukowski and Matheson suggested that prolonged sawing action of the permanent sutures could damage the tissue, and they therefore recommended slowly absorbed suture material – polydioxanone, rather than polypropylene. Another explanation for their findings is that in some patients, as we have shown previously [8], the rectus sheath is abnormal either at initial repair or becomes increasingly so over time. Support for such a possibility is provided by experience with patients undergoing surgery on the abdominal aorta.

43.4 Incisional Herniation After Resection of Abdominal Aortic Aneurysm

In 1986, Stevick et al. [9] presented their observations regarding incisional herniation following celiotomy, closed with continuous absorbable suture, after operations on the abdominal aorta. There were no wound infections, eviscerations, or dehiscences. Nevertheless, after a minimal follow-up of 1 year (average, 3 years), 21.2% had developed incisional herniation. Remarkably, 37% of the 27 aneurysm patients herniated, a figure almost four times as high as the 10% of the 39 suffering from Leriche's syndrome. In explaining their findings, which have been confirmed repeatedly [10,11], the authors speculated whether an inherent defect in healing exists in the patients suffering from aortic aneurysmal disease. They referred to my own work [8] regarding a twofold increase in the incidence of inguinal herniation in patients with abdominal aneurysm, which we ascribed to a shared response to cigarette smoking, metastatic emphysema. They also cited Tilson's suggestion [12] of a familial and genetic defect in certain patients with aortic aneurysm, leading to potential defects in collagen. This author also postulated an abnormality in copper metabolism, allowing the formation of lysyl-derived cross-links and thereby decreasing tensile strength [13]. Nevertheless, my laboratory could not confirm this possibility.

43.5 Personal Observations

In the late 1960s, during the development of a modified McEvedy posterior preperitoneal approach to the repair of groin herniation in late adult life, I [8] noticed that the rectus sheath was attenuated. Samples of constant size weighed significantly less than controls. Collagen showed decreased amounts of the mature insoluble polymeric component. Fibroblasts proliferated poorly, and uptake of radioactive proline was inhibited. Electron microscopy showed irregularity, variable diameters, and some ultracellular positioning of the fibers. Similar findings were present in skin and pericardial biopsies.

Thus veterans, almost all of whom smoked heavily (many having already suffered the consequences, e.g., emphysema, lung cancer, accelerated atherosclerosis), were presenting in late middle age with a surprisingly high incidence of primary inguinal herniation, almost half having direct or bilateral defects. They showed evidence of widespread damage to connective tissue (in particular in the abdominal wall) different to that seen in lathyrism because cross-linking of collagen was unaffected. Since the damage to collagen demonstrated in the rectus sheath, skin, and pericardium resembled that seen in patients with pulmonary emphysema, it seemed likely that the changes in the abdominal wall were secondary to the systemic effects of smoking, i.e., metastatic emphysema. Uninhibited proteolytic activity, activated neutrophils, and macrophages, all derived from the lungs along with products of tobacco consumption, were envisaged as causing collagenolysis and inhibiting repair, the process being analogous (and the inverse) of the metastatic damage to the lung and skin seen in acute pancreatitis or visceral and extremity ischemia [14]. Similar changes in collagen have recently been described, using immunohistochemistry, in the fascia transversalis of patients with inguinal herniation [15, 16].

43.6 Supporting Data

In these patients with inguinal herniation, 18% of whom had pulmonary emphysema, leukocytosis was observed with elevated circulating elastolytic activity and a reduced antiproteolytic inhibitory capacity was confirmed in 1985 even after aneurysmectomy [17]. Neutrophils showed enlarged zymogen granules that were primed for proteolysis. The age distribution of 2500 groin hernia patients admitted to our surgical service resembled that of 500 patients treated for lung cancer and 3000 seen with cardiovascular disease. In 1988, the use of tobacco was reported to be significantly more common in patients presenting with hernia, especially women [18]. A similar finding was reported recently in patients whose defect recurred following groin herniorrhaphy [18].

In 1987, Weitz and his colleagues provided independent support for the metastatic emphysema hypothesis when they unequivocally recovered the "fingerprints" of free active neutrophil elastase (increased fivefold) from the plasma of cigarette smokers by measuring a specific fibrinopeptide cleavage product of fibrinogen identified by radioimmune assay. They concluded that their "findings raise the possibility that other systemic complications of cigarette smoking (for example, atherosclerotic disease) may be the result of uncontrolled neutrophil elastase activity."

43.7 Congenital and Genetic Influences

Not all patients with incisional herniation are or have been smokers. Obviously other factors are involved. Deak et al. [20] provided evidence regarding the importance of gene expression in patients with hernias. Nine men, 17–67 years of age, with either indirect or direct inguinal defects were studied. Few smoked, some had a familial history, and a third group demonstrated hypermobility. Isotopically labeled skin fibroblasts secreted twice as much type III collagen (one of two common forms among the 29 types) as controls. The altered ratio to type I collagen led to a decrease in insoluble (polymeric) fibrils and changes in fibrillogenesis, fibril diameter, and bundle architecture (confirming our original observations). They commented than an "increase in type III collagen (a metabolic abnormality of production) may predispose certain individuals to the development of herniation and recurrence after corrective surgery."

43.8 Tissue Reinforcement

Concern regarding the strength of hernial ring closure began soon after the modern era of herniology was introduced by Bassini in the 1880s. Imbrication was introduced to the groin by Andrews and for ventral herniation by Mayo in 1901 [21]. This technique has been applied to incisional herniation even though underlapping increases tension. Unfortunately, experimental and clinical results have been less than expected [22]. This has been explained by a failure of the layers to bind satisfactorily without extensive abrasion.

43.9 Plastic Reinforcement

Usher, who pioneered polypropylene mesh prostheses, in his original work [23] recommended extensive underlap of the edges of hernial defects with "tension-free" repair, relying on the prosthesis to span the neck of the protrusion. If sutures were to be used, he was concerned that they would tear out of the hernial ring. To prevent this, he advised reinforcement of the inner and outer surfaces with a plastic mesh cuff, thus providing selvage [24]. This latter technique has not been widely accepted because of the fear of infection. Nevertheless, Usher's original introduction of large prosthetic replacements of the abdominal wall has now, by its low recurrence rate, essentially replaced suture repair of incisional herniation: "incisional hernia repairs using suture techniques are based on the unsound principle of approximation of the defect edges which leads to excessive tension and subsequent repair failure. Prosthetic mesh allows defects of any size to be repaired without tension with a reported lower recurrence."

In conclusion, replacing suture repair with wide, deep, tension-free, prosthetic coverage of the abdominal defect in incisional herniation is recommended.

43.10 Summary

Historically, suture repair of incisional herniation has been beset by complications, most of which have been eliminated by continuous, single-layer mass suturing, but the recurrence rate remains too high. The problem is that modern sutures continue to cut out. The question of tissue normality has therefore been reviewed.

The presence of a muscular aponeurotic scar, with or without infection, plays an important role equivalent to that in recurrent inguinal herniation. Buttonhole herniation demonstrates the poor quality of the rectus sheath in many of these patients, particularly those operated on for abdominal aortic aneurysm, but surprisingly not Leriche's syndrome. Previous metabolic studies are reviewed, supporting the concept of metastatic emphysema in smokers. Independent data confirming uncontrolled neutrophil elastase activity is cited, along with congenital and genetic factors.

Possible solutions are mentioned, including tissue reinforcement by imbrication, which has proven to be disappointing and prosthetic selvage, which has not been widely adopted for fear of infection. In conclusion, Ellis' (1986) suggestion of replacing suture repair with wide, deep, tension-free, prosthetic replacement of the abdominal wall defect (Usher) is recommended.

43.11 Discussion

Amid: Abramson from Israel has a rather plausible theory for the mechanism of hernia formation; according to him, the sutures apply pressure on the tissue, and as a result of ischemic changes, the patient develops microherniation, and the same mechanism continues and eventually evolves into a real incisional hernia.

Kingsnorth: I think in incisional herniation the concepts are a little bit different. I am quite sure that it is tension free, because I think we have seen this week that what most of us are doing is freeing up the fascial layers, the lamina, and the skin flaps and then we are reapproximating the wound edges. In fact, it has been said by some people that we are doing this under a certain amount of tension. But I think the main principle is reinforcement with very large sheets of mesh, and I do not think that we are in the business of leaving large wounds open and tension free and blocking a hole with a mesh. I think that the main principles of incisional hernia repair are very careful preparation of the tissues and the layers, bringing them all together and approximating them, and then reinforcing those suture lines with the big sheets of mesh. I do not know whether you would agree with that?

Read: I think I would agree in a way, although we do believe that with the mesh present, even if that original suture line breaks down as a result of tension, as you say there is tension, we do believe that we have something that is a reinforcement perhaps, a buttress. Filipi has indicated that he has done tension-free repairs, in other words he leaves a hole in his repairs. The majority of us do not.

Schumpelick: Do you think that from your point of view there is an indication for a reinforcement of the abdominal wall in certain cases primarily after aortic aneurysm, for example? Is the risk so defined that we can say yes, and are these patients in which we would do primary mesh enforcement, or is it not so proven?

Read: That is an important suggestion, and there have been some indications that people may well be going towards that idea. I think that the problem is that a number of people do not follow up their cases, that they are not too concerned about the recurrence rate. I think we have become concerned as herniologists, but a number of vascular surgeons are so concerned about the aorta, the vascular system, hemorrhage, and problems like that, that they are not so worried about the wounds as some of us are. So I think that is important, because the incisional rate with aneurysm, for instance, is persistently high.

Filipi: Read, I want to mention that I am going to abandon my technique!

Bendavid: With all due respect to Frances Usher, the first recorded use of tension-free repair, or at least the concept, goes back to 1944 by Don Aquaviva of Marseilles in France, so I think that is a correction that should be made.

Read: I appreciate that information, but it was perhaps in the English language that the first report of tension-free repair was by Usher, but I stand corrected.

Bendavid: In fact, it is very interesting to see that the actual shape of the prosthesis that he used, which was made of nylon, looks like the bottom of an iron, with holes for the cords. Very interesting to discover.

Jeekel: I think tension-free repair is not the only thing; it is important of course, but there are also the tissues and it is important how you stitch the tissues and how wide your bite is etc. What is important about healthy tissue? You said that scar tissue should be excised. I would like to have information on that. I do not know of any good information that we should remove scar tissue at the edges of the area where you try to repair the incisional hernia. Is there any good information about that?

Read: I do not think there is any information about that. I know of no surgeon who, in repair of incisional herniation, excises the muscular aponeurotic scar. I know of nobody who has done that. I do not think we have any information on that.

Bendavid: There is definitely information; it was published by Flament and also by Travolini of Italy. Whenever they have studied the concept of incisional herniation, they have analyzed tissues away from the incision and defect, and you will see changes that are degenerative, decreasing of course the further away you are from incision. They have also suggested that the very medial portion should be resected and not used, and this is really degeneration that extends laterally.

Read: I do not know of any randomized studies in which people have studied excision of the muscular scar.

Flament: No, our work was not about the scar tissue, but about disease of the muscles, and we took biopsies of the muscles when operating on huge incisional hernias, away from the defect. We showed there was a fatty degeneration, sclerosis of the muscles, and we called that muscle disease of the huge incisional hernias, but we did not do any work on the scar tissues.

Israelsson: There are several reports of a higher rate of incisional hernia after abdominal aortic aneurysm surgery, and this has been interpreted as delayed or somewhat impaired wound healing in these patients. Some cases are related to their aneurysmatic disease. In our series, we looked for this effect; we have well over 200 patients with abdominal aneurysms who were operated on by two vascular surgeons, and there are no increased hernia rates whatsoever in our series. In fact, the herniation rate in these patients is lower than the average herniation rate at our clinic. We have had an overall hernia rate of 15%, and certain individual vascular surgeons achieve hernia rates of about 4%. The reason in our series is quite obvious, because our vascular surgeons perform a meticulous suturing of the midline incision. There may be impaired wound healing in patients with abdominal aneurysms, but if there is this can readily be compensated for by a meticulous suture technique.

Greenburg: I would certainly like to support what my colleague from Sweden just said about aortic aneurysm surgery. We have well over 400 aneurysms done in Providence at the Miriam since 1986, and I do not think any of these have recurred as ventral hernia in these incisions. We have not seen them, and I do not know why that is, because we certainly have an incidence of ventral hernia following general surgery. That almost fits with something I wrote about many years ago; in terms of acute wound failure in a series of 40, only one was in a patient with an aneurysm, and that patient had other risk factors. That leads me to the common question of who is at risk of developing a wound failure. Certainly there are technical factors that we have to address, and these patients who are at risk probably need some form of primary prevention. We have not quite got a standardized mechanism today for taking care of these hernias once they occur. How can we move from that to going to a preventative method if we do not know who is at risk?

Schumpelick: I enjoyed the comment from Israelsson, because we all have the same problem with cardiac surgery. We have a high rate of incisional hernias after cardiac surgery; we heard this some days ago. If you look at the operating team that closes the abdomen in these cases, they are usually in their first year, the cardiac surgeon has gone, and there is an intern doing the job.

Amid: One short comment about excising the scar tissue with the retromuscular repair that is very popular now, i.e., excising the scar tissue from the edge of the herniated defect; it seems to be counterproductive, because it makes the final closure over the mesh, which is important for a temporary external support, almost impossible.

Read: I would reply to the point that Greenburg made. The interesting finding in these papers that I presented is that, with the same surgeons, the same mobilization of the abdomen, and the same size wound, their results with aneurysm were different from their results with Leriche's syndrome. We have previously shown that if you examine the blood elastase concentration in these patients, it is distinctly elevated in aneurysm patients but it is not elevated in Leriche's syndrome; the elastase changes have been confirmed by other physicians, so I would agree with you that, after a long aneurysm operation, for instance, vascular surgeons are not particularly meticulous. Perhaps they are worn out and concentrating on the cardiovascular system. But the fact that they had a different result between aneurysm and Leriche's syndrome is an interesting finding.

Filipi: I would like to ask Flament a question. You mentioned that you had two deaths after ventral hernia repair. I wondered if you could tell us a little more about them. Were they related to respiration? And what have you learnt from those deaths to prevent them in the future?

Flament: We had three in the last 500 patients. One had necrotizing enteritis, and we could not explain why. I think the death was not related to the treatment of incisional hernia. The second one was due to myocardial infarction and was not related to the procedure. The third one was a deep wound sepsis. We have not have any recent patients who have died of respiratory insufficiency, but in the first part of our experience before we had these very careful respiratory preparations we had two patients who died of respiratory insufficiency. This is what we pointed out in our paper, the importance of respiratory preparation. The deaths in our last cases were related to external causes and not related to our treatment of incisional hernias. Our only one that was related was caused by infection.

Gislason: In the study I presented on Tuesday, there were 78 patients with burst abdomen, and eight of them had been operated on for aortic aneurysm, and of these eight, six were operated on by the same surgeon, so I think it has a lot to do with the technique.

Bennett: Discussing the possibility of repairing those patients at risk of primary wound dehiscence with a buttressing mesh, one of the commonest causes is wound infection, and we know that many emergency procedures are performed for peritonitis, and those are the very patients who are going to be at risk of having a wound dehiscence. Do we feel it is safe to put the buttressing mesh into the abdomen of a patient who is being operated on for acute peritonitis? Do we feel it is safe to primarily buttress a laparotomy which has been performed for a peritonitis, using a mesh?

Read: I think all of us would agree that it is not safe for peritonitis, but I think we were wondering whether the vascular surgeons have got a high incidence of incisional herniation, perhaps related to technique. We do not know the exact reasons, but if they do have a clean wound in the first instance, then I think one could consider using a prosthetic mesh to reinforce that repair.

References

1. Jones, T. E., Newell, E. T., Brubacker, R. E.: The use of alloy steel wire in the closure of abdominal wounds. S.G.O., 1941; 72:1056.
2. Andrews, Edmund and Bissell, Arthur D.: Direct Hernia: A Record of Surgical Failures. 8.G.O., 1934; 58:753–761.
3. Pollock, A.V., Greenall, M. J., Evans, Mary: Singe-layer mass closure of major laparotomies by continuous suturing. J R 5 Med, 1979; 72:889.

4. Lamont, P. M. and Ellis, H.: Incisional hernia in re-opened abdominal incisions: An overlooked risk factor. Br. J. Surg., 1988; 75:374.
5. Krukowski, Z. H. and Matheson, N.A.: Buttonhole incisional Hernias: A late complication of abdominal wound closure with continuous non-absorbable sutures. Br. J. Surg., 1987; 74:824–825.
6. Read, R. C. and Yoder, Gordon: Recent Trends in the Management of incisional Herniation. Archives Surg, 1989; 124:485–488.
7. Ellis, H., Grajraj, H., George, C. D.: Incisional hernias: When de they occur. Br. J. Surg., 1983; 70:290–1.
8. Read, Raymond C.: Metabolic factors contributing to herniation. Presented at the 1st Scientific Meeting of the American Hernia Society, Miami Beach, Florida, February 6–8, 1998; the Suvretta Symposium, St. Moritz, Switzerland, March 8–14, 1998; Submitted for publication to the journal "Hernia".
9. Stevick, C. A., Long, J. B., Jamasbi, B. and Nash, Martha: Ventral hernias following aortic reconstruction, The American Surgeon, 1988; 51:287.
10. Hall, Kevin A., Peters, Brian, Smyth, Stephen H., et al.: Abdominal wall hernias in patients with abdominal aortic aneurysma versus aortoiliac occlusive disease. Am. J. of Surg., 1995; 170:572.
11. Holland, A. J., et al: Incisional hernias are more common in aneurysma arterial disease. Eur. J. Vasc. Endovasc. Surg 1996; 12:196–200.
12. Tilson, M.D., Seashore, M.R.: Human genetics of the abdominal aortic aneurysm. 8.G.O. 1984:158:129–32.
13. Tilson, M.D., Davis, G.: Deficiencies of copper and a compound with ion-exchange characteristics of pyridinoline in 5 km from patients with abdominal aortic aneurysms. Surg., 1983; 94:134–41.
14. Lee, P.C., Howard, J.M.: Fat necrosis. Surg Gynecol Obstet 1979; 148:786–789.
15. Pans, A., Pierard, G. E., Albert, A., et al: Adult groin hernias: new insight into their biomechanical characteristics. Dur J of Clin Invest, 1997; 27:14.
16. Pans, A. and Pierard, G. E.: lmmunohistochemical study of the rectus sheath and transversalis fascia in adult groin hernias. Presented at the 1~ Annual Scientific Meeting of the American Hernia Society, Miami Beach, Florida: Feb., 1998.
17. Brown, S.L., Buckstrom, B., Busuttil, R. W.: A new serum proteolytic enzyme in aneurysm pathogenesis. J. Vasc. Surg., 1985; 2:393499.
18. Scott, J. Stephen: Causes of groin hernia recurrence following open repair. Presented at the 1Annual Scientific Meeting of the American Hernia Society, Miami Beach, Florida: Feb., 1998.
19. Welt, J. 1., Crowley, K. A., Landman, S. L., et al: Increased neutrophil elastase activity In cigarette smokers. Ann Intern Med 1987; 197:680482.
20. Deak, Susan B., Ricotta, John J., Mariana, Thomas J., et al: Abnormalities in the Biosynthesis of Type III Procollagen in Cultured 8 km Fibroblasts from Two Patients with Multiple Aneurysms. Matrix Vol. 12, Gustav Fischer Verlag: Stuttgart 1992; 92–100.
21. Mayo, W. J.: An Operation for the radical cure of umbilical hernia. Ann. Surg., 1901;34:276–280.
22. Luijendijk, R. W., Lemmen, M. H., Hop, W. C., et al: Incisional hernia recurrence following vertical Mayo repair (vest over pants) for primary hernias of the midline. World J of Surg 1997; 21:62–66.
23. Usher, F. C.: The repair of incisional and inguinal hernias. S.G.O., 1970; 131 :525.
24. Usher, F. C., Cogan, J. E. and Lowry, T. 1.: A new technique for the repair of inguinal and incisional hernias. A.M.A. Arch. Surg., 1960; 81:847454.
25. George, C. D. and Ellis, H.: The results of incisional hernia repair: A twelve year review. Ann. R. Coll. Surg. Engl., 1986; July 68(4):185–7.

CHAPTER 44

Pitfalls and Complications in Open Recurrent Hernia Repair

R. Bendavid

The successful treatment of hernias does not depend on prefabricated gadgetry, but on the understanding of anatomy and pathology. It is paradoxical that such a common surgical problem still baffles the general surgeon at large. I would like to identify ways and means whereby pitfalls may be flagged and complications avoided.

44.1 Clinical Setting

It is a significant advantage to be familiar with the surgical terrain. For example, the recurrence rate for femoral hernias is much higher than the reported 10% and ranges from 11.8% to 75%, while for inguinal hernia the rate is from 2.3% to 20% [10]. Our own statistics at the Shouldice Hospital reveal that 13% of patients have a second, simultaneous hernia which of itself will require surgery [7]. These recurrences have been referred to as "missed" or "overlooked" hernias and can be a source of embarrassment.

Whenever possible, operative notes of a previous operation can be of help in anticipating difficulties: in this respect, previous McVay repairs imply a tedious dissection near the ligament of Cooper and hence the femoral vessels.

It is relevant to keep a patient's age in mind, as the incidence of sliding hernias increases with advancing age: 6% for all patients, but 20% over the age of 70 [3].

Whenever incisions are present from other operations (Pfannenstiel, low midline, or paramedian incisions), a careful distinction must be made between inguinal and incisional hernias. The so-called parapubic hernia can mislead a surgeon and even several surgeons into performing an irrelevant operation [2]. The previous use of mesh may dictate a different approach such as a suprapubic preperitoneal access. In short, no information can ever be detrimental.

44.2 Surgical Setting

Surgery must be seen as a two-stage procedure: the dissection and the reconstruction.

The dissection begins with a skin incision, which must allow an optimal exposure. If it is a transinguinal preperitoneal approach, then the incision must be made along a line joining the anterior superior iliac spine to the pubic crest and preferably 2 cm medial to the latter. Following the incision of the external oblique aponeurosis, it is of value to recall some facts that practice and experience have provided:

1. All surgical maneuvers must begin in normal tissues and proceed towards scarred areas; planes are more easily found and the spermatic cord protected.
2. The spermatic cord is often best identified at the internal ring or at the pubic crest; the vas deferens is most often adherent in a different position from the spermatic vessels.
3. When dissecting the spermatic cord, a sleeve of scar tissue or mesh is desirable to prevent injury to the spermatic vessels.
4. If an indirect hernia is not found, it must be confirmed by the presence of a peritoneal protrusion on the medial aspect of the deep inguinal ring.
5. The posterior inguinal wall must be incised to gain access to the preperitoneal space of Bogros to rule out femoral, prevesical, interstitial, and Laugier hernias.

The reconstruction must consider the quality of tissues. Unfortunately, this quality cannot be measured, and hence ones personal judgement is called for. If in doubt, do not hesitate to reinforce the repair with the use of prosthetic materials. If mesh is to be used, then it should cover an area beyond the immediate recurrence site, since evidence points to the fact that hernia disease is a systemic problem [26]. The use of fascia transversalis, whether imbricated or as a layer, must be discouraged; an incision from the internal ring to the pubic allows exposure of the proper anatomical structures for repair (lateral edge of rectus, transversus abdominis, and internal oblique). Relaxing incisions must be relied upon more frequently to create a tension-free pure tissue repair.

The nerves of the inguinal region (iliohypogastric, ilioinguinal, and genitofemoral) should never pose a problem. If they cannot be retained intact or if imbedded in scar, they should be divided. The sensory loss is minimal and never exceeds 3–4 cm in diameter about the pubic crest. The sensory loss affects superficial touch, but not deep touch or pin prick.

44.3 Complications

Despite the most careful technique, unexpected complications do occur. These complications can be seen to form four classes, which will be dealt with as follows: (1) organ involvement, (2) infections, (3) prostheses, and (4) recurrences.

44.3.1 Organ Involvement

44.3.1.1 Testicles

Two clinical situations must be differentiated, namely transient orchitis and ischemic orchitis. Transient orchitis is self-limited and consists of mild edema of testicle and scrotum with a resolution within 1 week to 10 days. However, it can take on the aspect of an ischemic orchitis in its full clinical form, with a threatened loss of testicle. Color Doppler ultrasound, however, demonstrates an intact circulation and hence the prediction that the testicle will remain normal [14].

Ischemic orchitis implies the eventual loss of the testicle. The symptoms range from mild scrotal discomfort to severe pain requiring aggressive analgesia. The testicle is usually enlarged, two to three times the original size, becoming woody, hard, and associated with low-grade fever. I have seen instances where no testicular pain or swelling were manifested [14].

In a study covering more than 52,000 patients at the Shouldice Hospital, the incidence of testicular atrophy was identified to be 0.036% (or one in 2768 operations) following primary repair and 0.46% (or one in 217 operations) following recurrent hernia repair.

Vas Deferens

Transection of the vas deferens can occur with every technique, especially when scar tissue or mesh encases the structure. When desired, reconstruction can be carried out with a 0 Prolene as a stent. The latter can be removed in 72 h.

The vas deferens can also be accidentally crushed with forceps or be scarred down in a tortuous position, resulting in a clinical syndrome recently reported as dysejaculation. This syndrome is characterized by a burning and painful sensation during ejaculation. The clinical picture may last up to 5 years [9].

Lymphatics

Hydroceles and seromas may complicate hernia repair. Seromas, predictably, are commoner following the use of prosthetic materials. Here, caution must be exercised, as needle drainage can create an infection and jeopardize the repair. The incidence of hydrocele is 0.7% [20], and of seromas, 0%–17.6% [11].

44.3.1.2 Vessels (Artery, Vein)

Superficially, hematomas and ecchymoses may result from careless ties or cautery of sizable vessels (external pudendal, circumflex iliac, and superficial epigastric). The deep inferior epigastric artery (one) and veins (two) must be carefully identified when splitting the floor of the canal. These vessels, if need be, can be divided with impunity. Within the space of Bogros, the iliopubic, rectusial, and rectusio-epigastric veins must be visualized [8]. The presence of an aberrant obturator artery must always be remembered when sutures are placed through the ligament of Cooper, always under direct vision and never through an intact fascia transversalis.

This same careful step will prevent laceration to the femoral vein, an injury which has jeopardized many a McVay repair [3, 11], leading to its demise as a technique.

Laceration of the femoral vein can also occur when incorporating the shelving edge of Poupart's ligament during a repair.

When inserting a mesh in the space of Bogros, one must remember that the iliac artery is barely 1 cm deep to the internal ring.

All control of bleeding must be under direct vision, while deep suture ligatures and blind clamping must be proscribed.

Delayed complications are seen as stenoses, false aneurysms, and arteriovenous fistulas [12].

44.3.1.3 Nerves

The innervation of the inguinal region is so varied that only 60% of dissections show a "normal" ilioinguinal nerve [19]. Neuropraxia and hypesthesia have been reported in 15%–20% of patients following open hernia repair [15, 16, 18, 22], while chronic pain was seen in 5% [13, 25, 32].

44.3.1.4 Visceral

Laceration of the urinary bladder is uncommon and is easily managed when recognized. The mishap can occur as the bladder may "slide" into a direct inguinal hernia. Two cases were reported in a series of 3229 hernioplasties [24].

Large and small bowel lacerations are observed during the freeing of incarcerated or strangulated segments of bowel at the superficial ring or femoral ring. The inadvertent laceration of large bowel may occur during dissection of an unrecognized sliding inguinal hernia. Whenever "sliders" are suspected, the hernial sac must simply be freed and reduced without opening it [28, 34].

44.3.1.5 Bone

Osteitis pubis as a complication of hernia repair had almost completely disappeared until the introduction of staples in laparoscopic surgery, where they are inserted into the ligament of Cooper and underlying pubic ramus.

44.3.2 Infections

In general, infection rates are significantly increased in females, 2.1 times compared to men [30] and in patients over the age of 70, a 3.2-fold higher incidence [30].

Particular to incarcerated, recurrent, umbilical, and femoral hernias, a higher rate of infection is noted: 7.8%, 10.8%, 5.3%, and 7.7% respectively [23].

In operations lasting 30 min or less, sepsis was seen in 2.7%, compared to 9.9% in operations lasting 90 min [30].

With prosthetic materials, the incidence of infection has ranged from 0% to 0.6% [1, 17, 27, 29, 31]. These infections should be differentiated into deep and superficial, as the latter should not affect the incidence of recurrence [33].

In the presence of prostheses, delayed infections can be seen, and I have witnessed two cases, 12 and 19 months after surgery, respectively.

44.3.3 Prostheses

Prosthetic materials are not entirely free from inherent complications. Because they are eventually "inhabited" by fibroblasts, they develop a rigidity and buckling that is uncomfortable. I have known a patient to request removal of the mesh.

Because of the fibrosis which permeates the interstices of a mesh, scar contraction will eventually shrink that mesh by 20% [3], meshes should therefore never be taut. Infection of a prosthesis should be treated aggressively by drainage and systemic antibiotics. Mesh removal should be a last resort, and this has occurred only twice in our 2500 cases at the Shouldice Hospital.

44.3.4 Recurrences

Ironically and unfortunately, recurrences remain the commonest complications of hernia surgery. The incidence ranges from 2.3% to 20% for inguinal hernias and from 11.8% to 75% for femoral hernias [10, 21]. Some of the reasons for such disappointing results need to be emphasized.

A review of 1057 recurrent inguinal repairs by Obney and Chan [21] revealed the following statistics: 37% were indirect hernias, 8% were femoral hernias, and 10% had more than one hernia. As so often emphasized, anatomy remains the essential discipline to be mastered by the surgeon who elects to do herniorrhaphies.

Corruption of established and proven techniques is often the cause of many failures, and in no small way the experience of the surgeon is a valuable asset, as can be ascertained from the results of specialized centers.

More importantly today, the pathology of hernia disease must be considered as one of collagen deficiency and accorded a treatment that goes beyond the "punched-out" lesion of the floor of the canal [26].

44.4 Conclusion

When all is said and done, good hernia surgery free from complications requires a good knowledge of anatomy and a sprinkle of common sense. To quote Hillel: "The rest is commentary."

44.5 Discussion

Jeekel: We found that, in our midline incisions, nylon gave less pain that other materials; the French have shown that steel in hernia surgery may be the best material to use. What in your opinion is the best material to use with the fewest complications and the best results?

Bendavid: We still use stainless steel at the Shouldice Hospital, but not for any particular reason other than that it was originally used. Shouldice himself, the father of the technique, started in 1945, and in those days they used cotton and silk. Some of the complications of the time were sinus formation and sinus tracks, and he found himself doing nothing but removing sinus tracks; one day, he got angry and said he did not want to see this material any more, and from now on nothing is to be used but stainless steel. We have used it since then with no difficulty whatsoever. I know that you can use any other material and the results can be just as good. I do not think the suture material itself (other than from the point of view of infection) should be a problem or should make any difference whatsoever to the results. I would certainly put more emphasis on the technique, good dissection, exposure of the proper layers; this will affect the results of the operation, and I would discard any notions of suture material being a factor.

Jeekel: I wonder whether the French now use steel after the publication that was done a few years ago?

Flament: No, I do not think that anyone uses steel, because everyone is concerned with twist of the strap. When we visited Bendavid in Toronto, we saw they used a small hook to prevent the twist of the steel strap.

Bendavid: The use of steel is fairly easy and you have to have a routine. In our case, because we have to use 30 cm of it, we have a simple hook that you can make out of anything, or even if it is missing the assistant can hook his or her finger and follow you while you are suturing. You do not want a kink. Once you have a kink in the wire, that will actually lessen its tensile strength and it will break very easily. As long as you make square knots, you should have no difficulty whatsoever. We use a gauge of about 32 or 34, which is 16/1000 of an inch, I think. It is thin enough, it is comparable to 2/0 or 3/0 Prolene, and it is in fact very easy to use. It is just a matter of doing it often enough, and certainly in the case of infection, you never have to take down a repair.

Schumpelick: We stopped using buttress suturing 8 years ago and will not do any more because I do not think that they work and are sometimes even dangerous. I would like to hear the opinion of those present about buttress sutures in the prevention of incisional hernia. Secondly, how should we deal with patients on a low dose (100–300 mg) of aspirin each day? Should we treat them normally? Should you wait for operation? How do you handle them?

Bendavid: It is interesting that when I started at the Shouldice Hospital about 20 years ago, they used to use aspirin as an analgesia, and I found that a lot of them did develop ecchymosis. We certainly do not use it any more, but if a patient is on aspirin and for a good reason (e.g., cardiac or cerebral reasons), I do not discontinue it; I would leave them on it and certainly we used to, so I never worry about it.

Schumpelick: What if it is a high dose, 1 g a day?

Bendavid: I still do not worry; I leave them on their aspirin personally. I know some would discontinue it, but we have done it very often and safely. I have only known of two patients over the past 20 years who have gone on to have a stroke, but certainly the pathology rather predicated that, one was sitting on a time bomb, and it would have happened anyway, because of an extremely narrowed carotid artery. I wanted to mention another fact: if you calculate and if you use Prolene, at the end of the year – certainly in our hands – you are looking at $25,000 worth of Prolene material; if you use stainless steel, you are looking at about $200 a year, because we have stainless steel that comes in bobbins of 400 yards and each bobbin is about $20, so if you are looking at statistics and looking at cost, this is a very important issue. We do not use buttress sutures; the bulk of our surgery, in fact 98% or 97%, are groin hernias, and that is where all the steel is used. We never use it for incisional hernias. I am sure that, at the beginning, the ten surgeons at the Shouldice Hospital were wondering whether I had any sexual problems looking for all these things. In fact it was information volunteered by the patient, and there is no doubt in our mind that this is a real syndrome. It is so classic; 1 month after surgery, they say that they have started having burning on ejaculation, and it can begin before or during or it can be afterwards, and it lasts. The worst case I have seen lasted about 5 years, but eventually it does clear up. We followed up all the patients involved originally; I reported 16 cases and now we easily have about 150 cases, and it has never been reported, but I do know that there are studies where even the application of soft forceps on the vas can actually create the disruption of the muscular layer with the vas and create some adhesions. There has to be some occlusion or some mechanism where there are adhesions within the lumen of the vas, because it happens just before or during, and I am sure you have all seen during recurrences that you have a loop of vas deferens that is so kinked or has curves and is plastered against the posterior wall or adjacent tissues, so that any ejaculation would have to overcome this detour. There is no doubt that it exists, and if you keep an eye open from now on you may see it. Then again, it has to do with the volume, and if you are only going to see 50 cases a year of hernias or 100 cases, you may not. We see over 7000 cases, so we have the volume. Has anyone ever seen it?

Wantz: We have one interesting case. The patient had pain on ejaculation immediately after operation and soon a pea-sized cyst, a mass, was noted and that was a spermoma; it was a little cyst filled with sperm. The duct was partially divided right where the duct had been in contact with the mesh, and that was repaired and the patient was cured. It was not my patient, but it happened at our hospital.

Bendavid: We have referred all these patients to a urologist to investigate, but they never came up with anything whatsoever, not even any infections to account for some discomfort.

Simmermacher: We heard quite convincingly from Israelsson that you should use a 4:1 ratio in closure of incisional hernias. Is there any kind of ratio in doing a Shouldice repair? What do you advise in the future?

Bendavid: Most of our incisional hernias are actually done by three of us at the hospital. We still use stainless steel in most of the cases; we have not systematically studied the ratio, but I have seen that ratio in the past. I certainly could not comment on it. Besides, the variation is so marked that we could extend the study to each inguinal hernia, because not so long ago Shouldice was curious about this factor and whether the light internal ring can in fact cause testicular atrophy, and he was walking around looking at all ten surgeons and the nature of their suturing. Some are very tight, while some very loose, so there really was a range of tightness and distance, and we do have a variable degree, at least an appreciable one, in testicular atrophy. The same would apply I would imagine in incisional hernia. I can look at it from now on; I have not paid any attention to it so far, but I do know the incidence of recurrence without mesh is elevated; we will have to look at it.

References

1. Amid, P.K; Shulman, A.G; Lichtenstein, I.L. The Lichtenstein open tension free hernioplasty. In inguinal hernia: advances or controversies. Oxford, England, Radcliffe Medical Press 1994: 107–16
2. Amid, P.K. Biomaterial and abdominal wall hernia surgery – in Arregui ME; Nagan RF, eds Inguinal hernia: Advances or Controversies? Oxford England: Radcliffe Medical Press 1994: 107–116
3. Amid, P. Biomaterials in hernia surgery. Presented at Suvretta II Hernia Conference given by Professor V. Schumpelick (Aachen), St. Moritz, Switzerland, March 8–14, 1998
4. Battochio, F. Chirurgia Delle Ernie, pp 69–2, Utet, 1994, Milan.
5. Bendavid, R. Femoral hernias: primary vs recurrence. Int. Surgery 1989; 74: 99–100.
6. Bendavid, R. Incisional para-pubic hernias. Surgery, 1990 Vol 1 of #5, pp 898–901.
7. Bendavid, R. in Hernia IV, 1995. Editors: L.M. Nyhus & R. Condon. Lippincott, pp 217–226.
8. Bendavid, R. The space of Bogros and the deep inguinal venous circulation. Surg Gynecol Obstet 1992; 174: 355
9. Bendavid, R Dysejaculation. Problems in General Surgery, Vol 12 #2, pp 237–238 1995 Lippincott-Raven Publishers, Philadelphia
10. Bendavid, R. Expectations of hernia surgery (inguinal and femoral) – in Principles and Practice of Surgical Laparoscopy, Paterson-Brown, S; Garden, J. (Eds), W.B. Saunders, 1994, pp 387–414
11. Brown, R; Kinateder, R.J; Rosenberg, N. Ipsilateral thrombophlebitis and pulmonary embolism after Cooper's ligament herniorrhaphy. Surgery 1980; 87: 230–2
12. DeBord, J. Vascular complications of hernia surgery – in Prostheses and Abdominal Wall Hernias; Ed. R. Bendavid; Chapter 38, pp. 357–366; R.G. Landes Company, Austin Texas, 1994
13. Gilbert, A.I. Reduced morbidity, recurrences and costs South. Med. J. 1979; 72:831
14. Hamilton, P; Murphy, J; Bendavid, R. Color Doppler Ultrasound in the Assessment of ischemic orchitis after inguinal herniorrhaphy. Problems in General Surgery, Vol 12 #2, pp 229–232 1995 Lippincott-Raven Publishers, Philadelphia.
15. Laha, R.K; Rao, S; Pidgeon, C.N; Dujovny, M. Genitofemoral neuralgia Surg. Neurol. 1977; 8: 280
16. Lyon, E.K. Genitofemoral causalgia Can. Med. Ass. J. 1945; 53:213
17. MacFayden, B.V. Laparoscopic Inguinal Herniorrhaphy: Complications and pitfalls – in Arregui ME; Nagan RF, eds Inguinal hernia: Advances or Controversies? Oxford England: Radcliffe Medical Press 1994: 284–296
18. Magee, R.K. Genitofemoral causalgia (a new syndrome) Can. Med. Ass. J. 1942; 46:326
19. Moosman, D.A; Oelrich, T.M. Prevention of accidental trauma to the ilioinguinal nerve during inguinal herniorrhaphy. Am. J. Surg. 1977; 133: 146–148
20. Obney, N. Hydrocoeles of the testicle complicating inguinal hernias. Can. Med. Ass. J. 1956; 75: 733
21. Obney, N; Chan, C.K. Repair of multiple time recurrent inguinal hernias with reference to common causes of recurrence. Contemp. Surgery, Vol 25, Dec 1984, pp 25–32
22. O'Brien, M.D. Genitofemoral neuropathy Br. Med. J. 1979; 1:1052
23. Olson, M; O'Connor, M; Schwarz, M.L. Surgical wound infections. Ann Surg 1984; 199:253–9
24. Phillips, E.H. Complications of laparoscopically guided inguinal hernioplasty – in Prostheses and abdominal wall hernias, Ed. R. Bendavid, Chapter 58, pp. 524–530, R.G. Landes Co., Austin Texas
25. Pollack, R; Nyhus, L.M. Complications of groin hernia repair Surg. Clinic. N. Am. 1983; 63:1363
26. Read, R.C. The role of protease-antiprotease imbalance in the pathogenesis of herniation and abdominal aortic aneurysms in certain smokers. Postgraduate General Surgery, April 1992, Vol 4 #2, pp 161–165

27. Rosin, R.D. A rational approach to laparoscopic hernia repair, with particular emphasis on herniotomy and/or ring closure – in Arregui ME; Nagan RF, eds Inguinal hernia: Advances or Controversies? Oxford England: Radcliffe Medical Press 1994: 229–232
28. Ryan, E.A. An analysis of 313 consecutive cases of indirect sliding inguinal hernias. Surg Gynecol Obstet 1956; 102:45
29. Schultz, L.S; Graber, J.N; Hickok, D.F. Transabdominal preperitoneal laparoscopic inguinal herniorrhaphy: lessons learned and modifications – in Arregui ME; Nagan RF, eds Inguinal hernia: Advances or Controversies? Oxford England: Radcliffe Medical Press 1994: 301–306
30. Simchen, E; Rozin, R; Wax, Y The Israeli study of surgical infection of drains and the risk of infections in operations for hernia. Surg Gynecol Obstet 1990; 170: 331–7
31. Tetik, C; Arregui, M.E.; Castro, D. Complications and recurrences associated with laparoscopic repair of groin hernias: a multi-institutional retrospective analysis – in Arregui ME; Nagan RF, eds Inguinal hernia: Advances or Controversies? Oxford England: Radcliffe Medical Press 1994: 494–500
32. Wantz, G.E. Complications of inguinal hernia repair Surg. Clin. N. Am. 1984; 64:287
33. Wantz, G.E Complications of synthetic prostheses in hernia surgery. Problems in General Surgery, Vol 12 #1, pp 79–83 Lippincott-Raven Publishers, Philadelphia
34. Welsh, DRJ Bilateral sliding inguinal hernias. Postgraduate General Surgery, 1992; 4:114

CHAPTER 45

Complications of the Laparoscopic–Endoscopic Approach in Recurrent Inguinal Hernia Repair

E. Schippers

Alhough there were isolated reports of laparoscopic repair of small inguinal hernias in the early 1980s, it was not until the laparoscopic revolution in general surgery stimulated by laparoscopic cholecystectomy that additional efforts were directed toward laparocopic hernioplasty. As early as 1989, at the 18th meeting of the American Society of Laparoscopic Gynecologists, Bogojavlensky presented a video demonstrating the laparoscopic repair of a inguinal and femoral hernia. Several basic techniques evolved.

45.1 Methods of Repair

The plug–patch technique was one of the first laparoscopic techniques performed. In the early version of this repair, mesh was inserted into the hernia defect and the peritoneum was closed over it. After early recurrences with unfixed mesh and after the development of a laparoscopic stapling device, the technique was modified. A patch was placed over the "plug" and it was anatomically stapled in place. However, the most popular laparoscopic technique that emerged was the transabdominal preperitoneal technique (TAPP).

The preperitoneal space is accessed through an incision in the peritoneum, and the mesh is fixed to Cooper's ligament or the iliopubic tract; the peritoneum is then sutured or stapled closed. Later on, a complete preperitoneal technique was described. Here, the preperitoneal space is developed between the abdominal wall and the peritoneum with blunt dissection and CO_2 insufflation or balloon dissection. A large piece of Prolene mesh is stapled to Cooper's ligament and the other side of the aponeurotic sling, covering the entire pelvic and inguinal floor. Another unique technique was the placement of an intraperitoneal onlay mesh (IPOM). Adaptation of the techniques of laparoscopic hernioplasty has been much slower than the adaptation of techniques of laparoscopic cholecystectomy. The reasons for this include the feeling that the laparoscopic hernia techniques were significantly more complicated than the open techniques. In addition, the open techniques were already well accepted by patients and surgeons, and the recurrence rate for the laparoscopic techniques were unknown.

45.2 Results

However, the incidence of complications and recurrences associated with endoscopic hernia repair in 4743 patients was reported in 1995 [1, 2]. The kind of repair was closure of the internal ring in 3.7%, the plug and patch technique in 7.6%, mesh prostheses using the IPOM technique in 14%, TAPP in 53.7%, and totally extraperitoneal prostheses (TEP) in 21.8%.

In these patients, the overall rate of minor complications was 10.6%. Leading in this group were hematomas, neuralgias, and testicular or thigh pain (Table 1). The total rate of major complications was 0.5%, including bleeding and colon, small bowel, and vascular-lesions (Table 2).

After a follow up of 13–22 months, the recurrence rate was 3% after closure of internal ring, 9%–22% with the plug and patch technique, 2%–2.2% after IPOM, 0.7%–1% after TAPP, and 0%–0.4% with the TEP technique. Phillips [3] analyzed in his patients (n=75) the reasons for early recurrence following laparoscopic hernioplasty. The main reason for recurrence was a small mesh (n=36), followed by mesh that had never been stapled (n=19), no repair (n=13), staples pulled through (n=5), and other reasons (n=10).

Numerous case reports with specific complications due to the laparoscopic placement of meshes in patients with groin hernias have been published since mentioning chronic inguinal pain [4] and ileocutaneous fistula, for example, after endoscopic repair with meshes [5].

Table 1. Minor complications in endoscopic inguinal hernia repair (n=4743) [1, 2]

Complication	Operations (n)
Testicular or thigh pain	72
Emphysema of the scrotum	15
Hydrocele	5
Hematoma	114
Urinary retention	60
Neuralgias	77
Migration of prosthesis	6
Trocar site infection	9
Pelvic ostitis	1
Total	359 (7.6%)

Table 2. Major complications in endoscopic inguinal hernia repair (n=4743) [1, 2]

Complication	Operations (n)
Bladder injury	3
Colon injury	2
Vascular injury	3
Small bowel obstruction	5
Mesh infection	2
Trocar site hernia	2
Total	16 (0.5%)

45.3 Repair of Recurrences

In addition to these complications, the endoscopic approach for groin hernia was recommended especially in the treatment of recurrences. It is emphasized that the laparoscopic view of the posterior wall not only avoids the scar tissue of any previous repair, but also gives a magnified panoramic view of all three potential hernia orifices.

Three reports on the results of the endoscopic repair of recurrent inguinal hernia are now available in a large number of patients [6–8]. In 1995, Sandbichler [6] reported on 192 patients who underwent a TAPP repair after a primary Bassini (n=134), Shouldice (n=47), or other kind of repair (n=19). The endoscopic type of repair was a TAPP procedure. Leibl [8] reported his results in 210 patients with a recurrent hernia after conventional hernia repair in 1996. His procedure of choice for the reoperation was a TAPP procedure. Felix [7] did not mention the primary repair in his 173 patients with a recurrent hernia. His type of endoscopic repair was a TAPP procedure in 72% and a TEP procedure in 28%.

The overall complication rate in these patients (n=583) was 16.8%. The analysis of the complications showed minor complications in 9%, and bleeding complications were hematoma and seroma (Table 3). Major complications included colon injury (n=1), mesh infection (n=1), persistent neuralgia (n=1), and bleeding (n=3), giving an overall rate of 1%. The recurrence rate after endoscopic repair of recurrent hernias was 0.5% after a follow-up of 16–24 months. A retrospective analysis of these patients revealed small meshes, the mesh slit, or unclear anatomy as potential reasons for the recurrences. However, the reoperation was done endoscopically in all patients (Table 4).

Table 3. Minor complications in endoscopic repair of recurrent inguinal hernias in the literature (n=583) [6–8]

Complication	Operations (n)
Hematoma/seroma	75
Neuralgias (transient)	8
Hydrocele	21
Chronic epididymitis	2
Total	106 (14.9%)

Table 4. Recurrence rate after endoscopic repair of recurrent inguinal hernias in the literature (n=583) [6–8]

Authot	Year	Operations (n)	Follow-up (months) Range	Mean	Recurrences (n)	Cause	Type of repair
Sandbichler	1995	200	9–31	18.4	1	Small mesh	Endoscopic
Leibl	1996	210	4–36	16	2	Small mesh slit	Endoscopic
Felix	1996	173	6–48	24	1	Anatomy	Endoscopic

45.4 Comments

From the data available in the literature, it is apparent that the endoscopic repair of recurrent inguinal hernia is feasible. The complication rate is low and comparable to the open procedure. In addition, numerous techniques have been described since the beginning of laparoscopic hernioplasty, although most of them have since been abandoned. Covering the myopectinal orifice with a large prosthesis appears to be the most widely used procedure and the most effective one in terms of complication rate and recurrences. In this group, the TEP approach seems to be the most promising.

These results indicate that the endoscopic prosthetic repair of recurrent inguinal hernia may be appropriate. The low recurrence rate of 0.5%, in particular, speaks for this technique. Arguments in favour of the endoscopic technique include the excellent panoramic view of the groin anatomy even after several previous repairs. The absence of extensive scar tissue allows proper preparation and prevents injuries of the spermatic duct structures. Tension-free repair can be combined with the benefits of the minimal-access technique, which are mild postoperative pain and full physical activity after only 1 week.

Arguments against the endoscopic repair are the reported complications and the recurrences due to the learning curve of an endoscopic surgeon who is not trained in the new anatomy. The transabdominal approach, in particular, carries the risk of adhesion formation. The TEP approach is technically challenging, especially for the repair of recurrent hernias. Gas leakage and scar tissue formation after primary mesh placement are troublesome in this technique.

The preliminary results after endoscopic repair of recurrent hernia are also promising, and it has to be remembered that the endoscopic technique is still evolving. The long-term observations will answer the remaining questions about this technique, including the late recurrence rate, the risk of adhesions, and especially the risk of implantation of foreign material into the abdominal wall. Up to now the endoscopic approach for the repair of the recurrent hernia can be recommended only in the hands of experts as the procedure of choice.

45.5 Discussion

Flament: We do not do laparoscopic hernia surgery but see patients referred to us after failures, and we feel that these complications are underestimated in the literature. I would like to show you four slides of complications we have observed over the past 2 years, which are only a part of the complications we have had to treat. First, after bilateral laparoscopic repair in a young man, we had to do orchidectomy; then, 6 months later, we found a sepsis on the opposite side. So the complication may be major for young people. Our main concern is the shrinkage of mesh, and major pain may lead to reoperation even in every young patients. This one was 27 years old, and when we removed the mesh you can see that there is real shrinkage and this leads to very major neuralgia. Reoperation, removal of the mesh, no more pain. Another example is a repair in a 45-year-old man in whom we had to remove a mesh with more than

20 staples. The last two slides are patients who we operated on in February 1998. I cannot show you any histological slides, because the pathologists told us that these processes are like rock and we cannot cut through them to give you a histological slide. A patient I operated upon just before coming here at the end of February had very disabling groin pain and I had to remove his two laparoscopic meshes. They had not fixed well enough and they shrunk, causing the patient very bad pain. One week after the removal of these two meshes, he did not feel any pain. So even with only the experience of one department of surgery, seven patients had to be referred for reoperation in 2 years. So I think the complications are underestimated in the literature.

Schippers: I totally agree with you that the rate of complications is underestimated. As a referral center in Germany, we have similar experiences with those kind of patients, but the slides you showed were complications mainly related to the mesh. I can show you similar slides after the open approach with mesh. Perhaps it is due to the technique of the surgeon and not the procedure?

Schumpelick: I am impressed that you have nearly the same slides as we have. The mesh has shrunk in the vertical direction, and not in the horizontal direction; I think that is because of flexing of the hip joint; the permanent flections of the hip joints cause a vertical shrinking or pulling together of the mesh.

Filipi: I would suggest that there is a possibility that the space created for the mesh was not adequate and it was not flattened properly at the time of surgery. I do not know and we will never know.

Bendavid: You have recorded some figures that also come from what I think is one of the nicest papers. I think you were involved with it 2 years ago in surgery, and it was most probably one of the most extensive and certainly one of the most thorough reviews of the complications. I will always admire Bob, because he made a list that was self-incriminating and in fact it showed complications amounting to about 33%, including the minor and major complications. It is interesting because, for the purpose of our own conference, I have taken your statistics and applied them to ours, and if we had the same complications we would have had to take on another two surgeons just to handle the complications alone. I would like to refer everyone to that paper, because it was an extremely honest and clear dissertation.

Filipi: I might however add that if we were to look at the complications at the Shouldice Clinic in the first 2 years of experience, the number would have been high as well.

Bendavid: I would disagree entirely, because the complications are the same today as they were 50 years ago, except perhaps for the fact that we had more problems with the suture material, but the basic nature of the surgery has not changed in 50 years. We had a recurrence at the beginning because we did not obey or follow Bassini's precepts, namely because there was no splitting of the floor of the canal and no resection of the cremaster. We consider that we started improving dramatically from 1945, and since 1952 it has been exactly the same for the last 43 years. So I do not think there was a learning period. It was a discovery period; we had a technique and as a matter of fact I do not like seeing recurrences of 30% associated with Bassini, as we saw yesterday, because if a Bassini procedure is done properly, the results would be as good as any operation anywhere.

Simmermacher: Just a short remark to be historically correct. I think we should give the credit of doing the first laparoscopic herniorrhaphy to Ralph Gere in1980.

Schippers: I was citing the first case which was published, and he published in 1990.

Simmermacher: He published as well, but he did it during other laparoscopic procedures in 1980.

Amid: One short comment. I think it is very important to make a distinction between shrinkage of the mesh due to folding as a result of poor fixation and shrinkage of the mesh as a result of contraction in the way I showed it, because in the shrinkage that I showed there is really no fault; it is just a uniform shrinkage as a result of scarring.

Schumpelick: Dr. Schippers, what do you think the learning curve of your figures is, and what are the systemic problems with the laparoscopic approach? Can you differentiate now or is to too early?

Schippers: With respect to the complications, the severe complications mean damage of the intestine and things like that. These are case reports. In one group it was case number 58 and another was case number 170, for example, so even after a long period of experience they had severe complications. However, there was a wonderful publication by Filipi's group together with Stoppa and Wantz, looking for the reasons for recurrence in mesh repair in general. As far as I understood it, but correct me if I am wrong, it was due to a failure of dissection of the anatomy, regardless of whether an open approach or a laparoscopic approach was used, so it is mainly the surgeon who is responsible for all kinds of complications; it is still a learning curve.

Schumpelick: In the paper by Liem and coworkers published in the *New England Journal of Medicine* last year, there was a remark that after 600 days no more recurrence can be expected because the mesh is placed. Is that your conclusion too?

Schippers: My knowledge from the literature is that, especially after the laparoscopic procedures and also in the open procedure, recurrence occurs in the first year or it will never occur, or at least it will not occur often, so the other reason is that it is a technical failure.

Berger: Could I add a remark about the shrinkage of the mesh. When the mesh is in a good position and when it is secured tightly, then you have a small amount of shrinkage only. These meshes are filled with fibroblast, collagen, and scar material. If you want to have better meshes or you want to change how you put them in and how you stitch them, just think about the normal split skin graft and you may come to a better solution.

Filipi: When we see a colon injury, just because of that one case alone, you might say that laparoscopic surgery is contraindicated. In our institution, we have found three unsuspected cancers at the time of laparoscopy for laparoscopic hernia repair using the TAPP repair, so perhaps these disasters can be counterbalanced by that unusual incidental finding.

Bendavid: When you speak to laparoscopic surgeons, they say that it takes about 100 cases before you feel comfortable. The average surgeon does about 50 cases a year, so does it mean that in the first 2–3 years these 100 first cases are failures or somebody may die from it? In Ontario we have had four deaths directly associated with laparoscopic surgery.

Filipi: There is no doubt that there have been deaths related to laparoscopic surgery; I am not sure what types of procedures these were.

Bendavid: They were usually vascular; one was a perforation of the large bowel, which was recognized about 48 h later. But I am not so concerned about a surgeon who is beginning to learn a new technique or is going to apply it. My real fear is with the experts. We have seen for example that in London, on two occasions, and certainly on one of them, one of the world experts in hernia surgery actually lost a patient on the table through laceration of a vessel and the patient dying on the table. This was no beginner, this was a world authority. It frightens me to go to someone who is an expert and fear that there is a possibility that really does not exist with an open technique, and when you are strictly dealing with a hernia, no one should die from a hernia operation or a femoral hernia operation; that is my real fear.

Amid: What was the nature of the laparoscopic operation for these four deaths you mentioned in Ontario?

Bendavid: I am only referring to hernias. These were four reported nationally and they were all hernia operations. In fact, there was an investigation into cholecystectomies, and there was a paper published in Ontario and analyzed in the news. The incidence of complications in cholecystectomy is really way out of proportion, and this is in fact an ongoing problem in Ontario being looked at by the papers, and as you know, once a paper gets involved with this sort of thing, it gets national coverage and the academics are now coming out trying to put forward all these arguments. But certainly, with reference to inguinal hernias, I know of four. I'm afraid I did not bring the clip from the national news; it would have been interesting.

Schippers: Concerning the learning curve and feeling comfortable, when did last ask your residents whether they feel confident with a Shouldice repair? How many have they done to feel comfortable? I think the Shouldice repair is difficult for beginners and they might even need 50 operations to feel comfortable. The second thing is, don't you think there is a bias concerning the new procedure? It is more spectacular to speak about death after laparoscopic repair than death after conventional repair. We might have deaths after conventional repair, but they have not been reported in hernia.

Bendavid: I have often heard this from surgeons that the Shouldice repair is complicated; actually, there is nothing complicated about the Shouldice repair that would not be as complicated in the Bassini or McVay procedure. The only different step in the Shouldice repair is also the very difficult step in the Bassini or McVay procedure, and that is the splitting of the floor of the canal. In any operation you do for an open technique, you open your external oblique fascia, and if you do not do that, you have not ever done an operation for hernia.

Kingsnorth: We discussed yesterday about efficacy and effectiveness; it is definitely efficacious in the Shouldice Clinic, but it is not as effective when it gets into the hands of general surgeons. I think one of your surgeons at the Shouldice Clinic has suggested a learning curve of perhaps 1000 cases.

References

1. Phillips, E.H., M. Arregui, B.J. Carroll, J. Corbitt, W.B. Craftin, M.J. Fallas, C. Filipi, R.J. Fitzgibbons, M.J. Franklin, B. McKernan, D. Olsen, A. Ortega, L.H. Payne jr., J. Peters, R. Rodriguez, P. Rosette, L. Schultz, A. Seid, R. Sewell, R. Smoot, F. Toy, R. Waddell, S. Watson: Incidence of complications following laparoscopic hernioplasty. Surg Endosc (1995) 9: 16–21
2. Tetik, C., M.E. Arregui, J.L. Dulucq, R.J. Fitzgibbons, M.E. Franklin, J.B. McKernan, R.D. Rosin, L.S. Schultz, F.K. Toy: Complications and recurrences associated with laparoscopic repair of groin hernias. Surg Endosc (1994) 8: 1316–1323
3. Phillips, E.H., R. Rosenthal, M. Fallas, B. Carroll, M. Arregui, J. Corbitt, R. Fitzgibbons, A. Seid, L. Schultz, F. Toy, R. Wadell, B. McKernan: Reasons for early recurrence following laparoscopic hernioplasty. Surg Endosc (1995) 9: 140–145
4. Schumpelick, V., G. Arlt, A. Schlachetzki, B. Klosterhalfen: Chronischer Leistenschmerz nach transperitonealer Netzimplantation (TAPP) Chirurg (1997) 68: 1297–1300
5. Miller, K., W. Junger: Ileocutaneous fistula formation following laparoscopic polypropylene mesh hernia repair. Surg Endosc (1997) 11: 772–773
6. Sandbichler, P., H. Draxl, H. Gstir, H. Fuchs, A. Furtschegger, G. Egener, E. Steiner: Laparoscopic Repair of Recurrent Inguinal Hernias. Am J Surg (1996) 171: 366–368
7. Felix, E. L., C. Michas, M. H. Gonzales jr.: Laparoscopic Repair of Recurrent Hernia. Inc. Am J Surg (1996) 172: 580–584
8. Leibl, B., J. Schwarz, P. Däubler, K. Kraft, R. Bittner: Endoskopische Hernienchirurgie (TAPP) – Goldstandard in der Versorgung von Rezidivhernien? Chirurg (1996) 67: 1226–1230

CHAPTER 46

Quality Control in Hernia Surgery: The Swedish Experience

E. Nilsson

When defining quality of hernia surgery, we have to consider recurrence rate, frequency and severity of complications, postoperative discomfort and rehabilitation [1]. For each of these variables or end points, we may define goals according to our own previous experience and best external results [2] and measure the extent to which these goals are reached. In this evaluation, there is a common denominator, economy. In today's industrialised world, in which facilities cannot meet demands, surgical quality may be defined as the fulfilment of aims at a minimum cost. In the management of groin hernia, surgery alone is responsible for frequency of recurrence and postoperative complications, whereas convalescence is to a large extent affected by advice given to patients [3–5] and socio-economic factors [6, 7]. When patients are asked whether they consider avoidance of recurrence of hernia or speed of recovery to be the most important outcome, the great majority regard avoidance of recurrence as the most important [8]. Hence surgeons should do their utmost to prevent recurrence following hernia surgery, while at the same time undertaking all efforts to make convalescence as short and free from discomfort and pain as possible.

46.1 Recurrence Rate: Obtaining Information

Since the time of Bassini [9], hernia surgeons have determined the quality of their surgery by examining their patients postoperatively. For a proper evaluation of recurrence rates in case series, information is required regarding the following variables:

- Definition of recurrence ("a weakness in the operation area necessitating a further operation or the provision of a truss" [14] or "the presence of an expansile cough impulse" [17])
- Method of follow-up
- Length of follow-up
- Completeness of follow-up

Other variables of interest include the setting of the investigation (teaching hospital or not, and the number, level of qualification and specific interest of participating surgeons) and case mix of operations (age and gender of patients, percentage of emergency procedures and operations for recurrent hernia). Very few non-specialised units have the capacity to follow up cohorts of hernia patients year after year with scientific rigour. An easily available outcome measure is the percentage of operations done for recurrent hernia, which in population-based studies varies between 12% and 18%. As pointed out [10], this is a measure of surgical quality of the past and is a very slowly changing index. Figure 1 illustrates the annual percentage of operations for recurrent hernia, assuming the incorporation of drastic improvements that would lower the re-operation rate at 25 years from 17% to 7% or 0% in a defined population. After 5 years of such drastic improvements in surgical quality, 11% and 7% of all hernia operations, respectively, would still be performed because of recurrence. Obviously, a more sensitive yardstick of outcome quality is needed in routine practice even in hospitals with defined catchment areas.

46.2 The Swedish Hernia Register

The Federation of County Councils and the National Board of Health and Welfare in Sweden have collaborated at the national level to create and support so-called national quality registers [11]. Today, more than 30 quality registers exist, all of which have undergone a gradual transition from serving local interests to becoming nationwide. To be eligible for funding, a register has to fulfill the following criteria:

1. Contains individual-based data on diagnosis, medical interventions and outcomes
2. Has professional support, e.g. involvement of professional bodies

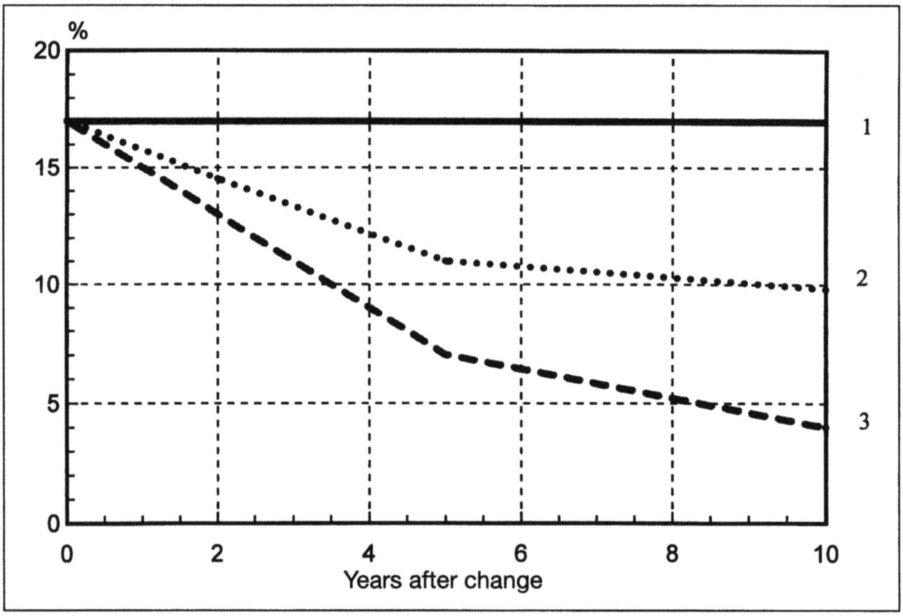

Fig. 1. Changes in reoperation rates in a defined population following drastic improvement in the quality of surgery. At year 0, the reoperation rate due to recurrence at 25 years has changed from 17% to 7% [2] or 0% [3]. It is assumed that the number of reoperations at a "steady state" in the population equals the number of reoperations at 25 years in the respective cohort and that, at 2 years, 25% of all reoperations have been done, at 5 years, 60%, and at 10 years, 75% [18]

3. Has permission from the Data Inspection Board
4. Is responsible for contact conferences and reporting
5. Involves several collaborating units
6. Includes relevant data from privately run health services

The importance of permission from the Data Inspection Board in Sweden to use personal identification numbers unique to each citizen cannot be overemphasised. It means that any re-operation can be linked to any previously registered operations. Furthermore, actuarial analyses may be adjusted for death of patients.

A quality register for hernia surgery was established in 1992. It was anticipated that such a register might contribute to quality and cost-effectiveness by enabling comparisons between the achievements of one unit and aggregated data for all participating hospitals and by generating a basis for local audit. All hernia operations performed at a participating hospital are documented according to a protocol in which patient characteristics, type of hernia and previous hernia operations, if applicable, method of repair, anaesthesia, postoperative complications, further complaints and re-operation are stated. Initially, the register comprised eight hospitals. In March 1998, 39 hospitals were aligned to the register. According to the Register Board, a goal for each participating hospital should be to achieve a cumulative incidence of re-operation for recurrence 2 years after surgery of 2% or less. During the first few years of audit, the mean re-operation rate at 2 years for the initially participating hospitals amounted to 4% (see Fig. 2). The range between the hospitals was 1.5%–6.7% [12]. A follow-up study 3 years postoperatively was undertaken using a questionnaire and selective clinical examination of all patients aged 15–80 years old [13]. It was observed that the recurrence rate exceeded the re-operation rate by 39%. Recurrence rate at 3 years (using Marsden's definition of recurrence [14]) amounted to 150 of 1564 operations (10%) in

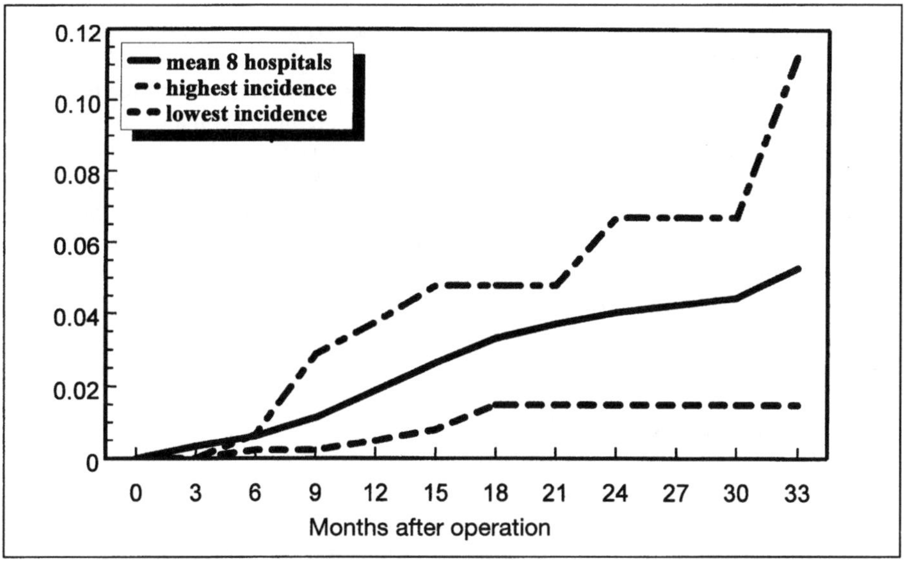

Fig. 2. Cumulative incidence of reoperation in 4879 hernia repairs. (From [12], with permission)

the study, with statistically significant variations between hospitals. Since the start of the register, the cumulative incidence of re-operation at these eight hospitals has decreased significantly (in fact it has been halved). The relative risk of being re-operated at the end of 2 calendar years was 0.55 (95% CI, 0.35–0.86) for operations performed in 1995 compared to operations performed during 1992. An analysis of re-operation risk using data from all hernia repairs of the first 3 years of the register audit is shown in Table 1. Postoperative complications, direct hernia, operation for recurrence and absorbable suture were variables associated with an enhanced risk for re-operation. Outcome of an analysis of this type represents knowledge extracted from operations performed during the study period. Consequently, the results may vary depending on the time and setting of the analysis due to adaptive changes taking place among participating hospitals and surgeons. For instance, being operated in a hospital with a catchment area greater than 100,000 inhabitants was associated with an elevated risk for recurrence at 3 years in the initially participating hospitals [13]. After presentation of this finding to participating surgeons, hospital catchment area disappeared as a risk factor in subsequent analyses.

Table 1. Relative risk of reoperation for recurrence, adjusted for methods of repair, in 4879 hernia repairs (modified from [12])

Variable type	Relative risk	95% CI
Postoperative complication	2.63	1.64–4.24
Direct hernia	2.23	1.56–3.19
Recurrent hernia	1.81	1.24–2.65
Absorbable suture	1.77	1.15–2.73

CI, confidence interval.

Since the start of the register, the use of methods of repair has changed dramatically. Conventional open repairs (Bassini, Marcy, McVay and other non-mesh open repairs) were used for 66% of all repairs in 1992 and for 18% of operations in 1996. The use of mesh has increased substantially in participating hospitals, from 7% in 1992 to 51% in 1996. No operation group (conventional open, Shouldice, mesh open and laparoscopy) has been associated with an increased risk for re-operation, although conventional open repairs come very close to being an elevated risk. As noted above, the percentage of hernia repairs done for recurrence is a very slowly changing index of outcome. Hence, it is not surprising to find that, from 1992 to 1996, the annual fraction of herniorrhaphies recorded in the Swedish Hernia Register because of recurrent hernias has remained constant at 16%–17%.

46.3 Register Data and Economics

Register data may provide some insight into the economy of Swedish hernia surgery. Firstly, one out of six hernia operations performed between 1992 and 1996 was due to a recurrent hernia. As 16,000–20,000 hernia repairs are performed annually in Sweden, this means that some 3000 operations each year are due to failures after previous surgery. Secondly, the percentage of operations done as day-case surgery is immediately available from the register. It has increased from 33% in 1992 to 52% in 1996. This has important implications for the overall hospital costs of hernia surgery. Thirdly, a register may provide data concerning "effectiveness" of techniques representing their use in common practice as opposed to "efficacy", i.e. the use of techniques in the hands of experts under optimal conditions [15]. For example, of the 4056 operations recorded in the Swedish hernia register in 1996, 835 were laparoscopic and 3221 open procedures. The operation time (mean ± SD) for laparoscopic and open operation was 69±27 and 54±23 min, respectively, with a difference between means of 15 min (95% CI, 13–17 min) [16].

46.4 Register Data and Randomised Controlled Trials

Whereas randomised controlled trials are necessary in order to obtain information concerning what is presumed to be a better technique in relation to standard methods, population-based register data is equally necessary in order to analyse the external validity of conclusions reached in randomised controlled trials. The internal validity of the Swedish hernia register has been studied by cross-checking register data with medical records. The external validity (generalisability of all Swedish hospitals) cannot be judged from register data alone. However, the register is open to all units and in 1998 comprised between one third and a half of all hospitals undertaking hernia repair in Sweden. Swedish hernia surgery needs to be improved as far as quality of outcome is concerned. In order to further this process, detailed knowledge concerning the current reality, including learning curves of methods and surgeons, is necessary. It is our ambition that the Swedish hernia register should provide this information.

46.5 Conclusions

The Swedish hernia register has demonstrated variations in outcome quality between participating units and has provided data for local audit and follow-up studies. Improvement of outcome has been demonstrated, but much remains to be done. The overall quality of hernia surgery is anticipated to increase in the future and differences between participating units to diminish. Less emphasis will therefore be placed on inter-hospital comparisons, and more on discussion of standards, on cost analyses and on using register data as a basis for randomised controlled trials.

46.6 Discussion

Simmermacher: You already talked before about a good example of what should be done in other countries, because I reported last year in Naples that an investigation in

Holland revealed that the official register told us that we had about 19% of recurrences in inguinal hernia and the hospital indicated it might be 14%–15%, so a large number of patients are lost to us and our figures to control our own quality.

Nilsson: We know the achievements of each hospital from the registry centre and we send back to each hospital their own data and figures. But it was also agreed upon from the start that the data are owned by the hospital; we do not make them public and have not done so far.

Schumpelick: The same is true in our country. For example, there was a study comparing local recurrence in rectal carcinoma in five different clinics, and it ranged from 2% to 31%. This data goes to the public and the public tries to get further information, because they want to know which hospital is so bad. It was very difficult to keep the public out. It's a little bit like George Orwell – we must be careful with this data.

Nilsson: I am aware of this paper and we have to draw a balance. We all want an open society. This data is produced to improve hernia surgery. When historical data is produced, the real surgery shown in this diagram is actually something that was produced 2, 3 or 5 years ago.

Devlin: Firstly, this was a very well produced paper. In looking at the population-based data, certainly in the United Kingdom, we are changing over to make the hospital responsible for collecting the data and validating it and checking up on that. Secondly, the interpretation and publication of the data is being made a professional responsibility, and whether we like it or not, in the current year we will have to publish the names of all the doctors involved. Whether doing this will improve hernia surgery and indeed any other surgery is open to debate in the profession, but undoubtedly it will happen, and certainly at the moment we publish day-case rates and re-operation rates for every condition under the sun. I think this will lead to better surgery in the future.

Bendavid: To make the study meaningful, you must have a quality control so that the surgeons who do a Lichtenstein or a Shouldice repair can rely on those statistics.

Nilsson: We have not done that so far. We used some meetings and have arranged conferences; we have tried to convey the message of what a Lichtenstein repair is and what a Shouldice repair is. We have made a few guidelines on it, but this should be improved upon. When we had in the protocol the Shouldice procedure, of course it is not done as it is in the Shouldice Clinic; we could define a few guidelines, but our way was to show the references and arrange meetings, and some of you have been to our registry centre.

Greenburg: I really enjoyed what you were saying; I have a long-standing interest in databases and have worked with the U.S. medical system through the peer review organisation to effect the kind of change that you may be able to do. I congratulate you on this nationwide approach, because you are collecting and validating very important data. I think what you are really about here is changing the behaviour of surgeons with this data. So the question would be, could you improve practice in terms of recurrences or lengths of stay or whatever are you trying to achieve – best practice across the system – to minimise the complications?

Nilsson: In short, it would be to change the middle portion of the curve, using the upper portions of the quality curve as best reference. Then I think the lower-quality hospitals would follow; they have to.

Read: In the United States, we have not got this process going with hernia surgery, but we do have it going with heart surgery. On New York state, for instance, hospitals are ranked in regard to mortality following open heart surgery, and doctors are even being named. I am not quite sure whether they are ranking individual surgeons, but I think the cardiac surgeons have set the way in the United States in this regard, and perhaps other areas such as hernia surgery will follow.

Simmermacher: If you are travelling by tube in New York from one place to another, we might soon see advertisements saying something like "the best place to get your cardiac surgery was Station Island, but now it is North Shore." Then you get those numbers as I told you before; I do not know whether that is what we are aiming for, but we probably have to face it.

Devlin: Could I stick to cardiac surgery for a moment and point out to you all that naming and the requirements for outcome data in cardiac surgery has led to a cardiac surgeon appearing before our General Medical Council and being punished for having a death rate higher than normal, and this will happen elsewhere. It is only a question of time.

Nilsson: Yes, I am aware of that as well. There are many issues involved here. First of all, it is the organisation of surgery, and I think the title of O'Connor's paper is both amusing and enlightening. Every system is designed to get the results it gets, and this opinion is that of course we can remove the bad apples, but that is not enough. We have to look at the organisation, education, and that is the issue in Swedish hernia surgery at the moment.

Flament: If we point out the result of every hospital and of every team, we have to have a good classification system, otherwise it makes no sense; it would be like comparing the results of colorectal surgery and mixing up Dukes A, B and C patients. We have to know which type of hernia we are talking about if we are listed with our results; no one will operate on big hernias because they will be afraid of complications.

Devlin: I agree entirely; we must avoid problems of case mix if we are going to do this, but if we have the problems of case mix sorted out properly, the evidence is that people will continue to tackle a challenging case. We found that in England, where we have every single death registered and reviewed. We found that challenging cases are still tackled. However, as Nilsson has said, we have managed to eliminate the bad apples, bad practice altogether and change things. Going on from that, if we go on to establish guidelines, there is clear evidence coming out of England that guidelines have changed practice.

Acknowledgements. The Swedish Hernia Register is supported by the National Board of Health and Welfare and the Federation of County Councils (Sweden). The authors thank surgeons in participating hospitals for their co-operation.

References

1. Rutkow IM. The importance of socioeconomic issues in surgical outcome: what is a relevant end point? Eur J Surg 1995;161:545–548.
2. Sackett DL, Rosenberg WMC, Gray JAM, et al. Evidence based medicine: what it is and what it isn't. BMJ 1996;312:71–72.
3. Shulman AG, Amid PK, Lichtenstein IL. Returning to work after herniorrhaphy: "take it easy" is the wrong advise. BMJ 1994;309:216–217.
4. Majeed A, Brown S, Williams N, et al. Variations in medical attitudes to postoperative recovery period. BMJ 1995;311:296–296.
5. Kehlet H, Callesen T. Recommendations for convalescense after inguinal herniorrhaphy: a questionnaire study. In Danish with English summary. Ugeskr Laeger 1998;160:1008–1009.
6. Barwell NJ. Recurrence and early activity after groin hernia repair. Lancet 1981;2:985–985.
7. Salcedo-Wasicek MC, Thirlby RC. Postoperative course after inguinal herniorrhaphy. A case-controlled comparison of patients receiving workers' compensation vs patients with commercial insurance. Arch Surg 1995;130:29–32.
8. Lawrence K, McWhinnie D, Goodwin A, et al. Randomised controlled trial of laparoscopic versus open repair of inguinal hernia: early results. BMJ 1995;311:981–985.
9. Bassini E. Ueber die Behandlung des Leistenbruches. Archiv für klinische Chirurgie 1890;40: 429–476.
10. Johanet H, Cossa JP, Marmuse JP, et al. Cure de hernie de l'aine par laparoscopie. Résultats à quatre ans de la voie transprépéritonéale. Ann Chir 1995;50:790–794.
11. Synnerman J, Mebius C, and Andersson G. National health care quality registers in Sweden 96/97. Stockholm. Federation of Swedish County Councils, National Board of Health and Welfare. 1997.
12. Nilsson E, Kald A, Anderberg B, et al. Hernia surgery in a defined population. A prospective three year audit. Eur J Surg 1997;163:823–829.
13. Kald A, Nilsson E, Anderberg B, et al. Reoperation as surrogate endpoint in hernia surgery: A three year follow-up of 1565 herniorrhaphies. Eur J Surg 1998;164:45–50.
14. Marsden AJ. The results of inguinal hernia repairs: a problem of assessment. Lancet 1959;i:461–462.
15. Institute of Medicine. Assessing medical technologies. National Academy Press, Washington 1985;71–71.
16. Nilsson, E. and Anderberg, B. Laparoskopisk operation för ljumskbråck. Operationstid, vårdtid, postoperativ smärta och analgetikakonsumtion samt konvalescens. 1997. Stockholm, The National Board of Health and Welfare, Sweden. http://www.sos.se/mars/kva002/kva002r.htm
17. Shuttleworth KED, Davies WH. Treatment of inguinal herniae. Lancet 1960;i:126–127.
18. Devlin HB, Kingsnorth AN. Management of abdominal hernias. London: Chapman & Hall Medical; 1998; p. 267–270.

Part X Conclusion

CHAPTER 47

Panel Discussion

47.1 Incision

Schumpelick: Now we come back to the talks and discussions of the past 5 days. Let's start with the question of how to close a laparotomy. We have discussed laparotomy from the anatomical point of view and the surgical point of view, and the first question is from the anatomical point of view: Which incisions are preferable?

Skandalakis: Personally, I like the transverse incision, despite the fact that it is more painful. In the literature in the United States, the results are the same, but I prefer the transverse incision for more than one anatomical reason. If we cut through nerves, let's say two lower thoracic nerves in the abdomen, they say that we are going to have a partial paralysis of the muscle involved, so perhaps a transverse incision may be better. However, I was happy with the midline incision despite the fact that Pascal told me emphatically and categorically that I should not do it. I was doing midline incisions and I was very happy.

Prescher: I want to make some remarks about the nerves. We have the costal arch and the xiphoid process, then the rectus muscle with its origins and nerves come from the side laterally. Below the costal arch from T6 to T12 and in the upper part they are running cranially, in the medial part they are often orientated horizontally, and in the caudal part they are descending. It is an important fact that in this side the nerves are lying above the transverse abdominus muscle and that communicating branches between these nerves exist. The nerves enter the rectus sheath on the dorsal side; they run behind the muscle and enter the rectus sheath in the lateral part of rectus muscle. This point should indicate the entrance. This line of entrance runs from a more medial site in the upper part to a more lateral site in the lower part. If the nerves have entered the sheath, they diminish and distribute in such a manner in the muscle, and it is important that these rami are also interconnected by anastomoses so that a sort of plexus innovating the rectus muscle results. If you make an incision in the lateral side of the rectus muscle over a long distance, several of these nerves will be disturbed, and such an incision is dangerous. If you make an incision within the muscle over and along, many of these nerves and the plexus will be destroyed; and if the muscle itself is mobilized within its sheath, it is dangerous to disrupt the nerves at the entrance points. Therefore I would prefer a horizontal incision, because then only some of the anastomosing rami are destroyed, which is I suppose not so important. If a long incision has to be made, I would prefer a midline incision. The midline incision does not destroy any vessels or nerves, but here we have another structure which is important, the linea alba, which extends from the xiphoid process and has a criss-cross architecture of a special nature. I will not discuss this point further. This linea alba is adherent at the anterior side of the xiphoid process. In this area, a special ligamentous architecture exists, and some ligaments from the ribs, from the sternum merge together with linea alba. If you make an incision in the linea alba and you detach the linea alba from the xiphoid process, it would be very difficult to reattach this stricture. Therefore I suggest that the midline incision should end 2 cm below the xiphoid process. The area is a dangerous area because the reattachment of the linea alba is very difficult. To sum up, transverse incisions are preferable from the anatomical point of view. For long incisions, I prefer the midline incisions.

Kingsnorth: The lateral paramedian incision is not an ordinary paramedian incision. The incision through the skin and the anterior rectus sheath is made 2 cm from the midline and then the muscle is reflected laterally, and the incision through the posterior rectus sheath is 2 cm further laterally so that there is protection from the muscle when you close the posterior sheath. That is why it is called a lateral paramedian incision, and it is the one we discussed earlier that shows exceptionally good results in terms of a small rate of incisional hernia.

Schumpelick: I suppose this kind of incision is a good one concerning the distribution of the nerves, but if the muscle is deflected strongly to the lateral side, it is dangerous to disrupt the entrance points of this nerves. What about the vascularization of the linea alba compared with the rectus sheath?

Prescher: The linea alba is bradytrophic tissue and there are perforating branches from the epigastric vessel system distributed. The linea alba has a low vascularization.

Read: That is from an anatomical point of view. Would anyone like to make a comment on that? We have two of the top anatomists from the United States and they can answer every question I ask. What about the lower abdomen, Dr. Prescher? Is it the same or do we have to think about other things because we do not have the posterior rectus sheath and so on? What do you propose on the lower abdomen, the midline or the transverse incision?

Prescher: I suppose in the lower abdomen there is the same consideration. But it must be kept in mind that the nerves are descending and therefore a transverse incision is more dangerous than in the middle parts of the abdomen.

Schumpelick: Some surgeons are doing pararectal incisions in gallbladder surgery or for right hemicolectomy in the upper and lower abdominal wall. What do you think about pararectal incisions?

Prescher: The pararectal incision over a long distance is a very dangerous procedure because many nerves are destroyed.

Schumpelick: We are only looking at the anatomical point of view and the problem of surgical access. What interests me is that sometimes there is a given incision and you have to do another one. There is a rule saying at least 2 cm distance, but sometimes I have seen a broad parallel line, e.g., beginning with a pararectal incision, then we have to do a midline because of rectal carcinoma and we have paralysis of the muscle in between. Can we have a consensus about the distance of two incisions in the abdominal wall that are parallel to each other. Is there anything in the literature?

Skandalakis: We have to avoid this by all means, because we not only destroy the blood supply but also the nerve supply. The best for me is the transverse incision. You have several anatomical layers to put together, and the gynecologists teach us about the Pfannenstiel incision, which is a very good incision if they try not to cut the 12 thoracic nerves. So I prefer the transverse incision, but my second incision is not the pararectal but the rectal incision through the interior rectal laminae.

Kingsnorth: An incision that used to be quite popular in England for appendicectomy was what we called the Battle incision; that was a right lower quadrant pararectal incision. It was an appalling incision, and it resulted in an enormous amount of problems, including incisional hernia.

Kingsnorth: Dr. Devlin, have you seen much of the consequences of the pararectal Battle incision?

Devlin: It is a terrible incision; many of the patients get incisional hernias, and it is not a good incision anyway.

Schumpelick: One thing I would like to say is that in newborn children, for example, with pylorospasm, I will not do a vertical incision. They will grow over time and then the man or women will have such a long incision. Do a horizontal one on children if you are obliged to do an operation.

Skandalakis: The other thing I would like to emphasize is that when we have a scar there, it is better to remove the scar than to make a new incision. If we have irradiation of the abdominal wall, this is a big problem – how to choose which is the healthy skin. The other thing we must not do is to form corners there to have an incision like that and make a thick incision, except if we have to do a thorough abdominal incision and we can go through the eighth, ninth, or seventh rib in the intercostal space.

Devlin: A vertical incision is not often needed in children; a horizontal one will do, the reason being that the pelvis is very small in children, the subchondrial region is very small, and all the organs are in the center of the abdomen, so a horizontal incision gives easy access to all parts of the abdomen.

Chevrel: I think for a long incision it is preferable to use a transverse incision, because when you repair the abdominal wall at the end of the operation you have two layers of suture with a good supply, and if you use a midline incision you have only one layer of suture and the blood supply is not very good. We always have more incisional hernias after midline incisions.

Israelsson: I do not think there are any clinical studies indicating that the midline incision is inferior to other incisions except for the muscle-splitting incisions; the Pfannenstiel incision and muscle-splitting incision for appendicectomy, for instance, have a low incidence of wound dehiscence and incisional hernia. Then there is one clinical study with excellent results with a lateral paramedian incision, but these results have not been reproduced and they can be criticized because equal surgery was not performed through the midline and paramedian incision. That will always be a problem in these studies; you cannot use the midline access when you do major surgery. Surgery with a high rate of wound complications is another thing which forces the surgeon to choose the midline incision; we need a place to put the ileostoemy, the colostomy. If we have used the pararectal lateral paramedian or the skin incision is even outside the midline, then we will have problems with our ostomies and again for repeated surgery; that is one strong reason to keep to the midline incision, because you do not divide the anatomical structures. Now we have a concept of bad arterial circulation in the midline, but that derives from the surgeon not dividing any blood vessels. Now we think that a transverse incision is perfuse because we have to divide a lot of arteries and veins and they are not in the midline.

Schumpelick: I think I agree that you cannot say transverse or median or paramedian are always possible or useful. Except for low rectal carcinoma, you cannot reach the top of the rectum by transverse incision. It can be very difficult, but generally speaking if you have to choose, I would say you could agree that, if you have the choice, the transverse incision is slightly superior to all vertical incisions, and among the vertical ones, the paramedian incision seems to be a little better than the median.

Read: We learnt from Dr. Scott in this meeting that the linea alba is broad and that it is not really a line, it is a band in the upper abdomen. I think it is important how you make a midline incision, because if above the umbilicus you can avoid seeing the rectus muscle when you make your incision, I think you have a better chance of getting a strong closure if you preserve the medial portion of the rectus sheath on both sides.

Conze: From the mechanical point of view, there is a study mentioned in the book by Chevrel from Greenal in 1980 about the tear-out forces in the horizontal or vertical direction, and it shows in the horizontal direction you have a much better resistance to tearing out the suture, about twice or three times as high as in the vertical direction.

47.2 Closure

Kingsnorth: The next point to discuss is closure, and the options are: interrupted, continuous, mass, or layered and what suture materials should be used: absorbable, long-term absorbable, or permanent; and finally, should catgut be obsolete for laparotomy closure? I think we probably have a consensus here for that. So we will finish that question. Could we have some discussion then on the question of interrupted versus continuous closure. I think Dr. Israelsson probably helped us more with this topic than anyone else. Could you just summarize again and give us your bottom line on this, interrupted versus continuous for laparotomy closure?

Israelsson: Continuous suture is faster, it takes less time, it is equally safe, and I do not think there is much more to say about it.

Kingsnorth: Is it equally safe or is it better?

Israelsson: It is equally safe as the interrupted technique.

Kingsnorth: Couldn't push you anymore?

Israelsson: It is enough, if it is equally safe and faster.

Kingsnorth: Do we have agreement on that, that interrupted and continuous are equal but continuous is easier for the surgeon? Again, we have recognised that convenience is one of the things that guides most of us.

Wantz: It is virtually impossible to tie an interrupted suture any other way but too tight unless someone puts a clamp inside and spreads it apart for you, so I think the interrupted suture is just gone. The only way to make a loose closure is with a continuous one.

Kingsnorth: Interrupted sutures from my observations of operating in a few departments around Europe is still very popular for closing laparotomy wounds. You leave the residents to close them laboriously with interrupted sutures.

Israelsson: The suture rarely breaks. In 1023 midline incisions, the suture broke in one instance. That was failure of suture to me. I do not think that the suture can be too loose. You can put too much tension on the suture and have necrosis due to too much tension.

Gislasson: I think that the continuous suture is better; it is associated with a lower rate of burst abdomen. Both the French study and the literature show less risk of burst abdomen with continuous sutures.

Kingsnorth: The next question is: mass closure versus layered suture; this is possibly going to be more difficult. I think we defined mass as all layers except the skin, so that means subcutaneous, all the fascial layers and the peritoneum.

Greenburg: Midline incisions or all incisions including transverse?

Kingsnorth: It includes all incisions; mass closure of a transverse incision would include all those layers. If you are going to close it with a mass suture.

Schumpelick: It is not necessary to close the peritoneum. I think that is very well demonstrated, and we know when you put stitches into the peritoneum, it is a disadvantage to the patients because it can cause adhesions, so you should avoid closing the peritoneum. It is not necessary and you leave stitches in the abdomen, which is not good.

Kingsnorth: I think then perhaps we could return to the fat, because Dr. Israelsson said in an obese patient where you have a lot of subcutaneous fat, the stitch then becomes loose and you go over to the 5/1 suture length and you increase the rate of incisional hernia. So are we saying a mass closure in an obese patient should be avoided?

Israelsson: There are several clinical studies that clearly show that mass closure is superior to a layered closure because you have a low rate of wound adhesions. There is a problem with this mass closure. The description of a mass closure was included all of the abdominal wall except the skin. This is a very old description, and I am not really sure whether that is how we do it personally. I only suture the linea alba and the upper aponeurosis, the upper umbilicus. I do not think we should place sutures in muscle, and we definitely should not place them in the peritoneum.

Schumpelick: It is also true in the paramedian incision; where you have two layers of rectus sheath and the muscle in between, you make a muscular closure or you make a layered closure, and you have to avoid the peritoneum.

Israelsson: The theory is to close both upper aponeuroses separately.

Kingsnorth: It looks to me as if we are saying that mass closure as originally defined is not a good method of closure. I think most of us are in favor of layered closures, which obviously in the midline incision is just one layer, but excluding fat and excluding peritoneum, only fascia. Is that correct?

Chevrel: I think the choice of the closure depends on different factors, and for a young patient I would use a continuous suture, but in elderly patients or for reoperation for incisional hernia, I prefer to use interrupted suture with permanent sutures. They are not the same patients, and they do not have the same possibility of healing.

Kingsnorth: Can we move onto the type of suture as Chevrel has taken us onto that. His preference is absorbable, not meaning catgut, but one that absorbs in a matter of months: Let's say absorbable, continuous for young patients, and interrupted nonabsorbable for older patients. Have we got any advise on that in the auditorium here?

Devlin: I agree.

Osther: Having abandoned the catgut suture, I think we should look at what has been shown in fully randomized studies and not just what we feel. It has been shown in every fully randomized study that the suture does not make much of a difference. You have the same rates of wound dehiscence using slowly or rapidly absorbable PDS or permanent sutures, so what is really important here is the surgical technique.

Kingsnorth: Should Vicryl be used to close a laparotomy wound?

Osther: It has been shown in randomized studies comparing a PDS type of suture with PGS, Vicryl or Dexon, and there were no differences in these studies.

Kingsnorth: So we can give the surgeons a wide choice with this one?

Osther: Yes. But if we are going for a continuous suture, I think the monofilament suture PDS is more appropriate, because these multifilament sutures have this sawing effect.

Carlson: I just want to qualify that last statement. The literature on absorbable versus permanent suture in laparotomy closure is not uniform. There are a couple of randomized studies which show there is a higher hernia rate using Dexon or PGA for closure of laparotomy.

Kingsnorth: That is an important point, because I think we decided that acute wound failure is not suture dependent, it is surgeon dependent, so we are looking at late wound failure. And if you are telling us that there are some studies showing that absorbable sutures increase late wound failure, then we should perhaps be deciding upon nonabsorbable sutures.

Schumpelick: That means that at the moment we cannot decide whether PGS or nylon or PDS is superior in every type of patient. I think the studies by Osther are convincing.

Kingsnorth: I think you told us PDS is alright and with Vicryl we are undecided.

Schumpelick: In an infected area, PDS or PGS is better than any nonabsorbable suture.

Gislasson: I studied the literature and found 11 clinical studies; we did not find any difference between Dexon, Vicryl, PDS, and the nonabsorbable suture, but I think that PDS is at least theoretically the best, so I think we should make the safest choice.

47.3 Suture Bites

Israelsson: When I talk about this suture to wound ratio, I always end up with surgeons asking me how wide the suture bites should be, what the distance between the bites should be, and I always refuse to answer, because I had expected in my study to find some correlation between the suture bites and distances but I did not. Surgeons with quite different techniques – one taking very large bites but few, the other taking very small bites and very close to each other – produce equal results as regards wound infection and late incisional hernia provided that the suture to wound length ratio is above 4.

Conze: What is your personal type of operation?

Israelsson: I think you should be at least 10 mm away from the fascia edge.

Jeekel: And the vertical distance between two bites?

Israelsson: Well, it should not be too long. You have got to have a ratio of at least 4.

Israelsson: The problem with the abdominal wall is that it is not a piece of paper and you cannot treat it like a piece of paper. The only way to achieve a ratio is to suture the wound, measure the ratio, and adapt or change your technique for the next time until you have a proper ratio.

Klinge: You told us that you do not mind whether the bites are small and frequent or big and less frequent and you stated that the results were equally good as long as the ratio is correct, but you did not study that, did you?

Israelsson: Of course not.

Klinge: So why are you sure you can say it?

Israelsson: Because the stitch length is an indirect measure of the amount of tissue you include into the stitch. You do not know if there is a significant difference between the surgeons in small and big bites.

Kingsnorth: You cannot take a slide rule into the operating theater and so I think you have got to have some rough and ready guidance. A 1-cm bit from the wound edge and a 1-cm stitch interval is a rough guidance, I think, without having to take your slide rule and your calculator.

Flament: Science must not let us forget what we have learnt for many years or even centuries of surgery. In France there is a rule that the distance between two stages is equal to the bite. I learnt that 30 years ago.

Schumpelick: That was in interrupted sutures. It was in continous sutures, too. Dr. Israelsson is it your rule in Norway too?

Israelsson: I would have expected that we are here because we need science. I think you may very well have these instructions 1 cm from the edge, 1-cm intervals, but my point is that surgeons should not rely on these instructions; they should measure, and they should calculate the ratio. That is very important.

Schumpelick: I think the message is clear. Now to the suture material. We are talking about a median incision of the abdominal wall, and we heard that 2/0 can be enough from the physical strength of the suture. But I do not think that any of us would use 2/0, because it is too thin and it cuts through. What is preferred in this field 0, 1, 2?

Greenburg: I use number 1 most of the time.

Schumpelick: May I ask who uses 1? The majority. I think that is nearly a consensus.

47.4 Postoperative Activities

Kingsnorth: We will now discuss postoperative activities. Any restrictions required? Any indications for the abdominal belt? Can we take the activities first? Dr. Amid, you are keen on putting people on bicycles and getting them jogging, will you start the discussion?

Amid: As you know, I have not done general surgery for about 10 years now; in hernia surgery this is only relevant when I do an incisional hernia. Because my incisional hernias have mesh in the retromuscular area, closure of the midline is not so important as primary closure of the laparotomy, but I use either 0/1 or 0/2 with a 1-cm bite.

Kingsnorth: So are we saying that there is a difference, that we should restrict patients differently whether they have mesh or just the primary closure? Is there any difference in advice about physical activity?

Simmermacher: I think we should not restrict the patient because I think if you are going to restrict the patient after laparotomy, then we have doubts about our closure technique, and if you have consensus on the closure technique, then there should be no restrictions. In my view an abdominal belt should be abandoned.

Kingsnorth: I think we have had some information on the bursting strength of wounds and coughs, how many kilopascals of cough we generate, and I think we have decided that a cough can generate 20 kPa, but the closure should be able to withstand pressures of up to 100. I do not think we worry about acute wound failure in terms of activity. Is that correct? If we close the wound properly, patients should be able to recover from their abdominal surgery without restriction. Is that correct?

Amid: Many years ago, Lichtenstein did a wound healing study which is now a classic in practically every surgical textbook, because the strength of the wound takes 2 months to become 80%, so during the first 2 months the strength of the wound depends on the suture, so there should be no difference between day 1 and day 60 as far as activity is concerned.

Kingsnorth: So I think that question we can pass on then. No restriction. Does anybody want to speak in favor of abdominal belts?

Schumpelick: We give our patients abdominal belts if they want them because it decreases the pain when coughing and standing up sometimes. I do not think it works in anyway as protection, but it helps better respiration in my experience.

Kingsnorth: Professor Schumpelick, I think you should give your patients proper analgesia rather than a belt.

47.5 Primary Closure of Incisional Hernia

Schumpelick: Primary closure of incisional hernia. Is there a place for it now? Does it depend on the defect size, on the location, on the size of sac protrusion in the supine position, and on the number of recurrences? Is there any place anymore for primary closure of incisional hernia, or should we use meshes in all patients?

Jeekel: I think we need data to express our thoughts, and there is no data to answer this question. We did a prospective randomized study on all incisional hernias less than 6 cm, one group with mesh and one with primary closure, and we have to await the results of prospective randomized studies to give the answers. Even in small incisional hernias of 2–3 cm, I still wonder whether you may need support by a mesh, but we will have to wait for the answer.

Simmermacher: I think an even more important point is how long the incisional hernia exists, because an incisional hernia lasting for a long time is going to act like a tissue defect and then things are again different. So I agree with Dr. Jeekel that we need data from good clinical studies.

Schumpelick: In the literature, there is a lower risk of recurrence from small hernias. Less than 4 cm is absolutely safer. Any other opinions? Who closes small hernias directly? Please hold up you hands – that is nearly the majority. I think there are some studies to be done. What about location? Does it make a difference in your decision, upper abdomen, lower abdomen, right, lateral?

Herszage: It is easier to talk about small defects or medium defects. It is easier to close in the midline, but when bone is one of the limits of the defect, it is an absolutely different technique. A small to medium defect with a bone limit will be transformed in a bigger defect in the technique.

Simmermacher: Your question was whether we close incisional hernias primarily or whether we use mesh. I was a bit disappointed that our Argentinean friend did not mention that there was a third possibility by a kind of relaxing incision according to Ebaneezer and Ramirez, which appeared to give good results.

Schumpelick: We came to relaxing incisions. We only asked about the style of closure of small incisions. That means that in the small hernias it is left open. We could do a prospective trial on the bigger ones. Is there confirmation that we have to use mesh? Dr. Herszage, you have only a few cases of mesh in big hernias.

Herszage: If we cannot use a mesh, we use a lot of relaxing incisions.

Schumpelick: Dr. Greenburg, you are a little bit reluctant to use mesh in the preperitoneal approach for recurrent inguinal hernias. Are you reluctant to use mesh in incisional hernias?

Greenburg: I tend to agree with my South American colleague that if I can make relaxing incisions in the fascia, I will move them together up to the 10- to 12-cm range.

Schumpelick: Dr. Wantz, is that the traditional American style?

Wantz: The traditional American way of fixing hernias seems to be to inlay a piece of mesh, then to have four or five recurrences, and then to find a way to fix them. I use mesh in all major incisional hernias.

Flament: When we looked for the monograph of the French Association of Aurgery, we did what is usual for this kind of work, an enquiry for 1 year of surgery to send to all French surgeons. We had answers from many people and collected 1265 cases of treatment of incisional hernias. The recurrence rate for primary closure was more than 30%.

Bendavid: I cannot see any advantage of such generous relaxing incisions, I would simply use a mesh. Where you need extensive relaxing incisions, why not use mesh? I cannot see how, by making a relaxing incision on the anterior rectus sheath, you are going to get the next two layers, the muscular layer and posterior rectus sheath, to come together.

Schumpelick: Let's talk now about location, size of infiltration, and number of recurrences. Is that a factor influencing your decision for or against mesh, the number of recurrences? I think not. A big hernia is a big hernia even in a recurrent case. What about multiple recurrences?

Flament: To err is human, but to persist in error is of the devil.

Kingsnorth: So what you are saying is that a recurrent incisional hernia of any size should be repaired with mesh. I agree with that.

Schumpelick: Do we all agree that recurrent hernias should get a mesh? Hold up your hands. What about multiple defects? We often have multiple defects, small bridges of tissue between, and sometimes these tissues are weak, sometimes strong. How do you handle multiple defects?

Greenburg: I convert all of them to a single incision and then close the wound as a primary wound or with mesh as necessary.

Schumpelick: Even if the bridge is strong?

Greenburg: Yes.

Schumpelick: Even if the bridge is 8 cm?

Greenburg: For multiple defects, yes.

Schumpelick: Dr. Flament, even if it is a big, strong bridge, you want you put them together.

Flament: Yes.

Schumpelick: What about the Mayo procedure? Is it still justified? We have seen a lot of studies here showing no difference to direct suture. We know that the Mayo procedure is a very honest operation, but is it justified to do this operation?

Filipi: I use the Mayo technique for umbilical hernias less than 2 cm in diameter, and I think it is appropriate for that.

Schumpelick: You think it is superior to direct suture or is it only convention?

Filipi: I do not know whether it is superior.

Schumpelick: We used to do it, but since seeing our figures we have stopped doing it. I think there is no difference at all. There was a question from Kingsnorth about the size of eventration with the patient in the supine position. Is that important for your decision to use a mesh or not?

Greenburg: I need to have a definition of eventration, because I think that is one of the softer signs we have.

Schumpelick: That is a good question, we do not know.

Kingsnorth: Yes, a multilingual translation of bulge, the amount of abdominal contents outside the abdominal wall. We tried to translate it so everyone could understand it.

Greenburg: If you really want to look at what we have said about normal defect and size, that is a very important measurement. We know that from the imaging studies and we know that there are different quantities, volumes of things that are outside of that, that are part of the sac. My definition of eventration is a weakness in the wall that is attached to the defect.

Kingsnorth: I think what we were trying to get across is the contents of the sac when the patient is lying down. If they reduce completely, would it influence the method of repair? If it is irreducible, let's say, and a bulge still remains, does that affect the way you approach the operation?

Schumpelick: I think we will come back to that when we discuss how to classify incisional hernia.

47.6 Relaxing Incisions

Herszage: A surgeon who manages relaxing incisions must never have a problem closing an abdominal wound.

Kingsnorth: Could you tell us at what point you would not use a relaxing incision and would prefer a mesh?

Herszage: When the posterior wall, the transverse area is so weak that I cannot do this; in these cases I use a mesh.

Kingsnorth: So you are talking about the quality of the tissues having nothing to do with size of defect. I think we would find that very difficult to define as a group, the quality of the tissues. You say that you use relaxing incisions and flaps if the quality of the tissue is good.

Herszage: Yes, normally we find excellent flaps, not in all patients but in the majority of the patients who we use relaxing incisions in. But if in surgery we see that this is a weak tissue, then we use a mesh.

Kingsnorth: Can Dr. Read help us with a definition of a weak tissue? Or are we unable to define that?

Read: I think with the previous speaker it is one of these things that if you see it you can recognize it, and I think it does take judgement, but I think with experience the surgeon can decide whether the tissue is good stuff or not.

Kingsnorth: I think we are probably going to decide that mesh is applicable on size of defect not on quality of tissue, because quality of tissue is very hard to define. Is that agreeable? Relaxing incisions are not used often in Europe or North America.

Simmermacher: The Ramirez procedure was described by Ramirez in the *Journal of Plastic Surgery* in 1990. It appears in our hands to be quite an effective method, and although we have not done a prospective randomized trial on it, we normally try to close incisional hernias first by relaxing incisions.

Kingsnorth: What about the quality of the tissue?

Simmermacher: We do not say the quality of tissue is bad and therefore we use a mesh, but I do have the impression that we are misjudging in one or two cases the quality of the tissue and get the problem of bulging on the lateral side, where the relaxing incision is done?

Herszage: I understand Dr. Simmermacher, because the Ramirez technique is similar to our technique, but it was published 40 years later. We have a lot of experience with this kind of technique. De Alto, who is 93 (and still alive), has never used a mesh, but we use mesh when the posterior layer is too weak.

Kingsnorth: The answer to this is there is no controlled data so we cannot answer the question, but I think it is largely because it cannot be answered and most of us do not have experience with these relaxing incisions. The majority are probably using mesh. It may be that flaps are equally good, but we do not have any data to answer the question so we are using mesh. But there could be situations where someone could do a study where we could use relaxing incisions and flaps.

Schumpelick: I think in hernia surgery there are signs besides controlled trials. We cannot do everything in a controlled trial. If the French group have managed more than 2000 cases with success, that is a message. Therefore I would like to ask whether relaxation incisions are necessary?

Flament: There was one paper by our friend Trevelini on relaxing incisions. He made relaxing incisions depending on the pressure of insufflation by the anesthetist. When he closed the abdominal wall, he measured and calculated the abdominal compliance and, according to the result, he made long or short relaxing incisions. From that there is a good indication that when the patients are under general anesthesia and relaxed, if our anesthetists say that the pressure is going up in the respirator, we know that the pressure might be too high in the abdomen, so we use relaxing incisions.

Devlin: Could I just make an observation on what Schumpelick has just said. He asked whether we need a controlled trial. The answer must surely be no. What we need is evidence; the evidence may come from a controlled trial, from a cohort study, or history. So we should not get hung up on controlled trials all the time.

Kingsnorth: I agree totally with you. But we have to operate, and we cannot always say there is no controlled trial and do the old mistake.

Stoppa: I want to complete what my friend Flament said, because before the opinion of the anesthetists you have the problem of the gap to reduce to close the wall in front of the prosthesis. That is an indication, so when you say always on demand, the demand is sometimes evident.

Kingsnorth: Could we have Dr. Wantz' views, because I think you have most probably seen more recurrent incisional hernias than many people. Have you seen a lot of problems after people have used relaxing incisions and flaps?

Wantz: The only relaxing incisions we use are to close the anterior rectus sheath when we cannot get it together, and we do not always use that. More often than not, we put another piece of mesh in place. I do not think that relaxing incisions are very popular in the United States. I say again I think it is a sorry statement that in the United States surgeons just inlay a piece of mesh and call that a hernioplasty.

Schumpelick: But sometimes it could be a substitute for using a mesh?

Wantz: Yes, if we cannot get it together, we put a secondary piece of mesh in just to make us feel better to close the anterior exit that we are counting as the main mesh, which is of course rectomuscular.

Kingsnorth: Maybe our recommendation should be that they are used infrequently, but should only be used by experienced surgeons who know what they are doing and who have considerable experience of using them. They should not just be used as an excuse to relieve tension just because you think that is the right thing to do.

Amid: When Flament makes a relaxing incision, it is not for the sake of the security of the repair. It is to improve the pulmonary function. We also use a second piece of mesh if we cannot bring the midline together, because if you want to make a relaxing incision, the price you have to pay is making an extensive skin flap, and that can be the source of a problem, a seroma formation, hematoma, or infection, so a second piece of mesh is better in my opinion than making a relaxing incision of any kind.

47.7 Mesh Repair for Incisional Hernia

Schumpelick: Let's talk about pneumoperitoneum. Who uses this routinely in big hernias? Five, so a minority. What about weight reduction? Is there anyone who favors weight reduction, and is there anyone who says it is not possible because people do not reduce their weight?

Greenburg: People not only do not reduce their weight, but I think you run the risk of taking a nutritionally incompetent individual who is obese and by putting them on a diet making them even more nutritionally incompetent. You then operate on them, subjecting them to a stress which is an operation with an increased risk of infection and a host of other problems. I have never seen the Rhode Island wide body able to loose weight before an operation.

Filipi: I would not agree with that. I think their chances of having a lower albumin or prealbumin level after attempted weight loss is unlikely. Clearly many patients will not loose weight, but I think it is appropriate to give them a 2- to 3-month period to try to loose weight. Some of them in fact do, at least that is my experience.

Schumpelick: Perhaps I should try the question the other way around. I think all of us propose weight reduction but only a few succeed. Would you do the operation even though the patient had not succeeded with weight reduction?

Greenburg: Yes, I would proceed but they need to be informed.

Kingsnorth: I think a lot of this depends on the health care system in which you are working. I think possibly in the United States your patient might run along to another surgeon, but in the United Kingdom, where we have waiting lists and a patient might have been waiting 6 months, 1 year or even 2 years for an incisional hernia repair, you can closely supervise weight loss, but it only happens in the minority. Some very successfully shed 20, 30, 40 kg, and others are completely resistant. With those between, I go ahead and operate.

Schumpelick: Is there anyone who is reluctant about smoking? Trying to turn someone into a nonsmoker? I think it is more difficult than closing a hernia. Now we come to the technique of mesh. Who favors inlay mesh? Can we say it is obsolete or is there anyone uses it sometimes in small hernias? Can we first define inlay?

Kingsnorth: Blocking the hole, just suturing the mesh around the defect without any attempt to close the hole, no underlap, no overlap.

Simmermacher: I think this is one of our tasks. We should define these words, because I know in my thesis I used the word inlay meaning on the dorsal side of the abdominal wall. Inlay from inside against the wall, and by inlay you mean just bridging the defect without any overlap. So we should define inlay, sublay, and onlay.

Schumpelick: I think any overlap is onlay.

Simmermacher: On the outside?

Schumpelick: Yes. The inlay is without any overlap, and sublay is underlay.

Simmermacher: We should agree on that because that is also important.

Schumpelick: Does anybody favor onlay? I think Chevrel favors onlay. Do you want to say why you favor it?

Chevrel: I think it is very easy to place the mesh, but the mesh needs to be wide, overlapping, and fixed immediately by fibrin glue. It is easy to avoid faults; this mesh is fixed with a little tension, so that is different to the reconstruction of the linea alba, which is tension free. The mesh will reinforce the reconstruction of the linea alba if placed with a little tension.

Amid: I definitely do not favor onlay, but when you are dealing with a frozen abdomen and you cannot find a plane to put sublay, I have done about six operations where I put a very large onlay of at least 8 cm overlap beyond the edge of the defect. I then sutured the edge of the defect to the body of the mesh and then two or three more circular sutures around it. I usually end up with four rows of sutures, four circles. The innermost one is right at the edge.

Schumpelick: I showed my slides 2 days ago. We had bad results with onlay. Does anyone routinely favor?

Read: There are a number of surgeons in the United States favoring onlay at the moment, and I think they do not seem to have seen the light as you have.

Schumpelick: It is the same in my country. Who favors onlay in the routine case of large incisional hernia? Dr. Flament. Sublay? Dr. Filipi, the majority. What is the extent of overlapping that is best. We talk about 5 cm. Is there anyone who says 2 cm is enough, or 5 cm is not enough, it should be 8 cm?

Devlin: Four.

Schumpelick: Who says 4 cm? Is it typically English?

Devlin: We cannot make a definition like this; it depends on the size of the defect.

Kingsnorth: Going back to Dr. Flament, your technique is to put the mesh so as to cover the whole of the area behind the rectus muscle?

Flament: Yes. So the lateral limit of the prosthesis is the line of the rectus sheath. It depends how wide the rectus muscle is, but we go as far as we can without cutting the insertion of the transverse muscle.

Kingsnorth: So the mesh occupies the entire space behind the rectus muscles.

Schumpelick: I think the message is: as far as possible. Is that right?

Kingsnorth: Let's say a minimum.

Schumpelick: The minimum is 5 cm.

Stoppa: What Dr. Flament said just now is a practical thing to be considered. The overlapping depends on the dimension of cleavage space. Above the line of Douglas, you can measure only the width of the rectus, but below or laterally you can expand the overlapping more, so I think the minimum is 5 cm.

Schumpelick: The question can become very important if we have, for example, a pararectal hernia in the lateral point of the rectal sheath. Should you open up the rectal sheath laterally or can we make a 2-cm overlap? I think we should open up the rectus sheath and go to the lateral.

Devlin: I understand that we are planning to publish this meeting, and to do that we have to get something said that will carry the message to our colleagues, the general surgeons, and the message to them is surely that inlay is obsolete, putting it just 1 cm around is obsolete; it must overlap depending on the anatomy. If we can get that message over, we have succeeded a lot.

Schumpelick: What else? Huge incisional defects that cannot be closed directly. Mesh is underlay. How should we handle huge defects? Sandwich, composite mesh, or what else?

Chevrel: I think it is preferable to use a sandwich mesh with absorbable mesh deeply and nonabsorbable mesh only with a wide overlapping.

Stoppa: That is acceptable.

Schumpelick: Your way of doing it?

Stoppa: Yes, with double mesh.

Schumpelick: Outside nonabsorbable, inside absorbable? Other suggestions?

Herszage: We used to close incisional hernias up to 30 cm without any kind of relaxing incision, using the technique I showed. If we cannot close it, we use the sac in some instances. We resect the sac only as a last step to make a natural barrier to the intestine.

Kingsnorth: Tell me, Dr. Herszage, are your reasons for doing this economic ones, or are they because you prefer natural tissues to synthetic mesh?

Herszage: No, not for economic reasons. I think if we think in economic terms, a lot of graft surgery or organ replacement cannot be done. Economic reasons for surgery are not important, we do it because we believe in biology. It is better for the patient to use his or her own tissue if we can do excellent reconstruction.

Stoppa: Is that an indication to make a plasty, a muscle plasty, as shown by Dr. Berger, or to make a corium plasty, or cutis plasty, dermis plasty on top of the hole.

Greenburg: There are times in the acute situation when you may have to be creative in the presence of infections or if there is no other tissue. I do not think they should be necessary as a routine, but the good general surgeon should understand how to do that.

Stoppa: I think the abdominal muscle plasty in malignancy is a different topic. It is only in routine use now.

Greenburg: I do not do it in routine use, only under very unusual circumstances.

Schumpelick: Other comments. Well what should we do? May I ask if you have a situation tomorrow morning and there is a big hole not to be closed, and you have a mesh as sublay, who would use a Vicryl mesh to close this hole? Who would not close this hole at all and would leave it open? (Majority indicate Vicryl).

Chevrel: Some people did not put their hands up.

Kingsnorth: Composite mesh or Gore-Tex?

Amid: There is really no place for composite mesh in this situation. If I understand you correctly, you have enough peritoneum to close, then you put a sublay mesh over the closed peritoneum, and now you cannot close the defect. Your question is how to handle this defect, either by inlay or Vicryl, or an inlay of nonabsorbable mesh.

Schumpelick: Or by dermis or muscle plasty?

Amid: I guess some people prefer the absorbable meshes. I have used absorbable mesh on three occasions and all three times I have had massive seroma. I am not sure, but I think the seroma was caused by an inflammatory response to the product and hydrolysis of the absorbable mesh. Since then, I have been using nonabsorbable mesh in the superficial layer, and that has not given me any problems at all. But in these cases, I put drainage tubes over the deep mesh and over the superficial mesh.

Chevrel: If the defect is in the upper part of the midline, at this level the width of rectus muscle is 10–12 cm and it is possible to use a wide flap with the anterior rectus sheath. You have 10 cm and you use this flap with an onlay mesh. I have done this in two cases.

Schumpelick: I think it is a good suggestion.

Kingsnorth: How should we handle the overlapping at the rib cage? And how should we handle the overlapping laterally to the rectus? This is going to be in a very small number of incisional hernias. I guess there are not a lot of us here who have a vast experience with this. It is probably Dr. Herszage and Dr. Chevrel who are going to help us answer these questions.

Herszage: I prefer to apply the mesh to the limit of the rib cage, over the transverse plane, and to the xiphoid and pubic bone, of course. They are excellent places to fix meshes.

Schumpelick: Is the rib cage a better fixation point than Cooper's ligament?

Herszage: No, we use Cooper's ligament too. We have two recurrences in hernia, and one big incisional hernia in the middle of the abdomen, so we use one mesh like a racket and we prolong the mesh up to the xiphoid and the edge of the rib cage. Then we fix it laterally to the external line of muscle of the spigelian line and the upper part to the xiphoid bone, and inferiorly to the pubic bone, to Cooper's ligament, to the iliac fossa etc.

Kingsnorth: Does anyone do more than the occasional operation for this? I think you have got to be versatile, haven't you? I think you have written about this, haven't you, Dr. Bendavid?

Bendavid: The so-called parapubic hernia, which results from radical prostatectomy, is number one, and it also results from a lot of the rectus-splitting incisions. Unfortunately, some surgeons make their incisions extremely low, so that there is really no chance of ever healing the recti back. So you are stuck and you have to be very careful, because it is a kind of a hernia that can occur. I had a patient who had 12 operations, because what happens is that you have a defect that you close, and it seems closed at the time of surgery with the patient lying flat, but you always have separation between muscle and bone, and this is where it sneaks under. So you have to insert the mesh deep to the posterior aspect of the pubis, and you have a good infrapubic ligament that will hold both sides and of course Cooper's ligament.

Schumpelick: How do you fix it, with wire?

Bendavid: You have to insert a wide piece of mesh. It is a wide piece that you anchor inferiorly to the inferior pubic ligament and to Cooper's ligament.

Schumpelick: Should we fix the mesh to the rib cage?

Bendavid: To the rib cage. It has never been a problem, because you lay it as high as you can. I have never found any problems with this. It is close to the defect where you have to have the good sutures; the remainder really remains flat and you hope that in time it will be incorporated with scar tissue. Otherwise you also run the risk of neuralgias.

Kingsnorth: Now laterally to the rectus. I think Dr. Stoppa gave us the answer to that: you put the mesh in the preperitoneal space.

Stoppa: The principle is to rub widely the hernial sac in every case, so you have to make a space for the placement of the mesh. You make this room as deep and simple as possible. Above the line of Douglas for medium incision; the best place of course is anterior to the posterior sheath of the rectus muscle. The other area you can place it easily is the preperitoneal space. Laterally to the rectus sheath there is no question. You get the posterior sheath of the rectus and you fall into the preperitoneal space.

47.8 Mesh Fixation

Schumpelick: Next we will talk about the fixation of the mesh. We have transcutaneous fixation, absorbable fixation (fibrin glue). How should we fix our mesh?

Stoppa: I agree with Dr. Flament, to answer your question: absorbable, interrupted, 1/o no trans-subcutaneous. Fibrin glue is probably good, and recently we have used another glue, which was not very easy to handle.

Schumpelick: Dr. Flament, would we agree that trans-subcutaneous fixation is not always necessary?

Flament: Yes, we have never tried it any other way, so I cannot comment on the best way. We have used transcutaneous in 1000 cases, so we feel comfortable with it.

Schumpelick: Let's start with the questions of suture material. You changed from non-absorbable to absorbable.

Flament: Yes, only because we had complaints of patients who felt the knot beneath the skin. We observed no change in our results, changing from nonabsorbable to absorbable.

Schumpelick: We went the same way because of this problem of the palpable knots. Now we use 3/0 PDS.

Wantz: We always fix Mersilene mesh to the anterior abdominal wall with absorbable sutures and we never fix polypropylene because it does not need to be fixed.

Schumpelick: Can I ask what the rational of fixation is? Is it only to keep it in one place for appearance until it is fixed by the scar? Do we then need nonabsorbable sutures? Dr. Filipi, you used to fix your mesh in inguinal hernia repair laparoscopically with clips. Is it easier?

Filipi: For incisional hernias, I have always used nonabsorbable sutures and I have not had patients complain of pain from the sutures, at least with these repairs, so I do not have a preference. But I do not have that much experience.

Amid: Our series is about 200 and it does not include these gigantic hernias that we saw from France. In the first half of our series we used transcutaneous buttonholes, and in the second half we sutured with staples, and there are three advantages with staples. Firstly, you do not have to have very precise measurements of the mesh because you can tailor it as you go; secondly, it is much easier to apply, it may only take 5 min to do it; and thirdly, it has a better cosmetic effect.

Schumpelick: What about continuous or single stitches? Some people said they used continuous stitches.

Kingsnorth: Are you worried about nerve entrapment with all these staples? Many nerves enter from the lateral side of the rectus, and staples may cause neuralgias.

Amid: It is very easy to avoid that because when you complete your dissection, you visualize every neurovascular bundle of intracostal nerves. They are quite visible; in fact they will show you the extent of your dissection.

Kingsnorth: Are you looking at them through the mesh? Can you see a nerve through the mesh?

Amid: You do not have to look at it through the mesh. First, when you do your dissection, you see all those neurovascular bundles. Then when I put the mesh in it is a little larger than the pocket I have made and as a result the edge of the mesh folds. Then I put the stapler into that fold and I can easily see the vascular bundles not through the mesh, just directly, because the mesh has folded. Then the tip of the stapler pushes the mesh through the line and you fire the staple there. You need only two or three staples.

47.9 Mesh Material

Simmermacher: As far as the mesh material is concerned, I think that polytetrafluoroethylene (PTFE), Teflon mesh, is obsolete, and so far there are no positive findings to show that expanded PTFE (ePTFE) would be any better than other prosthesis in a sublay way.

Kingsnorth: Let's move on then to views about polyester and polypropylene. Dr. Wantz has got some pretty strong views.

Wantz: The only mesh that is elastic enough to conform to the curves of the belly is Mersilene; all the polypropylene meshes will kink when they are bent in two directions, and they are just not suitable for any long service. Now we have used polypropylene, usually above the umbilicus, about 20 times, but we much prefer Mersilene. I am an American surgeon and when I started this, I used polypropylene mesh, mainly Marlex, but we do not use Marlex anymore, as it is too expensive. I learned my lesson; you just cannot use polypropylene mesh because when the mesh gets put down into the iliac fossa, it is going to fold on itself. We have already had to repair blank hernias attempted to be repaired by polypropylene mesh, and they fail. American surgeons will put in an aortic graft of Dacron in the same damned space and not think anything of it, so why are you so scared of using Mersilene mesh?

Kingsnorth: I think this is going to be a difficult question to answer, because we have Chevrel who uses an onlay mesh, and he has moved from polyester to polypropylene. I guess we could take a poll. How many people actually use polyester mesh? I think it is most probably the majority, isn't it? Six for polyester. Polypropylene users? That is a majority.

Devlin: Is it possible to say which polypropylene?

Amid: There are six polypropylene meshes on the market.

Schumpelick: I do not think we should use trade names here. They are not so different.

Amid: That is right; except for surgical multifilament, the rest of the polypropylene meshes are monofilament and they can be used interchangeably. I would say whichever is less expensive.

47.10 Bowel Protection

Schumpelick: When do we have to do something about bowel adhesions in our sublay mesh repair? Is it a small hole, is it a big hole? Is it generally done because we are afraid of adhesions forming? Dr. Flament, when do you do something to protect the bowel?

Flament: Always, omentum if it is available, and absorbable mesh if there is no more omentum.

Schumpelick: But if the peritoneum is closed, if you have closed the peritoneum, would you do something to prevent adhesion formation?

Flament: No.

Schumpelick: When would you use the omentum? If you have a small hole, would you suture the hole? Is that enough? When would you use omentum, when you cannot close the hole?

Flament: We try to put the omentum flat every time, even when we close the primary incision.

Schumpelick: If you decide to use bowel protection, what is best? Omentum or absorbable mesh with a small pore size, Gore-Tex, or composite mesh? If you have to protect the bowel, what should be the choice? Everyone agrees that the first choice is omentum, and the second choice is absorbable mesh with a small pore size, that means Vicryl, or what else? Gore-Tex or composite mesh? Who favors Vicryl? Eight. Gore-Tex? One. Composite mesh? Two. The majority is for absorbable mesh.

Amid: There are at least two studies that agree that absorbable mesh does not work, that it prevents neither adhesions nor fistulae formation.

Schumpelick: Is there agreement that we have to drain all sublay meshes at the beginning? Is it more that 2 days usually? Is there a risk of infection with drainage to your knowledge?

Flament: Yes, if you leave the drains in too long.

Schumpelick: How long is too long?

Flament: I do not know, because we never leave the drains in for more than 4–5 days.

Kingsnorth: Let's clarify that. I think we said yesterday that drains should be left in until the drainage volume went below a certain level. I sometimes leave them in for longer than 5 days.

Schumpelick: Now we come to a very important topic, how to treat or handle infection.

Herszage: We open the wound and we use sugar over the mesh.

Schumpelick: Should we favor the method of removing the mesh. Is there anyone who says it is bad to leave it in situ? I am not talking about PTFE – this has to be removed – but polypropylene or Mersilene mesh should stay in situ.

Schumpelick: Opening the wound is most important.

Filipi: I do not think we answered the question about a persistent seroma, i.e., you have removed the drain and now you have a seroma that is obvious clinically.

Kingsnorth: I think that we image them. We usually ask a radiologist to do this under aseptic conditions, and that may have to be repeated.

Bendavid: But when?

Kingsnorth: When they become troublesome to the patient, no particular size.

Schumpelick: I would suggest doing it yourself by ultrasound; otherwise it is a big event for the patient.

Wantz: Mind you, you can use doxycycline. We have used it twice in these big seromas.

Kingsnorth: That is anecdotal. We cannot take it as a general recommendation.

Wantz: I think you can, because if you have a persistent seroma that lasts more than 1 month, you had better do something about it, either operate on it, or get it sealed off. That is the kind of seroma I am talking about, and if you have not seen these then, maybe you should let them go the other side, but if a patient has a seroma for 2 months, I think you are obliged to do something about it.

Kingsnorth: We will try it.

Wantz: The treatment is doxycycline.

47.11 Mesh Migration

Kingsnorth: Is mesh migration preventable? Are polypropylene meshes without any risk in the long term (we are talking about malignancy)? Are there any age limitations? Do we need new materials? I think we have answered the question about preventing mesh migration in that it has been said that polypropylene mesh does not need suturing, but other meshes do.

Bendavid: Again, we have to identify what you mean by migration, because you can also have migration through bowel, through prosthesis, or when you are talking about a mesh being loose, and becoming displaced, so displacement may be a better term.

Kingsnorth: As for the long-term risk, do we believe that these meshes carry a risk of malignancy, and is it worth telling our patients?

Schumpelick: Dr. Stoppa, why do you limited the use of mesh according to the patient's age? You used to say mesh only above 50 years. What do you say now?

Stoppa: For hernias not before 40.

Schumpelick: Why is that so?

Stoppa: It is a safety rule, because we have no experimentation, and no studies on long-term mesh results. Therefore we should be cautious in young patients.

Kingsnorth: Let's hear it from the laparoscopic surgeons, you are putting loads of mesh into lots of young patients. Do you have any worries about malignancy?

Klaiber: No, I do not. My age limit is 35 because of the tissue. As you get older, the tissue gets weak, and that starts at about 35, I am sorry to say.

Kingsnorth: Dr. Filipi, do you agree with that?

Filipi: We do not operate on primary hernias, so most of the patients we operate on laparoscopically are older and it is not really an issue. Occasionally, you see a younger person with a bilateral hernia, but that is not very often.

Kingsnorth: So we are agreed at the moment that malignancy is not a concern. What about age limitations? Are we going to say a magic number? No magic numbers. Do we need new mesh materials? Hands up. Yes, everybody wants them, so we will just say yes for that.

47.12 Classification

Schumpelick: If we want to do multicenter trials, and we need trials, we must talk about classification, and I therefore favor making the Suvretta classification of hernias a simple one, so that we can talk in the future about the same size of hernia. We have had a lot of literature presented here, talking about incisional hernias done this way and that way, so we cannot compare the literature. Is a consensus possible on a classification of incisional hernia from the group?

Flament: I did not see the ratio between the quantity of bowel in the sac and the capacity of the abdominal cavity. This is what Reeve called the second abdominal cavity. This must be taken into account.

Flament: Size of eventration, that means the size of the bowel outside the abdominal cavity. The words have to be very precise.

Kingsnorth: Loss of domain has been used for some time, and it is a good term, so can we define the percentage of the abdominal contents that has lost its domain.

Schumpelick: I fully agree with what Flament said. We probably have to measure the circumference of the abdomen at the place where there is no hernia and where there is hernia. You can do this with some kind of tape measure.

Simmermacher: No, just in a transverse direction, so you get an impression of how big the original abdominal cavity is and then the place where the biggest eventration is so that you have an idea.

Kingsnorth: Is there any specific indications for doing computed tomography (CT) scan? I certainly do CT scans in the giant incisional hernias, but can we have a recommendation? I am talking about specific indications in giant incisional hernia. Should we know the contents there? Do we need to know sometimes whether there is bladder, liver, stomach?

Amid: Why don't we just say that if the fascial defect is over 15 cm – I do not know what the right dimension is – but if the largest diameter of the fascial defect is greater than, say, 15 cm, a CT should be done to determine the ratio of viscera outside the circumference.

Kingsnorth: Maybe it is simpler to say significant loss of domain and then leave "significant" to be interpreted, because we cannot be more specific than that. Significant loss of domain warrants a CT perhaps.

Devlin: If there is no loss of domain, you do not need a CT scan. If there is loss of domain, you are dealing with a hemodynamic problem of the whole patient, and therefore you need a CT and some estimate.

Schumpelick: Can we make loss of domain a good criteria?

Devlin: Yes.

Schumpelick: Is it international?

Kingsnorth: We could make it international. Perhaps we should say then that CT scan is rarely required, but where there is significant loss of domain it must be left up to the operating surgeon to decide.

Schumpelick: I have another question about the size of hernia. What is more important, the width, the length, or should we say the square width, the surface? Surface is better. How should we classify multiple defects? I think this classification should be intraoperative, so if we cut out the bridges, the resulting defect must be measured. I think below 10 cm^2, below 20 cm^2, and so on, is a good classification to begin with, and then we come to loss of domain and infection, which I think is very important. Should we talk about body mass index?

Truong: I think for classification of the incisional hernia, there should be two factors. The first one is the size of the defect, and the second is the relationship between the eventrated bowel and the lumen of the abdominal cavity.

Bennett: We have spent a lot of time talking about open repair of incisional hernia. Is there a role for laparoscopic repair of incisional hernia?

Scott: The main comment I would like to make about laparoscopic repair of incisional hernias is whether we are going to be able to follow the principles of open repair, if we can, we can do it, but if we cannot , it cannot be done. I think it is very simple, and we are working towards that goal.

47.13 Recurrent Inguinal Hernias

Kingsnorth: Recurrent inguinal hernias, a classification. I did fish out Campanelli's classification, so that might be something we can start on. There is R1, R2, and R3. First of all, do we need a classification of recurrence?

Stoppa: He showed me this classification before publishing it, so I know the principle of the classification, but this must be tried now to be confirmed. I think it is important to have a classification of recurrent hernia.

Kingsnorth: Do we accept this, or can it be defined?

Greenburg: I think I shared some data yesterday, which has held up since then, that 2 cm does not make much sense and 77% of these things are less than 4 cm, so I would say indirect less than 4 cm, direct less than 4 cm, the presence of an indirect hernia, multiple hernias, femoral hernias, all of these need to be looked at. The other issue would be in the Nyhus classification. Could you simply use the same descriptor and just add an R for recurrent and just work from that?

Kingsnorth: But the whole of the posterior inguinal wall is only 4 cm, so we have a debate here between 2 and 4 cm.

Scott: I was just going to say that one of the things the American Hernia Society is trying to do is to come up with a more accepted classification system, and when I say accepted, I mean one that will be used by surgeons, and we can get them to use this classification because it is not done very often in the United States. Obviously, the first thing you have to do is decide which factors are important factors in the repair or the recurrences of the repairs. I personally think that 2 cm is a pretty good size to work with, because as you said the groin is not that large.

Klaiber: I would suggest using the Nyhus classification. A, B, C, and D, and add 1, 2, 3, 4, or more centimeters in diameter, because we are already used to this classification; we just have to add the diameter.

Kingsnorth: I am not used to it because I use the Aachen classification. What is the Nyhus classification?

Klaiber: A is lateral, B is medial, C is femoral, and D is mixed, then you add 1, 2, 3, 4. The same as the last Suvretta classification.

Kingsnorth: The 1994 meeting took 4 days to settle on 1.5 cm, the finger and the open forceps for the laparoscopists. Perhaps we should modify this to make it 1.5 cm.

47.14 Treatment

Schumpelick: I would like to ask which treatment everyone uses here. For example, who uses the Shouldice repair in first recurrences? Who uses the Lichtenstein repair in the first recurrence? Who uses an umbrella?

Kingsnorth: I think we are getting very much into the classification, giving you the operation, so it depends on the type of recurrence for the type of operation you would do. I think an important recommendation might be to use the preperitoneal repair for recurrence.

Wantz: You are not just repairing a part of a myopecneal orifice. That is the value of the classification; if you can always put an appropriate peritoneal piece of mesh in, that will repair all hernias permanently and for good.

Kingsnorth: We have a strong case here for doing a preperitoneal repair for all recurrent inguinal hernias. Any objection to that?

Simmermacher: I wonder whether an indirect recurrent inguinal hernia exists.

Kingsnorth: Yes, we found it in all series, and it accounts for about 30%–40% of all recurrent inguinal hernias.

Bendavid: I do not think you should separate recurrences into first, second, third, fourth, and fifth; they should just be a recurrence, because some fifth recurrences are easier to repair than a first recurrence.

Schumpelick: I propose we drop this topic. I think we need a classification or else it is not sensible. Our last topic is about recurrent groin hernia, anesthesia, nerves, and epigastric vessels, that can be discussed here. What is the procedure and anesthesia of choice in a recurrent inguinal hernia, inguinal and femoral? Who is for local anesthesia?

Kingsnorth: If it is possible, yes.

Schumpelick: Who is for general anesthesia? Spinal anesthesia? Local seems to be a little bit ahead of spinal and general. Is that so?

Kingsnorth: I do not think we can really take anything from this straw poll, because people will use the type of anesthesia that is available in their hospitals. If you are not used to using spinal anesthesia, you will never use it. If you are used to using a lot of local anesthesia, you will use it very frequently. I think the type of anesthesia depends on your skill and the skill of your anesthesiologist.

Schumpelick: Yes, I agree, but if we make a suggestion saying that half of the people or one third use local anesthesia, then we favor this method in the hospitals. I know from my experience in Germany. We started with no clinics using local anesthesia, and now it is increasing because people have read books that say it works. This suggestion would therefore be helpful to introduce safer anesthesia; otherwise we will do it for the next 30 years with general anesthesia. Now, how should we handle nerves and epigastric vessels? Robert said yesterday that he cuts all nerves.

Bendavid: If they are in the way, certainly I do cut them off.

Schumpelick: Do the majority cut all nerves if they are in the way? In the recurrent hernia, that is five. Who tries to preserve nerves if they can be removed?

Kingsnorth: If they can be preserved.

Bendavid: These two questions have nothing to do with each other. If I can preserve them, I preserve them.

Kingsnorth: The message that I am trying to put forward is that if they get in the way, I cut them cleanly, and I do not damage or diathermy them.

Amid: It is important to know how you cut the nerve if you want to. Do you just cut it and let it go? I made asked my neurosurgical friends, and the consensus was that if you cut the nerve, you have to ligate it to prevent neuroma formation. Not only do you have to ligate it, but you also have to implant or bury the proximal end into the muscle, because if you do not do that, and the proximal end becomes attached to one of the upper neurotic layers, particularly to the external oblique aponeurosis, every time the muscle contracts, it will pull on the nerve, and it becomes painful. However, if you bury the proximal ligated end between the muscle fibers, you provide a soft cushion for the nerve and you prevent it from becoming adherent to the upper neurotic structure.

Schumpelick: Who does this?

Amid: I do it all the time. There is no study.

Kingsnorth: You never mentioned it before in any of your publications.

Amid. No.

Bendavid: The neurosurgeons have the same agreement. Another point is that anyone who has a third recurrence or more should not try it under a local anesthetic.

Appendix: Questionnaire: on the last day of symposion

Answers in % of participating herniologists on the Suvretta II meeting. March 1998 (Authors list see above).

1 Laparotomy

1. Which incisions are preferable?
   - Midline: 66.7%
   - Transverse: 33.3%
2. Which incisions should be avoided?
   - Pararectal: 50%
   - Paramedian: 25%
   - Midline: 15%
   - Transverse: 5%
   - Oblique lateral: 5%

2 Closure of Laparotomy

3. Continuous or interrupted suture?
   - Continuous suture: 96.3%
   - Interrupted suture: 3.7%
4. Mass closure or layered?
   - Mass closure: 52%
   - Layered: 48%
5. Absorbable or nonabsorbable sutures?
   - Long-term absorbable (PDS): 61.6%
   - Permanent suture: 23.1%
   - Absorbable (PGA): 15.4%
6. Are short-term absorbable (catgut) sutures obsolete?
   - Yes: 88.5%
   - No: 11.5%
7. Suture bites
   - 1 cm: 55.5%
   - 1.5 cm: 25.9%
   - 0.5 cm: 11.1%
   - 2 cm: 7.4%

8. Suture distance
   - 1 cm: 70.4%
   - 0.5 cm: 14.8%
   - 1.5 cm: 11.1%
   - 2 cm: 3.7%
9. Gauge of suture material
   - 0: 37.0%
   - 1: 37.0%
   - 1/0: 14.8%
   - 2/0: 11.1%
   - 2: 0%
10. Patients' postoperative activities
   - No restriction: 77.7%
   - Restriction for 2 weeks: 11.1%
   - Restriction for 4 weeks: 7.4%
   - Restriction for 6 weeks: 3.7%
11. Abdominal binder (support)
   - No: 69.2%
   - Yes: 30.8%
     2 weeks: 19.2%
     4 weeks: 7.7%

3 Incisional Hernia

3.1 Indication for Primary Closure

12. Depending on (multiple answers possible):
   - Defect size: 85.2%
     <2 cm: 30.4%
     4 cm: 26.1%
     8 cm: 4.4%
   - Number of recurrences: 51.9%
   - Location (upper/lower abdomen): 37.0%
   - Size of eventration in supine position: 29.6%
   - Never (always mesh): 14.8%
13. How should multiple defects be dealt with?
   - Combine to form a single one: 100%
14. Should the Mayo closure be avoided?
   - Yes: 88.8%
   - No: 11.2%

3.2 Requirements for Relaxing Incisions

15. Indication:
    - On demand: 88.0%
    - Never: 8.0%
    - Always: 4.0%
16. Which type of incision?
    - Vertical: 62.5%
    - Pararectal: 25.0%
    - Midline: 6.3%
    - Any: 6.3%
17. Multiple incisions: 59.2%
    - On demand: 22.7%
    - Single incision: 18.1%

3.3 Mesh Repair for Incisional Hernia

18. Indication for pneumoperitoneum
    - Giant hernia: 30.8%
    - No indication: 26.9%
    - Extreme eventration: 23.1%
    - Giant hernia and respiratory problems: 15.4%
    - 50% eventration on CT: 3.9%
19. Indication for weight reduction?
    - Always if possible: 60.0%
    - No, not realistic: 24.0%
    - Body mass index (BMI) >20: 16.0%
20. Is inlay mesh obsolete?
    - Yes: 96.2%
    - No: 3.8%
21. Mesh position
    - Sublay: 85.2%
    - Onlay: 7.4%
    - Does not matter: 7.4%
22. Extent of overlapping
    - 5 cm: 84.6%
    - 8 cm: 15.4%
    - 2 cm: 0.0%
23. Huge fascial defects (closure of linea alba impossible)
    - Sandwich mesh: 76.0%
    - Plastic reconstruction: 24.0%
    - Dermis plasty: 16.0%

24. How should the overlapping at the rib cage be dealt with?
   - Mesh sublay: 52.4%
   - Onlay position: 28.6%
   - Periosteum suture fixation: 14.3%
   - Suture around ribs: 4.8%
25. How should the overlapping at the xiphoid be dealt with?
   - Mesh sublay: 45.0%
   - Onlay position: 35.0%
   - Periosteum suture fixation: 20.0%
26. How should the overlapping at the pubic bone be dealt with?
   - Fixation to Cooper's ligament: 42.9%
   - Mesh sublay: 33.3%
   - Periosteum suture fixation: 14.3%
   - Onlay position: 9.5%
27. How should the overlapping lateral to the rectus sheath be dealt with?
   - Open lateral – preperitoneal position: 42.2%
   - Lateral between muscles: 15.8%
   - Suture fixation spigelian line: 15.8%
   - Fixation to m. transversus (8 cm): 10.6%
   - Onlay position: 10.6%
   - Complete abdominal wall fixation: 5.3%

3.4 Fixation of the Mesh

28. Absorbable or nonabsorbable?
   - Absorbable: 60.0%
   - Nonabsorbable: 40.0%
29. Interrupted or continuous?
   - Interrupted: 68%
   - Continuous: 16%
   - Alternating: 16%
30. Gauge of suture
   - 2/0: 62.5%
   - 0: 20.8%
   - 1: 12.5%
   - 3/0: 4.2%
31. Transcutaneous fixation?
   - No: 69.2%
   - Yes: 30.8%
32. Fibrin glue?
   - No: 79.2%
   - Yes: 20.8%

3.5 Mesh Material

33. Is polytetrafluoroethylene (PTFE) obsolete?
    - Yes: 73.1%
    - No: 26.9%
34. Preferred mesh
    - Polypropylene mesh: 69.2%
    - Reduced polypropylene mesh: 23.1%
    - Polyester mesh: 7.7%
35. What is the ideal bowel protection?
    - Absorbable mesh with small pore size: 62.5%
    - Composite mesh: 29.2%
    - Gore-Tex underlay: 4.2%
    - Onlay position (no protection needed): 4.2%
36. Is migration definitely preventable?
    - No: 53.8%
    - Yes: 46.2%
37. Are polypropylene meshes definitely without any risk in the long term?
    - No: 59.3%
    - Yes: 40.7
38. Is an age limit required?
    - No: 51.8%
    - Yes: 48.2%
39. Do we need new mesh materials?
    - Yes: 100%

4 Classification of Incisional Hernia

40. Do we need a classification?
    - Yes: 100%
41. A classification should include (multiple answers possible):
    - Location: 96.3%
    - Maximum size of defect: 92.6%
    - Size of eventration: 85.2%
    - Number of recurrences: 85.2%
    - Multiple defects: 77.8%
42. Classification to be done:
    - Intraoperatively: 40.8%
    - Preoperatively: 37.0%
    - Both: 22.2%

5 Classification of Recurrent Inguinal Hernia

43. Do we need a classification?
    - Yes: 81.5%
    - No: 18.5%
44. A classification should include (multiple answers possible):
    - Size of hernial orifice: 100%
    - Number of recurrences: 95.6%
    - Location: 90.9%
    - Previous mesh: 9.1%
    - Patient's age: 4.6%
    - Obesity: 4.6%

6 Recurrent Inguinal Hernia

45. How should a first recurrence be treated?
    - Wantz procedure: 25.9%
    - Shouldice technique: 14.8%
    - Lichtenstein technique: 14.8%
    - Totally extraperitoneal (TEP) technique: 7.4%
    - Opposite to previous (anterior/posterior): 7.4%
    - Repeat first operation better: 3.7%
    - Transinguinal preperitoneal prosthesis (TIPP)/Rives technique: 3.7%
    - Bassini or McVay technique: 3.7%
    - Transabdominal preperitoneal (TAPP) repair: 3.7%
    - Umbrella technique: 0%
    - Stoppa technique: 0%
46. How should a second recurrence be treated?
    - Wantz procedure: 37.0%
    - Shouldice technique: 14.8%
    - Lichtenstein technique: 14.8%
    - TIPP/Rives technique: 11.1%
    - Opposite to previous (anterior/posterior): 11.1%
    - TEP: 7.4%
    - Repeat first operation better: 3.7%
    - Umbrella technique: 3.7%
    - Stoppa technique: 3.7%
    - TAPP: 3.7%
    - Bassini or McVay technique: 0%

47. How should a third recurrence be treated?
    - Wantz procedure: 30.8%
    - Lichtenstein technique: 19.2%
    - TIPP/Rives: 11.5%
    - Opposite to previous (anterior/posterior): 11.5%
    - Stoppa technique: 11.5%
    - TEP: 7.7%
    - Umbrella technique: 3.9%
    - TAPP: 3.9%
    - Shouldice technique: 0%
    - Repeat first operation better: 0%
    - Bassini or McVay technique: 0%

7 Recurrent Femoral Hernia

48. How should a first recurrence be treated?
    - Wantz procedure: 32.0%
    - Suture: 24.0%
    - Plug: 16.0%
    - TEP: 12.0%
    - Umbrella technique: 8.0%
    - TIPP/Rives: 4.0%
    - TAPP: 4.0%
    - Stoppa technique: 0%
49. How should a second recurrence be treated?
    - Wantz procedure: 33.3%
    - Umbrella technique: 16.7%
    - Plug: 16.7%
    - TEP: 12.5%
    - TIPP/Rives: 8.3%
    - Stoppa technique: 4.2%
    - TAPP: 4.2%
    - Suture: 4.2%
50. How should a third recurrence be treated?
    - Wantz procedure: 33.3%
    - Plug: 16.7%
    - TEP: 12.5%
    - TIPP/Rives: 8.3%
    - Stoppa technique: 8.3%
    - Umbrella technique: 8.3%
    - TAPP: 8.3%
    - Suture: 4.2%

8
Recurrent Groin Hernia

51. Recommended anesthesia:
    - Local whenever possible: 51.6%
    - Spinal: 25.9%
    - General: 18.5%
    - Does not matter: 3.7%
52. Handling nerves:
    - Preparation and preservation: 96.2%
    - Routine transection: 3.8%
53. Handling epigastric vessels:
    - Preparation and preservation: 100%
    - Routine transection: 0%

Subject Index